Health Promotion and Disease Prevention in Clinical Practice

EDITORS

STEVEN H. WOOLF, M.D., M.P.H.
ASSISTANT CLINICAL PROFESSOR OF FAMILY PRACTICE
MEDICAL COLLEGE OF VIRGINIA
RICHMOND, VIRGINIA
FAIRFAX FAMILY PRACTICE CENTER
FAIRFAX, VIRGINIA
SCIENCE ADVISOR, U.S. PREVENTIVE SERVICES TASK FORCE
U. S. PUBLIC HEALTH SERVICE
WASHINGTON, DC

STEVEN JONAS, M.D., M.P.H.
PROFESSOR OF PREVENTIVE MEDICINE
STATE UNIVERSITY OF NEW YORK AT STONY BROOK SCHOOL OF MEDICINE
STONY BROOK, NEW YORK

ROBERT S. LAWRENCE, M.D.
PROFESSOR OF HEALTH POLICY AND MANAGEMENT
JOHNS HOPKINS SCHOOL OF HYGIENE AND PUBLIC HEALTH
BALTIMORE, MARYLAND

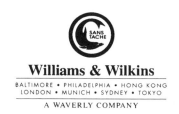

Williams & Wilkins

BALTIMORE • PHILADELPHIA • HONG KONG
LONDON • MUNICH • SYDNEY • TOKYO

A WAVERLY COMPANY

Editor: David C. Retford
Managing Editor: Kathleen Courtney Millet
Production Coordinator: Kimberly S. Nawrozki
Copy Editor: Bonnie Montgomery
Designer: Dan Pfisterer
Illustration Planner: Ray Lowman
Cover Designer: Tom Scheuerman
Typesetter: University Graphics, Inc.
Printer: Maple Press

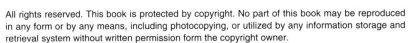

Copyright © 1996 Williams & Wilkins

351 W. Camden Street
Baltimore, Maryland 21201-2436 USA

Accurate indications, adverse reactions, and dosage schedules for drugs are provided in this book, but it is possible that they may change. The reader is urged to review the package information data of the manufacturers of the medications mentioned.

Printed in the United States of America

Library of Congress Cataloging in Publication Data

Health promotion and disease prevention in clinical practice /
    editors, Steven H. Woolf, Steven Jonas, Robert S. Lawrence.
        p.   cm.
    Includes index.
    ISBN 0–683–09270–7
    1. Health promotion.   2. Medicine, Preventive.   3. Clinical health
psychology.   4. Health promotion—United States.   5. Medicine,
Preventive—United States.   I. Woolf, Steven H.   II. Jonas, Steven.
III. Lawrence, Robert S., 1938–   .
    [DNLM: 1. Health Promotion—United States.   2. Preventive
Medicine.   3. Preventive Health Services—United States.   WA 110
H4345 1995]
RA427.8.H4923   1995
613—dc20
DNLM/DLC
for Library of Congress
                                                                    95–1212
                                                                    CIP

                                                            98 99
                                                    3 4 5 6 7 8 9 10

Reprints of chapter(s) may be purchased from Williams & Wilkins in quantities of 100 or more. Call Isabella Wise, Special Sales Department, (800)358-3583.

To Carol, Adrienne, and Cynthia,

whose love and support make all things possible,

and to all those who have dedicated themselves to the

promotion and practice of healthy living

Foreword

Health professionals value prevention. An ounce of it, we believe, is worth a pound of cure. For many years, however, we have been uncertain about effective strategies for implementing preventive care in clinical practice, unconvinced about the effectiveness of preventive interventions in reducing morbidity and mortality, and confused by the conflicting recommendations of different organizations. We have faced other barriers, such as lack of time for health promotion counseling in busy clinical settings, inadequate reimbursement for preventive services, and poor preparation in medical school and postgraduate clinical training for practicing health promotion and disease prevention. We had little or no hard evidence of the cost-effectiveness of some preventive measures.

During my tenure as U. S. Surgeon General, the Public Health Service took several important steps to address these problems. Chief among these was the establishment of the U. S. Preventive Services Task Force, an independent scientific panel that evaluated the evidence of effectiveness of over 200 screening tests, immunizations, and counseling interventions. The task force recommendations on which preventive services to include in the periodic health examination have been widely adopted by primary care clinicians, managed care programs, and other health care delivery systems. In *Health People 2000*, the federal government identified improving the delivery of clinical preventive services as one of the nation's top objectives for the year 2000. More recently, it launched the "Put Prevention Into Practice" campaign, a public-private partnership with professional societies, hospitals, and other health groups to provide clinicians with the tools for expanding preventive care in offices and clinics.

For individual clinicians, these promising developments at the national level have only begun to provide the practical advice needed to provide preventive care on the "front lines." Although recommendations of task forces and specialty societies are now widely available on the selection and frequency of screening tests, detailed instructions on how to perform them and interpret the results are often lacking. In-depth instructions on specific procedures are available in scattered publications, but few clinicians have the time to gather the information from the hundreds of journal articles, government reports, and specialty society documents in which they are contained, much less to integrate them into an overall approach to preventive care.

The timing could not be better for the publication of *Health Promotion and Disease Prevention in Clinical Practice.* This single reference brings together in one place the essential information that practitioners need in the office and at the bedside to provide high-quality preventive care. Written for clinicians by clinicians, this book is rich in practical advice, addressing the specifics of "what to do," based on current evidence and expert opinion, and directing the reader to appropriate primary sources for further details. The full scope of concerns faced by practitioners, ranging from how to take a prevention-oriented history to the design of office systems and computerized reminder systems, is addressed in detail in the pages that follow.

The reader will not get beyond the table of contents before noticing the hallmark of this work: its emphasis on modifying risk factors as the organizing framework for preventive care. One of my predecessors as U. S. Surgeon General, Dr. Luther Terry, was the first to call national attention to the health implications of personal behaviors in his 1964 report, *Smoking and Health.* Decades of subsequent research have not only confirmed the importance of smoking cessation, physical activity, healthy diet, safer sex, and other health behaviors in preventing disease, but they now suggest that efforts directed at improving these behaviors are more likely to reduce morbidity and mortality in the United States than anything else we do in medicine.

The implications of these findings to clinicians are obvious. If we are serious about promoting health and preventing disease, we must spend more of our time talking with patients about their health behaviors and less time subjecting them to tests and treatments. The time has come for a new approach to clinical practice in which the assessment and management of risk factors assumes as central a role in the doctor's office as the diagnosis and treatment of current complaints.

Our profession may have difficulty in making this transition. Medical schools do not train physicians to emphasize personal behaviors in taking a history, and even experienced clinicians have difficulty taking the next step once a problem has been identified. Few feel confident to answer patients' questions: "How do I stop smoking?" "Which foods should I eat?" "What's the right exercise program for me?" Clinicians traditionally trained to "tell patients what to do" may be unfamiliar with new approaches of shared decision-making and with helping patients to make choices that best suit their individual needs and personal preferences.

I urge clinicians who pride themselves on their clinical competence to acquire the most important clinical skill for the 21st century: learn how to answer these and similar questions. Read this book and the useful references it cites. Make excellence in the assessment and management of risk factors and the prevention of disease a central part of your daily routine.

Your efforts will result in better care for your patients and, when combined with similar efforts by your colleagues, will provide our nation's best hope for improving the health of Americans and reducing the exorbitant cost of rehabilitative and reparative medicine and surgery.

C. Everett Koop, M.D., Sc.D.

Preface

This book is intended for physicians, nurses, nurse practitioners, physician assistants, clinical social workers, and other clinicians who provide clinical preventive services as part of primary care. *Clinical preventive services* include counseling about personal health behaviors, screening tests for the early detection of risk factors and disease, immunizations, and chemoprophylactic regimens that are offered to patients before they develop clinical evidence of disease. These health maintenance interventions represent an important part of the daily activities of most clinicians, especially family physicians, pediatricians, general internists, nurse practitioners, and other health professionals who practice primary care medicine.

In recent years, major professional groups have issued guidelines on the periodic health examination and on specific clinical preventive services that should be offered to patients as part of ongoing personal health care. Groups such as the U. S. Preventive Services Task Force have summarized existing scientific evidence in support of clinical preventive services. Although these recommendations have helped define which preventive services should be offered to patients, they provide limited information about how the preventive maneuvers should be performed. The guidelines indicate, for example, how often women should receive a Papanicolaou test but do not explain how to obtain the specimen properly. Clinicians are advised to discuss tobacco use, exercise, and sexual practices, but the recommendations generally provide little information about how to counsel patients about these personal health behaviors.

The purpose of this book is to provide clinicians with practical information about how to perform clinical preventive services. The book is organized in the same sequence as the clinical encounter. The chapters in Section 1 explain how to gather information in the history, physical, and laboratory examination to evaluate the risk profile of the patient and to screen for early-stage disease. The chapters in Section 2 explain what to do with that information: how to talk to patients about specific health behaviors such as smoking or physical inactivity, how to immunize patients, and how to work up abnormal results from screening tests. The chapters in Section 3 offer practical suggestions about how to implement these recommendations in the office and in other health care settings: how to organize office and clinic systems to deliver preventive services; the use of computers, health maintenance schedules, and reminder systems; and ethics and social responsibility concerns in the delivery of preventive care.

The focus of this book on risk factors rather than target conditions is intentional. Most chapter titles address personal health behaviors (e.g., smoking, nutrition) rather than the prevention of specific disorders or disease categories (e.g., prevention of cancer or coronary artery disease). This emphasis on risk factors is important for three reasons.

First, unlike the care of symptomatic patients, for whom the "problem" requiring attention is a disease or symptom complex, the problems in preventive care are risk factors for disease (e.g., physical inactivity, rubella susceptibility), or the preclinical stages of a disease (e.g., asymptomatic cervical dysplasia, abnormal screening mammogram). Although clinicians and patients may share the broad goal of "preventing heart disease," the practical means to that end, with which they contend on a daily basis, are modifying dietary fat intake, serum lipids, physical activity, and blood pressure.

Second, individual risk factors often affect more than one disease category. For example, smoking, which increases the risk of heart disease, cancer, and other conditions, cannot be discussed exclusively under one disease category or another.

A third reason for emphasizing risk factors is that they provide the basis for designing a tailored health maintenance plan for the individual patient, rather than performing a standard battery of clinical preventive services. The adolescent who smokes cigarettes and has multiple sexual partners may require a different set of interventions than the adolescent who avoids these behaviors but is overweight and hypertensive. For the clinician, personal health behaviors assume the same role in the development of a treatment plan for preventive care as do presenting complaints for the management of a symptomatic patient. Just as abdominal pain triggers a series of focused questions, examination techniques, and laboratory tests to establish a diagnosis and prevent complications, a history that identifies health behaviors and other risk factors for disease should initiate a focused clinical approach tailored to the risk factors and the disorders with which they are associated.

This book is designed to help in that task. It is organized to provide guidance to the clinician on how to collect risk factor information in the history, physical, and laboratory examination; how to help patients modify risk factors; and how to use risk factor information to structure decisions about follow-up testing, treatment, and immunizations. The recommendations in this book generally conform with those of evidence-based groups, such as the U. S. Preventive Services Task Force. Wherever appropriate, the recommendations of the U. S. Preventive Services Task Force, government agencies, medical specialty societies, and private groups (e.g., American Cancer Society) are summarized.

The book is not designed to "sell" clinicians on the idea of practicing health promotion and disease prevention. Its emphasis on providing clinicians with practical information on how to provide preventive services leaves little space for discussing the scientific rationale for the recommendations or for citing relevant individual studies. Most references in the book are to publications that provide clinical practice guidelines and not to original research. An understanding of the scientific background for preventive care recommendations is, however, essential for the well-informed clinician. Detailed descriptions of the supporting evidence for clinical preventive services are available in the U. S. Preventive Services Task Force's *Guide to Clinical Preventive Services*, other similar reviews, and the references to which readers are referred in individual chapters.

In the United States, many, if not most, clinical preventive services are provided by physicians. Primary care physicians, in particular, engage regularly in the practice of health promotion and disease prevention and are the principal target audience for this book. Medical terminology and concepts familiar to physicians are therefore often used without further explanation. Nonetheless, the editors have, wherever appropriate, intentionally used the word "clinician" rather than "physician" to speak directly to non-physician health professionals who also provide clinical preventive services. In certain clinical settings and in many rural areas of this country, nurses, nurse practitioners, physician assistants, and other health professionals are the only primary care providers and have lead responsibility for the delivery of clinical preventive services. Even in other settings in which primary care physicians are available, non-physician health professionals are often more skilled in educating and counseling patients about specific prevention issues and can devote more time to these efforts than many physicians.

Preventive services for pregnant women are not discussed in this book, in part because space limitations preclude an adequate discussion of the details of clinical implementation. Nonetheless, most chapters in Section 2 provide information of direct relevance to pregnant women, especially those who smoke tobacco, use alcohol or other drugs, or engage in other health behaviors that threaten the health of both mother and fetus. The health and nutritional habits that are important during pregnancy often differ little from those that apply during other times of life. The chapters in this book do not discuss, however, the special factors that clinicians should consider when counseling pregnant women or when selecting screening tests and immunizations during pregnancy. Preventive services that are unique to pregnancy (e.g., screening for neural tube defects with amniocentesis or prenatal ultrasound) are also not addressed. Recommendations on these topics are available in the *Guide to Clinical Preventive Services*.

This book is not intended as a substitute for other medical textbooks. It is oriented toward preventive care and does not emphasize discussions of the treatment of existing disease. For example, discussions of cancer screening describe how to detect early-stage disease and do not provide recommendations on staging, chemotherapy, and other treatment measures once the cancer is detected. The range of conditions reviewed in this book is broad and includes many diseases for which new data and research findings are published regularly. The contents of this book are current as of 1995. Readers in subsequent years are encouraged to update the information by reviewing recent journal articles and publications that discuss current advances and new recommendations.

This book is targeted to health professionals in the United States; listings of epidemiologic data and the official recommendations of major groups generally refer to this country. This exclusion is made only for practical purposes; information from other countries is too extensive to include in one book. Moreover, health promotion and disease prevention priorities differ considerably in other countries, especially in developing nations, where many of the costly preventive technologies discussed in this book are of less importance than basic public health services. The same concerns about limited resources apply to the practice of preventive medicine at clinics in the United States that are located in disadvantaged communities and neighborhoods, where many of our uninsured population live. By selecting elements of this book that are appropriate for their specific practice setting, it is hoped that primary health care practitioners will find this publication useful in enhancing the quality of preventive care and the overall health status of their patients.

STEVEN H. WOOLF, M.D., M.P.H.
STEVEN JONAS, M.D., M.P.H.
ROBERT S. LAWRENCE, M.D.

Acknowledgments

We begin by thanking our contributors for the excellent chapters that they prepared for this book and for their patience and cooperation throughout the production process.

The editors also thank the following content experts for their helpful review comments on draft chapters: William L. Atkinson, M.D., M.P.H., Centers for Disease Control and Prevention; Patricia E. Bailey, M.D., Tufts University School of Medicine; Roger H. Bernier, M.D., Centers for Disease Control and Prevention; Trudy Bush, M.D., Johns Hopkins University; Robert W. Carr, M.D., M.P.H., SmithKline Beecham; Victoria Champion, D.N.S., R.N., Indiana University School of Nursing; Craig C. Clark, M.D., Fairfax Family Practice Center; Stephen B. Corbin, D.D.S., National Institute of Dental Research; James W. Curran, M.D., Centers for Disease Control and Prevention; Suzanne Dandoy, M.D., Virginia Department of Health; Carolyn G. DiGuiseppi, M.D., M.P.H., Office of Disease Prevention and Health Promotion (U. S. Preventive Services Task Force); Thomas P. Ehrlich, M.D., Fairfax Family Practice Center; Alan L. Engelberg, M.D., Monsanto Company; Paul S. Frame, M.D., Tri-County Family Medicine; Louis Francescutti, M.D.; Robert J. Friedman, M.D., New York University School of Medicine; Judy Gantt, Centers for Disease Control and Prevention; Marthe Gold, M.D., Office of Disease Prevention and Health Promotion; Lawrence W. Green, Dr.P.H., Institute of Health Promotion Research, University of British Columbia; Stephen C. Hadler, M.D., Centers for Disease Control and Prevention; Charles H. Hennekens, M.D., Dr.P.H., Harvard Medical School; Jan Howard, M.D., National Institute on Alcohol Abuse and Alcoholism; Douglas B. Kamerow, M.D., M.P.H., Office of Disease Prevention and Health Promotion; Neal D. Kohatsu, M.D., California Department of Health Services; Thomas E. Kottke, M.D., Mayo Clinic; Linda D. Meyers, Ph.D., Office of Disease Prevention and Health Promotion; Angela D. Mickalide, Ph.D., National Safe Kids Program; Marion Nestle, Ph.D., M.P.H., New York University; Steven M. Ornstein, M.D., University of South Carolina; Susan Palsbo, Ph.D., Group Health Association of America; Abigail L. Rose, Office of Disease Prevention and Health Promotion; Stephen C. Schoenbaum, M.D., Harvard Community Health Plan of New England; Leif I. Solberg, M.D., Group Health Foundation; Ray Strikas, M.D., Centers for Disease Control and Prevention; Walter Williams, M.D., Centers for Disease Control and Prevention. The reviewers

xv

cited here do not necessarily endorse all recommendations made in this book.

The work of the U. S. Preventive Services Task Force contributed greatly to the recommendations in this book, and the editors are therefore indebted to the members of the task force and to its skilled scientific advisors at the Office of Disease Prevention and Health Promotion (Washington, DC). Fairfax Family Practice Center (Fairfax, VA) is acknowledged for forwarding communications and correspondence from contributors and reviewers and for providing general clerical support.

The production of this book would not have been possible without the able assistance of the staff at Williams & Wilkins. The editors are particularly grateful to the managing editors, Kathleen C. Millet and Molly L. Mullen, their editorial assistant, Leah Hayes, the production coordinator, Kim Nawrozki, and the copy editor, Bonnie Montgomery. David C. Retford and Jonathan W. Pine, Jr. provided important leadership on this project. Finally, we thank Michael G. Fisher for his original suggestion that we write this book.

Contributors

Henrietta N. Barnes, M.D.
Assistant Professor of Medicine
Harvard Medical School
Boston, Massachusetts
Department of Medicine
The Cambridge Hospital
Cambridge, Massachusetts

David H. Bor, M.D.
Assistant Professor of Medicine
Harvard Medical School
Boston, Massachusetts
Chief of Medicine
The Cambridge Hospital
Cambridge, Massachusetts

Willard Cates, Jr., M.D., M.P.H.
Adjunct Professor of Epidemiology
University of North Carolina School of
    Public Health
Chapel Hill, North Carolina
Corporate Director of Medical Affairs
Family Health International
Research Triangle Park, North Carolina

Bruce V. Davis, M.D.
Associate Medical Director
Group Health Cooperative of Puget Sound
Seattle, Washington

Paul S. Frame, M.D.
Clinical Associate Professor of Family
    Medicine and Community & Preventive
    Medicine
University of Rochester School of
    Medicine and Dentistry
Rochester, New York
Tri-County Family Medicine
Dansville, New York

Dorian L. Gravenese, M.D.
Chief of Dermatology
Community Health Plan—The Medical
    Group
Attending Physician

Department of Medicine
    Long Island Jewish Medical Center
New Hyde Park, New York

Alan R. Greene, M.D., F.A.A.P.
Clinical Instructor of Pediatrics
Stanford University School of Medicine
Attending Pediatrician
Lucile Salter Packard Children's Hospital
Palo Alto, California
Attending Pediatrician
Mills-Peninsula Hospitals
Private Pediatrician, ABC Pediatrics
San Mateo, California

John C. Greene, D.M.D., M.P.H.
Professor and Dean, Emeritus
School of Dentistry
University of California, San Francisco
San Francisco, California

David A. Grimes, M.D.
Professor and Vice Chairman
Department of Obstetrics, Gynecology and
    Reproductive Sciences
University of California, San Francisco
Chief of Obstetrics, Gynecology and
    Reproductive Sciences
San Francisco General Hospital
San Francisco, California

Tee L. Guidotti, M.D., M.P.H.
Professor of Occupational and
    Environmental Medicine
University of Alberta Faculty of Medicine
Edmonton, Alberta, Canada

Hilliard Jason, M.D., Ed.D.
Clinical Professor of Family Medicine
University of Colorado Health Science
    Center
Denver, Colorado
Executive Director
Center for Instructional Support
Boulder, Colorado

Mark B. Johnson, M.D., M.P.H.
Assistant Clinical Professor of Preventive
    Medicine and Biometrics
University of Colorado Health Science
    Center
Denver, Colorado
Director
Jefferson County Department of Health
    and Environment
Lakewood, Colorado

Steven Jonas, M.D., M.P.H.
Professor of Preventive Medicine
State University of New York at Stony
    Brook School of Medicine
Stony Brook, New York

William J. Kassler, M.D., M.P.H.
Medical Epidemiologist
Division of STD/HIV Prevention
Centers for Disease Control and
    Prevention
Clinical Instructor
Department of Medicine
Emory University
Atlanta, Georgia

John M. Last, M.D., D.P.H.
Professor Emeritus
Department of Epidemiology and
    Community Medicine
University of Ottawa
Ottawa, Ontario, Canada

Robert S. Lawrence, M.D.
Professor of Health Policy and
    Management
Johns Hopkins School of Hygiene and
    Public Health
Baltimore, Maryland

**Perrianne Lurie, M.D., M.P.H.,
F.A.C.P.M.**
Public Health Physician
Division of Communicable Disease
    Epidemiology
Pennsylvania Department of Health
Harrisburg, Pennsylvania

Marc Manley, M.D., M.P.H.
Chief
Public Health Applications Research
    Branch

Cancer Control Science Program
Division of Cancer Prevention and Control
National Cancer Institute
Bethesda, Maryland

Thomas A. Mayer, M.D.
Professor of Emergency Medicine and
    Pediatrics
Georgetown University School of Medicine
George Washington University School of
    Medicine
Washington, DC
Chairman
Department of Emergency Medicine
Fairfax Hospital
Falls Church, Virginia

Marion Nestle, Ph.D., M.P.H.
Professor and Chair
Department of Nutrition and Food Studies
New York University
New York, New York

Julian B. Orenstein, M.D., F.A.A.P.
Assistant Professor of Pediatrics
George Washington University School of
    Medicine
Attending Physician
Department of Emergency Medicine
Fairfax Hospital
Falls Church, Virginia

Michael D. Parkinson, M.D., M.P.H.
Chief of Preventive Medicine
Office of the Surgeon General
U.S. Air Force
Washington, DC

Thomas H. Payne, M.D.
Clinical Computing Project
Group Health Cooperative of Puget Sound
Affiliate Assistant Professor
Department of Health Services
University of Washington
Seattle, Washington

Michael E. Stuart, M.D.
Director of Provider Education and
    Guideline Development
Group Health Cooperative of Puget Sound
Seattle, Washington

Stephen H. Taplin, M.D., M.P.H.
Associate Director, Preventive Care
Research
Department of Preventive Care
Group Health Cooperative of Puget Sound
Associate Professor of Family Medicine
University of Washington
Seattle, Washington

Robert S. Thompson, M.D.
Director
Department of Preventive Care
Group Health Cooperative of Puget Sound
Clinical Professor
Health Services Research and Pediatrics
University of Washington
Seattle, Washington

Edward H. Wagner, M.D., M.P.H.
Director
Center for Health Studies
Group Health Cooperative
Professor of Health Services
University of Washington
Seattle, Washington

Judith N. Wasserheit, M.D., M.P.H.
Director
Division of STD/HIV Prevention
Centers for Disease Control and
    Prevention
Atlanta, Georgia

Jane Westberg, Ph.D.
Clinical Professor of Family Medicine
University of Colorado Health Sciences
    Center
Denver, Colorado
Director
Center for Instructional Support
Boulder, Colorado

Steven H. Woolf, M.D., M.P.H.
Assistant Clinical Professor of Family
    Practice
Medical College of Virginia
Richmond, Virginia
Fairfax Family Practice Center
Fairfax, Virginia
Science Advisor, U.S. Preventive Services
    Task Force
U.S. Public Health Service
Washington, DC

Table of Contents

section one
Gathering Information

section two
What to Do with the Information
DESIGNING A HEALTH MAINTENANCE PLAN TARGETED TO
PERSONAL HEALTH BEHAVIORS AND RISK FACTORS

section three

Putting Prevention Recommendations into Practice

Introduction

STEVEN H. WOOLF, STEVEN JONAS, and ROBERT S. LAWRENCE

There is an inherent logic to health promotion and disease prevention.[a] It has always seemed more sensible to prevent the occurrence of diseases, or to stop them early in their natural history, than to delay treatment until the process of pathogenesis has resulted in irreversible damage to body tissues, organ systems, and physiologic processes. Clinicians know too well how ineffective medical and surgical interventions become at this late stage in the process, when controlling symptoms and forestalling progression, rather than curing the disease itself, are often all that can be offered to patients.

Yet thousands of Americans suffer from chronic diseases, such as heart disease, cancer, renal failure, stroke, chronic obstructive pulmonary disease, and diabetes mellitus. The burden of suffering has forced the health care system to invest heavily in caring for complications from these conditions, rather than in preventing the disease processes that caused them. On any given day in America, health care for end-stage diseases dominates the activities of doctors, hospitals, emergency departments, and nursing homes. These late-stage treatments are also largely responsible for the high cost of health care in this country. The United States spends more on health care than any other nation; in 1990, it spent $690 billion (13% of its gross domestic product), or about 41% of world health care expenditures (3). The most expensive, high-technology elements of American medicine are consumed in providing intensive care for late-stage conditions. Treatments in the last year of life account for nearly 30% of all Medicare expenditures, and about 40% of this expense is incurred in the last month of life (4). In contrast, prevention accounts for only 3% of health care expenditures in the United States (5), lying in the shadow of the sophisticated diagnostic and therapeutic technologies that dominate medicine.

[a]*Health promotion* is defined as "any combination of educational, organizational, economic, and environmental supports for behavior and conditions of living conducive to health" (1). Modifying personal health behaviors to reduce the risk of disease and injury is often described as health promotion. *Disease prevention* encompasses primary, secondary, and tertiary prevention. "*Primary preventive measures* involve entirely asymptomatic individuals (e.g., routine immunization of healthy children), whereas *secondary preventive measures* identify and treat asymptomatic persons who have already developed risk factors or preclinical disease but in whom the disease itself has not become clinically apparent. Obtaining a Papanicolaou smear to detect cervical dysplasia . . . is a form of secondary prevention. Preventive measures in symptomatic patients, such as antibiotic therapy to prevent wound infections, . . . are considered *tertiary prevention*" (2).

Prevention offers individuals and society a more rational strategy for dealing with disease and promoting health. The logic behind prevention is obvious. It is far more effective to prevent the occurrence of heart disease by modifying cardiac risk factors (e.g., avoiding tobacco use, increasing physical activity) than to attempt, years later, to regain the function of stenosed coronary arteries or ischemically damaged myocardium. It is better to administer a vaccine to a healthy infant than to care for the child who subsequently develops poliomyelitis. It is more rational to screen for and treat asymptomatic persons with high blood pressure than, years later, to provide hemodialysis therapy to patients with hypertensive renal failure or rehabilitative services to victims of stroke.

Despite this logic, the critical role of health promotion and disease prevention was not well-recognized as a priority area of national health policy until the early 1970s. At that time, a seminal Canadian document, the Lalonde Report, presented a new model for promoting public health that raised awareness about the importance of an integrated health promotion policy in improving the health status of the population (6). The Lalonde Report signaled the transformation of health promotion from the preceding "wellness" movement, a succession of vitamin and stress-reduction fads with little supporting scientific evidence, to a well-recognized epidemiologic and clinical science linking behavioral risk factors to specific disease outcomes. The incorporation of these principles into national health policy was formalized in the United States in 1979–1980, when the federal government published *Healthy People: The Surgeon General's Report on Health Promotion and Disease Prevention* (7) and *Promoting Health/Preventing Disease: Objectives for the Nation* (8), setting specific goals to be achieved by 1990. By the time that new objectives for the year 2000 (*Healthy People 2000*) were released in 1990 (9), health promotion and disease prevention had become a well-accepted component of national health policy. To date, 41 of the 50 states and the District of Columbia have issued their own *Healthy People 2000* plans, reflecting the diffusion of health promotion policy to the regional and local level (10, 11).

THE CURRENT SCOPE OF HEALTH PROMOTION AND DISEASE PREVENTION

Society can practice health promotion and disease prevention through several channels: (a) controlling communicable diseases, (b) protecting the environment, (c) modifying personal behaviors that affect health, and (d) preventing, or reducing the severity of, noncommunicable and chronic disabling conditions (12). The past century has witnessed achievements in health promotion and disease prevention in each of these areas. Infectious diseases that were the leading causes of death and disability in the United

States at the beginning of this century have become uncommon through improved public sanitation, housing, immunization programs, and nutrition. Poliomyelitis, for example, caused paralysis and death in hundreds of thousands of Americans before the polio vaccine was introduced in 1954 and the incidence of the disease declined; since 1991, no new cases of disease caused by wild-type polio virus have been reported in the Western hemisphere (13). Government and industry have worked to improve the cleanliness of air, water, soil, and food supplies and to increase the safety of products and transportation services, thereby reducing the incidence of infectious diseases, environmental and occupational illnesses, and injuries. Between 1988 and 1993, the proportion of Americans living in communities with clean air increased from 50% to 77% (10).

Health consciousness has been integrated into daily American life. Joggers and power walkers became common sights on residential streets in the 1970s. Concerns about nutrition and the importance of lifestyle in preventing infection with human immunodeficiency virus (HIV) grew in the 1980s. Now, other examples of health promotion have become evident in society: print and television advertisements feature messages about healthy, low-fat products and physical fitness; motorists routinely fasten their seat belts; children are protected by car safety seats and bicycle helmets; no-smoking policies have been adopted by employers, airlines, restaurants, and other public facilities; celebrities, advertisers, and public service announcements encourage cancer screening, safe sex, and avoiding drug and alcohol abuse and drunk driving. The personal health behaviors of Americans have changed. Since 1964, the proportion of Americans who smoke cigarettes has fallen from 40% to 25% (10, 14). Per capita tobacco consumption in the United States fell from 3.8 kg in the mid-1970s to 2.6 kg in 1990 (3). About 34% of the population now eat lower fat diets, and 24% exercise regularly (10). Americans have become more conscientious about cancer screening. Between 1988 and 1993, the proportion of women over age 50 who received a recent mammogram more than doubled, and 75% of women over age 18 have had a recent Papanicolaou smear (10).

These changes have been accompanied by favorable trends in the incidence of death and disability in the United States. Between 1940 and 1992, age-adjusted death rates for Americans decreased from 1076:100,000 to 505:100,000, and life expectancy at birth increased from 63 to 76 years. Between 1950 and 1991, infant mortality rates fell from 30:1000 to 9:1000 live births (15). Between 1979 and 1992, age-adjusted death rates decreased significantly for heart disease (28% reduction), cerebrovascular disease (37% reduction), and injuries (32% reduction) (15). Many of these changes have been attributed to behavioral risk factor modification. Reduced stroke mortality, for example, is believed to be due to early detection and treatment of hypertension. Since the late 1970s, the proportion of hypertensive persons with controlled blood pressure increased from 11% to 21% (10). Age-adjusted mortality for lung cancer, following a more than six-fold increase between 1940 and 1982, has remained stable since 1982, due largely to decreased tobacco use (16). Between 1987 and 1993, the frequency of alcohol-related traffic deaths decreased by over 30% (10).

These achievements aside, far too many Americans continue to suffer from diseases and injuries that are largely preventable. The health status of the population is far lower than it should be, primarily because the full benefits of health promotion and disease prevention have yet to be realized. Heart disease remains the leading cause of death in the United States, killing over 700,000 Americans annually (15). Each year in the United States, there are over 500,000 deaths from cancer, 140,000 deaths from stroke, 90,000 deaths from chronic obstructive pulmonary disease, and thousands more from other chronic diseases (15). About half of such deaths are potentially preventable, caused by a short list of modifiable risk factors (e.g., tobacco use, unhealthy diet, physical inactivity) (7). Mortality from motor vehicle injuries (about 40,000 deaths each year) could be reduced in half if seat belt use was maximized and drinking and driving were curtailed (13). HIV infection, which, in 1993, claimed over 38,000 lives and became the leading cause of death among persons ages 25–44 (17), is almost completely preventable by altering sexual practices and exposure to blood products. Teen pregnancy rates remain high (about 74:1000), and 7% of newborns are of low birth weight (10).

The incidence, morbidity, and mortality of certain diseases are disproportionately higher among disadvantaged and minority populations. The life expectancy of a black infant at birth is about seven years less than that of a white infant (15), and the infant death rate is nearly double that of whites (10). Among African Americans, age-adjusted deaths rates for coronary heart disease and cancer are 35–37% higher than those for whites, and stroke mortality rates are 86% higher (10). Similar disparities are reported for other minorities, such as Hispanics, Native Americans, and Asians and Pacific Islanders, who suffer from increased rates of diabetes mellitus, HIV infection, overweight, tuberculosis, and other conditions. As summarized in Table 1, data on the receipt of clinical preventive services consistently report disproportionate gaps in preventive care among minorities and disadvantaged populations.

The reasons for these inadequacies in health promotion and disease prevention are multifactorial. Strategies available to society for preventing diseases are limited by logistical, political, financial, religious, and philosophical obstacles. Regulations to protect the safety of the environment place economic and administrative burdens on private industry and gov-

Table 1.

Receipt of Preventive Services By Persons in the United States

Preventive Services	Estimated Proportion of Persons in the United States Who Had Received Preventive Service, 1993
Children (age 19–35 months)	
Immunizations	
DTP (3 or more doses)	88%
Polio (3 or more doses)	79%
MMR (1 dose)	84%
HiB (3 or more doses)	55%
HBV (3 or more doses)	16%
4 DTP/3 Polio/1 MMR	67%
Adults (age 18 and older)	
Routine check-up[a]	78%
Cholesterol (ever checked)	**71%**
Low-income Americans	55%
African Americans	72%
Hispanic Americans	62%
Native Americans	60%
Papanicolaou smear (last 3 years)	**78%**
Women age 65 and older	58%
Asian Americans/Pacific Islanders	69%
Native Americans	78%
Disabled Americans	69%
Breast examination and mammogram at age 50 and older (last 2 years)	**55%**
Women age 65 and older	49%
Low-income women	39%
Asian Americans/Pacific Islanders	53%
Native Americans	38%
Disabled Americans	51%
Asked at least one screening question[b] at routine check-up (last 3 years)	**63%**
Adults age 65 and older	48%
Asian Americans/Pacific Islanders	60%
Td (last 10 years)	**57%**
Adults age 65 and older	34%
Hispanic Americans	48%
Asian Americans/Pacific Islanders	45%
Disabled Americans	51%
Pneumococcal vaccine (once at age 65 or older)	**28%**
Low-income Americans	18%
African Americans	14%
Hispanic Americans	13%
Asian Americans/Pacific Islanders	21%

Table 1—*continued*

Preventive Services	Estimated Proportion of Persons in the United States Who Had Received Preventive Service, 1993
Influenza vaccine (last 12 months at age 65 or older)	**52%**
Low-income Americans	41%
African Americans	33%
Hispanic Americans	47%
Asian Americans/Pacific Islanders	54%

From National Health Interview Survey, National Center for Health Statistics, 1995. *Legend: DTP,* diphtheria-tetanus-pertussis vaccine; *MMR,* measles-mumps-rubella vaccine; *HiB, Haemophilus influenzae* type b vaccine; *HBV,* hepatitis B vaccine; *Td,* tetanus-diphtheria booster.

[a]In the last 3 years for persons age 18–64; in the last year for persons age 65 and older.

[b]For persons age 18–64, a question regarding one or more of the following: diet, physical activity, tobacco use, alcohol use, drug use, sexually transmitted diseases, contraceptive use; for persons age 65 and older, a question regarding one or more of the following: diet, physical activity, tobacco use, alcohol use.

ernmental agencies. Vaccines and screening services are costly to society and often unavailable to persons with limited access to health care. The biologic efficacy of vaccines and antibiotics to control infectious diseases is threatened by the emergence of new organisms, antibiotic-resistant strains, and vaccine failure. Perhaps the most effective means of promoting health, convincing individuals to change personal behaviors, cannot work if individuals lack the motivation or resources to change behavior. To change behavior voluntarily is difficult because unhealthy behaviors are often enjoyable or deeply ingrained in lifestyle and culture. Forcing changes in behavior, such as requiring the use of seat belts, poses philosophical, ethical, political, and legal problems and generally conflicts with American sensibilities about individual freedom.

HEALTH PROMOTION AND DISEASE PREVENTION IN CLINICAL PRACTICE

It is in this context of societal efforts that this book explores the role of clinicians in promoting health and preventing disease. The limitations of health professionals in this effort are as immediately apparent as their capabilities. Clinicians cannot ensure the cleanliness of water and food supplies, cannot redesign motor vehicles to improve safety, and cannot control the behavior of their patients.

Nonetheless, the potential capabilities of clinicians in promoting health are substantial. Clinicians, perhaps better than anyone, know the consequences of allowing conditions to progress to their final stages and the futility of offering treatments late in the natural history of disease. Clinicians are therefore among the most persuasive advocates of health promotion. Clinicians also have special access to the population; about 78% of Americans have contact with a physician each year, averaging about three office visits per year (18). Patients value the advice of doctors and other health professionals. Studies suggest that patients' decisions to stop smoking, undergo a mammogram, or have their child immunized are often traceable to the encouragement of their doctor. The clinician is essential to the delivery of many preventive services (e.g., Papanicolaou smears, sigmoidoscopic screening, prescriptions for hormone replacement therapy).

Clinicians have therefore always tried to emphasize preventive services in clinical practice. Pediatricians and family physicians, for example, have, for decades, prioritized health promotion and disease prevention issues during well-baby and well-child visits. Nurse practitioners, nurses, physicians' assistants, and other health professionals have emphasized nutrition, exercise, and other aspects of wellness. Much of the prenatal care provided by obstetricians, family physicians, and nurse midwives is dominated by prevention topics. Many specialists also engage in preventive care. Cardiologists devote much of their time to encouraging patients to modify cardiac risk factors, gastroenterologists screen for colorectal cancer, dermatologists encourage the prevention and early detection of skin cancer, ophthalmologists and optometrists screen for glaucoma, and so on.

Most clinicians, however, do fall short in providing the preventive services that are recommended for their patients. Studies have consistently found that patients routinely receive checkups without being questioned about personal health behaviors or receiving other recommended clinical preventive services (19–21). Only 44–49% of patients who smoke report that their physicians have advised them to smoke less or stop smoking (22, 23). Table 1 documents the extent to which Americans have not received recommended clinical preventive services. Nearly half of American women have not undergone breast cancer screening in the past two years. One out of three two-year-old children have not received recommended childhood immunizations. As of 1991, the percentage of infants who had been adequately immunized by their physicians against diphtheria, tetanus, and pertussis was lower in the United States than in any other industrialized country, with the exception of Ireland and Greece (3).

BARRIERS TO THE DELIVERY OF CLINICAL PREVENTIVE SERVICES

There are many reasons for inadequate attention to preventive services in the clinical setting (24). A fundamental barrier is that health professionals may lack motivation to practice prevention, for several perceived reasons. First, health promotion and disease prevention activities are often less "interesting" than curative medicine. Talking to healthy patients about personal behaviors is thought to provide less intellectual stimulation and to offer fewer dramatic clinical challenges than contending with full-blown dis-

eases.[b] Discussing low-fat diets, performing Papanicolaou smears, and injecting vaccines offer less professional excitement than performing crash resusci-
tations, transluminal angioplasty, laser surgery, joint reconstruction, and
other high-technology medical procedures. The latter provide an opportunity to apply more fully the advanced scientific knowledge acquired during
clinical training and from keeping abreast of current research. The scientific
principles of preventive medicine, by comparison, receive relatively little emphasis in most training curricula and seem less captivating to many clinicians.

A second disincentive to providing clinical preventive services is skepticism about their effectiveness. Uncertainty about the ability of screening
tests, counseling, and immunizations to reduce morbidity and mortality has
been a longstanding obstacle to preventive care for many years. It was this
skepticism that prompted the U.S. Public Health Service to establish the U.S.
Preventive Services Task Force (USPSTF) in 1984 (see "U. S. Preventive Services Task Force" at the end of this introduction). The USPSTF carefully examined the evidence for over 200 clinical preventive services. Although it
found that many preventive services lacked sufficient evidence to reach conclusions about their effectiveness or ineffectiveness, it was able to identify a
core package of clinical preventive services for which there was compelling
evidence of significant health benefits (13). The USPSTF findings have been
reinforced by other expert panels and medical groups, providing a strong scientific argument for emphasizing these measures in daily patient care (25).

A third, more practical, disincentive for clinicians interested in providing preventive services is uncertainty about exactly what to do: which preventive services to provide, how often, and on which patients. The USPSTF
and other expert panels, government agencies, medical specialty societies,
and private groups have responded to this need by issuing practice guidelines that specify the proper indications for a variety of clinical preventive
services (Table 2). Although there is some disagreement among groups
about certain recommendations, there is a growing consensus around a
core package of clinical preventive services (see Figure 22.1) of proven effectiveness that should be offered to patients.

The strength of the consensus about effective preventive care has not
been fully appreciated because of highly publicized controversies about
relatively narrow areas of disagreement (e.g., screening mammography for
women ages 40–49, the optimal age for the second measles vaccination).
Unfortunately, these marginal debates have distracted clinicians from the
many important recommendations about which there is little disagreement. For the busy practitioner, the areas of consensus provide more than

---

[b]The inaccuracy of these perceptions often does not become apparent until one begins to practice
health promotion and disease prevention as part of daily patient care. As any primary care provider
can attest, the practice of health promotion and disease prevention can be among the most challenging and gratifying aspects of medicine.

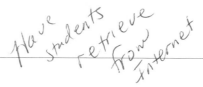
Table 2.

Examples of Groups Issuing Practice Recommendations on Clinical Preventive Services[a]

Groups	Publications Containing Guidelines	Clinical Preventive Services Topic Areas
Federal Government Agencies		
Agency for Health Care Policy and Research	Agency guideline booklets; journal articles	Clinical practice guidelines on selected clinical preventive services
Centers for Disease Control and Prevention	*Morbidity and Mortality Weekly Report* (j) (often reprinted in *JAMA* [j])	Recommendations on immunizations and screening tests for infectious diseases and selected chronic diseases
National Institutes of Health	National Cholesterol Education Program and National High Blood Pressure Education Program publications; *JAMA* (j) and other journals (NIH Consensus Development Conference reports)	Recommendations on screening and follow-up for high blood cholesterol and dietary guidelines, developed by National Cholesterol Education Program; screening and follow-up for high blood pressure and lifestyle interventions, developed by National High Blood Pressure Education Program; recommendations developed by NIH Consensus Development Conferences
Medical Specialty Societies		
American Academy of Pediatrics	*Pediatrics* (j) (committee reports); *Report of the Committee on Infectious Diseases* (bk) ("Red Book" on childhood immunizations); *Recommendations for Preventive Pediatric Care* (fs); other organizational publications	Recommendations regarding screening tests, anticipatory guidance, health promotion, and immunizations developed by committees in specific topic areas (e.g., Environmental Health, Genetics, Infectious Diseases, Practice and Ambulatory Medicine); immunization guidelines developed as part of the Immunization Practices Advisory Committee

Table 2.—*continued*

Groups	Publications Containing Guidelines	Clinical Preventive Services Topic Areas
American Academy of Family Physicians	*Age Charts for Periodic Health Examination* (fs); other organizational publications	Recommended clinical preventive services during the periodic health examination, developed by Commission on Public Health and Scientific Affairs
American College of Obstetricians and Gynecologists	*ACOG Committee Opinions, ACOG Technical Reports* (fs)	Recommendations on selected screening, counseling, immunizations, and chemoprophylaxis during prenatal and well-woman care
American College of Physicians	*Annals of Internal Medicine* (j) (individual policy statements of Clinical Efficacy Assessment Project committee); *Common Screening Tests* (bk) (compendium of Clinical Efficacy Assessment Project policy statements); *Guide for Adult Immunization* (bk) (report of Task Force on Adult Immunization)	Recommendations on screening tests and chemoprophylaxis, developed by the Clinical Efficacy Assessment Project; immunization guidelines developed as part of the Immunization Practices Advisory Committee
Independent Panels		
U.S. Preventive Services Task Force	*Guide to Clinical Preventive Services* (bk); articles in *JAMA* (j) and other journals	Recommendations on over 200 screening, counseling, immunization, and chemoprophylactic interventions
Canadian Task Force on the Periodic Health Examination	*Canadian Guide to Clinical Preventive Health Care* (bk); articles in *Canadian Medical Association Journal* (j) and other journals	Recommendations on screening tests, counseling, immunizations, and chemoprophylactic interventions
Immunization Practices Advisory Committee	*Morbidity and Mortality Weekly Report* (j), *Report of the Committee on Infectious Diseases* (bk) (American Academy of Pediatrics, see above), *Guide for Adult Immunization* (bk) (American College of Physicians, see above)	Immunization guidelines developed under the auspices of the Centers of Disease Control and Prevention, usually with endorsement by the American Academy of Pediatrics, American Academy of Family Physicians, and/or American College of Physicians

Table 2.—*continued*

Groups	Publications Containing Guidelines	Clinical Preventive Services Topic Areas
	Private Advocacy Groups	
American Cancer Society	Articles in *CA Cancer Journal for Clinicians* (j)	Recommendations on cancer screening and nutrition
American Heart Association/American College of Cardiology	Articles in *Circulation* (j) and *Journal of the American College of Cardiology* (j); organizational publications	Recommendations on screening tests for heart disease and cardiac risk factors, nutrition and other cardiac risk factor modification

Legend: j, journal; *bk*, book; *fs*, fact sheet or pamphlet.

*This list is not exhaustive. Many other government agencies, specialty societies, and private organizations publish recommendations on specific types of clinical preventive services. Listed publications include only those that provide clinicians with instructions on how to deliver clinical preventive services. Most organizations have other publications on related topics.

enough work, without even taking on the controversial elements of preventive care. Ensuring the delivery of the core package of clinical preventive services that is supported by all groups (e.g., ensuring that all patients who smoke receive counseling, that women over age 50 undergo mammography screening every 1-2 years, that childhood immunizations are up-to-date) presents, by itself, a formidable challenge for most busy clinicians. If this alone could be achieved, most of the deficiencies in the current practice of preventive medicine would be remedied.

Which specific clinical preventive services should be provided? The recommended clinical preventive services for patients in specific age and risk groups have been specified by the USPSTF (see *Guide to Clinical Preventive Services* [13]) and other groups (see Table 2). The USPSTF recommendations are summarized in the appendix of this book. The scientific evidence on which the recommendations are based is examined in detail in the USPSTF *Guide* (13) and in the corresponding *Canadian Guide to Clinical Preventive Health Care* (26). The details of how to perform the recommended clinical preventive services are the principal focus of this book. As noted in the preface, Section 1 describes how to collect risk factor information during the history, physical, and laboratory examination. Section 2 presents the ways and means of using that information to help patients modify risk factors and to determine appropriate follow-up tests, treatments, immunizations, and counseling. Section 3 addresses implementation systems, which are necessary to achieve comprehensiveness and efficiency in providing complete preventive care to all patients.

Unfortunately, even the well-motivated provider encounters many additional barriers related to delivering clinical preventive services (28). Practice organization and health care systems often present obstacles in busy clinical settings. Chief among these are lack of time, especially for counseling; lack of self-confidence in professional skills to provide preventive care, often due to inadequate emphasis on prevention during clinical training; and simply forgetting about prevention in the midst of other clinical responsibilities. Provider reimbursement for clinical preventive services has, for many years, been inadequate under traditional indemnity (fee-for-service) health insurance plans. Although support for prevention under capitated plans is increasing with the growing role of managed care in primary care medicine, it remains unclear whether this trend will result in wider delivery of clinical preventive services. Other barriers to preventive care involve patients: people in need of clinical preventive services often do not receive them because they are disinterested, fearful, or lack access to health care. Over 15% of Americans, or about 40 million persons, currently lack health insurance (10).

Recent years have witnessed efforts by government agencies, medical organizations, and health care delivery systems to address many of these implementation barriers. Government agencies, medical specialty societies, and medical journals have worked to disseminate clinical preventive services recommendations to health professionals through journal articles, conferences, and organizational publications aimed at preventive care. A national campaign, "Put Prevention Into Practice," was launched in 1994 by the federal government (with cooperation from the American Academy of Pediatrics, American Academy of Family Physicians, American Nurses Association, American Academy of Nurse Practitioners, American Hospital Association, American Cancer Society, managed care organizations, and other groups) to provide practitioners with implementation tools for providing preventive services in the primary care setting. Computerized reminder systems have been designed to help clinicians remember which preventive services are indicated. Public education campaigns have used print and broadcast advertisements and programs, magazine articles, and other media (e.g., online services) to encourage Americans to visit their doctor to obtain screening tests, immunizations, and other recommended preventive services.

Problems with patient access to, and provider reimbursement for, clinical preventive services have also received attention from policy makers. *Healthy People 2000* (9), the national health objectives laid out in 1990, made access to clinical preventive services an explicit priority for the country. National health care reform discussions in 1992–1994, which ultimately failed to produce final legislation, were consistent in emphasizing the need for Americans to have access to effective clinical preventive services. Similar recommendations are now being made in discussions of health care reform at the state level. Private market forces also appear to be expanding access to preventive care. Health insurers, employers, and managed care programs have widened coverage of clinical preventive services as part of their efforts to control the rising costs of health care. Preventive services are popular with consumers, and many plans compete for patient enrollment by advertising their respective preventive services packages.

THE IMPORTANCE OF PATIENT EDUCATION AND COUNSELING IN PREVENTIVE MEDICINE

The clinical preventive services that practitioners should provide are classified by the USPSTF as (a) counseling interventions, (b) screening tests, (c) immunizations, and (d) chemoprophylaxis. *Counseling interventions* refer to efforts to educate patients about the consequences of personal health behaviors (e.g., tobacco use, diet, physical activity, sexual practices, injury prevention) and to work in a collaborative fashion on strategies for risk factor modification. *Screening tests* are special tests or standardized examination procedures for the early detection of preclinical conditions (e.g., cervical dysplasia) or risk factors (e.g., elevated serum cholesterol) in asymptomatic persons. *Immunizations* include the use of vaccines and immunoglobulins to prevent infectious diseases. *Chemoprophylaxis* refers to the use of drugs, nutritional and mineral supplements, or other natural substances by asymptomatic persons to prevent future disease.

This book gives special emphasis to counseling patients about risk factors. Modifying personal health behaviors is probably the most effective way for patients to prevent disease. One of the key findings of the USPSTF, based on its extensive review of the evidence, is that clinicians are more likely to help their patients prevent future disease by asking, educating, and counseling them about personal health behaviors than by performing physical examinations or tests. In other words, talking is more important than testing:

> The data suggest that among the most effective interventions available to clinicians for reducing the incidence and severity of the leading causes of disease and disability in the United States are those that address the personal health practices of patients. (2, p. xxii)

Despite the relative superiority of talking over testing, one is more likely to see the opposite in clinical practice. As in other areas of medicine, preventive care is dominated by procedures and testing. Patients seeking preventive care are more likely to undergo a rectal examination or cholesterol test than to be asked whether they smoke, what they eat, or whether they exercise. To some extent, the disaffection with counseling is due to factors already mentioned, such as lack of time, inadequate reimbursement, and skepticism about effectiveness. More broadly, however, the emphasis on testing is a generic phenomenon in medicine, owing to medicolegal concerns about the risks of not ordering tests, test-ordering habits acquired during clinical training, fascination with high technology, skepticism about the potential harms of testing, intellectual curiosity about test results, and patient demand (28). Patients feel that their doctor is more competent and that they are receiving better care if they undergo extensive testing.

There are, however, additional reasons for the reluctance of practitioners to emphasize personal health behaviors and other risk factors during patient assessment. First, clinicians are accustomed to dealing with the here and now. Clinical training and the pragmatic realities of patient care encourage attention to current problems and not to risk factors for future disease. Their distant impact in the future gives health behaviors the perception of being less serious than "real" pathology in the present, in part because of the universal human tendency to discount future events. Such perceptions often conflict with the facts. A patient's discomfort from reflux esophagitis, for example, may *seem* more important than a discussion of health behaviors. But if the patient smokes cigarettes, failure to have this discussion will allow the patient's most likely cause of death (heart disease) to escape attention at a time in life when it might be preventable. In the final analysis, dyspepsia is less important than death, and yet in practice it may receive more attention.

A second reason for the tendency of clinicians to emphasize testing over talking is the perception that screening tests are more effective than counseling. Once again, this perception is often erroneous. The extensive review of the literature performed by the USPSTF determined that, although routine screening can lower mortality for selected conditions (e.g., breast, cervical, and colon cancer, hypertension), routine screening for most other diseases appears to have little or no effect on health outcomes (13). In contrast, unhealthy personal behaviors are the leading causes of death in the United States. In 1990 in the United States, there were 400,000 deaths attributable to tobacco use, 300,000 deaths from unhealthy eating habits and physical inactivity, 100,000 deaths from alcohol use, 35,000 deaths from firearms, and 30,000 deaths attributable to sexual practices (29). Given the magnitude of these effects, even if a clinician has only modest success in convincing patients to change behavior, the effort is far more likely to prevent disease than administering tests.

The general ineffectiveness of screening tests stands to reason. If one considers the time line of the natural history of disease (Fig. 1), it becomes apparent that screening tests cannot detect a disorder until the disease process has produced a measurable pathophysiologic abnormality. Treat-

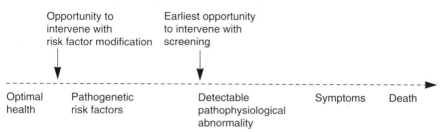

Figure 1. "Time line" for pathogenesis of preventable disease, which begins with modifiable risk factors that, over time, can lead to pathophysiological abnormalities. Once these abnormalities develop, screening tests may be able detect the problem before the patient develops symptoms but not until the disease process has progressed to the point of producing a detectable pathophysiological disorder. Through modification of personal health behaviors, the patient can intervene much earlier in the process and is therefore more likely to be effective.

ment interventions at this stage are often of limited effectiveness because the pathophysiologic process has usually already advanced to the point of producing irreversible disease. Personal health behaviors that cause disease, on the other hand, play a key etiologic role much earlier on the time line. Modifying such behaviors early in the natural history can prevent (or, in some cases, reverse [30]) progression of the disease many years before it would be detectable by physical examination or screening tests. Attention to these causes of disease and injury can accomplish real prevention, whereas the inherent nature of screening requires one to wait for the disease process to begin.

PRINCIPLES OF EXCELLENCE AND QUALITY IN PREVENTIVE MEDICINE

Basic to the practice of good preventive medicine, as to the practice of all medicine, is taking a thorough history. The clinician cannot determine which preventive services are indicated for a particular patient without first considering the patient's risk factors. It is self-evident that the clinician cannot recognize the need to advise a patient to stop smoking without first inquiring whether he or she smokes. The need to advise an adolescent about sexual practices will not become apparent until the clinician determines whether the teen is sexually active. The need to begin colorectal screening at an earlier age because of hereditary polyposis will not become apparent unless the clinician inquires about the family history. A diagnostic approach to risk factors is of as much importance in designing a plan for prevention as is a diagnostic approach in determining how to treat symptomatic patients. Proposing a uniform health maintenance plan for all patients is as inappropriate as suggesting a single treatment plan for all patients with chest pain. The history, physical, and laboratory examination must be used to construct an individual risk profile. Only then can one determine which preventive services are indicated and which deserve priority.

The risk factors identified in the evaluation should be treated as real problems, recorded on the patient's "problem list" along with diseases, physical findings, and symptoms. Unhealthy personal behaviors, inadequate screening, and overdue immunizations represent problems that require as clear and as determined a follow-up plan as atrial fibrillation, rectal bleeding, a palpable spleen, or a new systolic murmur. Indeed, the fact that a patient does not exercise, has multiple sexual partners, drinks and drives, or has not had a mammogram in five years may represent a more serious threat to the patient's health than most conditions that appear on conventional problem lists. Certainly they require as much attention if the patient is to reduce the risk of adding new diseases to the problem list in future years. The bulk of this book (Section 2) is devoted to advising the clinician on how to address risk factors once they are identified.

Preventive medicine cannot be practiced properly without a seamless integration with other aspects of health care. Providing preventive services in isolation from the patient's primary health care often limits their effectiveness. Appropriate counseling about personal health behaviors, such as advising safe exercise levels, requires an awareness of the patient's past history and coexisting medical problems. Screening tests performed in isolation from the primary care provider (e.g., screening at community health fairs) can leave the patient without a means for acting on the results. Clinicians who prescribe preventive therapies (e.g., who start antihypertensive medications on a patient noted to have high blood pressure) without consulting the primary care provider may be unaware of other medications and medical problems that need to be considered and may duplicate or complicate efforts undertaken by the primary care provider. This book is therefore targeted to primary care providers, who are most knowledgeable about the patient's complete medical history, have the skills to diagnose and manage the broad array of clinical problems that arise in health promotion and disease prevention, and have a relationship with the patient that facilitates continuity in the health maintenance program. The primary care provider is best suited to coordinate the patient's referrals to specialists, ensuring that patients receive necessary expert care in categorical areas without allowing other problems to "fall through the cracks."

Clinicians who are not primary care providers, such as specialists (e.g., cardiologists, ophthalmologists), emergency department clinicians, and hospital nurses, should also provide preventive services. It is important, however, that their focused contribution to the patient's preventive care be integrated into a comprehensive health maintenance plan under the coordination of the primary care provider. A dermatologist who performs a skin cancer screening examination, a gastroenterologist who performs a screening sigmoidoscopy, or an emergency department nurse who administers a vaccination, for example, should notify the primary care provider and should forward copies of their findings to be included in the patient's primary care medical record.

Discussions in this book about patient education and counseling emphasize a shared decision-making model (31) and a respectful style of discourse between clinicians and patients. This approach differs from the old-fashioned paternalistic counseling style in which the doctor "tells the patient what to do." The philosophy espoused in this book is that patients are entitled to make informed decisions about how they live their lives and about their health care. Clinicians have a professional responsibility to ensure that patients' decisions are based on complete and accurate health information but do not have a right to force the outcome of decisions. Once they have given the patient the necessary information about benefits and harms, they must respect the patient's preferences, even if the patient decides against doing what the clinician recommends. An authoritarian approach to promoting personal behavior change is rarely effective. Instead, this book encourages a collaborative model for decision-making, which permits the clinician and patient to work together to determine the best choice for that individual. The book speaks of choices, not "orders"; patient initiative, not "compliance"; and partnership, not "prescription."

Although this trend in patient empowerment in decision-making is occurring throughout medicine, it is especially appropriate in the practice of preventive health care. In health promotion, the "locus of control" lies more so with the patient than with the clinician. In curative medicine, the clinician can often perform a procedure to solve the patient's problem (e.g., by placing a cast, removing an infected gallbladder, suturing a laceration). In health promotion, only the patient can solve the problem. Stopping smoking, changing eating habits, increasing physical activity, and other changes in lifestyle are under the control of the patient and occur outside of the doctor's office or clinic. The clinician can, and should, provide information about the health risks associated with the behavior, encourage change, and suggest strategies for doing so, but the ultimate determinant of whether change occurs is the patient and not the clinician. The patient's feelings and attitudes about these health issues therefore require the full attention and respect of the clinician.

This book's emphasis on patient education is reflected in the "Resources" sections at the end of most chapters, which include a list of organizations, government agencies, and federal clearinghouses that make brochures, counseling services, and other information resources available to the public. Characteristic of the current "information age" and the growth of medical consumerism, the scope of health information available to patients and the technologies for obtaining it are expanding rapidly. This information can supplement and reinforce the counseling provided by the clinician and can help the patient frame new questions, as well as identify the resources for answering them. It is the clinician's responsibility to ensure that patients are aware of these information resources and how to obtain them. Of all the services that clinicians can provide in the practice of health promotion and disease prevention, information is certainly the most valuable.

Finally, excellence in the practice of health promotion requires a holistic approach to understanding "health." The biomedical paradigm that dominates modern medicine has a tendency to be reductionist, to measure health in terms of blood test results, radiographic findings, and electrocardiographic changes. Clearly, health is more than the absence of disease, and it comprises more than the discrete biophysical entities that we are currently capable of measuring. The interconnections between the mind and body are only beginning to be understood. It seems clear that health is influenced not only by biophysical factors but also by emotional and spiritual life, family dynamics and relationships, work satisfaction, income, food security, educational status, personal achievements, and social support.

Busy clinicians can easily overlook these issues, especially if these problems are not perceived as "medical" concerns. Failure to consider the broader context of health can limit or undermine the clinician's efforts to help patients. A clinician who is preoccupied with a patient's "noncompliance" in getting a mammogram, without considering her personal life, may never discover that depression over her husband's death quells her interest in living longer. An overweight inner city youth concerned about basic survival and gang-related shootings will be helped little by a clinician preoccupied with weight management. Clinicians benefit from taking the time to consider these issues. By learning more about their patients' lives, clinicians can enjoy fuller and more satisfying relationships with their patients and their families. Their suggested strategies for behavior change are more likely to be relevant to their patients' living conditions and, accordingly, are more likely to achieve results. Defining health objectives more broadly gives clinicians the gratification of knowing that their efforts are directed toward goals that are meaningful to their patients and that relate directly to the overall quality of their lives.

U. S. PREVENTIVE SERVICES TASK FORCE

The U.S. Preventive Services Task Force (USPSTF) was established by the U.S. Public Health Service in 1984. It is an independent panel of nonfederal experts that uses a systematic methodology to review the evidence of effectiveness for clinical preventive services (screening tests, counseling interventions, immunizations, chemoprophylaxis), assigns ratings to the quality of the data, and issues clinical practice recommendations reflecting the strength of the supporting evidence. The USPSTF included 20 members in 1984–1989 and 10 members in 1990–1995. Preventive services are not recommended by the USPSTF unless there is compelling evidence of effectiveness and that the benefits outweigh the risks. The USPSTF works in close collaboration with primary care medical specialty societies (American Academy of Family Physicians, American Academy of Pediatrics, American College of Physicians, American College of Obstetricians and Gynecologists) and federal government health agencies (e.g., Centers for Disease Control and Prevention). USPSTF recommendations have been reviewed by hundreds of content experts in the United States, Canada, Europe, and Australia. The USPSTF also collaborates with a similar panel in Canada (Canadian Task Force on the Periodic Health Examination), which was established in the 1970s and which developed the original methodology on which the USPSTF approach was based. In 1989 and 1996, the USPSTF published the first (2) and second (13) editions of the *Guide to Clinical Preventive Services*, a summary of the evidence for nearly 200 screening tests, counseling interventions, immunizations, and chemoprophylactic regimens. The 1996 USPSTF recommendations, excerpted from the *Guide*, are listed in the appendix of this book. Other USPSTF reviews have been published in medical journals. Further details about the USPSTF and how its recommendations were developed are available in the *Guide* and in other reviews (32).

REFERENCES

1. Green LW. Prevention and health education. In: Last JM, Wallace RB, et al., eds. Maxcy-Rosenau-Last Public health and preventive medicine. 13th ed. Norwalk, CT: Appleton and Lange, 1992:787–802.
2. U.S. Preventive Services Task Force. Guide to clinical preventive services. Baltimore: Williams & Wilkins, 1989.
3. World Bank. World development report 1993. Washington, DC: World Bank, 1993.
4. Lubitz JD, Riley GF. Trends in Medicare payments in the last year of life. N Engl J Med 1993;328:1092–1096.
5. U.S. Centers for Disease Control and Prevention. Estimated national spending on prevention—United States, 1988. MMWR 1992;41:529–531.
6. Lalonde M. A new perspective on the health of Canadians. Ottawa: Information Canada, 1974.
7. Healthy People: The Surgeon General's Report on Health Promotion and Disease Prevention. HEW Publication No. 79-55071. Washington, DC: U.S. Department of Health, Education, and Welfare, 1979.
8. Promoting health/preventing disease: objectives for the nation. Washington, DC: U.S. Department of Health and Human Services, 1990.
9. U.S. Public Health Service. Healthy people 2000: national health promotion and disease prevention objectives. Publication (PHS) 91-50212. Washington, DC: U.S. Department of Health and Human Services, 1991.

10. McGinnis JM, Lee PR. *Healthy People 2000* at mid decade. JAMA 1995;273:1123–1129.

11. American Public Health Association. Healthy communities 2000: model standards, guidelines for community attainment of year 2000 national health objectives. 3rd ed. Washington, DC: American Public Health Association, 1991.

12. Last JM, Wallace RB, et al., eds. Maxcy-Rosenau-Last Public health and preventive medicine. 13th ed. Norwalk, CT: Appleton and Lange, 1992.

13. U.S. Preventive Services Task Force. Guide to clinical preventive services. 2nd ed. Baltimore: Williams & Wilkins, 1996.

14. Fiore MC. Trends in cigarette smoking in the United States: the epidemiology of tobacco use. Med Clin N Amer 1992;76:289–303.

15. Kochanek KD, Hudson BL. Advance report of final mortality statistics, 1992. Monthly vital statistics report; vol. 43, no. 6, suppl. Hyattsville, MD: National Center for Health Statistics, 1995.

16. Garfinkel L, Silverberg E. Lung cancer and smoking trends in the United States over the past 25 years. CA 1991;41:137–145.

17. National Center for Health Statistics. Annual summary of births, marriages, divorces, and deaths: United States, 1993. Monthly vital statistics report; vol. 42, no. 13. Hyattsville, MD: National Center for Health Statistics, 1994.

18. Benson V, Marano MA. Current estimates from the National Health Interview Survey. Vital Health Stat 10(189). Hyattsville, MD: National Center for Health Statistics, 1994.

19. Woo B, Woo B, Cook EF, et al. Screening procedures in the asymptomatic adult: comparison of physicians' recommendations, patients' desires, published guidelines and actual practice. JAMA 1985;254:1480–1484.

20. McPhee SJ, Richard RJ, Solkowitz SN. Performance of cancer screening in a university general internal medicine practice: comparison with the 1980 American Cancer Society guidelines. J Gen Intern Med 1986;1:275–281.

21. Lewis CE. Disease prevention and health promotion practices of primary care physicians in the United States. Am J Prev Med 1988;4(suppl):9–16.

22. Anda RF, Remington PL, Sienko DG, Davis RM. Are physicians advising smokers to quit? The patient's perspective. JAMA 1987;257:1916–1919.

23. Frank E, Winkleby MA, Altman DG, Rockhill B, Fortmann SP. Predictors of physicians' smoking cessation advice. JAMA 1991;266:3139–3144.

24. Pommerenke FA, Dietrich A. Improving and maintaining preventive services, Part 2: Practical principles for primary care. J Fam Pract 1992;34:92–97.

25. Hayward RSA, Steinberg EP, Ford DE, Roizen MF, Roach KW. Preventive care guidelines: 1991. Ann Intern Med 1991;114:758–783.

26. Canadian Task Force on the Periodic Health Examination. The Canadian guide to clinical preventive health care. Ottawa: Canada Communication Group, 1994.

27. Frame PS. Health maintenance in clinical practice: strategies and barriers. Am Fam Physician 1992;45:1192–1200.

28. Woolf SH, Kamerow DB. Testing for uncommon conditions: the heroic search for positive test results. Arch Intern Med 1990;150:2451–2458.

29. McGinnis JM, Foege WH. Actual causes of death in the United States. JAMA 1993;270:2207–2212.

30. Ornish D, Brown SE, Scherwitz LW, Billings JH, et al. Can lifestyle changes reverse coronary heart disease? The Lifestyle Heart Trial. Lancet 1990;336:129–133.

31. Kasper JF, Mulley AG Jr, Wennberg JE. Developing shared decision-making programs to improve the quality of health care. QRB 1992;18:183–190.

32. Sox HC, Woolf SH. Evidence-based practice guidelines from the U.S. Preventive Services Task Force. JAMA 1993;269:2678.

section one

Gathering Information

1. Principles of Risk Assessment

STEVEN H. WOOLF

INTRODUCTION

Case 1. *A 21-year-old male college student was brought to the emergency department following a motor vehicle accident. He was the unbelted driver of an automobile involved in a high-speed collision. The patient was ejected from the vehicle on impact and thrown 50 yards, sustaining fatal head injuries. The blood alcohol concentration was 0.24%. Past medical history revealed that the patient had been seen for gastritis at the student health center on three occasions in the past year. The records revealed no discussion of the patient's alcohol use, which had been a problem since high school, or his regular practice of driving without using seat belts.*

Case 2. *A 52-year-old woman presented to a gastroenterologist with a three-month history of progressive left-lower-quadrant abdominal pain, weight loss, and fatigue. In the past few days she had noted bloody stool. A colonoscopic examination with biopsy revealed an obstructing adenocarcinoma of the sigmoid colon. The patient underwent a partial colectomy and colostomy placement. Past medical history was noteworthy for ulcerative colitis, which was diagnosed when the patient was 24 years old but which had not required extensive medical care. The patient's previous clinical encounters had been limited to preventive visits to her gynecologist, who had never discussed her ulcerative colitis and had not recommended periodic colonoscopy or sigmoidoscopy.*

Case 3. *A 49-year-old corporate executive was brought to the emergency department 45 minutes after clutching his chest and collapsing during a business meeting. The electrocardiogram revealed 3-mm ST-segment depression in the anterior leads. Thrombolytic therapy was attempted, but the patient developed ventricular fibrillation and could not be resuscitated. Post-mortem examination revealed a blood cholesterol level of 356 mg/dL and large stenotic plaques in the left main and anterior descending arteries. Family members indicated that the patient had been gaining weight and smoking more heavily in recent years but was otherwise healthy. His siblings were also healthy, but two sisters were being treated for high blood cholesterol. The patient's father and uncle had also died at a young age from unexpected heart attacks. The patient visited a physician only three times as an adult, primarily for treatment of joint injuries received during unsuccessful attempts at jogging. The physician's notes addressed the joint injuries but did not discuss the patient's to-*

bacco use, family history, eating habits, or physical inactivity. No prior record of the patient's blood cholesterol level could be found in the chart.

Case 4. *A 20-month-old girl was admitted to the hospital with a one-day history of fever, headache, and increasing lethargy. Physical examination was suggestive of meningitis, and culture of the cerebrospinal fluid grew* Haemophilus influenza *type b. After completion of intravenous antibiotic therapy, the patient was discharged from the hospital but was noted to have permanent hearing impairment. Review of the family physician's records revealed that the patient had received appropriate immunizations until nine months of age, but subsequent appointments for well-child examinations were canceled by the parents for unexplained reasons and thus* Haemophilus *vaccination was never completed. The patient's mother did see the family physician on two occasions for treatment of facial lacerations, but the child's immunization status and the conditions at home were not discussed. Six months later, a telephone call from a neighbor prompted an evaluation by the local child protective services agency, which revealed that both the child and mother were regular victims of beatings by the father.*

What these unfortunate cases have in common is that each patient suffered or died from conditions that were potentially preventable earlier in life. Diseases (e.g., coronary artery disease, colon cancer), injuries (e.g., motor vehicle accidents, physical abuse), and infections (e.g., meningitis) were preceded months, years, and decades earlier by risk factors or preclinical disease states that escaped detection and intervention.

Unfortunately, prevention failures of this magnitude are neither exceptional nor uncommon in the United States. Each day, thousands of Americans undergo treatment for conditions that could have been prevented earlier in their lives if the underlying causal risk factors had been identified. The failure to detect and treat those risk factors while patients are healthy often culminates years later in the need for aggressive medical interventions (e.g., chemotherapy, surgery, dialysis) and in the suffering of chronic impairment (pain, paralysis, mental illness, disability, death). The fact that such personally, socially, and financially costly consequences can be prevented through relatively simple interventions—counseling about harmful behaviors (e.g., smoking), immunizations, and screening for early disease—and the reality that so many Americans do not receive these services, have created a growing concern among both professionals and the public. Preventive care in the United States is inadequate for many reasons, including limited access to care, patient noncompliance, and costs. In many cases, however, the failure to receive preventive care is attributable to the failure of clinicians to include risk assessment in their routine care of asymptomatic and healthy patients. The purpose of this chapter is to review the importance of risk assessment and the theoretical principles that underlie the clinical risk assessment activities discussed in this book.

See Chapters 2–4 for details on how to perform risk assessment in patient care.

THE ROLE OF PREVENTION IN ILLNESS VISITS

In this book, the terms "asymptomatic" and "healthy" are not meant to describe patients without complaints; only a few patients visit their doctor without complaints for the sole purpose of obtaining preventive checkups. Rather, the terms refer to the absence of signs or symptoms of *target conditions*. For example, the executive who was seen on three occasions for joint injuries was "symptomatic" in the usual sense of the term—he had acute orthopedic complaints—but he was asymptomatic with respect to the target condition of coronary artery disease.

This, in fact, is the usual context of preventive care: the detection of risk factors in asymptomatic patients (with respect to target conditions) often occurs during clinical encounters that have been scheduled by the patient to address other, more immediate problems. For example, a patient schedules an appointment for sinusitis, but is found to be physically inactive and returns home with both an exercise and antibiotic prescription. A patient presents with a vaginal yeast infection but is noted to have not had a Papanicolaou smear for five years. A preschool boy with inadequate well-child care is rushed to the emergency department for treatment of acute otitis media and receives his second measles-mumps-rubella vaccination before being discharged.

The need to incorporate prevention practice into illness visits creates two obvious problems. First, patients, who are generally concerned about their current complaints, may be unprepared to address risk factors for unrelated, inapparent health problems that may or may not occur in the future. Second, clinicians can easily overlook the need for preventive interventions unless they are able to see beyond the patient's current complaints and begin identifying risk factors that threaten the patient's future health. They cannot wait for the patient to return to the office for a preventive visit devoted to this purpose, since most patients, especially high-risk individuals who face the greatest need for preventive services, rarely schedule such visits. To be part of regular medical practice, preventive medicine must be part of the daily routine and cannot be limited to annual physicals or well-person examinations. With the exception of visits for serious or painful health problems, which demand the complete attention of both clinician and patient, every clinical encounter in the office, hospital, and emergency department presents an opportunity for health promotion and disease prevention. The clinician must adopt the habit of looking beyond the patient's current complaints to address future disease, a process that begins with risk assessment.

WHAT IS RISK ASSESSMENT?

Risk assessment in the clinical setting refers to the collection of information about risk factors during the history, physical, and laboratory examination.[a] *Risk factors* are personal characteristics, physiological parameters, symptoms, or preclinical disease states that increase the likelihood that an individual has or will develop a particular disease. Examples of personal characteristics that can increase risk are health behaviors (e.g., smoking), family history, environmental exposures, and occupation. Examples of physiological risk factors include laboratory test results (e.g., serum cholesterol concentration), anthropomorphic measurements (e.g., weight), and other laboratory information (e.g., electrocardiographic abnormalities). Similarly, symptoms and past or present disease states may also increase a patient's likelihood of having disease. Chapters 2, 3, and 4 discuss how to perform risk assessment during the history, physical, and laboratory examination, respectively. Section II of this book discusses what to do with the findings.

Risk assessment should not be regarded as a unique clinical activity, separate from routine patient care. It is, after all, a well-established component of the thorough history, physical, and laboratory examination taught throughout clinical training. Personal characteristics that increase risk, such as smoking and family history, are commonly addressed in the social and family history sections of the history; preclinical disease states are sought in a careful physical examination; and physiological risk factors are often detected in conventional laboratory studies. Yet many physicians perform incomplete risk assessments when evaluating healthy patients for preventive care.

THE IMPORTANCE OF RISK ASSESSMENT

What accounts for incomplete risk assessments by clinicians? Why, for example, did the businessman's physician not investigate his family history and cardiac risk factors? In some cases, the oversights are due to *lack of knowledge* and the clinician's unfamiliarity with current guidelines. The gynecologist may not have remembered that ulcerative colitis is a risk factor for colon cancer and that periodic endoscopic surveillance may be necessary. In other instances, the oversight is due to *lack of time.* The physician in a busy student health center may have lacked the time to ask about the patient's drinking habits or seat belt use. In some cases, the oversight is due to *distraction* by the patient's current complaints. The family physician's concentration on suturing the mother's facial lacerations may have made him less attentive to the source of her injuries or her daughter's missed ap-

---

[a]Population-based risk assessment, such as the measurement of environmental and other health risks facing society, is not discussed here.

pointments. Sometimes the oversight is *attitudinal,* due to an inappreciation of the clinical importance of prevention. Problem drinking, seat belt use, unsuccessful exercise, eating habits, and missed appointments may have seemed unimportant at the time, and the serious consequences of overlooking them may have been inapparent.

Perhaps the most important reason for incomplete risk assessments is neither lack of time or knowledge but rather the reluctance of clinicians to believe that preventive interventions are worthwhile. Many do not appreciate the linkage between the quality of preventive care and the thoroughness of risk assessment, despite its obvious logic: clinicians cannot provide patients with rational advice on health maintenance or intervene with early-stage disease without first identifying the risk factors and disease states that most deserve their attention. A standardized "prevention package" for all patients is rarely appropriate, effective, or well-received. The prevention priorities for a 55-year-old smoker with a family history of premature heart disease obviously differ from those of the health-conscious young athlete, the drug-using, depressed adolescent who talks of suicide, or the elderly nursing home patient. If the clinician is to have a meaningful and effective impact on the patient's risk of future disease, the prevention message must be tailored to the risk profile of that individual.

Risk assessment is also necessary for rational ordering of screening tests. For many years, physicians administered a standard battery of laboratory tests as part of annual checkups, such as screening blood counts and chemistries, urinalyses, chest radiographs, and electrocardiograms. Many physicians continue this practice today. The problem with this approach, aside from its enormous cost, is that it generates large numbers of false-positive results (see Chapter 4). This, in turn, leads to a "screening cascade" of unnecessary diagnostic workups and treatment interventions. Because these adverse effects are less likely when screening is targeted to patients with specific risk factors (in whom the pretest probability and positive predictive value are increased), expert panels, such as the U.S. Preventive Services Task Force, have recommended that physicians avoid routine test batteries and instead order selected screening tests based on the patient's individual risk profile. This recommendation obviously requires the physician to first identify the patient's risk factors. It also reinforces the need for physicians to return to the time-honored tradition of careful history-taking and to limit current overreliance on laboratory testing.

PSYCHOLOGICAL BASIS OF INCOMPLETE RISK ASSESSMENTS: ILLNESS-BASED VS. RISK FACTOR-BASED THINKING PROCESSES

The tendency of physicians to perform incomplete risk assessments may result from using the wrong thinking process when evaluating patients.

The commonly used thinking process when evaluating symptomatic patients identifies chief complaints as the primary problem and has as its objective the clarification of the diagnosis and treatment plan. This *illness-based thinking process* is, appropriately, oriented to the present and not the future. In such patients, risk assessment—the collection of risk factor information in the history, physical, and laboratory examination—is performed to explain the patient's *current* symptoms. In this task it plays a relatively minor role. Experienced clinicians know that the history of present illness and physical examination findings are usually all that are needed to make the diagnosis. Although risk factor information can occasionally enhance diagnostic accuracy, most clinicians discover over time that their diagnostic accuracy is rarely compromised by an incomplete social, family, or occupational history. Physicians accustomed to caring for symptomatic patients are therefore not driven to compulsive questioning about risk factors.

In preventive medicine, risk assessment has a different purpose, because the patient has not yet developed target conditions. Thus, a different *risk factor-oriented thinking process* is necessary. The patients' risk factors—not their current complaints—are properly viewed as the primary problem. In contrast to their minor role with symptomatic patients, risk factors constitute the primary problem in preventive care, and risk assessment is the essential starting point for addressing the scope of the problem. What follows in the thinking process is a problem-oriented examination of how to modify the identified risks. A patient with the risk factors of tobacco use, exposure to tuberculosis, and susceptibility to influenza requires a special program of smoking cessation counseling, tuberculin skin testing, and influenza vaccination. A patient with the risk factors of multiple sexual partners, intravenous drug use, and a history of dysplastic nevi requires a special program of sexual practices and substance abuse counseling, screening for malignant melanoma, and vaccination against hepatitis B. These interventions will not be carried out if the clinician does not first establish the risk factor "problem list" through risk assessment.

Physicians are more accustomed to the thinking process used for symptomatic patients than to the thinking process used for preventive care, and their tendency to use the customary illness-based thinking process in preventive care probably accounts for the frequency of incomplete risk assessments. To illustrate the consequences of this mismatch, consider the example of a physician accustomed to the illness-based thinking process who enters the examination room of the previously mentioned patient with sinusitis. Because the illness-based thinking process defines current complaints as the primary problem, the physician immediately identifies purulent rhinorrhea and maxillary tenderness as the matter at hand. With additional physical examination findings to confirm the diagnosis, there is little reason to pursue risk assessment. For a patient with obvious sinusitis, why should the physician obtain a social, family, or occupational history? The only risk factors to which the illness-based thinking process might direct the physician are those related to sinusitis. The patient would be sent home with an antibiotic prescription, but without a discussion of the need for increased exercise.

High-quality preventive care requires the clinician to adopt a risk factor-oriented thinking process that is independent of the evaluation of current complaints. Once the current complaints have been addressed, the next step is to switch to a risk factor-oriented thinking process, which begins a comprehensive search for silent risk factors. In a systematic process that takes less than a few minutes to complete, the clinician supplements the sinusitis history with information about the risk factors discussed in Chapter 2 and checks whether the patient is up-to-date on the recommended physical examination and laboratory screening procedures discussed in Chapters 3 and 4. (Flow sheets and other office systems discussed in Chapter 23 can speed this process.) In this example, questions from Chapter 2 would call attention to the patient's physical inactivity and would prompt a discussion of exercise or arrangements for a return visit devoted to this topic.

The risk factors identified through this process vary among patients. Each patient's risk factor "problem list" constitutes an *individual risk profile,* which provides global information on the patient's overall risk for future disease, as well as a framework for tailoring the patient's health maintenance plan. For example, consider a patient who makes an appointment with a physician to obtain a tetanus immunization, which has not been updated for over 10 years. Rather than simplistically responding to this request, the physician performs a brief but thorough risk assessment to review the individual's risk profile. This reveals that the patient has multiple risk factors, including a family history of premature coronary artery disease and a personal history of smoking, hypertension, overweight, and hypercholesterolemia, as well as delayed tetanus immunization. This "big picture" perspective enables the physician and patient to review the complete list of risk factors and to work together to "triage" the priorities. They first agree that the cardiac risk factors pose a greater threat to future health than susceptibility to tetanus, skip the tetanus immunization, and use the remaining time to devise a plan for cardiac risk factor modification. It is rarely appropriate or possible to address all risk factors at once. Health maintenance planning involves collaborative work with the patient: setting priorities by determining which problems the patient is willing and able to address first and agreeing on a follow-up plan for addressing other risk factors. See Chapter 5 for further details about this process.

SETTING REASONABLE LIMITS AND PRIORITIES IN RISK ASSESSMENT

There are at least hundreds of personal characteristics, physiologic parameters, environmental exposures, symptoms, and preclinical disease states that can increase an individual's risk for future disease. Practical and scientific reasons make it implausible for clinicians to screen for all risk factors during risk assessments. The most important practical constraint is lack of time; a typical office visit can accommodate a discussion of no more than two or three risk factors. Moreover, for many risk factors, there is insufficient scientific evidence that the risk factors pose significant risks or that attempts to modify them are effective in improving health. At its best, devoting time to these unproven measures may be useless and, at its worst, this practice can divert the clinician and patient away from more important risk factors that deserve their attention.

How, then, should the clinician select the factors to address in risk assessment? Consider the following questions: (*a*) how serious is the target condition? (*b*) how common is the risk factor? (*c*) what is the magnitude of risk associated with the risk factor? (*d*) how accurately can the risk factor be detected? (*e*) what is the evidence that potential interventions improve health outcomes? and (*f*) how does this information compare with other health priorities?

How Serious Is the Target Condition?

Risk factors for a trivial health problem may not deserve attention. The burden of suffering from the target condition is best judged by its frequency and severity. Frequency is typically measured in terms of incidence or prevalence. *Incidence*, a dynamic measure, is the proportion of the population that acquires the disease in a given period of time. *Prevalence*, a static measure, is the proportion of the population that has the disease at any given time. A variety of outcome measures are used to estimate the severity of a disease. Traditional measures include morbidity, mortality, and survival rates, but recent health services research has encouraged the use of more meaningful measures of quality of life, functional status, and overall well-being. In terms of mortality, a convenient ranking of the importance of diseases is the leading causes of death, which can be determined for the general population (Table 1.1) or stratified by specific risk groups. Table 1.2 lists the leading causes of death for specific age groups.

How Common Is the Risk Factor?

A risk factor that is extremely uncommon may not be worthy of routine screening, and some risk factors that are extremely common may be weak

Table 1.1
Leading Causes of Death in the United States

Rank	Cause of Death	Number of Deaths, 1991	Age-Adjusted Death Rate (per 100,000)	Percent of Total Deaths (%)
1	Heart disease	720,862	148.2	33.2
2	Malignant neoplasms	514,657	134.5	23.7
3	Cerebrovascular diseases	143,481	26.8	6.6
4	Chronic obstructive pulmonary diseases	90,650	20.1	4.2
5	Accidents	89,347	31.0	4.1
6	Pneumonia and influenza	77,860	13.4	3.6
7	Diabetes mellitus	48,951	11.8	2.3
8	Suicide	30,810	11.4	1.4
9	HIV infection	29,555	11.3	1.4
10	Homicide and legal intervention	26,513	10.9	1.2

Source: National Center for Health Statistics. Advance Report of Final Mortality Statistics, 1991. Monthly Vital Statistics Report, Volume 42, Number 2, Suppl. Hyattsville, MD: Public Health Service, 1993.

predictors of future disease. Like target conditions, the frequency of a risk factor in the population is generally measured by prevalence and incidence rates and may vary considerably in different segments of the population.

What Is the Magnitude of Risk Associated with the Risk Factor?

The magnitude of risk conferred by a risk factor can be defined in terms of relative or absolute risk. *Relative risk* is the ratio between the risk of disease among persons with the risk factor and the risk among those without the risk factor. A relative risk of 2.0 suggests that persons with the risk factor are twice as likely to develop the disease as persons without the risk factor. Such ratios, which are often used in both the medical literature and lay media to emphasize (and sensationalize) the magnitude of risk, can be misleading if not accompanied by information about the *absolute risk,* the actual proportion of persons with the risk factor who will develop the disease.

To clarify the distinction, consider hypothetical risk factors A and B.

Table 1.2
Leading Causes of Death, United States, by Age Group

1–4 Years	5–14 Years
1. Accidents	1. Accidents
2. Congenital anomalies	2. Malignant neoplasms
3. Malignant neoplasms	3. Homicide and legal intervention
4. Homicide and legal intervention	4. Congenital anomalies
5. Heart diseases	5. Heart diseases
6. Pneumonia and influenza	6. Suicide
7. HIV infection	7. Pneumonia and influenza
8. Perinatal conditions	8. Chronic obstructive pulmonary diseases
9. Septicemia	9. HIV infection
10. Benign neoplasms	10. Cerebrovascular diseases

15–24 Years	25–44 Years
1. Accidents	1. Accidents
2. Homicide and legal intervention	2. Malignant neoplasms
3. Suicide	3. HIV infection
4. Malignant neoplasms	4. Heart diseases
5. Heart diseases	5. Homicide and legal intervention
6. HIV infection	6. Suicide
7. Congenital anomalies	7. Chronic liver disease and cirrhosis
8. Pneumonia and influenza	8. Cerebrovascular diseases
9. Cerebrovascular diseases	9. Diabetes mellitus
10. Chronic obstructive pulmonary diseases	10. Pneumonia and influenza

45–64 Years	65 Years and Older
1. Malignant neoplasms	1. Heart diseases
2. Heart diseases	2. Malignant neoplasms
3. Cerebrovascular diseases	3. Cerebrovascular diseases
4. Accidents	4. Chronic obstructive pulmonary diseases
5. Chronic obstructive pulmonary diseases	5. Pneumonia and influenza
6. Chronic liver disease and cirrhosis	6. Diabetes mellitus
7. Diabetes mellitus	7. Accidents
8. Suicide	8. Nephritis, nephrotic syndrome, nephrosis
9. HIV infection	9. Atherosclerosis
10. Pneumonia and influenza	10. Septicemia

Source: National Center for Health Statistics. Advance Report of Final Mortality Statistics, 1991. Monthly Vital Statistics Report, Volume 42, Number 2, Suppl. Hyattsville, MD: Public Health Service, 1993.

Risk factor A is a risk factor for disease A, risk factor B is a risk factor for disease B, and both diseases are fatal. The relative risk of risk factors A and B are 2.0 and 1.1, respectively. Readers of the medical literature and lay media are likely to conclude at first glance that risk factor A is almost twice as dangerous as risk factor B. The missing information is the absolute risk. Suppose the absolute risk for persons with risk factor A is 1:50,000, whereas the risk is 1:100,000 for persons without risk factor A. Thus, although it is true that the relative risk is 2.0 (1:50,000 is twice the risk of

1:100,000), the patient's absolute risk of developing disease A is increased by only 0.001% (1:100,000 subtracted from 1:50,000) by having risk factor A. Put differently, 99.998% of persons with risk factor A will not develop the disease.

Absolute risk helps to clarify the distinction between risk factors and real disease, a common source of confusion among both health professionals and the public. Once the relationship between a risk factor and a disease is established and public education campaigns are launched to raise awareness of the risk factor, there is a tendency for both clinicians and patients to feel that a disease has been discovered when they detect a risk factor. A good example of this phenomenon is the successful effort of the federal government in the 1980s to expand public awareness of the importance of blood cholesterol levels. Although there were important health benefits to this program, an unfortunate consequence was that too many Americans with borderline cholesterol levels (200–239 mg/dL) became anxious that they had a disease and rushed to specialists for help. This "cholesterol scare" would have been less likely if patients understood that cholesterol levels in this range increased their 10-year absolute risk of dying from heart disease by only about 0.5–1.5%. That is, over 98% of persons with these cholesterol values would not die of heart disease within the following decade (1).

Next consider the situation for risk factor B, which has a lower relative risk (1.1) than risk factor A (2.0). Suppose, however, that the absolute risk for disease B is 1:10 (0.1) among persons with this risk factor and 1:11 (0.0909) for persons without this risk factor. Thus, although it is true that the relative risk associated with risk factor B is 1.1 (0.1/0.0909), it increases the absolute risk for disease B by 0.9% (0.1–0.0909). Recall that the absolute risk for disease A was increased 0.001% by risk factor A. Thus, although the relative risk of risk factor B (1.1) is nearly half that of risk factor A (2.0), the absolute risk data tell us that persons with risk factor B are 900 times (0.9/0.001) more likely to develop disease B than are persons with risk factor A to develop disease A. (Note that, even with this higher risk, 90% of persons with risk factor B will not develop the disease).

Unfortunately, it is all too common for the public, policymakers, and health professionals to overlook these details when they make arguments for or against health interventions. For example, based on the above information, is it appropriate for a newspaper headline to claim that risk factor A or B is a more serious problem? The answer is that neither relative nor absolute risk data provide sufficient information to answer the question. The analysis is incomplete without considering the *population attributable risk*, the proportion of the population affected. Suppose that one million Americans have risk factor A, but only 1000 have risk factor B. Reducing

the absolute risk of disease A by 0.001% will save 1000 (1 million ×
0.001%) lives, whereas reducing the absolute risk of disease B by 0.9% will
save only nine (1000 × 0.9%) lives. Thus, whether in the government or
clinic, the importance of a risk factor requires consideration of relative,
absolute, and population attributable risk.

How Accurately Can the Risk Factor Be Detected?

Even if the target condition and risk factor are serious, efforts to detect
risk factors may be ineffective or harmful if the screening test is inaccurate. Inaccurate screening tests can produce *false-positive* results, which suggest incorrectly the presence of the risk factor, or *false-negative* results,
which suggest incorrectly the absence of the risk factor. False-positive results can generate unnecessary anxiety, follow-up testing, and treatment.
False-negative results can lead to delays in the detection and treatment of
the risk factor. The accuracy of a screening test is measured in terms of *sensitivity, specificity,* and *predictive value.* In general, a screening test is more
likely to produce false-positive results if the risk factor is uncommon in the
population. See Chapter 4 for definitions of these terms and for further
discussion of these concepts.

What Is the Evidence that Potential Interventions Improve Health Outcomes?

Even if the risk factor and target condition are important and the available
screening tests are accurate, there is little point in screening if there is inadequate evidence that available interventions improve outcomes. The
best evidence to this effect are intervention studies demonstrating that patients who undergo risk factor modification achieve better health outcomes than those without the intervention. More often, however, all that is
available is epidemiologic evidence suggesting that the risk factor causes
the disease. In such cases, proponents of risk factor modification may use
this evidence of causality to infer that interventions will be effective. Unfortunately, such assumptions are not always valid. For example, there is
considerable evidence of an association between dietary fat and cancer,
but no study has yet demonstrated that lowering dietary fat intake reduces
the incidence of cancer. In exceptional cases, the effectiveness of risk factor modification can be inferred from the strength and consistency of the
evidence. For example, there has never been a controlled intervention
study demonstrating that smoking cessation reduces the incidence of cancer—and the performance of such a study is unlikely for ethical reasons—
but the enormous strength and consistency of the evidence and the lower
rates of disease in persons who stop smoking are considered adequate evidence to infer that such measures are effective.

How Does This Information Compare with Other Health Priorities?

Individual risk factors and diseases do not exist in a vacuum. In deciding whether to devote limited time and energy to a particular risk factor or health problem, the conscientious clinician must also consider its relative importance in relation to the other risk factors and health problems that also require attention. Advising patients about dietary fiber intake may be important, but is it more important than using the same time to discuss dietary fat consumption, tobacco use, the need for breast cancer screening, or blood pressure monitoring? Advocates of prostate cancer screening may emphasize that 40,000 American die each year from this disease but, by examining the data in Table 1.1, the clinician can put these numbers in perspective as they relate to other serious diseases the patient and clinician must consider.

HEALTH RISK APPRAISALS

One tool for summarizing risk information in the office is the health risk appraisal (HRA), a tool introduced in the 1970s to collect risk data from patients and generate epidemiologically-based, personalized risk projections for future illness. The HRA has evolved into a variety of formats over its 25-year history, beginning with hand-tallied instruments and now largely involving interactive software. The typical HRA asks the individual to answer questions about personal health behaviors, family history, and other risk factors; some HRAs also input current clinical data, such as blood pressure and serum cholesterol values, or ask individuals to remember their most recent measurements. The output of the conventional HRA is a list of risk factors that warrants the individual's attention and a quantitative estimate of the overall risk of disease. The hallmark of the HRA is a composite personal health risk score that is calculated by comparing the individual's risk profile with epidemiologic and actuarial data; many HRAs generate an *appraisal age*, a "health" or "physiological" age that can be contrasted with the individual's chronological age. Some HRAs also provide qualitative risk information on such topics as environmental exposures, safety practices, nutrition, mental health, and the need for screening tests and immunizations.

Most HRAs conclude with educational messages that advise individuals on how to reduce their risk, often specifying the "achievable health age" that will result from such a change, or that encourage individuals to obtain further instructions from a health professional. For example, an HRA might indicate that, "if you adhere to an exercise program, you will extend your useful life expectancy by 0.1 years." Additional innovations in HRA products include individualized instructions, attractive on-screen and print graphics, support materials (e.g., videotapes, compact disc/read-only

memory systems to access background information), expanded risk assessments of environmental and medication-related risks, data linkages to
other medical information systems, on-screen modeling of the effects of
making specific lifestyle changes, and software for analyzing population
risk information and forecasting economic costs for employers.

HRAs are widely used in the public and private sectors. At least 30 organizations sell HRA products, and several of these vendors are believed to
market tens of thousands of HRAs per year (2). One popular HRA product is *Healthier People*, an instrument first developed by the Carter Center of
Emory University and the Centers for Disease Control in the 1980s (3).
HRAs are generally used to encourage individuals to participate in health
promotion programs (primarily at worksites), to give employers data about
the major health risks faced by their workers, and to measure the health
behavior patterns of large populations. They were first developed by physicians, however, for use in the clinical setting to collect risk information
and facilitate patient education. The HRA risk factor printout was seen as
a tool for alerting physicians to health behaviors that need attention and
for encouraging patients to change their lifestyle. Increasingly, managed
care organizations and large practice groups with a contractual responsibility for preventive care are using HRAs to monitor the effectiveness of
health promotion programs.

HRAs are not without their methodological problems, however, which
are reviewed in detail elsewhere (2, 4). Individuals completing HRAs may
not provide accurate information, because they cannot understand the
questions (often due to ethnically or culturally biased wording), are uncomfortable answering them, or make mistakes in recalling data. The
quantitative estimates generated by HRAs may be invalid if they are based
on inapplicable epidemiological data (e.g., data may not be generalizable
to minorities or the elderly) or flawed risk calculations. Statistical methods
may be inadequate to handle missing data or adjust for confounding variables. HRAs can have poor reliability, generating inconsistent results
among different instruments, or the same instrument may produce different results when the questions are repeated. HRA products may recommend different lifestyle changes for individuals with the same risk profile.
HRAs are more likely to be misunderstood by blue-collar workers, and risk
estimates are generally unpersuasive or invalid among the young, old, or
minority groups. Other clinical concerns have also been raised, including
the possibility that quantitative estimates can give patients an inflated impression of the precision of risk projections and that HRAs might be mistakenly accepted as a substitute for visits with a physician. HRA products
vary in quality and the degree to which they inform consumers of these
methodological problems.

For the clinician, the most fundamental question about HRAs is
whether they are effective in helping patients to change behavior or in

helping providers to examine risks more systematically. The question is salient because of the sizable investment and time commitments required by practices that routinely use HRAs. Several controlled trials have examined the effectiveness of HRAs, and some have reported positive results (4). Although the studies clearly suggest that the combination of patient education and HRAs is associated with behavior change, it remains unclear, due to the study designs, whether the same results could have been achieved by patient education alone. There is little evidence to support the use of HRAs without patient education and good arguments to discourage the practice, including the possibility that patients will misinterpret the validity and implications of the results. The unique feature of HRAs, the presentation of quantitative, personalized risk projections, is intended to motivate behavior change by tailoring counseling to the individual and by supporting the recommendations with data. Aside from statistical concerns about their validity, it remains unclear whether these risk estimates are persuasive to lay persons, given the abstract relationship of absolute risk to distant events. Statistical facts may have a limited role in stimulating new health habits. Moreover, the predominant use of mortality projections in HRA relies to some extent on fear (of premature death) as a motivating force, whereas other, more positive objectives (enhanced well-being, appearance, productivity) are often more persuasive in lifestyle counseling.

THE BOTTOM LINE FOR THE PRACTITIONER

Fortunately for the practitioner, the risk factors and screening tests that usually deserve attention in the clinical encounter have already been identified by several expert panels, which have devoted years of research to examining the above issues. Chief among these is the U.S. Preventive Services Task Force (5), an independent panel established by the federal government in 1984 to develop evidence-based recommendations on which preventive services to include in the periodic health examination. Comprehensive preventive care recommendations have also been issued by medical specialty societies, and more specific recommendations on screening tests, immunizations, and health behaviors have been issued by government agencies, medical groups, and private organizations (6). These recommendations form the basis for the risk factor evaluations and screening tests discussed in Chapters 2–4.

Although the risk factors to address are therefore well-defined, clinicians have the daily opportunity to apply the risk assessment principles discussed in this chapter when counseling patients and when setting policy in their practice. When counseling patients about the meaning of risk factors, the conscientious clinician will provide information about both relative and absolute risk, allowing the patient to make a more informed decision about the importance or unimportance of the risk factor and limiting unnecessary anxiety. For example, providing only relative risk information to patients with risk factor A—telling them that they are twice as likely to develop a fatal disease than persons without the risk factor—is more likely to generate anxiety than if the absolute risk is also described. Patients who realize that their absolute risk of disease is only 0.002% will put this information in proper perspective and will be less likely to abandon more important health concerns to address this risk factor. Also, the realization that 99.998% of persons with risk factor A will not develop disease will also help them avoid the pitfall of confusing risk factors with disease.

The principles of risk assessment can also be applied when developing policy for one's practice. Although national guidelines are available to define important health priorities, local practice conditions or the emergence of new information following publication of the guidelines may prompt the need to supplement or modify recommendations for local practice. For example, although routine screening for diabetes mellitus might not be indicated for the general population, clinicians caring for Native Americans, in whom the prevalence of diabetes mellitus is high among certain tribes, might need to examine whether a different policy is indicated in their practice. Local news reports may heighten a community's concern over a particular risk factor (e.g., radon exposure) or health problem (e.g., Lyme disease) and may exert pressure on clinicians to screen for this condition. Finally, the medical literature may provide new information about the importance of a risk factor or the availability of a new screening test before national expert panels have had an opportunity to publish recommendations.

In each of these cases, the clinician should use the principles discussed in this chapter to determine the relative importance of the risk factor and its relationship to other established health priorities. How serious is the target condition? How common is the risk factor? What is the magnitude of risk associated with the risk factor? How accurately can the risk factor be detected? What is the evidence that potential interventions improve health outcomes? How does this information compare with other health priorities? Clinicians should also examine the source of articles advocating increased clinical attention to a particular risk factor. Such recommendations often originate from individuals, medical organizations, or government agencies that have a specialized interest in the topic. If an individual's research or an organization's mission is devoted to the eradication of a particular disease or risk factor, it may advocate full attention to this problem without first considering the effect of its recommendations on other serious health problems outside its focus of concern. Practitioners, who have the responsibility to address all of the patient's health needs, must be careful to use independent judgment before adding such topics to their risk assessment protocol.

Finally, the clinician must decide whether attention to the risk factor is a feasible activity for the practice. The practice must be capable of providing follow-up when the risk factor is identified. For example, before adopting exercise as a priority to address with all patients, the clinician should ask the following questions. (*a*) Is the promotion of exercise important to the practice and, if so, for which patients? (*b*) What are the objectives of exercise promotion, for patients and the practice? (*c*) Which clinicians in the practice should do the counseling, or will it be necessary to involve outside professionals (e.g., physical therapist, sports trainer)? (*d*) Should patient group counseling or community resources be considered? (*e*) How much time should physicians and other staff invest in education and training to provide the counseling? (*f*) Is there sufficient time to devote to the effort and how will it be paid for? (*g*) Should the practice formally encourage staff to exercise, both for their own health benefit and to serve as models for patients? See Chapter 23 for further details about the important decisions to make before implementing patient education and other preventive services in the office or clinic.

CONCLUSION

What follows in Chapters 2–4 are the details of how to perform risk assessment during the history, physical, and laboratory examination. Section II of this book contains chapters devoted to the risk factors that clinicians are most likely to encounter during risk assessments. These chapters are designed to provide the clinician with detailed information about what to do when a particular risk factor is discovered, including further questions for completing the risk assessment, screening tests for related disorders, counseling, and treatment. These efforts are clearly necessary if the clinician is to have a meaningful impact on helping patients to reduce their risk of developing diseases in later life.

REFERENCES

1. National Cholesterol Education Program. Second report of the Expert Panel on Detection, Evaluation, and Treatment of High Blood Cholesterol in Adults (NIH Publication No. 93-3095). Bethesda, MD: National Institutes of Health, 1993.
2. DeFriese GH, Fielding JE. Health risk appraisal in the 1990s: opportunities, challenges, and expectations. Ann Rev Public Health 1990;11:401–418.
3. Amler RW, Moriarty DG, Hutchins EB, eds. Healthier people: the Carter Center of Emory University Health Risk Appraisal Program Guides and Documentation. Atlanta: The Carter Center of Emory University, 1988.
4. Schoenbach VJ, Wagner EH, Beery WL. Health risk appraisal: review of evidence of effectiveness. Health Serv Res 1987;22:553–579.
5. U.S. Preventive Services Task Force. Guide to clinical preventive services, 2nd ed. Baltimore: Williams & Wilkins, in press.
6. Hayward RSA, Steinberg RP, Ford DE, Roizen MF, Roach KW. Preventive care guidelines: 1991. Ann Intern Med 1991;114:758–783.

2. The History

WHAT TO ASK ABOUT

STEVEN H. WOOLF

INTRODUCTION

Most of the leading causes of death and disability in the United States are caused by a small group of risk factors (1). Risk factors are personal characteristics, physiological parameters, environmental conditions, symptoms, or preclinical disease states that increase an individual's probability of having or developing a disease (see Chapter 1). The primary task of health promotion and disease prevention in clinical practice is to identify modifiable risk factors during the history, physical, and laboratory examination and to recommend preventive interventions that can help the patient decrease those risks. Preventive interventions include the modification of personal health behaviors (e.g., physical activity) or other risks, early detection of disease (e.g., cervical dysplasia), immunizations, and chemoprophylaxis. This chapter discusses how to collect risk factor information during the history. Chapters 3 and 4 discuss how to obtain further evidence of risk during the physical and laboratory examination, respectively.

This chapter does not discuss how to perform a conventional medical history. The conventional history taken when evaluating symptomatic patients includes questions about chief complaints, history of present illness, past medical and surgical history, current medications, drug allergies, and a review of systems, all of which relate to the *current* situation. This chapter discusses questioning patients about risk factors for *future* disease or injury. Although these questions are meant to be included in the social, family, and occupational history sections of the conventional medical history, they are often omitted or addressed superficially when clinicians evaluate symptomatic patients. As discussed in Chapter 1, the questions are generally not stressed in the evaluation of chief complaints because risk factor information is less important than eliciting symptom patterns in making a diagnosis.

Instead, many clinicians reserve detailed questions about risk factors for special visits, such as when they first meet a patient or when the patient presents for a periodic health examination (i.e., annual physical, preventive checkup). The problem with this practice, however, as explained in

Chapter 1, is that most patients, especially those in high-risk groups who have the greatest need for preventive care, typically do not schedule general checkups when they are asymptomatic. And, due to the physician's tendency to apply a thinking process that is better suited for symptomatic patients than for preventive care (see Chapter 1, "Psychological Basis of Incomplete Risk Assessments: Illness-Based vs. Risk Factor-Based Thinking Processes"), many physicians overlook important risk factors, even when they are attempting to be complete, because they lack a systematic approach to asking about risk factors.

This chapter reviews the risk factors that clinicians should ask about. The purpose of the questions is to identify which risk factors require further evaluation, either during that visit or at a subsequent appointment. These questions should be integrated into the regular clinical encounter, whether patients are being seen for the first time, for a periodic health examination, or for an illness visit. Illness visits comprise the majority of patient encounters at the office, clinic, emergency department, hospital, or nursing home. If risk assessments and preventive interventions are omitted from illness visits and offered only during well-person examinations, only a small percentage of a clinician's patients will benefit from preventive care. Conscientious clinicians therefore become accustomed to incorporating preventive medicine into routine illness visits. Except when examining patients in pain or those suffering from serious health problems, illness visits provide an appropriate opportunity to address the patient's risks for more serious health problems in the future (see Chapter 1).

It is obviously unrealistic, however, for clinicians to address all risk factors whenever a patient is seen. The average primary care office visit lasts 17 minutes (2), and most of that time must be devoted to the patient's chief complaints. Investing more than a few minutes in risk assessment is rarely feasible. These minutes provide enough time, however, to ask a few primary screening questions. *Primary screening questions* are brief questions that determine whether more detailed, *exploratory questions* are necessary at the present or on a future visit. An example of a primary screening question is, *"Do you smoke?"* More detailed, exploratory questions include *"At what age did you start smoking?"*, *"How many packs do you smoke each day?"*, *"What is your brand?"*, etc. Although risk assessment during illness visits is often limited to a few primary screening questions because of lack of time, well-person examinations and other preventive checkups allow more detailed exploratory questions.

Since all of the questions listed in this chapter cannot be addressed in a single visit, clinicians should establish a system for determining which questions are most important and a follow-up mechanism for ensuring that the remaining questions are asked at future visits. Clinicians who have time for only one question should probably ask whether the patient smokes (the same question should be asked of parents when children or adolescents are being seen). See Chapter 1 for further information about how to prioritize risk factor questions, and see Chapters 23 and 26 for suggestions on how to use reminder systems to add such questions to the office practice routine. For questions that cannot be addressed at the present visit, clinicians should schedule a return visit to address additional risk factors or should at least record reminder notes in the medical record about specific risk factors to address at a later date (e.g., "ask about eating habits when patient returns for cast removal"). The latter may be the best option for patients who only come to the doctor for illness visits.

When is the right time during an illness visit to ask questions about risk factors? One approach is to insert the questions into the history obtained for the presenting problem. Another approach is to first address the presenting problem and then bring up the patient's risk factors at the conclusion of the visit. Both models are illustrated below for a hypothetical patient who has visited the physician for treatment of influenza:

DURING THE HISTORY

Physician: *". . . So, to summarize, you've had a fever since Friday, and for the past two days you've had muscle aches, a sore throat, and fatigue. In a few minutes, I want to examine you but, before I do, let me ask you a question that also relates to your health. Do you smoke?"*

AT THE END OF THE CLINICAL ENCOUNTER

Physician: *". . . and remember to drink plenty of fluids. Call me if you feel that you are getting worse or if you notice new symptoms. Before you leave, I want to address an unrelated issue that also affects your health. How much exercise do you get?"*

Once a risk factor is identified, exploratory questions are often necessary to understand better the patient's individual risk profile and to offer meaningful recommendations about how to modify risk. See the other chapters in Section 2 of this book, which discuss exploratory questions and other techniques for learning more about a patient's risk factors and the interventions that should be recommended once a risk factor is identified. In this chapter, only primary screening questions are discussed. (The questions suggested in this chapter assume that the patient is asymptomatic, i.e., lacking signs or symptoms of the target condition. Patients who have already developed the target condition often require different risk assessment questions.)

This chapter provides sample language for screening questions, but the wording in clinical practice is best determined by the clinician, who can identify the optimal communication strategy for his or her patient.

Moreover, for most risk factors, research has not yet determined the "correct" wording for such questions nor tested their sensitivity and specificity. (See discussion of screening questionnaires later in the chapter.) The wording that clinicians use when asking risk factor questions should reflect their practice style and their relationship with the patient. The questions also need to be sensitive to the patient's age, educational background, primary language, culture, and health belief model. Because questions about risk factors often address sensitive aspects of personal behavior, the clinician should avoid judgmental or directive questions. Patients who are asked *"You aren't homosexual, are you?"* or *"I assume that you don't drink and drive"* may be reluctant to answer honestly. Similarly, facial expressions (e.g., raised eyebrows) and other nonverbal communication that suggest the clinician's disapproval are also inappropriate.

GETTING STARTED

Preferably before entering the room, the clinician should briefly review the patient's medical record to determine which risk factors have been discussed at previous visits, to recall the patient's previous successful or unsuccessful attempts at risk factor modification, and to determine which risk factors deserve attention at the current visit. A risk factor "problem list" on the inside cover of the medical record or reminder notes from prior visits (see Chapters 23 and 26) can often speed this review. If the patient has successfully changed a risk factor (e.g., smoking cessation) in the past, the clinician will want to offer positive reinforcement during the current visit and to verify that the patient has not relapsed. Other risk factors that have not been addressed should then be identified, and the clinician should determine which deserve attention in the current interview. See Chapter 1 for guidelines on how to determine which risk factors are most important.

As with any clinical encounter, the clinician should follow the basic principles of greeting patients (correct introductions and seating arrangements) and medical interviewing (determination of the patient's agenda, initial use of open-ended questions, maintenance of eye contact). Additional principles apply, however, when patients, or their parents, are being questioned about personal health behaviors. Unless patients are being seen for a preventive checkup that they have scheduled, they are often psychologically unprepared for a detailed discussion of their lifestyle. When risk assessment questions are introduced at the end of the history or at the conclusion of the visit, patients (or parents of young patients) may be surprised by the sudden change of subject or may be disturbed or offended by the personal nature of the questions. Transition statements serve an important role in laying the groundwork for such questions:

"Well, Mrs. Jones, I'm glad you've agreed to see Dr. Smith for an opinion on having gall bladder surgery. It will be good to get that resolved. You know, sometimes we can get so preoccupied with a specific medical problem—like your gall bladder—that we lose sight of other important health matters. I'd like to run through a short list of questions to make sure we aren't overlooking something important that also needs our attention. Is that all right with you?"

"So, Mr. White, I anticipate that your back pain will ease up if you follow the plan that we discussed, but I want you to let me know next week if it still bothers you. By the way, there are some personal health matters we haven't discussed in the past that, although they have nothing to do with your back, might some day affect your health in other ways. I'd hate for something important to fall through the cracks. For example, you once mentioned that you had been dating several people. As you know, there can be important health implications to sexual activity. How many sexual partners have you had in the last year?"

"Mrs. Jackson, I think your daughter's ear infection will respond well to the antibiotic I'm prescribing today. I'd like to see her again in a few weeks to reexamine her ear. Before you leave, though, I want to ask you a few questions about Tracy, double-check her shot record, and go over some conditions at home that might affect her risk of future illness or injuries. Is that all right?"

During both the introductory statement and the question period, the clinician should monitor the patient's emotional reactions. The patient's comments, vocal quality (tone, pitch, tempo), and nonverbal communication may signal discomfort, impatience, or a reluctance to discuss certain lifestyle issues. Recognizing these reactions and sharing the observations with the patient through reflection (e.g., *"You seem uncomfortable talking about this."*) are important for several reasons. First, if patients do not bring these emotions to the surface, they may suppress them or develop feelings of resentment or anger toward the clinician. Second, open discussion of the emotions and the clinician's validation of the feelings can often reduce patient anxiety. Third, although some patients use their discomfort or impatience as an excuse for changing the subject, the clinician's open acknowledgment of their feelings gives many patients the strength to return to the topic in greater detail. Often these patients will "open up" with disclosures that would not have been mentioned if the clinician were less empathic.

The clinician should also monitor the patient's choice of words, which may disclose important information about risk factors. Clues are often deeply imbedded in dialogue about other problems. The clinician may obtain more information by carefully listening to these subtle comments than from the patient's answers to routine screening questions:

"The chest pains seem to occur after meals, although lately I've wondered whether it's because of the way my life is going. Anyway, I tried antacids . . . "

"Doctor, you know it's got to be bad for me to come in—I haven't been to a doctor in years—I hate all those tests—but I just can't stand this shoulder pain anymore."

"I didn't start the baby on the medicine yet because I needed John to pick it up for me. He's been on a short string lately and I'm afraid to push him, with the way he gets. Now the baby has a fever and pulls on her ears . . ."

"No, my stomach pain isn't any worse after fatty meals. Lately, with my schedule, I've been getting a daily dose of french fries and greasy food, but that has never brought on the pain. It's only when I don't eat . . ."

"I doubt the headaches are due to the birth control pills. I stopped taking those things two months ago. My boyfriend thinks I've got migraines, which do run in our family . . ."

WHAT TO ASK ABOUT

Table 2.1 lists the type of primary screening questions that clinicians should employ on a routine basis to begin constructing an individual's risk profile. These questions address a fundamental set of risk factors: tobacco

Table 2.1
Sample Primary Screening Questions about Key Risk Factors

Note: See text for complete wording of questions. Different questions are indicated for patients in specific age or risk groups and for parents of infants and small children (see text).

1. Do you smoke cigarettes or use other types of tobacco?
2. How much exercise do you get?
3. What foods have you eaten in the past 24 hours?
4. Do you have sex with men, women, or both? How many partners do you have now, and how many were there in the past? Are you interested in getting pregnant, or are you using some form of birth control?
5. Do you drink alcohol? Have you ever used cocaine or other drugs?
6. Do you always fasten your seat belt when you are in a car? Do you ever drive after drinking, or ride with a driver who has been drinking?
7. Do you protect yourself from the sun when you are outdoors?
8. How often do you brush your teeth and how often do you floss? When did you last visit the dentist?
9. How are your spirits these days?
10. Have you ever been told that you had heart trouble, cancer, diabetes or a serious infectious disease?
11. Is there a family history of heart trouble, cancer, or diabetes?
12. What sort of work do (did) you do?
13. Have you ever been in other countries, or are you planning a trip to one?
14. When was your last _____?
    (recommended screening test)
15. When was your last _____?
    (recommended immunization)
16. Are you taking estrogen? Are you taking daily aspirin?

use; physical activity; dietary intake; sexual practices; alcohol and other drug use; injury prevention; exposure to ultraviolet light; dental hygiene; mental health and functional status; risk factors from past medical and family history; occupational and environmental exposures; travel history; and the status of recommended screening tests, immunizations, and chemoprophylaxis. Questions for pediatric patients need to be tailored to the patient's age to determine the content of the question and whether the patient or parents should be asked. Some sample primary screening questions for parents are included in the following discussion.

Tobacco Use

Sample Primary Screening Question: *"Do you smoke cigarettes or use other types of tobacco?"*

Exploratory Questions and Follow-Up: See Chapter 6.

If there is only one risk factor that a clinician can address in a clinical encounter, it should be tobacco use. Tobacco use accounts for 400,000 deaths each year in the United States (1). All adults, adolescents, and, occasionally, older children should be asked whether they smoke or use smokeless tobacco. If they do not currently use tobacco, the clinician should inquire whether they used tobacco previously and, if so, when they quit. Exposure to side stream smoke (passive smoking) should also be addressed in visits with infants, children, and pregnant women. Because patients who stop smoking often relapse, tobacco use should be readdressed periodically throughout the clinician's relationship with the patient. The topic also needs to be revisited regularly with children and adolescents, who are always at risk of starting to smoke or use smokeless tobacco for the first time.

Physical Activity

Sample Primary Screening Question: *"How much exercise do you get?"*

For Parents: *"How much exercise does your child get?"*

Exploratory Questions and Follow-Up: See Chapter 7.

Physical inactivity, an important risk factor for coronary artery disease, hypertension, obesity, and other chronic diseases, should be addressed with adults (including the elderly) and with children and adolescents, for whom the question may also need to be directed to the parents. Both the clinician and patient should have a clear understanding of what they mean by the term "exercise." *"Well, doc, what I mean by 'exercise' is that I have to take several walks through the factory each day to inspect production lines. I also have a flight of stairs at my apartment."*

Dietary Intake

Sample Primary Screening Question: *"What foods have you eaten in the past 24 hours?"*

> For Parents of Infants: *"Does the baby breast-feed or bottle-feed? How often does the baby take the breast (bottle) and how many minutes does he/she suck on each breast (how many ounces does he/she take)?"*

> For Parents of Older Children: *"What foods does he (she) eat during regular meals and snacks?"*

Exploratory Questions and Follow-Up: See Chapter 8.

The range of nutritional issues that can be addressed by the clinician is broad, including dietary intake of calories, saturated and unsaturated fat, cholesterol, fiber, sodium, iron, calcium, and vitamins. As discussed in Chapter 8, health professionals cannot offer meaningful counseling about these nutrients without first performing a dietary assessment of the foods that the patient typically eats. A complete dietary assessment for each food category is usually beyond the scope of a single visit. Of all the nutrients in the patient's diet, those that most affect the patient's future health are fat, cholesterol, fiber, and total calories. Clinicians with limited time should consider exploring these topics. *"Could you tell me about your consumption of meat? dairy products? fried foods? fruits and vegetables?"*

Infants and Children

Nutritional questions are essential during well-baby and well-child examinations, but primary screening questions about nutrition should also be considered during other visits, especially if compliance with well-child examinations is not anticipated or poor feeding practices are suspected. The most important nutritional priorities during childhood are to ensure that the diet is appropriate for healthful growth and development and that intake of dietary fats and sweets is limited.

Older Adults

In addition to the nutritional risks that face all adults, older adults face the added risks of nutritional deficiencies and malnutrition. They also face potentially harmful interactions between their dietary practices and their medical conditions and medications. The need for greater attention to the diet of older adults led to the launching of the Nutrition Screening Initiative (3), an interdisciplinary project of the American Academy of Family Physicians, the American Dietetic Association, and the National Council on Aging. This program recommends that, as a first step, clinicians should assess whether the patient suffers from impaired functional status and whether this impairment is caused by or results from nutritional deficiencies. (See "Mental Health and Functional Status" later in this chapter.) In patients who cannot provide reliable dietary histories, additional information about eating habits should be obtained from family members or caregivers.

Sexual Practices

Sample Primary Screening Questions: *"Do you have sex with men, women, or both? How many partners do you have now, and how many were there in the past? Are you interested in getting pregnant, or are you using some form of birth control?"*

Exploratory Questions and Follow-Up: See Chapters 11–12.

The U.S. Preventive Services Task Force and other groups advise clinicians to take a complete sexual history on all adolescent and adult patients. Due to the sensitive nature of this topic, clinicians often need to introduce questions about sexual behavior by explaining its relevance to their health; see Chapter 12 for suggested language. This introduction is especially important if the patient is being seen for an unrelated health problem. Clinicians also frequently need to overcome their own discomfort with discussing sexual behavior. Even in urban practices with many high-risk patients, less than 40% of physicians obtain a sexual history from their patients (4).

Depending on the patient's answers to screening questions about sexual practices, further questions are often necessary regarding the use of condoms, birth control methods, duration of current sexual relationships, current or prior sexual practices (e.g., anal or oral sex, association between alcohol or drug use and sexual activity, prostitution), and sexual contact with partners who used intravenous drugs, had multiple partners, or had known sexually transmitted diseases. See Chapter 12 for suggested language for addressing these issues. The sexual history may reveal evidence of dysfunctional relationships (e.g., *"I don't need birth control because we hardly make love anymore," "Don't tell my wife, but I've been with other women in the past year."*). Such findings deserve further exploration for psychosocial reasons (see "Mental Health and Functional Status" later in this chapter).

Adolescents

Surveys suggest that over half of students in grades 9–12 report having had sexual intercourse (5). The usual discomfort that patients experience when asked about sexual behavior is magnified further for adolescents, who are often reluctant to admit to sexual activity or are afraid that their discussions will not be kept confidential. A commonly used approach is to begin by normalizing and depersonalizing the practice (e.g., *"A lot of high school students are having sex these days."*) and assuring the patient of confidentiality before asking about sexual habits (*"Have you ever had sex?"*). Some clinicians ease the transition by first inquiring about peers (*"How about your friends?"*) and showing a nonjudgmental demeanor as the patient describes his or her sexual activity. Many adolescents then become comfortable enough to discuss their own sexual histories. See discussion of talking with adolescents under "Special Considerations" later in this chapter.

Alcohol and Other Drug Use

Sample Primary Screening Question: *"Do you drink alcohol? Have you ever used cocaine or other drugs?"*

Exploratory Questions and Follow-Up: See Chapter 13.

The U.S. Preventive Services Task Force, Canadian Task Force on the Periodic Health Examination, Institute of Medicine, American Academy of Pediatrics, and other groups recommend screening all adult and adolescent patients for evidence of alcohol dependence, problem drinking, or excessive alcohol consumption. As discussed in Chapter 13, however, patients' self-reports of the quantity and frequency of their alcohol use may not provide accurate information to identify problem drinking; the reported sensitivity of historical inquiry is only 10–50%. Similarly, patients with a current or past history of illicit drug use may be reluctant to discuss the subject. Clinicians must often rely on clues in the patient's responses and to other aspects of their medical history and lifestyle to detect a problem. For example, the answer, *"I just drink socially,"* requires further exploration. Commonly used questionnaires for alcohol abuse include the CAGE questionnaire (Table 2.2), the AUDIT questionnaire (Table 2.3), and the Michigan Alcoholism Screening Test (Table 2.4) (see also "Screening Questionnaires" later in the chapter). Alcohol and other drug use is discussed further in Chapter 13. Patients with a history of drug use or sexually trans-

Table 2.2
CAGE Questionnaire

_____	Have you ever felt you ought to **C**ut down on your drinking?
_____	Have people **A**nnoyed you by criticizing your drinking?
_____	Have you ever felt bad or **G**uilty about your drinking?
_____	Have you ever had a drink first thing in the morning (**E**ye opener) to steady your nerves or get rid of a hangover?

A positive response to two or more questions is generally considered positive.

From Ewing JA. Detecting alcoholism: the CAGE questionnaire. JAMA 1984;252:1905–1907. Copyright 1984, American Medical Association.

Table 2.3
Alcohol Use Disorders Identification Test (AUDIT)

1. How often do you have a drink containing alcohol?
   _____ Never (0 points)
   _____ Monthly or less (1 point)
   _____ Two to four times a month (2 points)
   _____ Two to three times a week (3 points)
   _____ Four or more times a week (4 points)
2. How many drinks containing alcohol do you have on a typical day when you are drinking?
   _____ 1–2 (0 points)
   _____ 3–4 (1 point)
   _____ 5–6 (2 points)
   _____ 7–9 (3 points)
   _____ 10 or more (4 points)
3. How often do you have six or more drinks on one occasion?
   _____ Never (0 points)
   _____ Less than monthly (1 point)
   _____ Monthly (2 points)
   _____ Weekly (3 points)
   _____ Daily or almost daily (4 points)
4. How often during the last year have you found that you were not able to stop drinking once you had started?
   _____ Never (0 points)
   _____ Less than monthly (1 point)
   _____ Monthly (2 points)
   _____ Weekly (3 points)
   _____ Daily or almost daily (4 points)
5. How often during the last year have you failed to do what was normally expected from you because of drinking?
   _____ Never (0 points)
   _____ Less than monthly (1 point)
   _____ Monthly (2 points)
   _____ Weekly (3 points)
   _____ Daily or almost daily (4 points)
6. How often during the last year have you needed a first drink in the morning to get yourself going after a heavy drinking session?
   _____ Never (0 points)
   _____ Less than monthly (1 point)
   _____ Monthly (2 points)
   _____ Weekly (3 points)
   _____ Daily or almost daily (4 points)
7. How often during the last year have you had a feeling of guilt or remorse after drinking?
   _____ Never (0 points)
   _____ Less than monthly (1 point)
   _____ Monthly (2 points)
   _____ Weekly (3 points)
   _____ Daily or almost daily (4 points)
8. How often during the last year have you been unable to remember what happened the night before because you had been drinking?
   _____ Never (0 points)
   _____ Less than monthly (1 point)
   _____ Monthly (2 points)
   _____ Weekly (3 points)
   _____ Daily or almost daily (4 points)
9. Have you or someone else been injured as a result of your drinking?
   _____ No (0 points)
   _____ Yes, but not in the last year (2 points)
   _____ Yes, during the last year (4 points)

Table 2.3—*continued*

10. Has a relative or friend, or a doctor or other health worker, been concerned about your drinking or suggested you cut down?
    _____No (0 points)
    _____Yes, but not in the last year (2 points)
    _____Yes, during the last year (4 points)

The scoring key (in parentheses) should not appear on the form completed by patients. A score of 8 or more indicates a strong likelihood of hazardous or harmful alcohol consumption.

Adapted from Saunders JB, Aasland OG, Babor TF, et al. Development of the Alcohol Use Disorders Identification Test (AUDIT): WHO collaborative project on early detection of persons with harmful alcohol consumption. Addiction 1993;88:791–804.

Table 2.4
Michigan Alcoholism Screening Test Questionnaire

1. Do you feel you are a normal drinker? (2 points)
2. Have you ever awakened the morning after some drinking the night before and found that you could not remember a part of the evening before? (2 points)
3. Does your spouse (or parents) every worry or complain about your drinking? (1 point)
4. Can you stop drinking without a struggle after one or two drinks? (2 points)
5. Do you ever feel bad about your drinking? (1 point)
6. Do friends or relatives think you are a normal drinker? (1 point)
7. Do you ever try to limit your drinking to certain times of the day or to certain places? (0 points)
8. Are you always able to stop drinking when you want to? (2 points)
9. Have you ever attended a meeting of Alcoholics Anonymous? (5 points)
10. Have you ever gotten into fights when drinking? (1 point)
11. Has drinking ever created problems with you or your spouse? (2 points)
12. Has your spouse (or other family member) ever gone to anyone for help about your drinking? (2 points)
13. Have you ever lost friends or girlfriends or boyfriends because of drinking? (2 points)
14. Have you ever gotten into trouble at work because of drinking? (2 points)
15. Have you ever lost a job because of drinking? (2 points)
16. Have your ever neglected your obligations, your family, or your work for two or more days in a row because you were drinking? (2 points)
17. Do you ever drink before noon? (1 point)
18. Have you ever been told you have liver trouble? Cirrhosis? (2 points)
19. Have you ever had delirium tremens (DTs), severe shaking, heard voices, or seen things that were not there after heavy drinking? (2 points)
20. Have you ever gone to anyone for help about your drinking? (5 points)
21. Have you ever been in a hospital because of drinking? (5 points)
22. Have you ever been a patient in a psychiatric hospital or on a psychiatric ward of a general hospital where drinking was part of the problem? (2 points)
23. Have you ever been seen at a psychiatric or mental health clinic or gone to a doctor, social worker, or clergyman for help with an emotional problem in which drinking played a part? (2 points)
24. Have you ever been arrested, even for a few hours, because of drunk behavior? (2 points)
25. Have you ever been arrested for drunk driving or driving after drinking? (2 points)

Scoring key (in parentheses) should not appear on the form completed by patients. Score points for negative answers to questions 1, 4, 6, and 8 and for positive answers to all other questions. A total score of 5 or more points is highly suggestive of alcohol abuse.

Adapted from Selzer ML. The Michigan Alcoholism Screening Test: the quest for a new diagnostic instrument. Am J Psychiatr 1971;127:1653–1658.

mitted diseases should be asked specifically about past or present intravenous drug use. Patients who use either alcohol or other drugs should be
asked about driving while intoxicated, as discussed in the next section.

Adolescents

As with sexual behavior, adolescents may be reluctant to admit to alcohol
or other drug use for fear of disapproval or disclosure to parents, teachers,
or others. Nonetheless, because intoxication accounts for about half of
adolescent deaths in motor vehicle crashes and because substance abuse
often begins at this age, broaching this subject with teens is especially important. Again, it is often useful to first depersonalize the practice (e.g., *"A
lot of high school students drink or use drugs these days."*), assure confidentiality,
inquire about peers (*"How about your friends?"*), and then ask about the patient's habits (*"Have you ever used drugs?"*). See the discussion of talking
with adolescents under "Special Considerations" later in this chapter.

Injury Prevention Practices

Sample Primary Screening Question: *"Do you always fasten your seat belt when
you are in a car? Do you ever drive after drinking, or ride with a driver who has
been drinking?"*

> For Parents of Infants and Small Children: *"Is your child always secured
> in a safety seat when you or others transport him (her) in the car?"*

> For Parents of Older Children: *"Does your child fasten his (her) seat belt
> whenever he (she) is transported in a car?"*

Exploratory Questions and Follow-Up: See Chapter 10.

Many clinicians believe that a patient's driving habits are not a clinical concern, and yet motor vehicle accidents account for 50,000 deaths and five
million injuries each year in the United States. They are the leading cause
of injury-related deaths among persons under age 45 (6). Other causes of
unintentional injuries are also important, such as fires, burns, drowning,
sports activities, falls, and firearm accidents; primary screening questions
can address these risks by asking about smoke detectors, smoking in bed,
alcohol use during water sports, use of safety helmets, firearm security, and
other measures (see Chapter 10). Motor vehicle injury prevention, however, clearly has the highest priority. (Motorcyclists should be asked about
their use of safety helmets.)

Infants and Children

Motor vehicle injury is the leading cause of injury-related death in children over one year of age; therefore, questions about car seats and seat

belt use are essential. Other common causes of unintentional injuries during childhood include burns, fires, drowning, falls, poisoning, and firearm accidents. Thus, depending on the child's age, questions about hot water heater temperature, smoke detectors, swimming pool fences, stairway and window protectors, bicycle safety helmets, syrup of ipecac, access to poison control center telephone numbers, and firearm security may also be indicated (see Chapter 10).

Older Adults

Falls are a common cause of injury in older adults, especially among those over age 75, in whom falls are the leading cause of injury-related deaths (due largely to the complications of hip fractures and head trauma). The clinician should ask the patient, family members, or caregivers whether the home has been inspected for fall hazards. A sample screening question is, *"Have you gone through the house to look for bad lighting; things that could cause you to trip or slip on the floor, steps, or bathtub; or sharp corners or hard floors that could hurt you if you fell?"* The clinician should also review the patient's medications, which may increase the risk of falls (see Chapter 10).

Exposure to Ultraviolet Light

Sample Primary Screening Question: *"Do you protect yourself (your child) from the sun when you are outdoors?"*

Exploratory Questions and Follow-Up: See Chapter 14.

See discussion later in this chapter regarding questions about occupational or environmental exposure to sunlight.

Dental Hygiene Practices

Sample Primary Screening Question: *"How often do you brush your teeth and how often do you floss? Do your gums bleed? When did you last visit the dentist?"*

For Parents: *"How often does your child brush his (her) teeth? When was he (she) last taken to the dentist?"*

Exploratory Questions and Follow-Up: See Chapter 15.

Parents of infants should be asked about baby bottle-feeding practices that may increase the risk of caries (see Chapter 15). See later discussion in this chapter regarding questions about fluoride content in the local water supply.

Mental Health and Functional Status

Sample Primary Screening Question (Mental Health): *"How are your spirits these days?"*

Sample Primary Screening Question (Functional Status):

For Parents: *"What has your child learned to do recently?"*

For Older Adults: *"Are you having any trouble taking care of things at home, like getting your meals or cleaning yourself?"*

Exploratory Questions and Follow-Up: See Chapter 16.

Mental Health

As discussed in Chapter 16, the scope of potential problems and complications that fall under this category is broad, ranging from poor self-esteem, depression, and abuse (as victim or perpetrator) to violence and suicidal behavior. A single primary screening question is often inadequate to detect these problems. Thus, in order to detect a problem, the clinician must be alert to clues in the patient's behavior, affect, family dynamics, and physical examination findings, not only during the risk assessment visit but throughout the relationship with the patient. Patients who have recently experienced an important loss (e.g., death, divorce, loss of job) are at increased risk of depression. If there is evidence of depression, the patient should be asked whether he or she has considered suicide (e.g., *"Have you ever thought of hurting yourself?"*). Commonly used screening instruments for depression include the Zung Self-Rating Depression Scale (Table 2.5), Center for Epidemiological Studies Depression Scale, and the Beck Depression Inventory (see "Screening Questionnaires" later in this chapter). Routine screening for suicide risk is not recommended; see Chapters 10 and 16 for further details.

The clinician must also remain alert for signs of interpersonal conflict, domestic violence, or other risk factors for intentional injuries (e.g., child abuse, spouse abuse, sexual violence, homicide). Because patients and family members often display their "best behavior" during clinical encounters, the clinician must be able to see past this presentation to unmask signs of escalating tensions in a relationship, an individual's inability to resolve conflicts nonviolently, or the physical findings of abuse or neglect. A patient or family member's grimace, shrug, or hesitation in answering a screening question, such as, *"How are things at home?"* or their responses to open-ended questions, such as *"What are the good things and bad things about your relationship?"* are often the clinician's best clues in detecting an important problem at home. In responding to such questions, patients may give clues to the misuse of alcohol or other drugs or to the presence of other codependent behaviors. Although unproven, acting on these findings by arranging psychotherapy, marital counseling, substance abuse treatment, or social services may improve family dynamics and the emotional well-being of its members. In more advanced cases, these interventions may

Table 2.5
Zung Self-Rating Depression Scale

	A Little of the Time	Some of the Time	Good Part of the Time	Most of the Time
1. I feel down-hearted, blue, and sad.	(1 point)	(2 points)	(3 points)	(4 points)
2. Morning is when I feel the best.	(4 points)	(3 points)	(2 points)	(1 point)
3. I have crying spells or feel like it.	(1 point)	(2 points)	(3 points)	(4 points)
4. I have trouble sleeping through the night.	(1 point)	(2 points)	(3 points)	(4 points)
5. I eat as much as I used to.	(4 points)	(3 points)	(2 points)	(1 point)
6. I enjoy looking at, talking to, and being with attractive women/men	(4 points)	(3 points)	(2 points)	(1 point)
7. I notice that I am losing weight.	(1 point)	(2 points)	(3 points)	(4 points)
8. I have trouble with constipation.	(1 point)	(2 points)	(3 points)	(4 points)
9. My heart beats faster than usual.	(1 point)	(2 points)	(3 points)	(4 points)
10. I get tired for no reason.	(1 point)	(2 points)	(3 points)	(4 points)
11. My mind is as clear as it used to be.	(4 points)	(3 points)	(2 points)	(1 point)
12. I find it easy to do the things I used to.	(4 points)	(3 points)	(2 points)	(1 point)
13. I am restless and can't keep still.	(1 point)	(2 points)	(3 points)	(4 points)
14. I feel hopeful about the future.	(4 points)	(3 points)	(2 points)	(1 point)
15. I am more irritable than usual.	(1 point)	(2 points)	(3 points)	(4 points)
16. I find it easy to make decisions.	(4 points)	(3 points)	(2 points)	(1 point)
17. I feel that I am useful and needed.	(4 points)	(3 points)	(2 points)	(1 point)
18. My life is pretty full.	(4 points)	(3 points)	(2 points)	(1 point)
19. I feel that others would be better off if I were dead.	(1 point)	(2 points)	(3 points)	(4 points)
20. I still enjoy the things I used to.	(4 points)	(3 points)	(2 points)	(1 point)

Scoring key (in parentheses) should not appear on the form completed by patients. In the original study, depressed patients had a total raw score of 50–72 (mean of 59) and controls had a total score of 20–34 (mean of 26).

prevent physical illnesses and injuries, emotional morbidity from abuse or neglect, unwanted pregnancies, family disintegration, unintentional firearm injuries, and even homicide. See Chapter 10 for further discussion of the questions clinicians should ask when exploring the possibility of abuse.

Functional Status

As discussed in Chapter 16, functional status refers broadly to an individual's ability to perform age-appropriate tasks of self-care and self fulfillment. In childhood, this is often affected by abnormal physical or mental growth and development. In old age, functional status can be impaired by both physical and mental illness. The consequences affect other health behaviors, such as nutrition and injury prevention.

Infants and Children. When examining children, clinicians should ask parents whether the child is performing tasks and has reached developmental milestones expected for that age. They should be asked whether problems have been noted in the child's social relationships with playmates or learning skills at school. A variety of screening instruments have been developed for detecting developmental disorders. One of the oldest is the Denver Developmental Screening Test (7); its new revision, the Denver II (Fig. 2.1), was restandardized in 1989 (8). The Revision of Denver Prescreening Developmental Questionnaire (9) can be used to compare a child's performance to Denver Developmental Screening Test norms. Other questionnaires that have been highly rated by an expert panel (10) include the Batelle Developmental Inventory Screening Test (11), Infant Monitoring System (12), Developmental Indicators for Assessment of Learning—Revised (13), Screening Children for Related Early Educational Needs (14), and Developmental Profile II (15). The effectiveness of developmental screening is uncertain, however, since there is little scientific evidence that screened children experience better cognitive or behavioral outcomes than children who are not screened.

Older Adults. When examining older adults, clinicians should remain alert for evidence of difficulty performing the activities of daily living. Screening for cognitive impairment is more difficult, since a lengthy mental status examination is often impractical in a brief clinical encounter and may lack accuracy as a screening test. The clinician must often seek clues in the patient's speech, ability to understand medical instructions, and behavior in the office (see Chapter 16). The Mini-Mental State Examination is a screening instrument for cognitive impairment (Table 2.6). (See additional discussion about screening questionnaires later in this chapter and in Chapter 16.)

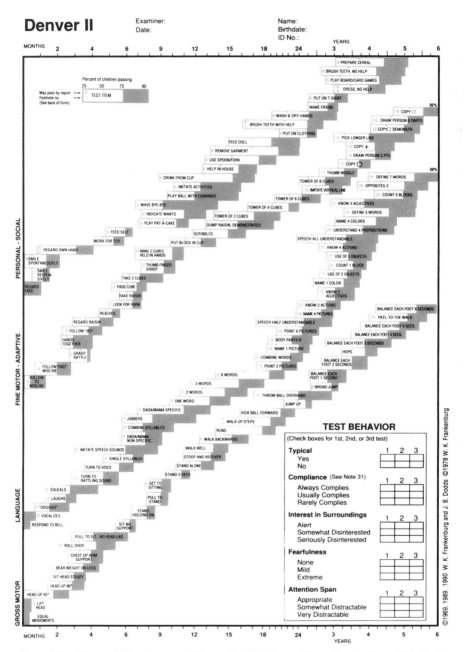

Figure 2.1. Denver II Developmental Screening Test form. (From Frankenburg WK, Dodds J, Archer P, Shapiro H, Bresnick B. The Denver II: a major revision and restandardization of the Denver Developmental Screening Test. Pediatrics 1992;89:91–97.)

Table 2.6
Mini-Mental State Examination

Orientation
1. What is the
    Year? (1 point)
    Season? (1 point)
    Date? (1 point)
    Day? (1 point)
    Month? (1 point)
2. Where are we?
    State? (1 point)
    County? (1 point)
    Town/city? (1 point)
    Floor? (1 point)
    Address/name of building? (1 point)

Registration
3. Name three objects, taking one second to say each. Then ask the patient all three after you have said them. Repeat the answers until the patient learns all three. (3 points)

Attention and Calculation
4. Serial sevens: give one point for each correct answer. Stop after five answers. (Alternative: spell *world* backward.) (5 points)

Recall
5. Ask for names of three objects learned in question 3. Give one point for each correct answer. (3 points)

Language
6. Point to a pencil and a watch. Have the patient name them as you point. (2 points)
7. Have the patient repeat "No ifs, ands, or buts." (1 point)
8. Have the patient follow a three-stage command: "Take the paper in your right hand. Fold the paper in half. Put the paper on the floor." (3 points)
9. Have the patient read and obey the following: "Close your eyes." (1 point)
10. Have the patient write a sentence of his or her own choice. (The sentence should contain a subject and an object and should make sense. Ignore spelling errors when scoring.) (1 point)
11. Show the patient a picture of two overlapping pentograms. Ask the patient to copy it. (Give one point if all the sides and angles are preserved and if the intersecting sides form a quadrangle.) (1 point)

A total score of less than 24 out of 30 points is generally considered abnormal.

Adapted from Crum RM, Anthony JC, Bassett SS, Folstein MF. Population-based norms for the Mini-Mental State Examination by age and educational level. JAMA 1993;269:2386–2391.

Risk Factors from Past Medical History

Sample Primary Screening Question: *"Have you ever been told that you had . . .*

Cardiac Module: *". . . heart trouble, high blood pressure, cholesterol problems, or diabetes?"*

Cancer Module: *". . . cancer, polyps or growths in your colon, ulcerative colitis, skin cancer . . ."*

For men: *". . . prostate problems?"*

For women: *". . . breast problems, an abnormal Pap smear, or trouble with your cervix?"*

Infectious Disease Module: *". . . sexually transmitted diseases? Have you ever had contact with someone who had a sexually transmitted disease, HIV or AIDS, or tuberculosis? Did you receive a transfusion during 1978–1985?"*

Mental Health Module: *". . . an alcohol or drug problem? Have you ever been treated for depression or a mental illness?"*

For Parents: *"Did your child have any complications during the pregnancy, when he (she) was born, or before leaving the hospital; were you ever told that he (she) had a birth defect, a behavioral or developmental problem, diabetes, or another disease; and have you (or anyone else with whom your child has had close contact) ever had a sexually transmitted disease, HIV or AIDS, or tuberculosis?"*

Exploratory Questions and Follow-Up. These are only some of the questions that could be asked in a thorough assessment of past medical history. These questions, however, provide critical information for determining whether patients fall within risk groups requiring special screening tests, immunizations, or other preventive services (see Chapters 3, 4, 18, and 19). Other questions are obviously necessary for the evaluation of patients with specific presenting complaints. These questions about prior illnesses may be too numerous for a single visit, unless the patient completes a medical history form before the interview (see later under "Screening Questionnaires"). If time is limited, a shorter screening question may be necessary, such as *"Have you ever been told that you had heart trouble, cancer, diabetes, or a serious infectious disease?"*

Risk Factors from Family History

Sample Primary Screening Question: *"Is there a family history of heart trouble or cancer, especially cancer of the breast, colon, prostate, or skin? Is there a family history of diabetes, cancer of the uterus, or skin moles called dysplastic nevi?"*

Exploratory Questions And Follow-Up: A number of additional questions are typically included in the "family history" section of the conventional medical history. The above questions address familial conditions that place patients in risk groups requiring special screening tests (see Chapters 3–4).

Occupational and Environmental Exposures

Sample Primary Screening Question: *"What sort of work do (did) you do? Does (did) your job or other activities expose you to loud noise, the sun, harmful chemicals, or other hazardous materials?"*

For Parents: *"Where do you live, how old is your home, and what is the source of your drinking water?"*

Exploratory Questions And Follow-Up: A thorough occupational or environmental history requires more detailed questions about risks of occupational illnesses and injuries than can be addressed within the scope of this book. The above questions are intended to screen for selected exposures that place patients in risk groups requiring routine screening tests and immunizations (see Chapters 3, 4, and 18). For example, skin and hearing screening are required for patients with occupational or recreational exposure to excessive sunlight or noise, respectively. Health care workers are at increased risk of being exposed to or transmitting nosocomially tuberculosis, hepatitis B, human immunodeficiency virus, and other harmful organisms (e.g., rubella). Questions for determining a worker's need for occupational screening tests (e.g., air sampling, pulmonary function testing, serum organophosphate measurement), however, are addressed in standard occupational medicine and environmental health texts.

Questions about living conditions can also provide important environmental risk information for tailoring the patient's health maintenance plan. Crowded or unsanitary living conditions, for example, increase the risk of tuberculosis, influenza, and other pathogens. Determining that a patient lives in a homeless shelter, correctional institution, nursing home, or migrant worker camp suggests the need for tuberculosis screening (see Chapter 4). Other questions may be important for children. Although a number of environmental factors are potentially relevant, some of which (e.g., passive smoke exposure) have already been addressed, characteristics of the home, such as its age (dwellings constructed before 1960 often contain lead-based paint) and the presence or absence of fluoride in the water supply, have special relevance to a child's risk of developing disease. As discussed in Chapter 4, the Centers for Disease Control and Prevention has developed a questionnaire (16) to screen for lead exposure and recommends that it be administered at each routine office visit.

Travel History

Sample Primary Screening Question: *"Have you (or your child) ever been in other countries, or are you planning a trip to one?"*

Exploratory Questions And Follow-Up: See Chapters 3, 4, and 18.

The risk of certain target conditions (e.g., hemoglobinopathies) or of exposure to infectious diseases (e.g., tuberculosis, hepatitis, human immunodeficiency virus infection) is increased for immigrants from certain countries in Asia, the Pacific Islands, Africa, Central and South America, and the Mediterranean. Patients traveling to developing countries or other regions in which malaria and other preventable infectious diseases are endemic require certain immunizations and chemoprophylaxis prior to their departure (see Chapter 18).

Screening Status

Clinicians should ask patients whether they have received the screening tests that are recommended for individuals in their age and risk group. For example, women over age 50 should routinely be asked, *"When was your last mammogram?"* See Chapters 3–4 for guidance on how to determine which screening tests are indicated for a particular patient.

Immunization Status

Clinicians should ask patients (or the parents of infants and children) whether they have received the recommended immunizations for their age and risk category (see Chapter 18). For most adults, the primary screening question is *"How many years has it been since your last tetanus shot?"* Older adults and patients with selected risk factors also require inquiries about influenza and pneumococcal vaccinations. For children and adolescents, the clinician must consult with the parents or review medical records to determine whether immunizations for measles, mumps, rubella, polio, diphtheria, tetanus, pertussis, *Hemophilus influenza* type b, and hepatitis B are up-to-date. See Chapter 18 for more details.

Chemoprophylaxis

Sample Primary Screening Question (For Women): *"Are you taking estrogen?"*

Sample Primary Screening Question (Primarily for Men): *"Are you taking daily aspirin?"*

Exploratory Questions and Follow-Up: See Chapter 19.

SPECIAL CONSIDERATIONS

Parents and Children

Information about the risk factors of infants and small children is obtained almost entirely from their parents or primary caregivers. Although it is generally preferable to have the child present in the room while the history is obtained (to help allay the child's anxiety and to observe the relationship between the child and parents), difficult topics that the parents cannot discuss openly in front of the child should be addressed in the child's absence. Questions about a child's risk factors may be misinterpreted by parents as an indictment of their parenting skills. The clinician must make a special effort to speak positively about the child's care and to maintain a nonjudgmental demeanor in asking about risk factors. *"Is Billy ever exposed to cigarette smoke?"* is a more neutral statement than *"I hope that you don't smoke in front of Billy."*

Adolescents

It is common for adolescents to have distant, rebellious, or even hostile attitudes when talking with adult authority figures. Clinicians who are surprised or disturbed by adolescent resistance often have difficulty in obtaining detailed risk factor information or an accurate history. The first step in overcoming this problem is for clinicians to understand their own feelings of anger or annoyance over the patient's uncooperative behavior, recognize that resistant behaviors are common among adolescents, and not take their reactions personally. The next step is to try to establish rapport with the adolescent by communicating a genuine interest in the patient as an individual (and not as a set of symptoms) by chatting initially about "real life," nonmedical topics and by emphasizing the confidentiality of the relationship.

> *"I'm glad to have finally met you, Wayne. Your mother has mentioned your name on several occasions, and it's finally nice to meet you in person. I understand that you go to Bishop High School. What kind of a school is Bishop?"*

The questions can gradually be directed to more personal concerns (e.g., *"Do you have good friends at Bishop?"; "How do you like living here after moving from Chicago?"; "Is it difficult to be the oldest brother in the family?"*) before the discussion acquires a medical focus.

> *". . . Wayne, I want to ask you some medical questions to see whether there are any things about the way you live that you might want to change to make yourself healthier. You need to know that whatever we say in this room is completely confidential. I am mainly concerned about your health, and I'm not interested in telling you what is right or wrong. Is that ok with you?"*

Although the clinician should appear relaxed and use language and terminology that are understandable to adolescents, there is little value in trying to "act cool" by using the expressions, terms, or nonverbal body language of young people. The artificiality of this practice is usually obvious to adolescents and sends a message of insincerity. Due to the emotional developmental stage of most adolescents, certain history-taking techniques that are effective with adults (e.g., silence, confrontation, and, occasionally, reflection) are often unsuccessful and anxiety-provoking when attempted with adolescents. As noted earlier in the chapter, the confidence of the adolescent patient can often be strengthened by "normalizing" behaviors, i.e., mentioning that the practice is common among other teens. Clinicians must pay close attention to the comments and nonverbal communication of adolescents to know when to probe further and when to change the subject.

Older Adults

Obtaining accurate risk factor information from older adults can be difficult for organic and attitudinal reasons. Organic barriers in the elderly include the patient's difficulty in understanding questions or providing co-
herent answers due to hearing loss, cognitive impairment, or other
medical factors. Clinicians often need to accommodate these limitations
through special measures, such as speaking more slowly in a loud, low
voice; writing the questions on paper; or obtaining the information from
caregivers. Attitudinal barriers include the patient's hesitation to identify a
risk factor as a problem because of a belief that it is a natural consequence
of aging (e.g., hearing loss), it is something that should not be complained
about (e.g., depression), or it is too late in life to benefit from risk factor
modification (e.g., smoking cessation after decades of tobacco use). Clinicians often need to spend time with the patient to correct these misconceptions, educate them about healthy aging, and encourage open
discussion.

Patient Privacy

Asking about risk factors with other individuals in the room is generally inappropriate for several reasons. First, the presence of other individuals
often makes patients uncomfortable and reluctant to discuss personal behaviors. The patient may give inaccurate or incomplete information, such
as denying or minimizing their involvement with behaviors that might be
judged negatively by others (e.g., the adolescent who denies sexual activity
or substance abuse because the parents are present). Second, taking a history under these conditions violates patient confidentiality. Third, if the
visit includes a physical examination, the visitors must leave the room anyway to respect the patient's privacy.

On the other hand, family members, caregivers, or friends who accompany patients can often provide important information about risk factors
that may not be volunteered by the patient. For example, a teenage patient denies tobacco use, but the mother tells the clinician that she routinely sees a cigarette package in his shirt pocket. A wife complains about
her husband's drinking problem even though he denies such behavior.
The children of an older adult, who denies problems at home, inform the
physician that they have witnessed frequent episodes of disorientation and
memory loss. It is therefore useful to ask individuals who have accompanied a patient whether they have any health concerns that they would like
to discuss. They should then be asked to leave the room.

Most individuals accompanying patients, once given an opportunity to
express their concerns, are quite agreeable to leaving the examination

room. Some parents of adolescents or older children may be surprised by or resistant to the request, in part because this practice was unnecessary when their children were younger, but a brief explanation will usually suffice to ease their anxieties. The adamant refusal of family members to leave the examination room or the tendency to dominate the interview should raise the clinician's index of suspicion that there are issues of abuse, neglect, or other problems that they do not want disclosed.

Interview Problems and Techniques

Silence, which frequently makes both clinicians and patients uncomfortable, is nevertheless often helpful in collecting risk factor information. Patients may introduce silence themselves, pausing after mentioning a risk factor to collect their thoughts or to marshal the courage to bring up a difficult topic. Rather than breaking the silence with another question, clinicians who wait for the patient to break the silence often are rewarded with additional information. *"No, I don't use any drugs, and I hardly touch alcohol . . .* (silence introduced by patient) *. . . Did I ever tell you, doctor, that I was once in a rehab program? I was using crack and heroin back then . . ."* Even if the patient does not introduce silence, the clinician may intentionally pause to see how the patient fills the silence. *"Things at home are fine, I guess . . .* (silence introduced by clinician) *. . . I do wish things were better between my husband and the kids, though . . ."*

Resistance is often manifested by a patient's hesitation in answering questions, vagueness, or an abrupt change of subject. Only a few patients express anger or hostility when asked questions about lifestyle. As noted earlier, the clinician's reflection and validation of the patient's feelings will often overcome this resistance. It is, however, the patient's right to terminate discussion of difficult topics. The clinician should respect those preferences and move on to other subjects.

Communication barriers can include deafness, language barriers, cognitive limitations, and cultural differences. Information about risk factors can be obtained from deaf patients by relying on lip reading, written questionnaires, handwritten notes, or sign language. Patients who cannot speak the clinician's language may require the aid of a translator to answer questions. If patients have partial command of the clinician's language, it easy to assume mistakenly that the patient understands questions or instructions. A patient may nod in response to a yes/no question without truly understanding what was asked. For example, a Vietnamese-speaking patient who says "no" when asked whether she has ever had "hepatitis B" might answer "yes" if the disease was named in her language. Patients with cognitive limitations, due either to inadequate education or limited intelligence, may have difficulty in understanding complex words or sentences.

The clinician should be careful to avoid sophisticated terminology (e.g., *saturated fats, hypertension, monogamous relationships*) and should verify that the patient truly understands the questions.

Patients with different *cultural backgrounds*, even if they have complete command of the clinician's language, may assign different meanings to risk factors or may be offended by certain questions. It is therefore important for the clinician to be familiar with and sensitive to the attitudes and health belief model of the patient's culture. For example, the very concept of prevention may not be meaningful if patients believe that diseases develop from sinful behavior, rather than medical risk factors, or that suffering from disease leads to spiritual growth. Patients from certain ethnic or minority communities may be confused by the clinician's choice of words. For example, they may view a "*negative* test result" as unfavorable news. They may deny a history of "diabetes" or "hypertension" but admit to having "sugar" or "high blood."

Screening Questionnaires

Many practices ask patients to complete a medical history form at their first visit. If they ask questions about relevant risk factors, these forms can provide the clinician with useful risk assessment information and save time during the interview by identifying which topics require further investigation. They can also stimulate the patient's thinking, prompting the patient to bring up certain issues with the clinician that would otherwise be forgotten. One limitation of such forms is that patients may not answer the questions honestly or may leave the questions unanswered. The forms may not be understandable, especially if the patient speaks a different language or has difficulty reading. Finally, the information can easily become outdated. Risk factor data from forms that were completed several years earlier are often useless. Thus, clinicians must be careful to supplement and update risk factor information obtained from medical history forms (see Chapter 23).

As noted earlier, screening questionnaires, standardized instruments that have been validated as screening tools for specific conditions, have been developed for the detection of depression, alcohol abuse, cognitive impairment, and other health problems. These instruments have been designed because of concerns that routine questions by clinicians have poor sensitivity and specificity in detecting these conditions. Unfortunately, most screening questionnaires also have limited sensitivity and specificity (Table 2.7). That is, a patient with an abnormal score may not have the condition (false-positive) and a patient with a normal score may have the condition (false-negative). For example, the Mini-Mental State Examination has a reported sensitivity and specificity of 87% and 82%, respectively

Table 2.7
Reported Sensitivity and Specificity of Common Screening Questionnaires

Screening Questionnaire	Sensitivity	Specificity
Zung Self-Rating Depression Scale	97%	63%
CAGE Questionnaire	49–89%	68–96%
AUDIT Questionnaire	61–92%	90–94%
Michigan Alcoholism Screening Test	84–100%	87–95%
Mini-Mental State Examination	87%	82%
Denver Developmental Screening Test	5–29%	89–99%

Adapted from U.S. Preventive Services Task Force. Guide to clinical preventive services. Baltimore: Williams & Wilkins, 1989; Canadian Task Force on the Periodic Health Examination. Canadian guide to clinical preventive health care. Ottawa: Canada Communications Group, 1994; Anthony JC, LeResche L, Niaz U, Von Korff MR, Folstein MF. Limits of the "Mini-Mental State" as a screening test for dementia and delirium among hospital patients. Psychol Med 1982;12:397–408.

(17). This means that, in a person with a 5% probability of having dementia, an abnormal score on the questionnaire has a positive predictive value of 20%: four people without dementia will score falsely positive on the questionnaire for every true case detected. An expert panel judging the accuracy of 19 screening questionnaires for childhood developmental delay gave its highest rating to instruments with a sensitivity and specificity approaching 80% and 90%, respectively. This means that the best performance of such instruments (assuming a sensitivity and specificity of 80% and 90%, respectively, and a 5% pretest probability of a developmental disorder) would be to falsely label two children as developmentally delayed for every true case detected; if the pretest probability is 1%, 12 children would be mislabeled for every true case detected.

In addition to their poor predictive value, completion of questionnaires is often too time-consuming to be done during the clinical interview. Common solutions are to ask patients who are at risk for the problem to complete the questionnaires before meeting with the clinician or, if the need for using the questionnaire first becomes apparent during the clinical interview, to ask the patient to complete the form while the clinician moves on to another patient. The clinician can then return to the patient's room to discuss the results. Another solution is to send the patient home with the questionnaire with instructions to mail it to the clinician.

A more comprehensive approach is to have the patient complete a health risk appraisal (HRA). HRAs, which are discussed in more detail in Chapter 1, provide the patient with personalized estimates of risk for future disease and recommend specific strategies for risk reduction. The potential advantages of using these instruments in the clinical setting are that the printouts provide the clinician with a list of behaviors that deserve attention and that the conclusions and calculations of HRAs can be a powerful motivator in convincing patients to change their lifestyle. The process of reviewing the HRA gives the clinician and patient an opportunity for health promotion counseling. As noted by Schoenbach and colleagues, "HRA provides in one 'package' a rationale, a framework for presentation of health information, an exercise that engages the client, and personalized feedback which serves both as a 'gift' from the counselor and a printed summary of the information to improve client recall." (18) The risk projections generated by HRAs may not be valid, however, and there is little direct evidence that combining patient education with HRAs is more effective in changing behavior than patient education alone (see Chapter 1). HRAs should certainly not be administered alone without accompanying patient education, in which a health professional explains the results and integrates the activity into an overall health maintenance program. More details about HRAs can be obtained from the Society for Prospective Medicine, P.O. Box 55110, Indianapolis, IN 46205-0110.

CONCLUDING THE RISK ASSESSMENT INTERVIEW

Discussions about risk factors should be concluded with the courtesies that are extended at the end of any clinical interview. Patients should be asked whether they have any additional concerns that they would like to discuss. They should also be told what to expect next. If the interview is to be followed by a physical or laboratory examination, a transition statement is often helpful. *"I want to talk with you further about the health issues that we have discussed. But before we do that, I'd like to examine you and perform a few tests so that we will have a complete picture of your risk factors. I'll step out for a few minutes so that you can change into this gown. Is that ok?"*

Risk factors and preclinical disease states to check for in the physical examination are discussed in the next chapter.

MEDICAL RECORD DOCUMENTATION

At a minimum, the clinician should document which risk factors were discussed in the notes for the visit. Preferably, the clinician should also maintain a risk factor "problem list" on the inside cover of the medical record. Entries on the problem list should indicate the dates when the risk factor information was obtained, previous attempts at risk factor modification, and the current status of the risk factor. Risk factors about which no information has been obtained should be flagged for attention at future visits. See Chapters 23 and 26 for further details on the use of alert stickers and other reminders in the medical record to call attention to specific risk factors during future office or clinic visits.

SUGGESTED READINGS

Bates B, Hoekelman RA. Interviewing and the health history. In: Bates B, ed. A guide to physical examination and history taking, 5th ed. Philadelphia: JB Lippincott, 1991:20–31.

Coulehan JL, Block MR. The medical interview: a primer for students of the art, 2nd ed. Philadelphia: FA Davis, 1992:101–113.

Golden AS, Bartlett E, Barker LR. The doctor-patient relationship: communication and patient education. In: Barker LR, Burton JR, Zieve PD, eds. Principles of ambulatory medicine, 4th ed. Baltimore: Williams & Wilkins, 1995:30–41.

National Institute on Aging. Working with your older patients: a clinician's handbook. Bethesda, MD: National Institute on Aging, 1995. Call 301-496-1752 to order.

REFERENCES

1. McGinnis JM, Foege WH. Actual causes of death in the United States. JAMA 1993;270:2207.
2. Schappert SM. National ambulatory care survey, 1991 summary. National Center for Health Statistics. Vital Health Stat 1994;13(116):21.
3. Report of nutrition screening I. Toward a common view. Washington, DC: Nutrition Screening Initiative, 1992.
4. Boekeloo BO, Marx ES, Kral AH, Coughlin SC, Bowman M, Rabin DL. Frequency and thoroughness of STD/HIV risk assessment by physicians in a high-risk metropolitan area. Am J Public Health 1991;81:1645–1648.
5. U.S. Centers for Disease Control and Prevention. Sexual behavior among high school students—United States, 1990. MMWR 1991;40:885–888.
6. Baker SP, O'Neill B, Ginsburg MJ, Li G. The injury fact book, 2nd ed. New York: Oxford University Press, 1992.
7. Frankenburg W, Dodds J. Denver developmental screening test-revised (DDST). Denver: DDM, 1975.
8. Frankenburg WK, Dodds J, Archer P, Shapiro H, Bresnick B. The Denver II: a major revision and restandardization of the Denver Developmental Screening Test. Pediatrics 1992;89:91–97.
9. Frankenburg WK, Fandal AW, Thornton SM. Revision of Denver Prescreening Developmental Questionnaire. J Pediatr 1987;110:653–657.
10. Glascoe FP, Martin ED, Humphrey S. A comparative review of developmental screening tests. Pediatrics 1990;86:547–554.
11. Newborg J, Stock JR, Wnek L, Guidubaldi J, Svinicki J. Batelle developmental inventory screening test. Allen, TX: DLM-Teaching Resources, 1984.
12. Bricker D, Squires J. Infant monitoring system (IMS). Eugene, OR: Center for Human Development, 1989.
13. Mardell-Czudnoswki C, Goldenberg D. Developmental indicators for assessment of learning-revised (DIAL). Edison, NJ: Childcraft Educational Corporation, 1983.
14. Hresko WP, Reid DK, Hammill DD, Herbert PG, Baroody AJ. Screening children for related early educational needs. Austin, TX: Pro-Ed, 1988.
15. Alpern G, Boll T, Shearer M. Developmental profile II (DP-II). Los Angeles: Western Psychological Services, 1986.
16. Preventing lead poisoning in young children. Atlanta: U.S. Centers for Disease Control and Prevention, 1991.
17. Anthony JC, LeResche L, Niaz U, Von Korff MR, Folstein MF. Limits of the "Mini-Mental State" as a screening test for dementia and delirium among hospital patients. Psychol Med 1982;12:397–408.
18. Schoenbach VJ, Wagner EH, Beery WL. Health risk appraisal: review of evidence of effectiveness. Health Serv Res 1987;22:553–579.

3. The Physical Examination: Where to Look for Preclinical Disease

STEVEN H. WOOLF and ROBERT S. LAWRENCE

The early detection of abnormalities on physical examination is an important part of disease prevention. In this chapter, *physical examination* refers to the inspection, palpation, percussion, and auscultation of the patient's body. It does not include taking a history (see Chapter 2), the performance of laboratory tests (see Chapter 4), or other components of the periodic health examination ("routine physical"). Some screening tests that are commonly performed at the time of the physical examination (e.g., Papanicolaou smears) are discussed in Chapter 4.

This chapter focuses on physical examination procedures to screen for asymptomatic disease rather than on the physical diagnosis of patients with symptomatic disease. Patients with presenting complaints or abnormal physical findings require careful, focused examination techniques to make the correct diagnosis. Physical examination procedures that qualify as preventive interventions are those that detect abnormalities in the absence of symptoms.

Although virtually any component of the physical examination (Table 3.1) can detect early-stage disease in the absence of symptoms, this chapter discusses only selected examination techniques. The comprehensive physical examination is beyond the scope of a single chapter, and there is considerable controversy as to whether such examinations are effective when performed for routine screening of asymptomatic persons. Moreover, there is little scientific evidence that healthy persons experience better outcomes as a result of head-to-toe physical examinations. Busy clinicians often have only a few minutes to spend with patients, and groups such as the U.S. Preventive Services Task Force have concluded that clinicians should invest most of that time in talking with patients about health behaviors (e.g., smoking) and lifestyle rather than performing physical examination procedures and tests.

This chapter therefore focuses on selected physical examination procedures for which there is at least some scientific evidence that routine screening may be beneficial. These include sphygmomanometry; routine measurement of height, weight, and head circumference; testing for ab-

49

Table 3.1
The Comprehensive Physical Examination

Skin
Head, scalp, face, nares
Pupils, sclera, conjunctiva, retina, extraocular muscles
Buccal mucosa, teeth, gums, tongue, pharynx
Ear, tympanic membranes
Neck, cervical lymph nodes, jugular veins, carotid arteries
Thoracic and lumbar spine
Posterior lung fields
Breasts, axillae
Precordial impulse, heart sounds
Shoulders, upper arms, elbows, forearms, hands, fingernails
Abdominal viscera
Genitalia, rectum, inguinal canal, femoral pulses
Hips, thighs, knees, lower legs, ankles, feet, toenails
Peripheral pulses
Mental status and central nervous system
Cranial and peripheral nervous system

normal hearing and visual acuity; oral cavity examination; clinical breast examination; digital rectal examination; and skin examination. The reader should consult the suggested readings at the end of this chapter for information about other preventive examination procedures not discussed here (e.g., auscultation of the heart or carotid arteries, palpation for abdominal aortic aneurysms or thyroid nodules, bimanual pelvic examination, testicular examination, newborn examination for pupillary light reflex or congenital hip dislocation). Other references should be consulted regarding examination procedures to screen for occupational illnesses and injuries.

The discussion of each examination procedure includes a brief introduction describing the target condition and the rationale for the screening test, guidelines on how often screening should be performed and on which patients, a summary of official guidelines issued by major organizations and agencies, and detailed instructions on patient preparation and technique. (The sources of the recommendations in the "Official Guidelines" sections are listed under "Suggested Readings" later in this chapter.) Because routine physical examination procedures usually detect no abnormalities, their most important value may lie in providing a setting for counseling patients about primary and secondary prevention of the target condition. Each section of this chapter therefore includes a "Standard Counseling" discussion of the reminders that clinicians should give all patients, even if no abnormality is detected, about how to prevent the target condition and when to return for additional screening. This section also refers readers to other relevant chapters in Section 2 of the book, which discuss in more detail how to counsel patients about specific health behaviors.

For those instances in which an abnormality is detected, "What to Do with Abnormal Results" refers the clinician to the appropriate section of Chapter 17 that outlines follow-up testing and treatment options. The discussion of each examination procedure also includes sections on the potential adverse effects of screening, the accuracy of the examination procedure, and suggestions on how to organize the office or clinic and maintain medical records for optimal screening. Data cited in the "Accuracy and Reliability as Screening Test" sections of this chapter and Chapter 4 are drawn from a large body of evidence. The hundreds of studies on which these estimates are based are not cited explicitly in these chapters due to space limitations. The reader interested in the source of the data is referred to other texts (1) that discuss the individual studies in more detail.

The screening procedures discussed in this chapter may leave patients with questions or heightened anxiety about their risk of disease. To help address these concerns, clinicians may wish to send the patient home with educational brochures, such as those listed in the "Resources" section at the end of this chapter, which can explain the meaning of a normal examination and encourage health behaviors for the primary prevention of the conditions for which they were screened. Patient education materials for patients in whom screening tests are *abnormal* are listed in Chapter 17 and elsewhere in this book. This chapter encourages clinicians to establish reminder systems in the office or clinic to ensure that patients receive recommended screening tests on time and return for repeat screening at the appropriate interval. See Chapter 23 for detailed recommendations on how to design office systems and routines for this purpose, and see Chapter 26 for specific suggestions for establishing manual and automated reminder systems. Finally, physical examination procedures in this chapter are discussed in reference to specific target conditions for which they are most beneficial rather than for all abnormalities that they can detect. Thus, clinical breast examination is discussed in reference to detecting breast cancer and not mastitis; digital rectal examination is discussed in reference to prostate and colorectal cancer and not hemorrhoidal disorders.

SPHYGMOMANOMETRY

Introduction

Nearly 50 million Americans suffer from hypertension (2). Studies have shown that the early detection and treatment of hypertension can reduce all-cause mortality as well as the incidence of cardiac and cerebrovascular events (2). Screening for hypertension is performed by periodic sphygmomanometry. In the physician's office or clinic, this measurement is typically obtained when routine vital signs are taken before the physician's examination.

Screening Guidelines. **All adults should undergo periodic screening for hyperten-**
sion. Blood pressure screening of children and adolescents is supported by weaker
evidence.

Official Guidelines. The American Academy of Pediatrics and the National Heart, Lung,
and Blood Institute recommend annual screening of children age 3 and older and adolescents. The American Academy of Family Physicians recommends periodic blood pressure
measurement after 18 months of age. The Canadian Task Force on the Periodic Health Examination and U.S. Preventive Services Task Force recommend periodic measurement of
blood pressure in adults and the latter also recommends periodic screening of childern.
The Joint National Committee on Detection, Evaluation, and Treatment of High Blood Pressure and the American Heart Association recommend that adults undergo screening every
two years if the previous diastolic blood pressure was below 85 mm Hg, every year if the
diastolic pressure was 85–89 mm Hg, and more frequently if the diastolic pressure was 90
mm Hg or greater. The American College of Physicians recommends that adults undergo
blood pressure screening every one to two years and at every visit for other reasons.

Patient Preparation

The patient should be relaxed and seated (or recumbent) for several minutes before blood pressure is measured. The arm should be at the level of
the heart, comfortably supported on a firm surface, and slightly flexed.
Clothing with constricting arm sleeves should be removed. The patient
should not have smoked or ingested caffeine for 30 minutes before measurement.

The examiner should select the proper cuff size to accommodate the
size of the patient's arm (Table 3.2). A normal-sized adult cuff will produce falsely elevated pressures on an obese arm and falsely low pressures
on a thin arm or on that of a child. Therefore, choose a cuff with a bladder
width that is 20% wider than the diameter of the arm or 40% of the circumference of the arm. The length of the bladder should be about 80% of
the circumference so that it does not completely encircle the limb. In children, the bladder width should not exceed two-thirds the length of the

Table 3.2
Proper Bladder Dimensions for Blood Pressure Measurement

Patient	Bladder Width (cm)	Bladder Length (cm)	Arm Circumference Range at Midpoint (cm)
Newborn	3	6	≤6
Infant	5	15	6–15
Child	8	21	16–21
Small adult	10	24	22–26
Adult	13	30	27–34
Large adult	16	38	35–44

Adapted from Human blood pressure determination by sphygmomanometry. Dallas, TX: American Heart Association, 1994.

upper arm and the bladder length should not encircle more than three-fourths of the circumference of the arm.

Technique

The cuff should be placed snugly around the upper arm, with the lower edge about one inch above the antecubital fossa, the bladder over the brachial artery, and the tubing over the medial aspect of the arm. Both the palpable systolic pressure and the audible Korotkoff sounds should be determined. (The level at which sounds are first heard, the systolic pressure, is phase 1 of the Korotkoff sounds, the level at which they become dampened is phase 4, and the level at which they disappear, the diastolic pressure, is phase 5.) If an abnormality is detected, the blood pressure should be compared in both arms in supine, sitting, and standing positions; in children, blood pressure should be measured in the lower extremities to rule out aortic coarctation. Differences of up to 10 mm Hg between arms are within the normal range, and the higher reading should be accepted as the patient's blood pressure.

Blood pressure is considered elevated if it exceeds the values listed in Table 3.3. Isolated blood pressure elevations can be due to anxiety and other factors (e.g., "white coat" hypertension), and the diagnosis of hypertension should therefore not be made until the patient has had three consecutive visits in which elevated blood pressure has been documented. Patients with an isolated blood pressure elevation should be informed that the elevation is not considered "high blood pressure" until repeat measurements are obtained, but the importance of returning for repeat measurements should be emphasized.

Table 3.3
Criteria for Elevated Blood Pressure

Age	Diastolic Blood Pressure (mm Hg)	Systolic Blood Pressure (mm Hg)
Newborn		96
8–30 days		104
0–2 years	74	112
3–5 years	76	116
6–9 years	78	122
10–12 years	82	126
13–15 years	86	136
>15 years	90	140

Adapted from Joint National Committee on Detection, Evaluation, and Treatment of High Blood Pressure. The fifth report of the Joint National Committee on Detection, Evaluation, and Treatment of High Blood Pressure (JNC V). Arch Intern Med 1993;153:154–183.

Standard Counseling

Patients should be reminded that exercise (Chapter 7) and weight management (Chapter 9) will help prevent hypertension and that their blood pressure should be measured again in one to two years.

What to Do with Abnormal Results

See Table 17.1.

Potential Adverse Effects

There are no direct adverse effects from measuring blood pressure, but the results can be inaccurate, producing psychological, behavioral, and even financial consequences if the results affect insurance or employment eligibility or require repeat office visits to rule out hypertension. Patients may experience anxiety over the possibility of having high blood pressure, and studies have confirmed higher rates of work absenteeism among persons who receive the label of "hypertension" (3). Inappropriately prescribed antihypertensive medications may also produce unnecessary adverse effects. Inaccurate sphygmomanometry can also produce false-negative results, allowing hypertensive persons to escape detection.

Accuracy and Reliability as Screening Test

Office sphygmomanometry is less accurate than invasive techniques for measuring blood pressure (e.g., intra-arterial monitoring), but its exact sensitivity and specificity are uncertain. Accuracy and reliability are affected by the type of instrument, the technique of the examiner, and the physiological state of the patient.

Office and Clinic Organization for Routine Screening

Intake procedures for obtaining vital signs should provide sufficient time to allow the patient to relax for several minutes before the blood pressure is measured. The office or clinic should be equipped with a variety of cuff sizes for adults and children. Aneroid manometers become inaccurate over time and should be recalibrated periodically. Reminder systems should be in place to ensure that patients return for routine screening, obtain consecutive repeat measurements for elevated values, and obtain appropriate counseling and treatment if hypertension is diagnosed.

Medical Record Documentation

In addition to the measured blood pressure, the size of the cuff (and site of auscultation if not the brachial artery) should be recorded. If blood pressure is measured in both arms, the arm and recorded values should be documented. Because blood pressure is often lower in the supine than in the sitting position, it may be useful to record the patient's position and to use the same position in future measurements. Until elevated blood pressure has been confirmed in three consecutive visits, the finding should be described in the medical record as "elevated blood pressure" and not as "hypertension" or even "high blood pressure." The follow-up plan for elevated blood pressure readings should be documented.

HEIGHT, WEIGHT, AND HEAD CIRCUMFERENCE

Introduction

Nearly 60 million Americans are overweight, a risk factor for diabetes mellitus, hypertension, coronary artery disease, other chronic diseases, and possibly higher mortality (4). Screening has been advocated as a means of detecting overweight and obesity and of initiating exercise and nutritional interventions to prevent complications (see Chapter 9). The principal screening tests for overweight and obesity are height, weight, and other anthropomorphic measurements. About 5–25% of children are obese, and about 4–5% of infants and children suffer from significantly delayed growth or failure to thrive (5). Frequent height, weight, and head circumference measurements are used to screen for abnormal growth velocity and to institute nutritional and social service interventions. Some screening tests for obesity (e.g., skinfold thickness, limb circumference) and abnormal growth (e.g., chest circumference) are not reviewed in this section.

Screening Guidelines. **The height and weight (and head circumference of infants and small children) should be measured at every pediatric visit (unless recent measurements have been obtained within the past few weeks) and should be plotted on an appropriate growth chart. The height and weight of adults should be measured periodically, but there is no scientific evidence regarding the proper interval.**

Official Guidelines. The above recommendations are similar to those of the U.S. Preventive Services Task Force and American Academy of Family Physicians. The American Academy of Pediatrics recommends that infants undergo screening at well-child visits at ages 0–24 months, annually from ages 2–6, and every two years thereafter. The American Heart Association recommends that adults obtain body weight measurements every five years. The Canadian Task Force on the Periodic Health Examination found insufficient evidence to recommend screening for obesity but did recommend serial measurement of height, weight, and head circumference in infants and children.

Patient Preparation

Patients should remove heavy clothing and shoes.

Technique

Height and weight are generally measured with a standing platform scale and a height attachment, although electronic scales are becoming more common. Most electronic scales do not require calibration, but platform scales should be calibrated to zero before the patient is weighed. When height is measured, patients should stand erect with their back against the scale or measuring wall and with their feet together. They should look straight ahead, with the outer canthus of the eye on the same horizontal plane as the external auditory canal.

Infants and small children should be weighed on an infant platform scale. The height of infants and small children is measured by placing the child in a recumbent position on a measuring board, holding the feet against a fixed footpiece, and moving the headpiece to touch the vertex. Head circumference should be measured by wrapping a measuring tape around the child's head at the level of the occipital protuberance and the supraorbital prominence.

Height and weight measurements are typically used to determine overweight and obesity by comparing the patient's height and weight with population norms for individuals with a similar height, weight, and body frame (Table 3.4). A weight that is 20% over the desirable range is typically defined as overweight. An alternative measurement method that may be more accurate is the body mass index, which is defined as the body weight in kilograms divided by the square of the height in meters. A body mass index of 27.8 or greater in men and of 27.3 or greater in women suggests overweight. The height, weight, and head circumference of infants and young children are used to detect abnormal size and growth velocity by plotting the data on age and gender-specific growth curves that reflect population norms (Fig. 3.1).

Standard Counseling

Patients should be counseled about the healthful benefits of exercise (Chapter 7) and weight management (Chapter 9).

What to Do with Abnormal Results

See Chapter 9.

Potential Adverse Effects

There are no direct adverse effects from measuring height and weight, but the results can produce psychological, behavioral, and even financial consequences if they affect insurance and employment eligibility and can incur inconvenience and costs to have the abnormality evaluated. False-positive results in measurements of infants and small children can create unnecessary parental anxiety about the possibility of a growth disorder. Some aggressive treatments for obesity, such as medications and very low calorie diets, are associated with some side effects and complications.

Table 3.4
Height and Weight Tables for Adults Age 25 and Over

Height (Without Shoes)	Weight in Pounds (Without Clothing)		
	Small Frame	Medium Frame	Large Frame
Men			
5'1"	105–113	111–122	119–134
5'2"	108–116	114–126	122–137
5'3"	111–119	117–129	125–141
5'4"	114–122	120–132	128–145
5'5"	117–126	123–136	131–149
5'6"	121–130	127–140	135–154
5'7"	125–134	131–145	140–159
5'8"	129–138	135–149	144–163
5'9"	133–143	139–153	148–167
5'10"	137–147	143–158	152–172
5'11"	141–151	147–163	157–177
6'0"	145–155	151–168	161–182
6'1"	149–160	155–173	168–187
6'2"	153–164	160–178	171–192
6'3"	157–168	165–183	175–197
Women			
4'9"	90–97	94–106	102–118
4'10"	92–100	97–109	106–121
4'11"	95–103	100–112	108–124
5'0"	98–106	103–116	111–127
5'1"	101–109	106–118	114–130
5'2"	104–112	109–122	117–134
5'3"	107–115	112–126	121–138
5'4"	110–119	116–131	125–142
5'5"	114–123	120–136	129–146
5'6"	118–127	124–139	133–150
5'7"	122–131	128–143	137–154
5'8"	126–136	132–147	141–159
5'9"	130–140	136–151	145–164
5'10"	134–144	140–155	149–169

From Clinician's handbook of preventive services. Washington, DC: U.S. Department of Health and Human Services, 1994:142–143.

Accuracy and Reliability as Screening Test

Although height and weight measurements are often accurate, there is considerable controversy as to whether height-weight tables for desirable weights, which are based on outdated actuarial data from insurance companies, are valid criteria for defining overweight. Body mass index appears to be a more accurate measure. (Concerns have also been raised about the validity of height, weight, and head circumference criteria for detecting growth disorders in infants and children.) Body fat content appears to correlate closely with skinfold thickness and waist-hip ratio, but measurement of the latter requires training and has greater variability than other screening methods.

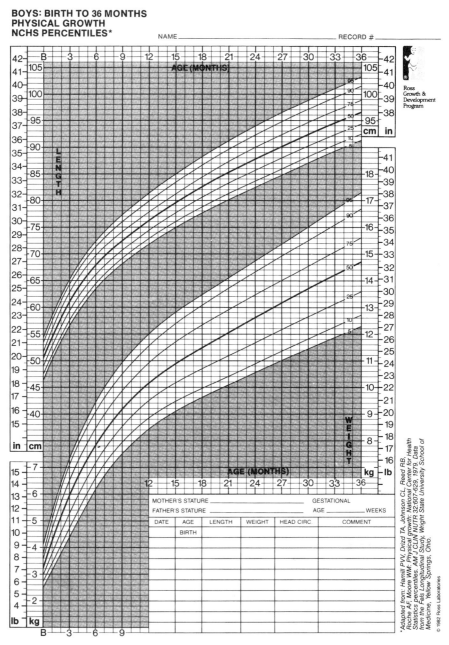

Figure 3.1. Weight-length chart for boys (age 0 to 36 months). (Used with permission of Ross Products Division, Abbott Laboratories, Columbus, OH. From NCHS Growth Charts, copyright 1982, Ross Products Division, Abbott Laboratories.)

Office and Clinic Organization for Routine Screening

Offices and clinics with pediatric patients should be equipped with infant platform scales, measuring boards, measuring tape, and a complete supply of pediatric growth charts for boys and girls of all ages. Height-weight tables for determining whether adult patients are overweight should be posted prominently in the chart or examining room. The office or clinic should have reminder systems in place to ensure that parents of children with abnormal growth velocity keep appointments for follow-up visits and that the children receive appropriate evaluation and treatment.

Medical Record Documentation

Height, weight, and other anthropometric data should be recorded in an area of the medical record that allows easy comparison with previous measurements and early detection of important trends. The appropriate age and gender-specific growth chart should be prominently displayed in the medical record of pediatric patients and should be filled out at each visit. The follow-up plan for abnormal height and weight should be documented in the medical record.

HEARING TESTING

Introduction

About 24 million Americans suffer from chronic hearing impairment, over one million of whom are under age 18 (6). About five million Americans cannot hear and understand normal speech, and about 10 million persons have noise-induced hearing loss. Screening for hearing impairment is performed because it has the potential to improve communication skills and functional status and because it may improve language development when detected in infants and young children. Hearing screening tests can include simple physical examination techniques, which are discussed in this section, and laboratory tests (e.g., audiometry, auditory evoked responses, otoacoustic emissions testing), which are discussed in Chapter 4.

Screening Guidelines. **Simple hearing screening should be performed at least once in young children (preferably before age 3) and periodically in the elderly, but there is no scientific evidence regarding the appropriate interval. Asymptomatic adolescents and young adults do not require routine hearing screening, unless they are exposed routinely to loud noise. See Chapter 4 for recommendations regarding electrophysiological and audiometric screening of newborns, children, and adults.**

Official Guidelines. The American Academy of Pediatrics recommends periodic historical inquiry about hearing during infancy and childhood and objective hearing testing by a "standard testing method" at ages 4, 5, 12, and 18 years. The Canadian Task Force on the Periodic Health Examination recommends hearing evaluation during the first two years of life, in adults attending for other reasons, and in the elderly. The U.S. Preventive Services Task Force found insufficient evidence to recommend for or against routine hearing screening of infants, children, and adults. Recommendations by the American Academy of Family Physicians are currently under review.

Patient Preparation

Hearing should be examined in a quiet area with little background noise.

Technique

Simple physical examination tests of hearing include the whispered voice, watch-tick, and tuning fork tests. In the whispered voice test, the examiner softly whispers words from a distance of one to two feet while the patient blocks the opposite ear by placing a finger on the tragus; the patient should be able to repeat at least half the words correctly. In the watch-tick test, the examiner checks high-frequency hearing by moving a ticking watch toward the patient's ear and noting the distance at which the sound is first heard.

Tuning forks (e.g., 512 Hz) are used to compare bone and air conduction. In the Weber test, the base of a vibrating tuning fork is placed on the midline vertex or forehead of the patient; lateralization of the sound is abnormal. In the Rinne test, the base of the vibrating tuning fork is placed on the mastoid bone and the examiner counts the number of seconds until the patient can no longer hear the sound. The vibrating tines are then rapidly moved to one to two centimeters from the auditory canal. The examiner counts the number of seconds until the patient can no longer hear the sound. The duration of air conduction should be longer than bone conduction. In the Schwabach test, the base of the vibrating tuning fork is placed on the mastoid bone. When the patient can no longer hear the sound, the base is rapidly placed on the examiner's mastoid bone to determine whether the sound is still audible.

The hearing of young children is tested qualitatively by observing their response to whispered voice or sounds and the progress of their developing speech skills (e.g., delayed vocalization). For example, the examiner can stand or crouch behind the child and whisper softly to determine whether the child turns to the sound or responds to a question (e.g., "Do you like ice cream?"). Children over age 3 or 4 can usually cooperate with tuning fork tests. See Chapter 4 regarding otoacoustic emissions and audiometry screening of newborns and young children.

Standard Counseling

Parents should be encouraged to contact the physician if they or teachers note that the child has poor hearing, speech, or language skills. All patients, especially adolescents and young adults, should be reminded that occupational or recreational exposure to loud noise increases the risk of hearing loss. Older adults should be counseled that, although loss of hearing is common with increasing age, it should not be accepted as "normal," can compromise their quality of life, and is often treatable with hearing aids.

What to Do with Abnormal Results

See Table 17.22.

Potential Adverse Effects

There are no known adverse effects from hearing testing, but inaccurate results may produce unnecessary anxiety, especially among the parents of young children; may affect insurance and employment eligibility; and may incur cost and inconvenience for appointments and testing to rule out a disorder. Inaccurate testing may produce false-negative results, allowing hearing impairment to escape detection.

Accuracy and Reliability as Screening Test

There are few data available regarding the sensitivity and specificity of physical examination techniques for hearing. See Chapter 4 regarding the accuracy of electrophysiologic testing and audiometry.

Office and Clinic Organization for Routine Screening

Examining rooms in which hearing screening is performed should not be located near loud working areas or noisy machines. The office or clinic should have referral and reminder systems in place to ensure that patients with abnormal screening tests receive appropriate diagnostic studies (e.g., audiometry, tympanometry) on site or through a referred specialist and that patients found to have hearing disorders receive proper treatment. Patient education literature about hearing aids and the need to treat presbycusis can be helpful to older adults.

Medical Record Documentation

The results of hearing tests should be recorded for each ear. The data can include the proportion of correctly heard words (whisper test), distance to hear watch sounds (watch-tick test), direction of lateralization (Weber test), ratio of air to bone conduction (Rinne test), or difference in examiner and patient conduction (Schwabach test). The follow-up plan for abnormal hearing should be documented.

VISUAL ACUITY TESTING

Introduction

Over nine million Americans have impaired visual acuity, and about 2–5% of American children suffer from amblyopia and strabismus (6). Screening for abnormal visual acuity is performed because the detection of visual impairment during early childhood may prevent abnormal eye development (e.g., amblyopia) and because poor vision at any age affects the patient's quality of life. Although there is little evidence that early detection of visual impairment reduces morbidity for school-aged children, adolescents, and young adults, detection in older adults may prevent injuries and improve functional status. Testing for abnormal visual acuity can range from simple acuity testing by primary care clinicians to sophisticated refraction measurements by eye specialists (see also Chapter 21 regarding glaucoma screening). This section discusses Snellen testing of visual acuity and screening tests for amblyopia and strabismus in young children. Inspection for a red reflex and the Bruckner test are not discussed.

Screening Guidelines.   **Visual acuity screening for amblyopia and strabismus is recommended at least once in young children (preferably before age 3 or 4). Periodic screening for impaired visual acuity is appropriate in older adults, but there is no scientific evidence regarding the optimal interval. Asymptomatic adolescents and young adults do not require routine visual acuity screening.**

Official Guidelines.   These recommendations are similar to those of the U.S. Preventive Services Task Force. The Canadian Task Force on the Periodic Health Examination recommends amblyopia screening in infancy and visual acuity testing in preschool children and the elderly (including funduscopy for elderly persons with diabetes mellitus). The American Academy of Family Physicians recommends an eye examination for amblyopia and strabismus at ages 3–4 and visual acuity screening in the elderly. The American Academy of Ophthalmology recommends an ophthalmological examination of newborns who are premature or at risk for eye disease; an examination of fixation preference and ocular alignment by age 6 months; an examination of visual acuity, ocular alignment, and ocular disease at ages 3–4; annual screening of schoolchildren for visual acuity and ocular alignment; occasional examinations from puberty to age 40; and an examination at age 40, every 2–4 years until age 65, and every 1–2 years thereafter. Similar recommendations have been issued by the American Optometric Association. The American Academy of Pediatrics recommends subjective testing of vision from infancy through age 3 and objective testing by a "standard testing method" annually from ages 4–8 and at ages 12, 14, and 18 years. Vision screening of preschool and school children is also required by law in some states and in a number of federal programs; in 1992, 38 states required screening of elementary school age children.

Patient Preparation

Individuals with a known refractive error and prescribed corrective lenses should wear their glasses or contact lenses for the examination.

Technique

To test visual acuity, the patient should sit or stand 20 feet from a standard Snellen eye chart. With one eye covered, the patient should read the letters aloud, moving from top to bottom, and then the test should be repeated with the other eye covered. The last full row of letters that the patient can read correctly indicates the acuity level. If the upper row of large letters cannot be seen at 20 feet, the patient should step forward until they become visible; the distance should be recorded in the upper figure (at a distance of five feet, the notation would be "5/200"). An acuity of 20/30 or better is generally considered normal for adults. If a standard Snellen wall chart is unavailable, acuity can be tested with pocket eye charts (Rosenbaum or Jaeger charts) held at a distance of 14 inches or, more approximately, by comparing the patient's ability to read printed material with that of the examiner. Illiterate and non-English-speaking patients can be tested with the Snellen "E" chart (Fig. 3.2) by asking whether the letter faces up, down, to the left, or to the right.

In children, visual acuity can be tested with the Snellen "E" chart by ages 5–6. Children may not cooperate with keeping one eye covered, in which case an eye patch can be taped over the eye. Children who do not understand the instructions can sometimes participate if they are given a card with a large E and told to turn the card in the direction of the letter on the chart ("tumbling E" test). The tumbling E test is ideal for children ages 3–5. The tumbling E test and other visual acuity tests should be performed at a distance of 10 feet. Normal visual acuity is approximately 20/50 by age 3, 20/30 by age 5, and 20/20 by age 6. Visual acuity testing is performed qualitatively during infancy by observing the patient's ability to fixate on a target and, by 3 months of age, to follow a moving object. By 6 months of age, the child should be able to grasp objects and recognize faces.

Screening for strabismus is usually performed with the cover test and Hirschberg test. In the cover test, a light source is placed at the middle of the examiner's forehead and each of the patient's eyes is covered in sequence. The test is abnormal when the examiner notes movement of one eye to fixate on the light when the other eye is covered. In the Hirschberg test, the examiner points a light source at the eyes and checks for an asymmetric light reflex. Convergent strabismus may be seen in normal infants until 6 months of age, but divergent strabismus is usually pathological at any age. Screening for amblyopia is based on visual acuity testing. A two-row difference between the acuity of each eye may indicate amblyopia.

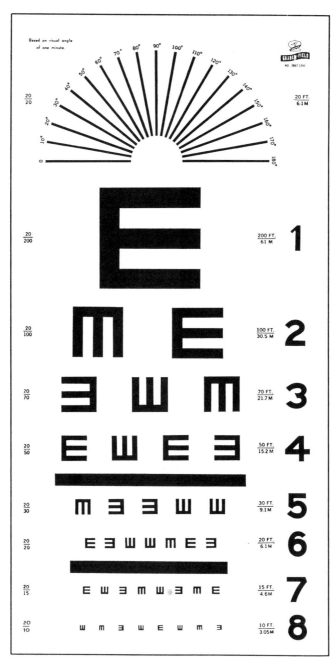

Figure 3.2. Snellen "E" chart. The patient can be asked in which direction the "legs of the table" point. (Reprinted with permission from Seidel HM, Ball JW, Dains JE, Benedict GW. Mosby's guide to physical examination, 2nd edition. St. Louis: Mosby-Year Book, 1991;38:389.)

Standard Counseling

Parents should be encouraged to contact the physician if they or teachers note that the child has difficulty seeing or has poor school performance. Older adults should be reminded that, although worsening vision is common with increasing age, it should not be accepted as "normal," can limit functional independence, increases the risk of falls and other unintentional injuries, and is often treatable with corrective lenses. Older adults may also benefit from routine examinations by an eye specialist, especially to screen for glaucoma (see Chapter 21).

What to Do with Abnormal Results

See Table 17.23.

Potential Adverse Effects

There are no known adverse effects from visual acuity testing, but inaccurate results can produce unnecessary anxiety, especially among the parents of young children; may affect insurance and employment eligibility; and may incur costs and inconvenience for visits to eye care specialists to rule out a disorder. Inaccurate screening may produce false-negative results, allowing visual disorders to escape detection.

Accuracy and Reliability as Screening Test

Few studies have examined the sensitivity and specificity of visual acuity testing. In children, Snellen letters are estimated to have a sensitivity of 25–79% and a specificity of about 85%. There is little evidence regarding the accuracy of the cover test or Hirschberg test.

Office and Clinic Organization for Routine Screening

Offices and clinics should be equipped with a Snellen wall chart (or pocket chart), a Snellen "E" chart, and eye covers. Visual acuity testing should not be performed in high-traffic areas, where the test is likely to be interrupted by the movement of staff or patients. A floor marker should identify the proper standing position. Nurses and physician assistants can perform visual acuity testing before the physician's examination. All staff who will perform the test should be trained in proper technique for performing the test and recording the results. The office or clinic should have referral and reminder systems in place to ensure that patients with abnormal visual acuity receive appropriate referrals to eye specialists and to verify that follow-up appointments are kept.

Medical Record Documentation

Visual acuity should be recorded for each eye. When the Snellen eye chart is used to determine the lowest row of letters that the patient can read correctly, indicate the number of letters from the next row that were read correctly (e.g., "20/25 + 2" means that the patient was able to read two letters from the 20/20 row). If strabismus is detected, indicate whether the eye is nasally deviated (esotropia) or temporally deviated (exotropia). The follow-up plan for abnormal visual acuity should be documented.

ORAL CAVITY EXAMINATION

Introduction

About 30,000 new cases of oral cancer occur annually in the United States (7). An estimated 8400 Americans died in 1995 from cancers of the buccal cavity and pharynx. Screening the oral cavity for cancer is advocated because of the potential to improve outcome through the detection of early-stage disease and because there is little harm or cost associated with the examination. There is little direct evidence, however, that screening for oral cancer results in improved outcomes.

Screening Guidelines. **Oral cavity screening of asymptomatic persons may be indicated in patients who use tobacco, drink excessive amounts of alcohol, or have found suspicious lesions on self-examination. There is little scientific evidence regarding the effectiveness of or optimal interval for oral cavity screening. See Chapter 15 regarding examinations for dental or periodontal disease.**

Official Guidelines. These recommendations are similar to those of the American Academy of Family Physicians. The U.S. Preventive Services Task Force and the Canadian Task Force on the Periodic Health Examination concluded that there is insufficient evidence to recommend for or against routine screening for oral cancer, but the Canadian Task Force recommended considering annual oral examination by a physician and/or dentist in patients over age 60 with risk factors for oral cancer. The American Cancer Society recommends including an oral cavity examination in the "cancer checkup," which they recommend performing every 3 years at ages 21–40 and annually thereafter. The American College of Obstetricians and Gynecologists recommends an oral cavity examination in all women every year or "as appropriate."

Technique

The oral cavity cancer examination begins with the lips, a potential site of both oral cavity and skin cancer. Dental appliances such as dentures should be removed. Using a tongue blade and a light source, the examiner should systematically inspect the buccal mucosa, gums, dorsum of the tongue, and hard palate. A nodule or growth on the palate, especially if it is not in the midline, should be evaluated further. The teeth should be inspected for plaque and carious lesions and the gums should be inspected for signs of inflammation, bleeding, or recession. The posterior pharynx should be inspected by depressing the tongue with a tongue blade and noting abnormalities in the tonsillar architecture. The hypopharynx can be viewed with a Number 5 mirror (or pharyngoscope).

Ask the patient to touch the tongue tip to the hard palate and inspect the floor of the mouth and the ventral surface of the tongue. Using a gloved hand, wrap the tongue with gauze, pull it to each side to inspect the lateral borders, and palpate the tongue for masses or nodules. White or red material should be scraped to distinguish between food particles and leukoplakia, a precursor to oral neoplasms. An ulcer, nodule, or thickened white patch on the lateral or ventral surface of the tongue may represent a malignancy. Leukoplakia should be suspected if an immovable white lesion resembling white paint is detected on the buccal mucosa, lower lip, tongue, or floor of the mouth.

Standard Counseling

Patients who use tobacco should be advised to stop smoking or chewing tobacco (Chapter 6), and those who drink excessive amounts of alcohol should receive appropriate counseling (Chapter 13). All patients should be counseled regarding preventive dental care (Chapter 15).

What to Do with Abnormal Results

See Table 17.8.

Potential Adverse Effects

The only direct adverse effects of the noninvasive oral cavity examination are the minor discomfort associated with the gag reflex and manipulation of the tongue. The detection of suspicious lesions can produce significant anxiety until a tissue diagnosis is obtained, however, and follow-up appointments with specialists may incur costs and inconvenience.

Accuracy and Reliability as Screening Test

Few studies have examined the sensitivity and specificity of the oral cavity examination, and the results have been variable, depending on the population, the skills of the examiner, and the study design: a sensitivity of 59–100%, specificity of 96–100%, and positive predictive value of 15–91% have been reported in different settings. Many believe that comprehensive examinations are more sensitive than the brief visual inspection of the oral cavity that is commonly performed by busy clinicians.

Office and Clinic Organization for Routine Screening

The examining room should be equipped with a good light source, tongue blades, and cotton gauze. Referral and reminder systems should be in place to ensure that patients with abnormal findings receive appropriate referrals to otolaryngologists, dentists, and other appropriate specialists; that the appointments are kept; and that patients with documented disease receive appropriate counseling and treatment.

Medical Record Documentation

The examiner should document that an oral cavity examination was performed and should describe the location, size, and appearance of abnormal lesions. The follow-up plan for suspicious findings should be documented.

CLINICAL BREAST EXAMINATION

Introduction

Over 180,000 new cases of breast cancer are diagnosed each year in the United States (7). It is the second leading cause of cancer deaths in women, accounting for an estimated 46,000 deaths in 1995 (7). Large clinical trials have demonstrated that mortality from breast cancer can be reduced by one-third in women aged 50–69 who receive routine screening consisting of an annual clinical breast examination (breast examination by a physician) and mammography every 1–2 years (1). Mammography is discussed in Chapter 4.

Screening Guidelines. **All women age 40 or older should undergo annual clinical breast examination. Women at increased risk of breast cancer (e.g., family history of premenopausally diagnosed breast cancer in a mother or sister) may benefit from routine clinical breast examinations beginning at an earlier age (e.g., age 35).**

Official Guidelines. These recommendations conform with those of the American College of Physicians. The Canadian Task Force on the Periodic Health Examination recommends annual clinical breast examinations in women ages 50–69, and the U.S. Preventive Services Task Force makes similar recommendations (if the clinical examinations are coupled with mammography). The American Academy of Family Physicians recommends clinical breast examination every 1–3 years in women ages 30–40 and annually thereafter. The American Cancer Society and American College of Radiology recommend clinical breast examination every 3 years from age 20 to 40 and annually thereafter. The American College of Obstetricians and Gynecologists recommends clinical breast examination in all women every year or "as appropriate."

Patient Preparation

The examination room should have adequate lighting. The patient should disrobe to the waist, remove her brassiere, and dress in a gown.

Technique

The clinician should be sensitive to the anxiety of patients undergoing this examination, who often have been sensitized to the risks of breast cancer through lay media or the illnesses of family or friends. A female chaperone may be advisable if the examiner is a man. The physician should inspect the breasts for size, symmetry, contour, skin color, and obvious lesions. Dimpling or retractions of the skin, edema resulting in peau d'orange texture (appearance of thick skin with large pores and accentuated markings), visible venous networks in one breast, or an abnormal nipple (e.g., bleeding, discharge, ulceration, inversion, retraction) may suggest carcinoma (Fig. 3.3). Breast inspection is best performed in different positions: first with the patient seated and arms at the side, then with the arms over the head, with the hands pressed against the hips (or palms pushed

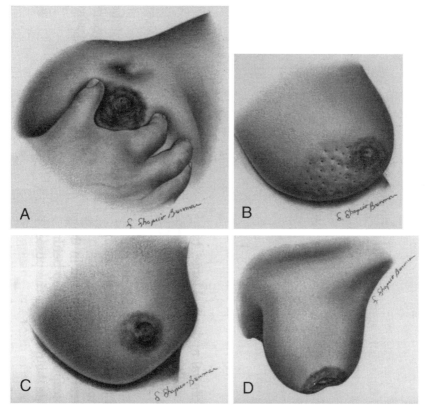

Figure 3.3. Physical findings on inspection of the breasts. **A.** Skin dimpling. **B.** Edema (peau d'orange). **C.** Abnormal contour. **D.** Nipple retraction and deviation. (Reprinted with permission from Bates B. A guide to physical examination, 5th edition. Philadelphia: JB Lippincott, 1991:336.)

against each other) to contract the pectoralis muscles, and, finally, with the patient leaning forward to place traction on the suspensory ligaments (Fig. 3.4).

The breasts (including the nipples and subareolar tissue), axillae, and supraclavicular areas should be palpated in a systematic fashion, feeling for lumps, nodules, or lymphadenopathy, with the patient in upright and supine positions. Concentric, rotatory, and other methods have been recommended for breast palpation (Fig. 3.5), but the most important re-

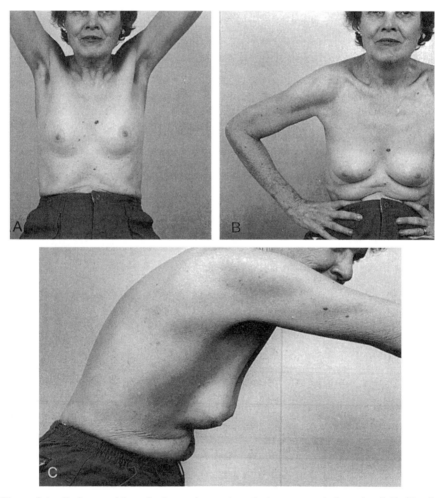

Figure 3.4.   Patient positions for breast inspection. **A.** Arms extended overhead. **B.** Hands pressed against hips. **C.** Leaning forward to place traction on the suspensory ligaments. (Reprinted with permission from Willms JL, Schneiderman H, Algranati PS. Physical diagnosis: bedside evaluation of diagnosis and function. Baltimore: Williams & Wilkins, 1994:226.)

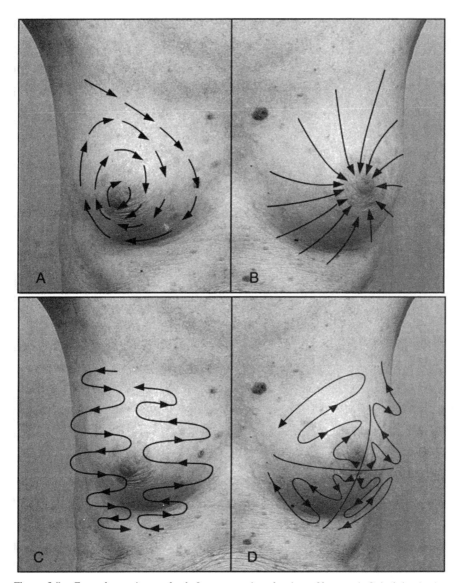

Figure 3.5. Four alternative methods for systematic palpation of breast. **A.** Spiral, beginning with the tail. **B.** Spokes, periphery to center. **C.** Back-and-forth method. **D.** Quadratic, i.e., palpation of each quadrant from areola to periphery. (Reprinted with permission from Willms JL, Schneiderman H, Algranati PS. Physical diagnosis: bedside evaluation of diagnosis and function. Baltimore: Williams & Wilkins, 1994:230.)

quirement is that each portion of the breast be fully examined in a system-atic fashion. Always palpate the tail of the breast, because most malignan-cies occur in the upper-outer quadrant. The tail is made accessible to pal-pation by having the patient raise her arms over her head. The entire axilla and supraclavicular areas should be palpated for lymphadenopathy, including the lateral portion along the under surface of the arm, the ante-rior wall along the pectoralis muscles, and the posterior portion along the scapular border. Supraclavicular nodes are best inspected by having the patient turn her head toward the side being examined while raising the shoulder and bending the head forward to relax the sternocleidomastoid muscle.

If a breast mass is palpated, the examiner should note its location, size, shape, consistency, tenderness, mobility, and borders. In pre-menopausal women, it is also important to note the stage of the patient's menstrual cycle. Breast carcinoma is more likely to be firm, nontender, and to produce dimpling or edema of the skin. Breast enlargement, nodularity, and tenderness that occur in monthly cyclical patterns and in different locations of the breast are often related to fibrocystic disease. These patterns are not consistent, however, and malignancy generally cannot be ruled out without careful documentation, repeat examinations, imaging studies, cyst aspiration, and/or tissue biopsy. Although small, 3–5 mm mobile axillary lymph nodes are common in adults, the examiner should note the location, size, consistency, and degree of fixation of any palpable nodes.

Standard Counseling

Women over age 50 should be advised to obtain a screening mammogram every one to two years (see Chapter 4). The clinical breast examination should be repeated annually. Women should be advised to notify the physician if suspicious masses or lesions are noted on self-examination. See Chapter 20 for further information about breast self-examination.

What to Do with Abnormal Results

See Table 17.4.

Potential Adverse Effects

The only direct adverse effects of the clinical breast examination are em-barrassment and discomfort during palpation. The detection of suspicious masses, however, can produce significant anxiety until a tissue diagnosis is obtained and can lead to invasive and uncomfortable procedures such as needle aspiration and biopsy. The costs and inconvenience associated with repeat office visits and appointments with specialists can be significant. In-accurate or incomplete examinations can produce false-negative results, allowing premalignant and malignant lesions to escape detection.

Accuracy and Reliability as Screening Test

Clinical breast examination alone, without mammography, has a reported sensitivity of 45–63% in detecting breast cancer. Studies using manufac-tured breast models report that the physician examination has a sensitivity of 87% in detecting masses greater than 1 cm in diameter. The reported specificity of the clinical breast examination is 98–99% but depends on the skills of the examiner and the age of the patient.

Office and Clinic Organization for Routine Screening

Examining rooms used for routine screening should offer complete pri-vacy, comfortable temperature, and good lighting. The clinical breast ex-amination provides an important opportunity for recommending mam-mography (see Chapter 4) and, if practiced by the physician, counseling how to perform breast self-examination (see Chapter 20). The office or clinic should therefore have systems in place to easily provide referrals for screening mammograms at the time of the breast examination and, if breast self-examination is recommended, to provide instructions and printed materials on proper technique (see Chapter 20). The office or clinic should have reliable referral and reminder systems in place to en-sure that women return for their next breast examination within one year; that patients with abnormal findings on breast examination return for fol-low-up evaluations and, when indicated, receive referrals to surgeons or ra-diologists; that appointments with outside specialists are kept; and that women found to have breast disease receive appropriate counseling and treatment.

Medical Record Documentation

The examiner should document that a complete breast examination was performed. If a breast lesion is found on examination, the clinician should document the location by noting the quadrant, its diagonal relationship to the nipple ("3 o'clock, 3 cm from the nipple"), its size in centimeters, and the consistency, mobility, and tenderness of the mass. The presence or ab-sence of skin, nipple, and lymph node findings should also be docu-mented. A diagram of the breast, indicating the specific location of the mass, may be helpful for future reference and for describing the findings to other examiners. The follow-up plan for abnormal findings should be documented in the medical record.

DIGITAL RECTAL EXAMINATION

Introduction

Colorectal and prostate cancers together account for over 95,000 deaths and over 380,000 new cases in the United States each year (7). Colorectal cancer is the second leading cause of cancer death among Americans, and prostate cancer is the second leading cause of cancer deaths among American men. Digital rectal examination is among the oldest screening tests that have been recommended to detect these malignancies. Other more sensitive tests (e.g., fecal occult blood testing, sigmoidoscopy, prostate-specific antigen) are discussed in Chapters 4 and 21. Scientific evidence that routine rectal examination can improve the outcome of colorectal or prostate cancer is limited, but many clinicians believe it should be performed because it has few direct adverse effects. The following explanation of how to perform routine screening digital rectal examination does not necessarily imply an endorsement of the practice by the editors.

Screening Guidelines. **Clinicians who advocate routine digital rectal examination recommend that the procedure be performed annually after age 40.**

Official Guidelines. The American Cancer Society recommends annual digital rectal examination of all adults beginning at age 40. The American Urological Association recommends annual rectal examinations for prostate cancer after age 50 (or after age 40 in African American men and men with a family history of prostate cancer). The American College of Obstetricians and Gynecologists recommends rectal examinations of all women every year or "as appropriate." The American Academy of Family Physicians recommends digital rectal examinations in persons 40 years of age and older but does not specify a frequency, noting that supporting scientific evidence is inconclusive. The Canadian Task Force on the Periodic Health Examination concluded that there was insufficient evidence to recommend for or against digital rectal examinations to screen for prostate cancer. The U.S. Preventive Services Task Force reached similar conclusions in reference to colorectal cancer but recommended against rectal examinations to screen for prostate cancer.

Patient Preparation

The examination can be performed in the Sim's (lying on left side with hips and knees flexed), supine lithotomy, knee-chest, or standing position. Explain to the patient why a digital rectal examination is indicated and acknowledge that it may be uncomfortable. The patient should be told that a cold-feeling lubricant will be used, that there may be a feeling of urgency for a bowel movement, but that the latter will not occur. Males should be told that palpation of the prostate gland may produce the urge to urinate. A chaperone may be advisable if the patient is the opposite sex of the examiner.

Technique

The gloved and lubricated examining finger is inserted through the anus, advanced along the anterior wall of the rectum, rotated to sweep circumferentially around the lateral and posterior rectum, and advanced superiorly to the rectovesical or rectouterine pouch. The examiner should feel uniformly for polyps, nodules, or other masses, as well as for narrowing or tenderness. Rectal carcinoma can present as plateau-like, nodular, annular, or cauliflower masses. The classic presentation is a sessile, hard, polypoid mass with irregular, nodular, raised edges and areas of ulceration. Many villous adenomas can be difficult to palpate.

When examining males, the examiner should palpate the prostate gland and seminal vesicles across the anterior wall of the rectum. The finger may feel more of the prostate if the examiner's body is turned slightly away from the patient. The examiner should feel the median furrow and middle lobe of the prostate and then sweep the finger across the lateral lobes, noting whether the surface is smooth or nodular, as well as the gland's consistency, shape, size, and mobility. The normal prostate gland is smooth, rubbery (consistency of a pencil eraser), and nontender, with well-defined borders. The normal size is about 3–4 cm in diameter (ordinarily twice the width of the examining finger), with less than 1 cm protrusion into the rectum; size generally increases with age. Prostatic carcinoma can present as one or more posterior nodules, which are often stony hard and painless. With more advanced disease, the entire gland may be stony hard and the median furrow may be obliterated.

After removing the finger, inspect fecal material on the glove for color, consistency, pus, or blood. Testing for occult blood is best performed on stool specimens obtained by the patient at home (see Chapter 4). To test for occult blood after the rectal examination, apply a smooth layer of the specimen to a guaiac card and apply a drop of developer. Blue coloration of the specimen is abnormal (see Chapter 17). The patient should be given tissues to remove the lubricant from the perianal area and should be invited to assume a more comfortable position.

Standard Counseling

Patients should be advised to notify the physician if they note blood in the stool; men should report urinary symptoms (e.g., urinary frequency or urgency, post-void dribbling). Digital rectal examination is often repeated on an annual basis after age 40. See Chapter 4 regarding supplying the patient with stool guaiac cards for fecal occult blood testing at home and for recommendations on screening sigmoidoscopy.

What to Do with Abnormal Results

See Table 17.5 and 17.7.

Potential Adverse Effects

The principal adverse effects of the digital rectal examination are discomfort and embarrassment. Generally, the discomfort is limited to the sensation of having to defecate or urinate, but some patients may experience painful mucosal irritation or spasm of the anal sphincter. Patients with hemorrhoidal disease or anal fissures may experience greater discomfort and may bleed after the procedure. If a suspicious mass or occult blood is detected, the patient may experience considerable anxiety until further testing is completed and may incur costs and inconvenience for follow-up office visits and procedures. Some follow-up tests, such as barium enema, colonoscopy, and prostate needle biopsy, have more substantial adverse effects (see Chapter 4). Inaccurate rectal examinations can produce false-negative results, allowing premalignant or malignant lesions to escape detection.

Accuracy and Reliability as Screening Test

The typical examining finger can reach only 6–10 cm into the rectum, making it possible to detect no more than 10% of colorectal cancers. Its sensitivity in detecting prostate cancer is also limited because the examining finger can only palpate the posterior and lateral aspects of the gland and because Stage A tumors are, by definition, nonpalpable. The reported sensitivity for detecting prostate cancer in asymptomatic men is about 55–68% in some studies but may be as low as 18–22%. About 6–33% of men with suspicious findings on digital rectal examination have histologic evidence of prostate cancer on needle biopsy.

Office and Clinic Organization for Routine Screening

Examining rooms used for routine screening should offer complete privacy and should be equipped with dressing gowns, gloves, lubricant, stool guaiac cards, and hemoccult developer. The office or clinic should have reliable referral and reminder systems in place to ensure that the rectal examination is repeated at the interval recommended by the physician, that patients with abnormal rectal examinations receive appropriate follow-up diagnostic studies and consultations with specialists, that appointments are kept, and that patients found to have documented disease receive appropriate counseling and treatment.

Medical Record Documentation

The examiner should document that a digital rectal examination was performed and, if guaiac testing was performed, the presence or absence of fecal occult blood. Prostatic enlargement can be graded on the basis of diameter in finger breadths (e.g., 1+ = three fingerbreadths, 2+ = four fingerbreadths, 3+ = five fingerbreadths, 4+ occupies most of the anterior outlet with encroachment of the rectal wall) or of depth of protrusion into the rectum: Grade I (1–2 cm), Grade II (2–3 cm), Grade III (3–4 cm), and Grade IV (more than 4 cm). The follow-up plan for abnormal findings should be documented.

SKIN EXAMINATION

Introduction

Over 700,000 new cases of skin cancer are diagnosed each year in the United States. About 34,000 of these cases are malignant melanomas, which accounted for an estimated 7200 deaths in 1995 (7). The outcome of malignant melanoma and other skin cancers can be improved significantly if detected early, and thus skin cancer screening examinations have been recommended. Direct evidence that complete skin examinations reduce the morbidity or mortality of skin cancer is limited, although the mean thickness of melanomas, a predictor of survival, appears to be lower in screened populations. The skin examination also provides an opportunity to detect signs of physical or sexual abuse.

Screening Guidelines. **Although clinicians should remain alert for malignant skin changes in all patients, comprehensive screening examinations of the skin are recommended primarily for persons with a personal or family history of skin cancer, clinical evidence of precursor lesions (e.g., dysplastic nevi, actinic keratoses, certain congenital nevi), and those with increased occupational or recreational exposure to sunlight. There is no scientific evidence regarding the optimal interval for skin screening.**

Official Guidelines. The Canadian Task Force on the Periodic Health Examination recommends against routine screening for skin cancer but suggests performing skin examinations in high-risk groups. Similarly, the American Academy of Family Physicians recommends complete skin examinations of adolescents and adults with risk factors for skin cancer. The American Academy of Dermatology and National Institutes of Health Consensus Panel on Early Melanoma recommend regular screening visits for skin cancer. The American Cancer Society recommends including the skin examination in the "cancer checkup," which it recommends performing every three years at ages 21–40 and annually thereafter. The American College of Obstetricians and Gynecologists recommends skin examinations for cancer in all women every year or "as appropriate." The U.S. Preventive Services Task Force found insufficient evidence to recommand for or against routine screening by primary care providers.

Patient Preparation

Patients undergoing a comprehensive skin examination should be asked to remove street clothing. The patient should wear a gown during the examination, and skin surfaces should be covered after they are examined.

Technique

For patients undergoing a comprehensive skin examination, the entire skin surface should be examined in a systematic fashion to ensure that all areas are inspected. Particular attention should be paid to sun-exposed areas (scalp, face, neck, shoulders, extensor surfaces of arms and hands) and to areas that are easily overlooked during routine self-examination (axillae, buttocks, perineum, backs of thighs, inner upper thighs, intertriginous surfaces). The skin cancer screening examination should search for evidence of basal cell carcinoma, squamous cell carcinoma, and malignant melanoma.

Basal cell carcinoma can be nodular, pigmented, cystic, sclerosing, or superficial, and it usually occurs on the head (especially the face), neck, and back. It may have a translucent, smooth, "pearly" appearance with a central depression (see Fig. 14.2A) but can also be pigmented or hyperkeratotic. Squamous cell carcinoma often presents as a soft, mobile, elevated mass with a surface scale or a crusting nodule or plaque (see Fig. 14.2B), but it can also have other appearances (e.g., the red-brown lesion of squamous cell carcinoma in situ, Bowen's disease). It usually occurs on sun-exposed areas such as the scalp, dorsal aspect of the hands, lower lip, and ear. Malignant melanomas include superficial spreading, nodular, lentigo, and acral-lentiginous forms. A pigmented lesion is more likely to be malignant if it is asymmetric, rapidly changes in size, or has irregulars borders, variegated colors, or a diameter greater than 6 mm (see Fig. 14.1, A–D). If suspicious lesions are discovered, the examiner should note the number, location, distribution, and physical characteristics of the lesion, including its size, shape, color, texture, and borders. See Chapter 14 for further details.

Patients with unusual bruises, lacerations, abrasions, or other signs of trauma with an unexplained etiology should be evaluated for a potential history of abuse (see Chapter 10).

Standard Counseling

Patients (and the parents of pediatric patients) should be reminded about the importance of limiting exposure to ultraviolet light (see Chapter 14). Patients should be counseled to advise the physician if a skin lesion changes in size, appearance, becomes tender, or starts bleeding; see Chapter 20 for further details about skin self-examination.

What to Do with Abnormal Results

See Table 17.10.

Potential Adverse Effects

The only adverse effect of the comprehensive skin examination is the embarrassment associated with being disrobed. Skin biopsies can be uncomfortable, may leave a scar, and may require a return office visit for suture removal. The patient may experience anxiety while awaiting the pathology report. Incomplete or inaccurate skin examinations may overlook important lesions and allow cancers to escape detection.

Accuracy and Reliability as Screening Test

Factors affecting the accuracy and reliability of the skin examination include the proportion of the body examined (only 20% of malignant melanomas occur on exposed skin surfaces), the frequency of the examination, the skills of the examiner, and the type of cancer being sought. Thus, studies have reported wide-ranging sensitivity and specificity estimates of 33–98% and 45–95%, respectively. The reported yield of total skin examinations in detecting cancer, even when performed by dermatologists, is about 3%. Dermatologists are about five times more likely to correctly identify malignant melanoma than clinicians who are not dermatologists.

Office and Clinic Organization for Routine Screening

Examination rooms used for routine skin cancer screening should offer complete privacy, dressing gowns, comfortable temperature, good lighting (preferably daylight or fluorescent lighting), and a magnifying lens or hand-held light source to closely inspect lesions. Since the skin examination provides an important opportunity to counsel patients about avoiding ultraviolet light exposure, patient education literature on this topic should be available (see "Resources" later in the chapter). In offices or clinics in which suspicious lesions are biopsied, equipment for performing biopsies and submitting pathology specimens should be easily accessible. Referral and reminder systems should be in place to ensure that patients return for repeat skin examinations at the interval recommended by the physician, that patients with suspicious lesions obtain skin biopsies on site or receive referrals to a physician who performs them, that the results of skin biopsies are obtained from the pathologist and documented in the medical record, and that patients found to have skin disease receive appropriate counseling and treatment.

Medical Record Documentation

The examiner should document that a skin examination was performed and should describe which skin surfaces were inspected. The location, size, color, distribution pattern, and other physical characteristics of suspicious lesions should be described. Standard terms for skin lesions should be used (e.g., macule, patch, papule, nodule, tumor, plaque). A body diagram may be useful in mapping the exact location of lesions. If a skin biopsy was performed, the clinician should describe the details of the procedure, including the size of the biopsy specimen (e.g., 3 mm punch) and the section of the lesion that was taken (e.g., border, full-thickness). The follow-up plan for suspicious lesions should be documented.

RESOURCES—PATIENT EDUCATION MATERIALS

Sphygmomanometry

National Heart, Lung, Blood Institute
Information Center
P.O. Box 30105
Bethesda, MD 20824-0105
301-251-1222
    "Facts About How To Prevent High Blood Pressure" (brochure 3281).

American Academy of Family Physicians
8880 Ward Parkway
Kansas City, MO 64114-2797
800-944-0000
    "What is High Blood Pressure?" (brochure 730).

Height, Weight, and Head Circumference

American Academy of Family Physicians
8880 Ward Parkway
Kansas City, MO 64114-2797
800-944-0000
    "Weight Control: Losing Weight and Keeping It Off" (brochure 1522).

American Academy of Pediatrics
Publications Department
141 Northwest Point Blvd.
P.O. Box 927
Elk Grove Village, IL 60009-0927
800-433-9016
    "Your Child's Growth: Developmental Milestones" (brochure HE0057).

American Heart Association
7320 Greenville Avenue
Dallas, TX 75231
214-373-6300
    "A Guide to Losing Weight" (brochure 50-1035).

Hearing Testing

American-Speech-Language-Hearing Association
10801 Rockville Pike
Rockville, MD 20852
800-638-8255, 301-897-8682
> "Can We Talk? A Guide to Your Child's Speech and Hearing" (pull-out information card); "How Does Your Child Hear and Talk?" (English, Spanish brochures); "Your Guide to Preventing Hearing Loss" (pull-out information card).

National Institute on Deafness and Other Communication Disorders Information Clearinghouse
1 Communications Avenue
Bethesda, MD 20892-3456
800-241-1044, 800-241-1055 (TRY)
> "Hearing and Hearing Loss" (Information packet DC-103); "Hearing and Older People" (fact sheet DC-24).

Visual Acuity Testing

American Academy of Pediatrics
Publications Department
141 Northwest Point Blvd.
P.O. Box 927
Elk Grove Village, IL 60009-0927
800-433-9016
> "Your Child's Eyes" (brochure HE0143).

American Optometric Association
243 North Lindbergh Boulevard
St. Louis, MO 63141
> "Family Guide to Vision Care" (brochure); "Answers to Questions About Common Vision Conditions" (brochure).

Krames Communications
1100 Grundy Lane
San Bruno, CA 94066-3030
800-333-3032
> "Total Eye Care" (brochure 1322).

National Institute on Aging
NIA Information Center
P.O. Box 8057
Gaithersburg, MD 20898-8057
800-222-2225
> "Aging and Your Eyes."

Oral Cavity Examination

American Cancer Society
1599 Clifton Road, NE
Atlanta, GA 30329
800-227-2345, 404-320-3333
> "Facts on Oral Cancer" (brochure, English 2630; Spanish 2706).

National Cancer Institute
Building 31, Room 10A24
Bethesda, MD 20892
800-4-CANCER
   "What You Need To Know About Oral Cancer" (brochure 93-1574).

Clinical Breast Examination

American Academy of Family Physicians
8880 Ward Parkway
Kansas City, MO 64114-2797
800-944-0000
   "Breast Cancer: Steps To Finding Breast Lumps Early" (brochure 1518).

American Cancer Society
1599 Clifton Road, NE
Atlanta, GA 30329
800-227-2345, 404-320-3333
   "Breast Cancer Questions and Answers" (brochure 92-750M); "Facts On Breast Cancer"
   (brochure, English 2003; Spanish 2701); "Special Touch: A Personal Plan of Action for
   Breast Health" (brochure 2095).

National Cancer Institute
Building 31, Room 10A24
Bethesda, MD 20892
800-4-CANCER
   "Take Care of Your Breasts" (brochure 93-3417).

Digital Rectal Examination

American Cancer Society
1599 Clifton Road, NE
Atlanta, GA 30329
800-227-2345, 404-320-3333
   "Facts on Colorectal Cancer" (brochure, English 2004; Spanish 2703); "Facts on
   Prostate Cancer" (brochure 2654).

American Institute for Cancer Research
1759 R Street, NW
Washington, DC 20069
800-843-8114, 202-328-7744
   "Reducing Your Risk of Colon Cancer" (brochure E2B-BHC); "Reducing Your Risk of
   Prostate Cancer" (brochure E42-BHP).

Krames Communications
1100 Grundy Lane
San Bruno, CA 94066-3030
800-333-3032
   "Colorectal Health" (brochure, English 1226; Spanish 1435).

National Cancer Institute
Building 31, Room 10A24
Bethesda, MD 20892
800-4-CANCER

"What You Need to Know About Prostate Cancer" (brochure 93-1576); "Cancer Tests You Should Know About: A Guide for People 65 and Over" (brochure 93-3256).

Skin Examination

American Academy of Family Physicians
8880 Ward Parkway
Kansas City, MO 64114-2797
800-944-0000
    "Skin Cancer: Saving Your Skin From Sun Damage" (brochure 1527).

American Cancer Society
1599 Clifton Road, NE
Atlanta, GA 30329
800-227-2345, 404-320-3333
    "Facts on Skin Cancer" (brochure 2049); "Fry Now, Pay Later" (brochure 2611); "Play it Safe . . . Beat Skin Cancer" (brochure 2675); "Why You Should Know About Melanoma" (brochure 2619).

National Cancer Institute
Building 31, Room 10A24
Bethesda, MD 20892
800-4-CANCER
    "What You Need To Know About Skin Cancer" (brochure 94-1563); "What You Need To Know About Moles and Dysplastic Nevi" (brochure 93-3133).

SUGGESTED READINGS

American Academy of Family Physicians. Age charts for the periodic health examination (Product No. 962). Kansas City, MO: American Academy of Family Physicians, 1994.

American Academy of Family Physicians, Committee on Practice and Ambulatory Medicine. Recommendations for preventive pediatric care (RE9224). Elk Grove Village, IL: American Academy of Pediatrics, 1991.

American Academy of Pediatrics. Vision screening guidelines. AAP News 1995;11:25. Reprinted in Am Fam Phys 1995;51:972.

American Cancer Society. Summary of American Cancer Society recommendations for the early detection of cancer in asymptomatic people. CA 1993;43:42–46.

American College of Obstetricians and Gynecologists. Routine cancer screening. ACOG Committee Opinion No. 128. Washington, DC: American College of Obstetricians and Gynecologists, 1993.

American College of Physicians. Common screening tests. Philadelphia: American College of Physicians, 1991.

Athreya BH, Silverman BK. Pediatric physical diagnosis. Norwalk, CT: Appleton-Century-Crofts, 1985.

Bates B. A guide to physical examination and history taking, 5th ed. Philadelphia: JB Lippincott, 1991.

Canadian Task Force on the Periodic Health Examination. The Canadian guide to clinical preventive health care. Ottawa: Canada Communication Group, 1994.

DeGowin RL, ed. DeGowin and Dewogin's bedside diagnostic examination, 6th ed. New York: MacMillan, 1994.

Hayward RS, Steinberg EP, Ford DE, et al. Preventive care guidelines, 1991. Ann Intern Med 1991;114:758–783.

Joint National Committee on Detection, Evaluation, and Treatment of High Blood Pressure. The fifth report of the Joint National Committee on Detection, Evaluation, and Treatment of High Blood Pressure (JNC V). Arch Intern Med 1993;153:154–183.

Judge RD, Zuidema GD, Fitzgerald FT, eds. Clinical diagnosis, 5th ed. Boston: Little, Brown & Co., 1989.

National Institutes of Health Consensus Development Conference. Diagnosis and treatment of early melanoma. 1992;10:1–26.

Oboler SK, LaForce FM. The periodic physical examination in asymptomatic adults. Ann Intern Med 1989;110:214–126.

Seidel HM, Ball JW, Dains JE, Benedict GW. Mosby's guide to physical examination, 2nd ed. St. Louis: Mosby Year Book, 1991.

Swartz MH. Textbook of physical diagnosis: History and examination, 2nd ed. Philadelphia: WB Saunders, 1994.

U.S. Preventive Services Task Force. Guide to clinical preventive services, 2nd ed. Baltimore: Williams & Wilkins, 1996.

REFERENCES

1. U.S. Preventive Services Task Force. Guide to clinical preventive services, 2nd ed. Baltimore: Williams & Wilkins, 1996.

2. Joint National Committee on Detection, Evaluation, and Treatment of High Blood Pressure. The fifth report of the Joint National Committee on Detection, Evaluation, and Treatment of High Blood Pressure (JNC V). Arch Intern Med 1993;153:154–183.

3. Haynes RB, Sackett DL, Taylor DW, et al. Increased absenteeism from work after detection and labeling of hypertensive patients. N Engl J Med 1978;299:741–747.

4. Kuczmarski RJ, Flegal KM, Campbell SM, Johnson CL. Increasing prevalence of overweight among U.S. adults: the National Health and Nutrition Examination Surveys, 1960 to 1991. JAMA 1994;272:205–211.

5. Boyle CA, Decoufle P, Yeargin-Allsopp M. Prevalence and health impact of developmental disabilities in U.S. children. Pediatrics 1994;93:399–403.

6. National Center for Health Statistics. Current estimates from the National Health Interview Survey, 1993. Vital Health Stat 1994;10 (190):94.

7. Wingo PA, Tong T, Bolden S. Cancer statistics, 1995. CA 1995;45:8–30.

4. Laboratory Screening Tests

STEVEN H. WOOLF

INTRODUCTION

Laboratory screening tests are blood tests, tests performed at the bedside (e.g., Papanicolaou smear), imaging studies, and other laboratory procedures (e.g., audiometry) performed on asymptomatic persons for the early detection of risk factors and preclinical disease. These tests are best used as an adjunct to the history and physical examination, but their role in screening, as in other areas of medicine, has been overemphasized. Until recently, both clinicians and patients equated the periodic health examination with a battery of screening tests: e.g., electrocardiogram, chest radiograph, spirometry, urinalysis, and comprehensive blood tests. Over time, this testing became the central activity of the prevention visit, minimizing the role of the history and physical examination. Even now, many patients judge the quality of their physicians by the number of tests that they order.

Several factors have contributed to the prominent role of laboratory screening in the periodic health examination. In some cases (e.g., mammography, Papanicolaou smears), studies have shown that periodic screening reduces morbidity and mortality. In many other cases, such evidence is unavailable but physicians have assumed, on the basis of personal or clinical experience, that screening is beneficial. Laboratory tests appeal to clinicians for other reasons. Although they are often no more accurate than a careful history and physical examination, test results may be perceived as more reliable because they are generated by sophisticated technologies or because the results are quantitative. Numbers *seem* more accurate than subjective impressions, even if the numbers are inaccurate. Practical factors also promote testing. These include concerns about malpractice liability if tests are not ordered, regulations and other requirements for screening, and potential financial gain. Laboratory tests are convenient: it is often easier to order tests than to perform a careful history and physical examination.

What is the harm of ordering laboratory screening tests? What is wrong with obtaining more information about a patient, other than the costs of the test? The costs certainly cannot be ignored. Nearly 670 million laboratory tests are ordered or performed in doctors' offices each year in the United States (1), and the resulting costs account for a large proportion of health care expenditures. At a time when the rising costs of health care have created a socioeconomic crisis in the United States, the unnecessary performance of costly laboratory tests is clearly inappropriate.

Aside from costs, however, laboratory screening tests can harm patients. Direct physical complications from screening tests (e.g., colonic perforation during sigmoidoscopy) are uncommon, but the information that the tests generate can lead to significant harm, especially if the results are inaccurate. Falsely positive screening tests can generate substantial anxiety while the patient awaits the results of confirmatory testing. Procedures performed to evaluate positive results (e.g., biopsies, colonoscopy, surgery) can be harmful. Although a simple blood test may seem innocuous, the results may set off a cascade of follow-up tests and procedures that carry substantial morbidity. Falsely negative tests can also be harmful, allowing the disease to escape detection, especially if the patient relies on the normal results to ignore warning signs and symptoms or to postpone appointments for repeat screening.

Falsely positive results are more common when laboratory tests are used for screening than when they are used for evaluating patients with symptomatic disease or special risk factors. This is true even when the sensitivity and specificity[a] are high. This is because the positive predictive value (PPV), the probability of true disease if a screening test is positive, depends on the prevalence, or pretest probability, of the disease. The PPV decreases, and the probability of producing falsely positive results increases, when patients at low risk of disease are tested, a common occurrence with screening. For example, if the pretest probability of disease is 1%, a test with a sensitivity and specificity of 90% has a PPV of 8.3%[b]: 11 patients will receive falsely positive results (and may require workups) for every true case of disease detected. If the probability is only 0.1%, the PPV falls to 0.9%: 111 patients will receive falsely positive results for every true case.

For many blood tests, the "normal range" is defined on the basis of population statistics. These tests are usually flagged as "abnormal" on laboratory printouts if they fall outside the 95% confidence interval (i.e., if less than 5% of the normal population would have the result), not because the result is necessarily pathological. Because "normal" is defined statistically, if the same test is repeated on 100 healthy persons, an abnormal result will occur an average of five times. For statistical reasons, the probability of

---

[a]*Sensitivity* is the proportion of persons with disease who correctly test positive. *Specificity* is the proportion of persons without disease who correctly test negative.

[b]The disease would affect 1000 persons in a population of 100,000 (prevalence = 1%), meaning that 900 (1000 × 90%) persons with disease would correctly test positive, and 9900 (1 − [99,000 × 90%]) persons without disease would incorrectly test positive. Thus, only 8.3% (900/9900+900) of positive test results would reflect true disease.

such results increases when multiple tests are performed at once, as in blood chemistry panels that combine over twenty tests at once. For example, when 20 independent variables are tested at once on a chemistry panel, there is a 64% probability of an "abnormal" result, even when no abnormality exists. When such tests are ordered routinely on healthy persons receiving periodic health examinations, the probability of falsely positive results is high and the clinician faces an ethical obligation to consider the potential adverse effects.

Given these concerns, what laboratory screening tests should physicians perform routinely in the periodic health examination? With advances in medical technology, physicians now have at their disposal hundreds of blood tests, imaging technologies, and other modalities that can detect diseases in asymptomatic persons. Since the late 1970s, authorities such as the Canadian Task Force on the Periodic Health Examination, the U.S. Preventive Services Task Force, and the American College of Physicians have used formal criteria and scientific evidence to weigh the benefits of such tests against their potential harms. In general, screening tests are not recommended unless there is (a) scientific evidence that the test can detect early-stage disease accurately (generating relatively few false-positive results) and (b) that early detection improves clinical outcome. If the false-positive rate is unacceptably high for universal screening (i.e., because of low disease prevalence, test specificity, or PPV), *selective screening* may be recommended for specific high-risk groups rather than for all patients. Although restrictive recommendations for targeted screening are often viewed as a cost-control policy, their most important benefit often lies in protecting healthy patients from the psychological and physical morbidity associated with inaccurate test results and unnecessary workups.

This chapter reviews the laboratory screening tests that are commonly recommended for asymptomatic persons (Table 4.1). These tests have been proven in clinical research to improve health outcomes (e.g., morbidity, mortality) or have other scientific support. They include tests that should be offered to all patients (Table 4.2) and tests that should only be performed selectively on patients with risk factors, due to poor PPV or other concerns (Table 4.3). Tables 4.2 and 4.3 generally conform with the recommendations of evidence-based groups such as the U.S. Preventive Services Task Force. The scientific evidence of the effectiveness of these tests and the arguments for why screening should be limited to selected populations or omitted completely are beyond the scope of this chapter. The reader should consult the references (especially the *Guide to Clinical Preventive Services*) (1) for more information about the scientific evidence for or against screening tests. The information in this chapter about screening tests of unproven effectiveness is provided as a guide for those physicians who choose to use them, but such tests are not necessarily advo-

Table 4.1
Laboratory Screening Tests

Screening Blood Tests
  Hemoglobin and hematocrit
  Hemoglobin electrophoresis
  Blood glucose and chemistry profiles
  Total cholesterol and lipid profiles
  Serologic tests for human immunodeficiency virus and syphilis
  Thyroid function tests
  Phenylketonuria screening
  Lead and erythrocyte protoporphyrin
Other Laboratory Screening Tests
  Papanicolaou smears
  Endocervical and urethral screening for gonorrhea and chlamydia
  Fecal occult blood test
  Sigmoidoscopy
  Mammography
  Electrocardiography
  Audiometry and newborn screening
  Tuberculin skin testing

cated by the editors. The editors specifically discourage the use of the screening tests discussed in Chapter 21.

The discussion of each screening test includes a brief introduction describing the target condition and the rationale for the test, a summary of official guidelines issued by major organizations and agencies, and detailed instructions on patient preparation and technique. (The sources of the recommendations in the "Official Guidelines" sections of this chapter are listed under "Suggested Readings" later in this chapter.) Although routine screening rarely detects clinically significant abnormalities, it does provide a setting for counseling patients about primary and secondary prevention of the target condition. Each section of this chapter therefore includes a "Standard Counseling" discussion of the reminders that clinicians should give all patients, even if no abnormality is detected, about how to prevent the target condition and when to return for screening. This section also refers readers to relevant chapters in Section 2 of this book, which discuss in more detail how to counsel patients about specific health behaviors.

For those instances in which an abnormality is detected, the following sections define the criteria for abnormal results and, in "What to Do with Abnormal Results," refer the clinician to the appropriate section of Chapter 17 that outlines follow-up testing and treatment options. The discussion of each screening test also includes sections on the potential adverse effects of screening, the accuracy of the test, and suggestions on how to organize the office or clinic and to maintain complete medical records for optimal screening. Data cited in the "Potential Adverse Effects" and "Accuracy and Reliability as Screening Test" sections are drawn from a large

Table 4.2
Laboratory Screening Tests for Asymptomatic Nonpregnant Persons

Laboratory Screening Test	Intended Target Conditions	Asymptomatic Patients to Screen	Optimal Frequency
		Newborns	
T$_4$/TSH	Congenital hypothyroidism	All newborns, age 1–7 days	Once
Phenylalanine	Phenylketonuria	All newborns, age 1–7 days	Once
		Adolescents and Young Adults	
Papanicolaou smear	Cervical cancer and dysplasia	All women who are sexually active or over age 18	q 1–3 yr
		Adults	
Total cholesterol	High blood cholesterol	Men age 35–65; women age 45–65	Unknown
Fecal occult blood test	Colorectal cancer/polyps	All persons over age 50	q 1 yr
Sigmoidoscopy	Colorectal cancer/polyps	All persons over age 50	Unknown
Papanicolaou smear	Cervical cancer/dysplasia	All women	q 1–3 yr
Mammography	Breast cancer	All women over age 50[a]	q 1–2 yr
		Older Adults	
Fecal occult blood test	Colorectal cancer/polyps	All older adults	q 1 yr
Sigmoidoscopy	Colorectal cancer/polyps	All older adults	Unknown
Papanicolaou smear	Cervical cancer/dysplasia	All healthy women	q 1–3 yr
Mammography	Breast cancer	All healthy women[b]	q 1–2 yr

[a]Many groups recommend beginning screening at age 40 years.

[b]Some groups recommend discontinuing screening at age 70, 75, or 79 years.

body of evidence. The hundreds of studies on which these estimates are based are not cited explicitly in these chapters due to space limitations. The reader interested in the source of these data is referred to other texts that discuss the individual studies in more detail, such as the U.S. Preventive Services Task Force *Guide to Clinical Preventive Services* (2).

As in Chapter 3, the screening tests discussed in this chapter may leave patients with questions or heightened anxiety about their risk of disease.

Table 4.3
Laboratory Screening Tests for Persons with Risk Factors[a]

Laboratory Screening Test	Special Risk Factors	Age Group	Frequency
Hemoglobin/hematocrit	Low birth weight or preterm birth, low socioeconomic status, history of drinking primarily cow's milk	Infants	Once
Hemoglobin electrophoresis	African or Mediterranean descent	Newborns; adolescents and adults of childbearing age	Once
Blood glucose[b]	Obesity, family history of diabetes mellitus, personal history of gestational diabetes	—	Unknown
VDRL/RPR Gonorrhea culture Chlamydial test HIV	Multiple sexual partners, history of sexually transmitted diseases, sexually active adolescent, partner of infected persons. See HIV risk factors (Table 4.4).	—	Unknown
Lead	Housing built before 1960, household members involved with lead-related occupations or hobbies, environmental lead sources in neighborhood, community with high or unknown lead prevalence	12–18 months of age	At least once
Electrocardiogram	Multiple cardiac risk factors, occupation affecting public safety, sedentary person beginning exercise program	Over age 40	Unknown
Otoacoustic emissions/ BAER	See Table 4.6	0–3 months	Once
Mantoux PPD	HIV infection, close contact with persons known or suspected of having TB, medical	—	Once

Table 4.3—*continued*

Laboratory Screening Test	Special Risk Factors	Age Group	Frequency
	condition associated with TB (e.g., chronic renal failure, diabetes mellitus, leukemia, Hodgkin's disease, condition requiring prolonged therapy with corticosteroids, immunosuppressive therapy), abnormal chest radiograph, immigration from high-prevalence country (e.g., most countries in Africa, Asia, and Latin America), medically underserved low-income population, alcoholism or intravenous drug use, residence in long-term institution (e.g., nursing home, correctional facility), work in health care facility (see text)		
Colonoscopy	Hereditary polyposis or nonpolyposis syndrome, ulcerative colitis, prior colonic polyps or cancer	—	Unknown

[a]Recommendations apply only to asymptomatic, nonpregnant persons. Cholesterol screening of children is recommended if their parents or grandparents have a history of premature coronary artery disease or elevated blood cholesterol (see text). The presence of screening tests in this table does not necessarily imply their endorsement by the editors of this book (or by the U.S. Preventive Services Task Force).

[b]Fasting blood glucose is more accurate than random glucose measurement.

To help address these concerns, clinicians may wish to give the patient educational brochures such as those listed in the "Resources" section of this chapter, which can explain the meaning of a normal examination and encourage health behaviors for the primary prevention of the conditions for which they are being screened. Patient education materials for patients in whom screening tests are *abnormal* are listed in Chapter 17 and elsewhere in this book.[c] Screening recommendations in this chapter apply only to

[c]This chapter encourages clinicians to establish reminder systems in the office or clinic to ensure that patients receive recommended screening tests on time and return for repeat screening at the appropriate interval. See Chapter 23 for detailed recommendations on how to design office systems and routines for this purpose, and see Chapter 26 for specific suggestions about manual and automated reminder systems.

asymptomatic persons[d] and therefore assume that the patient lacks clinical evidence of the target condition. Thus, for example, recommendations to limit chlamydia screening to persons with risk factors assume that the patient lacks signs or symptoms of infection. This chapter does not address laboratory tests performed in prenatal screening, occupational screening, preemployment screening, or screening for admission to schools.

SCREENING BLOOD TESTS

Hemoglobin and Hematocrit

Introduction

The complete blood count (CBC), which is often ordered as a routine screening test, can detect anemia, leukocytosis, thrombocytopenia, leukemia, and many other hematologic disorders. Of these, anemia is the only condition with sufficient prevalence for which early detection may be beneficial. Anemia is reported in nearly four million Americans (3). Iron deficiency, the most common cause of anemia in the United States, may be harmful in certain populations and age groups (e.g., young children, pregnant women) and is easily treated with iron supplements. Anemia may also be the first sign of occult diseases, such as colorectal cancer, for which early detection is beneficial. However, no studies have shown that routine screening for low hemoglobin or hematocrit results in improved clinical outcome in children, adults, or pregnant women.

Official Guidelines. The Canadian Task Force on the Periodic Health Examination recommended hemoglobin measurement of infants with low birth weight, low socioeconomic status, Chinese or aboriginal parents, or a history of drinking only cow's milk during the first year of life; it found insufficient evidence to recommend for or against screening in other infants. The U.S. Preventive Services Task Force recommends routine testing for anemia in high-risk infants and pregnant women. The recommendations of the American Academy of Pediatrics are currently under review. The American Academy of Family Physicians recommends measuring hemoglobin and/or hematocrit once during infancy. The U.S. Preventive Services Task Force, American Academy of Family Physicians, U.S. Centers for Disease Control and Prevention, and American College of Physicians do not recommend routine screening for anemia in asymptomatic adolescents and adults. The American College of Physicians recommends routine hemoglobin measurement in women who are recent immigrants from developing countries and in the institutionalized elderly.

---

[d]"Asymptomatic persons" refers to patients who lack signs or symptoms of the target condition, although they may be symptomatic for other reasons. Thus, a woman with ulcerative colitis may be asymptomatic with respect to hyperlipidemia. "Asymptomatic" also excludes persons with a prior history of the target condition, such as a healthy woman with a prior history of breast cancer.

Standard Counseling

All patients should be counseled to eat a healthful diet (see Chapter 8), and menstruating women should specifically be encouraged to eat iron-containing, low-fat foods. Parents should be counseled about healthful diets for their children (see Chapter 8).

Definition of Abnormal Results

In adults, anemia is defined in men as a hemoglobin concentration less than 13 g/dL or a hematocrit of less than 41% and in nonpregnant women as a hemoglobin less than 12 g/dL or a hematocrit of less than 36%. In children, normal values vary by age and sex. The normal hemoglobin is generally above 10.7 g/dL at one month of age, 9.4 g/dL at two months of age, 10.5 g/dL at six months of age, 11.5 g/dL at age two to six, and 13 g/dL at age 12. The normal hematocrit is above 33% at one month of age, 28% at two months of age, 33% at six months of age, 34–36% at age two to six, and 36% thereafter.

What to Do with Abnormal Results

See Table 17.15.

Potential Adverse Effects

Aside from the discomfort of venipuncture or capillary puncture, the principal adverse effect of screening is that patients with abnormal results often require additional blood tests (and, less frequently, imaging studies and invasive tests) to rule out an abnormality or identify its cause. Office or laboratory visits for these tests can incur costs and inconvenience. Patients, and the parents of young patients, can also experience considerable anxiety while awaiting the results. Iron supplements, which are often prescribed for iron deficiency anemia, can have adverse effects and may be prescribed unnecessarily if screening produces false-positive results or detects clinically insignificant iron deficiency or anemia.

Accuracy and Reliability as Screening Test

Capillary blood specimens are often more convenient to obtain than venipuncture specimens, especially in infants and young children, but the tests may be less accurate and reliable. Photometric analysis of microcuvette samples has a coefficient of variation of about 4% in measuring hemoglobin concentration. Automated analysis of the CBC using the Coulter system has a coefficient of variation of 3% or less for red blood cell concentration and 2% or less for hemoglobin concentration;

hemoglobin measurements are generally within 0.1 g/dL of the reference value.

Medical Record Documentation

The date and results of the hemoglobin and/or hematocrit measurement should be placed in the medical record, preferably on a health maintenance flow sheet.

Hemoglobin Electrophoresis

Introduction

Hemoglobin electrophoresis is the principal screening test for hemoglobinopathies, such as sickle cell disease and the thalassemias. Such screening is generally aimed at newborns, for whom early treatment of sickle cell disease has been shown to reduce the incidence of complications, and at adults of childbearing age, for whom genetic counseling can be helpful. Hemoglobinopathies occur primarily in specific racial and ethnic groups (e.g., African Americans and persons of Mediterranean, African, Middle Eastern, Asian, and Hispanic descent). Some experts, however, are concerned that screening targeted to these groups misses patients with sickle cell disease whose racial or ethnic background is not obvious, and have therefore recommended universal screening of all newborns.

Official Guidelines. The U.S. Preventive Services Task Force and Canadian Task Force on the Periodic Health Examination recommend hemoglobin testing of newborns at risk for hemoglobin disorders and offering testing to pregnant at-risk women at their first prenatal visit; the U.S. Preventive Services Task Force found insufficient evidence to determine whether newborn screening should be selective (infants at risk only) or universal. The American Academy of Family Physicians recommends testing high-risk newborns and discussing the test with young adults who have risk factors. In 1993, an expert panel convened by the Agency for Health Care Policy and Research recommended that all newborns should be screened for sickle cell disease, regardless of race or ethnic background. These recommendations were endorsed by the American Academy of Pediatrics, and similar recommendations were issued by a National Institutes of Health consensus development conference. The American College of Obstetricians and Gynecologists recommends testing women of reproductive age who are of Caribbean, Latin American, Asian, Mediterranean, or African descent. Newborn screening for hemoglobinopathies is mandatory in many states.

Definition of Abnormal Result

In patients with sickle cell disease (homozygous SS disease), hemoglobin typically consists of 80–100% hemoglobin S and 2–20% hemoglobin F. In hemoglobin SC disease, it consists of 30–60% hemoglobin S and 2–15%

hemoglobin F. Beta thalassemia is characterized by increased concentrations of hemoglobin A_2 and hemoglobin F.

What to Do with Abnormal Results

See Table 17.16.

Potential Adverse Effects

Aside from the discomfort of venipuncture or heel prick, there is little adverse effect from the test itself; however, screening (if done selectively) and positive results may be associated with stigmatization of the patient. Positive results may affect insurance and job eligibility and may disclose nonpaternity. Genetic counseling may be misunderstood and thereby affect adversely marital and reproductive decisions.

Accuracy and Reliability as Screening Test

The accuracy of hemoglobin electrophoresis depends on the type of test and which hemoglobin disorder is being detected. In most studies of screening for sickle cell disease, the sensitivity and specificity of hemoglobin electrophoresis, isoelectric focusing, and high-performance liquid chromatography are 88–100% and 98–100%, respectively. Accuracy is also potentially affected by red cell transfusion in the past four months, iron deficiency, polycythemia, and age less than three months.

Medical Record Documentation

The date and results of the hemoglobin test should be placed in the medical record, preferably on a health maintenance flow sheet. The clinician should also document the type of hemoglobinopathy and the nature of the counseling the patient or parents received.

Blood Glucose and Chemistry Profiles

Introduction

Multiple chemistry panels, such as the popular Sequential Multiple Analyzer (SMA) tests, can detect a variety of biochemical abnormalities and are often ordered as screening tests when patients undergo routine periodic health examinations. SMA panels typically include over 20 tests (e.g., sodium, potassium, uric acid, transaminases), which can potentially detect hundreds of medical problems. As noted earlier, however, the probability of falsely positive results in healthy persons is, for statistical reasons, quite common: over 60% if more than 20 independent variables are tested at once. These abnormal results (e.g., elevated liver function tests) often force physicians to order additional tests, even though the "abnormality" may be statistical rather than a true clinical disorder.

Of the conditions that can be detected with multiple chemistry panels, diabetes mellitus is the only common condition for which there is some evidence that early detection is beneficial. An estimated 14 million persons in the United States have diabetes mellitus (4). In detecting diabetes, the random glucose measurement that is typically obtained at periodic health examinations is less accurate than the fasting blood glucose or glucose tolerance test, but fasting measurements are sometimes impractical and glucose tolerance testing is costly when used for routine screening. No studies have shown that routine screening for diabetes mellitus results in improved clinical outcome. Studies suggest that glycemic control reduces progression of microvascular complications in persons with type I diabetes mellitus (5), but its effectiveness in persons with type II diabetes, which accounts for 90–95% of all cases, is uncertain.

Official Guidelines. The American Academy of Family Physicians and American College of Obstetricians and Gynecologists recommend periodic measurement of fasting plasma glucose in persons who are obese, have a family history of diabetes mellitus, or have a personal history of gestational diabetes. Although the American College of Physicians does not recommend routine screening for diabetes mellitus in asymptomatic persons, it does recommend selective screening with fasting plasma glucose in high-risk adults (diabetes mellitus in first-degree relative, overweight persons, history of gestational diabetes, member of ethnic group with high prevalence of diabetes mellitus) and screening once in obese adults over age 40 if knowledge of the diagnosis would motivate weight loss. It also recommends screening for gestational diabetes in pregnant women, noting that screening may also be indicated in high-risk women planning to become pregnant. The American Diabetes Association recommends screening high-risk asymptomatic individuals and pregnant women, noting that the fasting plasma glucose test is preferred over random glucose measurement. The Canadian Task Force on the Periodic Health Examination recommends against screening normal-risk nonpregnant adults but considered periodic testing of high-risk persons clinically prudent. The U.S. Preventive Services Task Force found insufficient evidence to recommend for or against screening for diabetes mellitus.

Standard Counseling

Patients should be counseled that the most effective ways to prevent adult-onset diabetes mellitus are exercise (see Chapter 7), a healthful diet (see Chapter 8), and weight management (see Chapter 9).

Definition of Abnormal Results

A random glucose $\geq$ 200 mg/dL or a fasting glucose $\geq$ 140 mg/dL on two occasions is suggestive of diabetes mellitus. The American Diabetes Association recommends further evaluation (oral glucose tolerance testing) of persons with a random plasma glucose level greater than 160 mg/dL.

What to Do with Abnormal Results

See Table 17.11.

Potential Adverse Effects

Aside from the discomfort of venipuncture, the principal adverse effects are that patients with abnormal results must often undergo further testing to rule out or confirm glucose intolerance or diabetes mellitus and can incur inconvenience and costs for office visits. Patients with falsely positive results may experience unnecessary anxiety. False-negative results can allow persons with occult diabetes mellitus to escape detection.

Accuracy and Reliability as Screening Test

A random blood glucose measurement has poor predictive value because there is wide overlap in glucose values among the normal population, persons with glucose intolerance, and those with diabetes mellitus. The reported sensitivity and specificity of a random plasma glucose measurement greater than 140 mg/dL are 45% and 86%, respectively. Fasting blood glucose, glycosylated proteins (e.g., hemoglobin A_1C), and glucose tolerance testing are more sensitive but can be impractical and costly for routine screening. As noted earlier, multiple chemistry panels have a high probability of producing falsely positive results.

Medical Record Documentation

The date and results of the glucose or blood chemistry measurement should be placed in the medical record, preferably on a health maintenance flow sheet.

Total Cholesterol and Lipid Profiles

Introduction

High blood cholesterol is a major risk factor for coronary artery disease, a leading cause of death in the United States. Early detection of high blood cholesterol allows the patient to use dietary fat reduction, exercise, and, if necessary, medication to reduce blood cholesterol to acceptable levels. The evidence that lowering cholesterol reduces the risk of morbidity and mortality from coronary artery disease comes primarily from pharmacologic trials involving middle-aged men with markedly elevated values. The generalizability of these data to children, adolescents, young men, women, and the elderly is controversial; questions about benefit, combined with concerns about the potential harms and costs of screening and treatment, have prompted some groups to discourage widespread screening.

Official Guidelines. The U.S. Preventive Services Task Force recommends periodic measurement of total cholesterol in men ages 35–65 and women ages 45–65 but states that there is insufficient evidence to make a recommendation regarding screening of older adults and younger persons, screening for other lipid abnormalities, or periodic screening if previous values have been normal. Cholesterol screening every 3–5 years is recommended by the American College of Obstetricians and Gynecologists. The Canadian Task Force on the Periodic Health Examination recommended "considering" screening in men ages 30–59 years but found insufficient evidence to recommend for or against the practice. The American College of Physicians recommends measuring total cholesterol in all persons at least once during early adulthood and at intervals of five or more years up to age 70. It recommends measuring LDL-cholesterol, HDL-cholesterol, and triglyceride levels in persons with an elevated total cholesterol. The National Cholesterol Education Program Coordinating Committee, which represents over 35 medical groups and government agencies, recommends that all adults 20 years of age and older undergo measurement of total cholesterol and HDL-cholesterol every five years. More frequent screening is recommended for persons with previously elevated values. The recommendations of the American Academy of Family Physicians are currently under review.

Recommendations to screen children for elevated blood cholesterol were issued in 1991 by an expert panel of the National Cholesterol Education Program. The panel recommended that screening be limited to children whose parents or grandparents developed cardiovascular disease by age 55 or whose parents have had cholesterol measurements of 240 mg/dL or greater. The American Academy of Pediatrics, American Academy of Family Physicians, and American Medical Association have issued similar recommendations. The U.S. Preventive Services Task Force found insufficient evidence to recommend for or against screening of children for hypercholesterolemia.

Standard Counseling

All patients should be advised to eat a healthful diet. Adults and children over two years of age should be counseled to limit their intake of dietary fat to less than 30% of total caloric intake and to limit cholesterol intake to less than 300 mg/day (see Chapter 8).

Definition of Abnormal Results

According to the National Cholesterol Education Program, borderline high blood cholesterol is defined in adults as 200–239 mg/dL and high blood cholesterol is defined as $\geq$ 240 mg/dL. In children and adolescents, the corresponding values are 170–199 mg/dL and $\geq$ 200 mg/dL, respectively. A growing body of evidence suggests the need to consider the ratio of HDL to LDL lipoproteins in interpreting the significance of total cholesterol measurements. LDL-cholesterol is considered elevated if it is $\geq$ 130 mg/dL in children and $\geq$ 160 mg/dL in adults (130–159 mg/dL is considered borderline elevated). HDL-cholesterol is considered low if it is < 35 mg/dL.

What to Do with Abnormal Results

See Table 17.2.

Potential Adverse Effects

Aside from the discomfort of venipuncture, the principal risk of cholesterol screening is unnecessary anxiety and the treatment of inaccurate or clinically insignificant cholesterol elevations. Cholesterol-lowering medications can have a variety of important side effects. Patients incur costs and inconvenience for periodic office visits to monitor lipid values and undergo testing. In children, excessive cholesterol-lowering diets may compromise nutritional requirements for healthy growth and development.

Accuracy and Reliability as Screening Test

A single cholesterol measurement may be misleading because of both laboratory variation (measurement error and variation between laboratories can skew values an average of 3–4%) and biologic variation (in some studies, repeated measurements on the same individual have a standard deviation of 18 mg/dL). Capillary blood specimens and desktop chemical analyzers may be less accurate. Cholesterol measurements should therefore be performed by an accredited laboratory that meets current standards for accuracy and reliability (bias and intralaboratory coefficient of variation less than 3%).

Medical Record Documentation

The date and results of the cholesterol or lipid profile should be placed in the medical record, preferably on a health maintenance flow sheet. Dietary counseling and prescriptions for cholesterol-lowering medications should be documented.

Serologic Tests for Human Immunodeficiency Virus and Syphilis

Introduction

Over 450,000 cases of acquired immunodeficiency syndrome (AIDS) have been reported in the United States and an estimated 0.8–1.2 million persons are infected with human immunodeficiency virus (HIV) (6). About 20,000 new cases of syphilis are reported each year in the United States (7). Early detection and treatment of infection with HIV or syphilis can reduce complications in the infected individual (e.g., rate of disease progression) and can prevent transmission to other members of the population.

Official Guidelines. Concerning HIV, the U.S. Centers for Disease Control and Prevention, American College of Physicians, American Academy of Family Physicians, American Medical Association, U.S. Preventive Services Task Force, and Canadian Task Force on the Periodic Health Examination do not recommend routine HIV screening of all asymptomatic persons but do recommend counseling and testing of persons with selected risk factors for HIV infection. The high-risk groups identified by the U.S. Centers for Disease Control and Prevention are listed in Table 4.4. The American College of Obstetricians and Gynecologists recommends offering testing to all women. HIV testing is currently mandatory for persons entering military service; donors of blood, organs, and tissues; federal prisoners; persons seeking immigration to the United States; and premarital couples in certain states.

Concerning syphilis, the U.S. Centers for Disease Control and Prevention, American College of Physicians, American Academy of Family Physicians, American Academy of Pediatrics, American College of Obstetricians and Gynecologists, American Medical Association, U.S. Preventive Services Task Force, and Canadian Task Force on the Periodic Health Examination recommend screening pregnant women and asymptomatic persons at increased risk of acquiring syphilis. These include sexual partners of known syphilis cases, persons with multiple sexual partners, homosexuals (American College of Physicians), prostitutes (U.S. Preventive Services Task Force, American Academy of Family Physicians), and sexually active adolescents (American Academy of Pediatrics, American Medical Association).

Table 4.4
High Risk Groups to Screen for HIV Infection[a]

Persons with a history of sexually transmitted diseases

Current or prior risk factors: intravenous drug users, homosexual and bisexual men,
hemophiliacs, sexual partners of persons in these categories or of persons with known
HIV infection, prostitutes, persons who received transfusion during 1978–1985

Persons who consider themselves at risk or request the test

Women at increased risk who are of childbearing age or pregnant. Risk categories are:
intravenous drug users; prostitutes; sexual partners of persons who were intravenous
drug users, bisexual, or HIV-infected; women living in communities or born in
countries with high HIV prevalence in women; and blood transfusions during 1978–1985

Patients with tuberculosis

Persons who were either recipients or sources of blood or other body fluids in cases of
accidental body fluid exposure

Health care workers who perform invasive procedures, dentists, and dental assistants

Donors of blood, semen, and organs

Adapted from U.S. Centers for Disease Control. Public Health Service guidelines for counseling and antibody testing to prevent HIV infection and AIDS. MMWR 1987;36:509-515; and Bartlett JG. Recommendations for the medical care of persons with HIV infection, 2nd ed. Baltimore: Critical Care America, 1992.

[a]Applies to asymptomatic persons with respect to HIV infection. HIV testing is also indicated for persons with signs of opportunistic infection or those with systemic symptoms or diagnoses associated with HIV infection or AIDS.

Standard Counseling

See Chapter 13 regarding pretest and posttest counseling for HIV testing. All sexually active patients should be counseled about the importance of maintaining monogamous relationships and of using condoms and spermicides (see Chapter 12). The benefits of abstinence should be emphasized when counseling adolescents. Patients who would benefit from hepatitis B immunization should be urged to receive the complete vaccine series (see Chapter 18). Patients who use intravenous drugs should be counseled about the use of clean needles, other methods to limit transmission of blood-borne diseases, and the need for drug rehabilitation therapy. All patients, especially those being tested for HIV infection, should be advised that a nonreactive test does not rule out recent infection, nor does it mean that they cannot become infected in the future.

Definition of Abnormal Results

Reactive enzyme-linked immunoassay (ELISA) tests for HIV antibody, and reactive Rapid Plasma Reagin (RPR) or Venereal Disease Research Laboratory (VDRL) tests for syphilis, are abnormal. Positive results require confirmatory testing (e.g., Western Blot, treponemal testing) to rule out false-positives.

What to Do with Abnormal Results

See Tables 17.17 and 17.20.

Potential Adverse Effects

Falsely positive results can generate anxiety, particularly for patients tested for HIV infection. Both testing and the disclosure of the results can stigmatize patients, damage personal relationships, affect job and insurance eligibility, and limit participation in social programs. HIV screening without appropriate counseling may leave patients with a false sense of security if the test is nonreactive.

Accuracy and Reliability as Screening Test

HIV testing by ELISA has a reported sensitivity and specificity of about 99%, but falsely positive results are possible. If the prevalence of HIV infection is 1%, an ELISA test with 99% sensitivity and specificity will have a PPV of about 50%, meaning that one false-positive case will be identified for every true case of HIV infection. Thus, a reactive ELISA test is typically repeated and, if the second ELISA test is reactive, a Western blot test is performed. Although the probability of falsely positive Western blot tests following sequential ELISAs is extremely low (about 0.001%), laboratories that do not adhere to quality control standards may have a higher rate of falsely positive or indeterminate results. The clinician should keep these concerns in mind in choosing a laboratory to which to submit the HIV specimen. Falsely negative HIV results can occur if the patient has been infected recently and not seroconverted; the median interval between infection and detectable antibody has been estimated at three months, and 95% of persons convert within six months. In screening for syphilis, the RPR and VDRL have lower sensitivity in primary (59–87%) and tertiary syphilis (70–73%) than in secondary syphilis (close to 100%). Because nontreponemal tests can also produce falsely positive results (specificity of 75–85% in persons with coexisting conditions, almost 100% in others), a treponemal test (e.g., fluorescent treponemal antibody test [FTA]) is ordered to confirm infection.

Medical Record Documentation

The date and results of the tests should be placed in the medical record, preferably on a health maintenance flow sheet. In the case of HIV screening, the physician should specifically document whether pretest and/or posttest counseling were provided. If patients are found to be infected with HIV or syphilis, the physician should describe whether the public health department was notified and whether partner notification or contact tracing was performed by the patient, office, or public health department.

Thyroid Function Tests

Introduction

Thyroid testing of newborns enables early detection of congenital hypothyroidism, a condition that affects one out of every 3600–5000 newborns and is associated with early mental retardation, growth failure, and neurologic disorders (8). These complications can be prevented by early initiation of thyroid hormone supplementation. About 2% of adults in the United States have goiter or other thyroid disorders (3). Thyroid testing of asymptomatic adults is performed to detect occult hypothyroidism and hyperthyroidism in patients unlikely to manifest conspicuous symptoms (e.g., the elderly). No studies have shown, however, that routine thyroid function testing of adults results in improved clinical outcomes.

Official Guidelines. Newborn screening for congenital hypothyroidism before hospital discharge is mandatory in all states and is recommended by most groups, including the U.S. Preventive Services Task Force, Canadian Task Force on the Periodic Health Examination, American Academy of Pediatrics, American Academy of Family Physicians, and

American Thyroid Association. The American Thyroid Association also recommends screening asymptomatic persons with a strong family history of thyroid disease, elderly patients (over age 60), postpartum women, patients with hypercholesterolemia or a prior history of thyroid disease, and patients with autoimmune diseases. The American College of Physicians and U.S. Preventive Services Task Force recommend against routine thyroid function testing of asymptomatic persons, and the Canadian Task Force on the Periodic Health Examination found insufficient evidence to make a recommendation. The recommendations of the American Academy of Family Physicians regarding adult screening are currently under review.

Definition of Abnormal Results

Congenital hypothyroidism is suggested by a T_4 of 6 $\mu g/dL$ or less, especially if combined with an elevated TSH (> 20 $\mu U/dL$). In adults, published normal values for total T_4 (5.0–13.0 $\mu g/dL$), free T_4 (0.7–1.8 ng/dL), total T_3 (80–230 ng/dL), and thyroid stimulating hormone (TSH, 0.4–10.0$\mu U/L$) vary with age and need to be verified with the local laboratory. Sensitive immunoradiometric or chemiluminescent TSH assays are often needed to detect the low TSH levels associated with hyperthyroidism.

What to Do with Abnormal Results

See Table 17.12.

Potential Adverse Effects

Aside from the discomfort associated with venipuncture or heel prick, there is little risk from the test itself. However, additional blood testing is generally required to evaluate abnormal results. In newborns, most abnormal results are falsely positive but parents may experience considerable anxiety until the disorder is ruled out. False-negative results can lead to delays in detecting and treating thyroid disorders.

Accuracy and Reliability as Screening Test

Isolated measurement of T_4 or T_3 can be misleading. Hyperthyroidism can be missed by a normal T_4 in the 5–25% of patients who have T_3 thyrotoxicosis. T_3 and T_4 levels can be spuriously elevated by high concentrations of thyroid hormone-binding proteins, pregnancy, or certain drugs. Medical conditions other than thyroid disease can cause low T_4 and T_3 levels ("euthyroid sick syndrome") or may raise T_4 and TSH levels. Studies have suggested that the PPV of an abnormal T_4, T_3, or free T_4 is 15–26%. The immunoradiometric assay for TSH has a reported sensitivity and specificity of

92–100% and 92–99%, respectively, in detecting hypothyroidism and of 86–95% and 92–95%, respectively, in detecting hyperthyroidism. Thyroid testing of newborns in the first two to six weeks of age has a sensitivity of about 84–89% and a specificity of about 99%, but sensitivity is lower in the first week of life.

Medical Record Documentation

The date and results of thyroid function tests should be placed in the medical record, preferably on a health maintenance flow sheet. In the case of newborn screening, the age of the patient at the time of testing should also be noted.

Phenylketonuria Screening

Introduction

Phenylketonuria is estimated to occur in one out of every 10,000–25,000 births (9). Phenylalanine levels are measured in newborns because dietary restrictions can prevent the severe mental retardation and neurologic and behavioral disorders associated with untreated phenylketonuria.

Official Guidelines.   Routine screening of all newborns for phenylketonuria is mandatory in every state. The American Academy of Family Physicians notes that the test is best performed at 3–6 days of age. The American Academy of Pediatrics recommends that a heel blood specimen be obtained before leaving the nursery and as close as possible to hospital discharge. Premature infants and those being treated for illness should be tested on or near the seventh day. The Academy recommends that infants who are tested before 24 hours of age receive a repeat screening test before the third week of life. Similar recommendations have been issued by the U.S. Preventive Services Task Force and Canadian Task Force on the Periodic Health Examination, but the latter recommends that repeat testing occur at 2–7 days of age.

Definition of Abnormal Results

A phenylalanine concentration of 2 mg/dL or greater is considered abnormal, but classical phenylketonuria requires a value of greater than 20 mg/dL.

What to Do with Abnormal Results

See Table 17.13.

Potential Adverse Effects

There is little risk from the test itself, aside from the discomfort of the heel prick. As explained in more detail later, however, infants with phenylketonuria may escape detection if a test performed in the first 24–48 hours of life is not repeated.

Accuracy and Reliability as Screening Test

Phenylalanine levels in affected infants are usually normal at birth and rise over the first few days of life. Newborns tested early in this period (e.g., newborns discharged within 24 hours of birth), are therefore more likely to have falsely negative results and require repeat testing. Early studies reported that the probability of falsely negative results was 2–31% on the first day, 0.6–2% on the second day, and 0.3% on the third day. Sensitivity may currently be higher due to the introduction of fluorometric assays and a nationwide laboratory proficiency program. The reported specificity of the test is 99.9%.

Medical Record Documentation

The date and results of phenylalanine testing should be placed in the medical record, preferably on a health maintenance flow sheet. The age of the patient at the time of testing should be noted.

Lead and Erythrocyte Protoporphyrin

Introduction

Recent national data suggest that 3% of preschool children in the United States have blood lead levels of 15 μg/dL or greater (10). Lead screening of asymptomatic children is performed because blood lead levels of 10–45 μg/dL rarely produce immediate symptoms or physical findings but may lead to abnormal neurobehavioral development. Children develop elevated lead levels through exposure to lead-containing paint, dust, water, air, and other environmental agents. The Department of Housing and Urban Development estimates that nearly four million homes in the United States with peeling paint or lead dust are inhabited by children under seven years of age. Early detection is thought to be beneficial by prompting the removal of environmental lead sources and, when necessary, the initiation of medical therapy (e.g., chelating agents) before irreversible neurologic damage occurs, but direct evidence that screening achieves these outcomes is currently lacking.

Official Guidelines. The U.S. Preventive Services Task Force recommends measuring the blood lead level at least once, at about 12 months of age, in children at increased risk of lead exposure (or those living in communities in which the prevalence of lead levels ≥ 25 μg/dL is either high or unknown). The American Academy of Pediatrics recommends screening all infants at age 9 to 12 months and, if possible, at about 24 months of age. The U.S. Centers for Disease Control and Prevention recommends that a questionnaire (Table 4.5) be used at each routine office visit to assess the risk status of the child. According to these recommendations, a child at low risk should receive a blood lead test at 12 months of age. If the result is less than 10 μg/dL, the child should be retested annually. If the result is 10–14 μg/dL, the child should be retested every 3–4 months. If two consecutive measurements are less than 10 μg/dL or three are less than 15 μg/dL, testing should be repeated in one year. If the questionnaire indicates that the child is at high risk, screening should begin at six months of age. If the first value is less than 10 μg/dL, testing should be repeated every six months; if two consecutive measurements are less than 10 μg/dL or three are less than 15 μg/dL, testing should be repeated annually. If the value is 10–14 μg/dL, the test should be repeated every 3–4 months. If two consecutive tests are less than 10 μg/dL or three are less than 15 μg/dL, testing can be performed annually. The U.S. Centers for Disease Control and Prevention recommends discontinuing routine screening at age six. The Canadian Task Force on the Periodic Health Examination recommends lead screening only in high-risk children. The recommendations of the American Academy of Family Physicians are currently under review. Universal or selective lead screening is required by law in a number of states.

Standard Counseling

Parents should receive information about the health effects of lead exposure and about common sources of lead in the environment (e.g., lead-based paint chips, soil, drinking water, parental occupations and hobbies, houses built before 1960).

Definition of Abnormal Results

According to the U.S. Centers for Disease Control and Prevention, a blood lead concentration ≥ 10 μg/dL is abnormal. The U.S. Preventive Services Task Force recommends using a threshold level for blood lead of 25 μg/dL. Erythrocyte protoporphyrin (EP) concentration is abnormal if it is greater than 35 μg/dL.

Table 4.5
Lead Screening Questionnaire

Does your child:
1. Live in or regularly visit a house with peeling or chipping paint built before 1960? This could include a day care center, preschool, the home of a baby sitter or a relative, etc.
2. Live in or regularly visit a house built before 1960 with recent, ongoing, or planned renovation or remodeling?
3. Have a brother or sister, housemate, or playmate being followed or treated for lead poisoning (i.e., blood lead ≥ 15 μg/dL)?
4. Live with an adult whose job or hobby involves exposure to lead?
5. Live near an active lead smelter, battery recycling plant, or other industry likely to release lead?

Adapted from Preventing lead poisoning in young children. Atlanta: U.S. Centers for Disease Control and Prevention, 1991.

What to Do with Abnormal Results

See Table 17.14.

Potential Adverse Effects

Aside from the discomfort of venipuncture, the principal risks of lead screening are parental and patient anxiety, the adverse effects of medical treatment, and the economic and familial disruption from activities to control residential lead hazards. Parents also incur costs and inconvenience for follow-up medical appointments for repeat lead testing.

Accuracy and Reliability as Screening Test

Blood lead is more accurate than EP in detecting low lead concentrations, but it is more expensive and may be subject to contamination from environmental lead. False-positive rates of 5–15% have been reported for capillary sampling. There is also significant laboratory variation in blood lead measurements. EP is less expensive and provides a better measure of chronic lead exposure, but it has less than 50% sensitivity in detecting levels below 50 $\mu g/dL$ and can be elevated due to other conditions (e.g., iron deficiency).

Medical Record Documentation

The date and results of lead testing and the type of test (blood lead, EP) should be noted in the medical record, preferably on a health maintenance flow sheet. If administered, the responses to the U.S. Centers for Disease Control and Prevention questionnaire should also be documented.

Office and Clinic Organization for Routine Blood Test Screening

Screening blood tests should be discussed with patients in areas of the office or clinic that permit patients to discuss confidentially their interest in specific tests (e.g., HIV). Reminder systems should be in place to ensure that the clinician receives test results; that patients with abnormal results receive proper follow-up testing, counseling, and treatment; that other affected persons (e.g., sexual contacts of infected patients, children of patients with high blood cholesterol or hemoglobinopathies) receive proper notification, testing, counseling, and treatment; that the public health department is notified of reportable diseases; and that the patient returns for repeat testing at the recommended interval. The office should have access to the performance record and certification status of the laboratories to which specimens are sent.

OTHER LABORATORY SCREENING TESTS

Papanicolaou Smears

Introduction

The Papanicolaou smear is performed regularly to detect cervical dysplasia, carcinoma *in situ,* and invasive carcinoma. An estimated 15,800 cases of cervical cancer were diagnosed and 4800 women died of this cancer in 1995 (11). Observational studies have shown that cervical cancer mortality can be reduced significantly through regular Papanicolaou testing. The optimal frequency for testing is uncertain, with most groups recommending an interval of every one to three years. There are few data to support more frequent screening, such as every six months. Colposcopy screening is discussed in Chapter 21.

Official Guidelines.   The American Cancer Society and American College of Obstetricians and Gynecologists recommend annual Papanicolaou smears for all women who are or have been sexually active, or who have reached age 18. They indicate that the test may be performed "less frequently at the discretion of the physician" after a woman has had three or more consecutive satisfactory normal annual smears. The American Academy of Family Physicians makes similar recommendations but notes that the "less frequent" interval should not exceed 3 years and recommends screening women over age 65 only if they have not had previous documented screening in which smears have been consistently negative. The American College of Physicians recommends that sexually active women undergo Papanicolaou testing every 3 years from age 20 until age 65, or until age 75 if they were not screened in the 10 years before age 66. Screening is recommended every 2 years for women at increased risk. The U.S. Preventive Services Task Force recommends screening at least every 3 years and discontinuing screening at age 65 only if the physician can document previous screening in which smears have been consistently normal. The Canadian Task Force on the Periodic Health Examination recommends annual screening after initiation of sexual activity or age 18 and, following two normal smears, screening every 3 years (or more frequently for high-risk women) until age 69.

Patient Preparation

The Papanicolaou smear is usually obtained during the pelvic examination. Patient preparation involves disrobing from the waist down and donning a gown or drape, lying supine on the examining table, and placing the legs in stirrups. A chaperone may be advisable if the examiner is a man. Papanicolaou testing should not be performed if the patient douched on the day of examination or if she is having moderate or heavy menstrual flow.

Technique

A speculum of appropriate size and shape for the patient's vagina should be lubricated and warmed with warm water; jelly lubricants may interfere with cytological studies. With two fingers placed at the introitus, the examiner should gently press down on the perineum and, with the other hand, slowly and gently introduce the closed speculum over the fingers (Fig. 4.1). The discomfort of pressing on the urethra can be minimized by holding the blades of the speculum obliquely and advancing them along the posterior vaginal wall. Once the speculum enters the vagina, the fingers of the other hand should be removed from the introitus and the blades rotated to a horizontal position. When the speculum is fully advanced, the blades of the speculum should be opened, and the speculum should be maneuvered until the cervix comes into view.

The examiner should inspect the cervix and external os for ulcerations, nodules, masses, bleeding, leukoplakia, or discharge. It is of special importance to the Papanicolaou test to visualize the squamocolumnar junction, the region from which 90–95% of cervical cancers arise. Current evidence is equivocal as to whether the detection of cervical cancer is increased by sampling endocervical cells, but many laboratories consider smears inadequate if these cells are absent. The squamocolumnar junction or transformation zone, which is located on the ectocervix or in the endocervical canal, often migrates inward with age, so that visualization in older women can be difficult. Any discharge obscuring the view of the cervix should be wiped away.

To maximize the likelihood of obtaining endocervical cells from the squamocolumnar junction, a complete Papanicolaou test requires two specimens, one from the endocervical canal and one from the ectocervix. The endocervical sample is obtained by inserting an endocervical brush or moistened cotton-tipped applicator into the canal and rotating it between the fingers. The ectocervical specimen is typically obtained with a wooden Ayre spatula. The longer end of the spatula is placed in the os, and the spatula is rotated in a circular fashion so that a full scraping of the squamocolumnar junction is obtained. Other devices for simultaneous sampling of endocervical and ectocervical cells (e.g., Cervex-Brush) have been less carefully evaluated. The specimens should be spread on one or more glass microscope slides and fixed immediately with either 95% ether-alcohol or a spray fixative. If an endocervical brush is used, the sample is obtained by rolling the brush across the slide. The patient should be told that the speculum will be removed; the speculum should be returned to the oblique angle before being gently withdrawn. Details about the patient's history (age, last menstrual period, type of contraception, previous cervical diagnoses or treatment) and relevant physical findings should be noted for the cytopathologist on the laboratory requisition form.

Standard Counseling

The patient should be advised to return for repeat screening at the recommended interval and should be encouraged to reduce risks of acquiring sexually transmitted diseases (see Chapter 12).

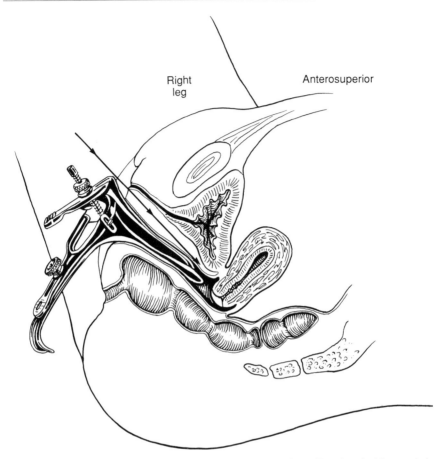

Figure 4.1. Introduction of the speculum through the introitus. (Reprinted with permission from Willms JL, Schneiderman H, Algranati DS, eds. Physical diagnosis: bedside evaluation of diagnosis and function. Baltimore: Williams & Wilkins, 1994:574–575.)

Definition of Abnormal Results

The Papanicolaou smear may suggest cancer or its precursors if the laboratory reports squamous intraepithelial lesions, atypia, dysplasia, cervical intraepithelial neoplasia, squamous cell carcinoma, or adenocarcinoma. The presence of human papilloma virus is also abnormal; several oncogenic forms (e.g., types 16 and 18) increase the risk of cervical cancer, but the natural history of their progression to cancer is poorly understood. Cervical samples that are identified by the laboratory as inadequate (e.g., due to absence of endocervical cells) may necessitate repeat testing, but there is little evidence regarding how many attempts should be made to obtain ad-

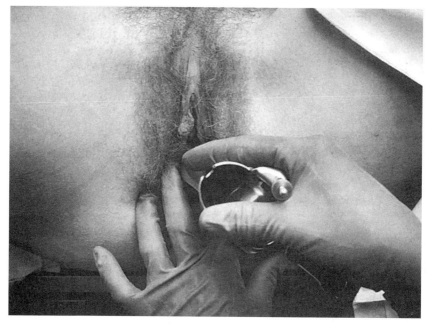

Figure 4.1. *continued.*

equate specimens or whether the effort will result in improved cancer detection.

What to Do with Abnormal Results

See Table 17.6.

Potential Adverse Effects

The pelvic examination and Papanicolaou smear can be both embarrassing and uncomfortable. Falsely positive results can generate unnecessary anxiety and follow-up testing, including colposcopy, endocervical curettage, and other procedures. Women incur costs and inconvenience for follow-up cervical examinations. Falsely negative results may allow women with preventable cancers to escape detection.

Accuracy and Reliability as Screening Test

In most studies, the Papanicolaou smear has a sensitivity of 20–45% and a specificity of 90–99%. Accuracy and reliability are affected by the skill of the examiner in obtaining a good specimen (e.g., obtaining endocervical cells) and of the cytopathologist in reviewing the smears. Physicians should submit Papanicolaou smears to cytopathology laboratories certified by the College of American Pathologists or the American Society of Cytologists.

Office and Clinic Organization for Routine Screening

The routine performance of cervical cancer screening requires examination rooms with comfortable examination tables equipped with stirrups, good lighting, specula of varying sizes and shapes (including both Graves and Pedersen specula), specimen collection equipment (e.g., spatulas, cytobrushes, cotton swabs), slides, fixatives, gloves, lubricant, and gowns or other coverings. Reminder systems should be in place to ensure that the physician receives a report from the cytopathologist, that patients return for repeat screening at the recommended interval, and that women with abnormal results receive appropriate follow-up and treatment.

Medical Record Documentation

The date and results of the Papanicolaou smear should be placed in the medical record, preferably on a health maintenance flow sheet. The physician should describe the appearance of the cervix and whether menstruation was noted. For future reference, it may be helpful to note in the medical record whether the uterus is retroverted and if a special speculum was required to visualize the cervix. The presence of cellular atypia, dysplasia, or carcinoma on the smear should be carefully documented, along with plans for follow-up and repeat testing.

Endocervical and Urethral Screening for Gonorrhea and Chlamydia

Introduction

Gonorrhea and chlamydial infections are among the most common of the sexually transmitted diseases, with over five million cases of infection reported annually in the United States (7, 12). These infections can cause urethritis and epididymitis in men and cervicitis, pelvic inflammatory disease, and infertility in women. Gonorrhea can also cause pharyngitis, proctitis, and other systemic illnesses. Infected persons are often asymptomatic or have nonspecific symptoms, which can delay diagnosis and treatment and increase the likelihood of transmitting the organisms to sexual contacts. Screening of high-risk groups has been recommended for early detection of such cases, partner notification, and prompt initiation of antibiotic therapy.

Official Guidelines.   The American Academy of Family Physicians, American Academy of Pediatrics, U.S. Centers for Disease Control and Prevention, American College of Obstetricians and Gynecologists, U.S. Preventive Services Task Force, and Canadian Task Force on the Periodic Health Examination recommend screening asymptomatic persons with specific risk factors. These include persons attending sexually transmitted disease, family planning, or adolescent health clinics; persons with multiple sexual partners; sexually active adolescents; prostitutes; persons with a history of sexually transmitted diseases; and recent partners of persons with gonorrhea or chlamydial infection. The U.S. Preventive Services Task Force made this recommendation only for women, finding insufficient evidence to make a recommendation for screening men. The American College of Physicians has not considered chlamydia screening but recommends gonorrhea culture in high-risk adults.

Patient Preparation

In women, the specimen is usually obtained during the pelvic examination. The patient must disrobe from the waist down, put on a gown or drape, lie supine on the examining table, and place the legs in stirrups. Men must lower their trousers and briefs and should sit or lie supine to prevent falls from vasovagal reactions. The patient should be cautioned that the procedure may be uncomfortable. A chaperone may be advisable if the patient is the opposite sex of the examiner.

Technique

For gonorrhea screening, a culture, nucleic acid probe, or Gram's-stain specimen is obtained from the urethra in men and from the endocervical canal in women. The specimen is obtained in men by advancing the culture swab about two to three centimeters into the urethra (or by sampling expressed urethral exudate). The specimen is obtained in women by inserting and rotating the swab or cytology brush in the endocervical canal. For culture specimens, the swab is streaked in a Z-pattern on a Thayer-Martin (chocolate agar) or Martin-Lewis plate. An enzymatic immunoassay test for gonorrhea is also available.

Both culture and nonculture tests (e.g., enzyme-linked immunoassay) are used for chlamydia screening, although the latter are generally more cost-effective for routine screening. Specimens can be obtained from the endocervix or urethra using a swab or cytology brush in the manner described for gonorrhea screening. Screening for chlamydia can be detected noninvasively in men by dipstick urinalysis of leukocyte esterase levels, but the test lacks accuracy (see below). For both gonorrhea and chlamydia screening, the clinician should refer to the manufacturer's instructions and consult with the medical laboratory to determine the proper type of swab, collection technique, and transport/culture medium. A nucleic acid probe that tests for both gonorrhea and chlamydia is available, and the use of polymerase chain reaction techniques is being explored.

Standard Counseling

All sexually active patients should be counseled to maintain monogamous relationships and should receive instructions on the correct use of condoms and spermicides (see Chapter 12). Women at increased risk should receive information about the early signs and symptoms of pelvic inflammatory disease. Adolescents should be advised that abstinence from sexual intercourse is the most effective preventive strategy.

What to Do with Abnormal Results

See Tables 17.18 and 17.19.

Potential Adverse Effects

Specimen collection can be uncomfortable, especially when obtained from the urethra, and can cause vasovagal reactions. False-positive results can cause unnecessary anxiety, concerns about infidelity, and unnecessary treatment. False-negative results can result in treatment delays and inadvertent transmission to other sexual contacts.

Accuracy and Reliability as Screening Test

The sensitivity and specificity of Gram's stain in detecting gonorrhea is about 50–70% and 95–100%, respectively. Gonorrhea culture has a reported sensitivity of about 80–95% and a specificity of 100%. The enzyme immunoassay has a sensitivity and specificity of 95% or more in men and 60–100% and 70–98% in women, respectively. The reported sensitivity and specificity of DNA hybridization is 95–97% and 99–100%, respectively. Douching within the previous 24 hours and vaginal lubricants or disinfectants may limit growth of gonorrhea.

In screening for chlamydia, the direct fluorescent antibody test has a sensitivity and specificity of 70–100% and 85–98%, respectively, in women. The enzymatic immunoassay has a reported sensitivity of 49–69% in men (urethra) and about 70–100% in women, and a specificity of about 95% in men and 85–98% in women. Office-based test kits, which can provide results in 10–30 minutes and are based on enzymatic immunoassay technology, have been less extensively evaluated and their accuracy is less certain. The reported sensitivity and specificity of the nucleic acid probe is 93–95% and 98–100%, respectively in men and women. Dipstick urinalysis for leukocyte esterase has a sensitivity and specificity of 70–80% and 70–85%, respectively, in detecting chlamydia in men and a PPV of 16% in a population with a prevalence of 7%. Cell culture for chlamydia is accurate (sensitivity and specificity of 75–90% and 100%, respectively) but requires special specimen preparation, storage, and handling and requires 2–6 days for results.

Office and Clinic Organization for Routine Screening

Offices and clinics participating in routine screening should be properly stocked with appropriate collection instruments (e.g., Dacron swabs), culture and transport media, and storage facilities (e.g., 3–10% CO_2 environment for gonorrhea cultures, freezer for some chlamydia transport media). Physicians and staff involved with the collection, plating, and handling of specimens should be trained in proper technique, and offices that send specimens to outside laboratories should maintain transport conditions that protect the quality of the specimen. Reminder systems should be in place to ensure that the physician receives the test results; that infected patients receive appropriate antibiotic therapy; that sexual contacts of infected patients are notified, tested, and treated; and that the public health department is notified of the case.

Medical Record Documentation

The date and results of the tests should be placed in the medical record, preferably on a health maintenance flow sheet. If patients are infected, the physician should describe whether partner notification or contact tracing was performed by the patient, office, or public health department. The physician should also document whether the public health department was notified of the case.

Fecal Occult Blood Test

Introduction

Fecal occult blood testing (FOBT) is a principal screening test for the early detection of colorectal cancers and adenomatous polyps. Colorectal cancer accounted for an estimated 55,000 deaths in the United States in 1995 (1). The FOBT can also be positive due to bleeding from lesions above the colon (e.g., peptic ulcer disease), nonmalignant colorectal lesions (e.g., hemorrhoids), and foods eaten by the patient. For many years, the effectiveness of FOBT was questioned, but randomized controlled trials have recently provided evidence of 33% lower colorectal cancer mortality in persons who undergo annual FOBT screening followed by colonoscopy for positive results. It is currently unclear to what extent the benefits seen in these studies are attributable to FOBT or to chance selection of persons for colonoscopic examination.

Official Guidelines. The American Cancer Society, American College of Physicians, U.S. Preventive Services Task Force, American College of Obstetricians and Gynecologists, American Gastroenterological Association, and American Society for Gastrointestinal Endoscopy recommend that all persons over age 50 undergo annual FOBT. The American College of Physicians recommends that annual FOBT begin at age 40 for persons with familial polyposis, inflammatory bowel disease, or a history of colon cancer in a first-degree relative. Revised recommendations of the American College of Physicians are currently in development. The Canadian Task Force on the Periodic Health Examination concluded that there is insufficient evidence to recommend for or against FOBT. The recommendations of the American Academy of Family Physicians are currently under review.

Technique

The FOBT can be performed in the examining room as part of the digital rectal examination (see Chapter 3), but it is considered less accurate (due to the single specimen, inadequate dietary preparation, and rectal trauma) than when specimens are obtained at home by the patient. Moreover, the studies that have demonstrated reduced mortality by performing FOBT have involved home testing. In home testing, patients are generally given three cards impregnated with guaiac (or other chemicals that detect peroxidase activity) and are asked to collect two specimens from three separate consecutive stool samples. The patient is given instructions to avoid eating red meat (beef, lamb, including processed meats and liver), fish, uncooked fruits and vegetables (especially melons, radishes, turnips, and horseradish), foods or supplements containing large amounts of vitamin C, nonsteroidal antiinflammatory agents, corticosteroids, and other medications that can cause gastritis during the week before the specimens are obtained. Evidence regarding the need for these restrictions is limited. Menstruating women and patients with active bleeding from rectal disorders (e.g., hemorrhoids) should postpone specimen collection until three days after the bleeding has ended. The cards are then mailed or delivered to the clinician's office.

When the slides are received, a drop of developer fluid is applied to the specimens, with blue discoloration representing an abnormal result. Rehydration of the dried specimens increases sensitivity at the expense of specificity, thereby increasing the likelihood of false-positive results. To date, however, the only study that has demonstrated a statistically significant reduction in colorectal cancer mortality from FOBT screening primarily used rehydrated slides.

Standard Counseling

The patient should be reminded to return for repeat screening at the recommended interval, to undergo sigmoidoscopy screening (if recommended by the physician), and to contact the physician if blood is seen in the stool.

Patients can also be advised that reducing dietary fat and/or increasing dietary fiber intake may reduce the risk of developing colon cancer.

What to Do with Abnormal Results

See Table 17.5.

Potential Adverse Effects

The FOBT can be distasteful and embarrassing and, when accompanied by the digital rectal examination, can be uncomfortable. Falsely positive results may generate anxiety and often require follow-up tests (e.g., colonoscopy, barium enema) with a greater likelihood of discomfort and complications. In some studies, one-third of persons undergoing FOBT received colonoscopy. Repeat office visits for these procedures may also incur costs and inconvenience. Falsely negative results may cause patients with disease to escape detection.

Accuracy and Reliability as Screening Test

The sensitivity and specificity of FOBT in clinical trials are 26–92% and 90–99%, respectively. Rehydration increases sensitivity at the expense of specificity. In healthy persons over age 50, the reported PPV of FOBT for cancer is 2–11%, or a ratio of 8–49 falsely positive results for each true case detected. The reported PPV for adenomas is 20–30%. Quantitative porphyrin tests may be more sensitive and specific than guaiac-based tests but have not undergone adequate evaluation of effectiveness.

Office and Clinic Organization for Routine Screening

Offices and clinics that encourage home FOBT should be equipped with self-addressed stool card packets that can be given to patients. In addition to three stool cards and a collection instrument (e.g., wooden spatula), the packet should include clearly written instructions on dietary restrictions and on how to collect the specimens. Special arrangements should be available for patients who do not speak English or who will have difficulty understanding the instructions. The envelopes used to mail the specimens must be approved by the U.S. Postal Service. Reminder systems should be in place to ensure that the packets are mailed or returned to the office, that patients return for repeat FOBT at recommended intervals, and that patients with positive results receive appropriate follow-up and treatment. Office systems should be in place to facilitate rapid processing of FOBT cards once received. See the discussion of digital rectal examination in Chapter 3 for FOBT requirements during that procedure.

Medical Record Documentation

The date and results of the FOBT should be placed in the medical record, preferably on a health maintenance flow sheet. The clinician should note whether the FOBT was a single test obtained during the digital rectal examination or three consecutive specimens obtained at home. The record should indicate whether specimens were rehydrated. The follow-up plan for abnormal results and for retesting should appear in the record.

Sigmoidoscopy

Introduction

Sigmoidoscopy is a principal screening test for detecting adenomatous polyps and colorectal cancer. Flexible sigmoidoscopes measuring 60–65 cm in length can inspect the distal third of the colon, the region in which colorectal malignancies are most likely to occur. Nonetheless, higher lesions (which have occurred more frequently in recent years) are not detectable by sigmoidoscopy, flat malignancies within reach of the sigmoidoscope can be missed, and the procedure is both costly and uncomfortable. For many years, the appropriateness of sigmoidoscopy has been questioned, with some groups recommending other forms of screening (e.g., barium enema, colonoscopy, FOBT) or no screening until better evidence of benefit became available. Recent case-control studies have suggested, however, that regular sigmoidoscopy screening significantly reduces the risk of dying from colorectal cancer.

Official Guidelines. The American Cancer Society, American College of Physicians, U.S. Preventive Services Task Force, American College of Obstetricians and Gynecologists, American Gastroenterological Association, and American Society for Gastrointestinal Endoscopy recommend that all persons over age 50 receive sigmoidoscopy screening (most groups recommend repeating the test every 3–5 years). The American College of Physicians supports the use of air-contrast barium enemas every 5 years as an alternative to sigmoidoscopy in certain circumstances. The American College of Radiology also recommends barium enema as an equivalent alternative to sigmoidoscopy but considers an interval of every 3–5 years appropriate. The American College of Physicians recommends that persons over age 40 with familial polyposis, inflammatory bowel disease, or a history of colon cancer in a first-degree relative should be screened with air-contrast barium enema or colonoscopy every 3–5 years. Similar recommendations for high-risk groups have been issued by other organizations, including the U.S. Preventive Services Task Force, although groups differ on whether colonoscopy screening should begin in early life for persons with hereditary polyposis and on the proper frequency for screening. The Canadian Task Force on the Periodic Health Examination concluded that there was insufficient evidence to recommend for or against sigmoidoscopy screening. The recommendations of the American Academy of Family Physicians are currently under review, and the recommendations of the American College of Physicians are currently being revised.

Patient Preparation

The patient should provide informed consent to the procedure after being advised of the potential benefits and risks. Preparation begins on the evening before the procedure, in which the bowel is evacuated. A variety of regimens are used, typically involving some combination of magnesium citrate, enemas, and fasting after midnight. Sedatives may be given to patients on the day of the procedure to reduce anxiety. Antibiotics are given to patients with prosthetic heart valves, congenital cardiac malformations, mitral valve prolapse with insufficiency, or other conditions requiring endocarditis prophylaxis. Before the examination, the patient dresses in a gown and lies in a lateral recumbent position with the lower leg extended and the upper leg flexed. Sigmoidoscopy is typically preceded by a digital rectal examination (see Chapter 3) and anoscopy.

Technique

The technique for performing flexible fiberoptic sigmoidoscopy, which is learned through supervised training and practical experience, is beyond the scope of this chapter. In brief, the procedure involves the gentle insertion of the sigmoidoscope tip through the anus and prompt, gentle advancement into the sigmoid colon. Careful inspection of the colonic mucosa, either through the eyepiece or a television monitor, typically occurs when the sigmoidoscope is slowly withdrawn. Advancement of the sigmoidoscope and the negotiation of sharp turns in the colon, particularly the sigmoid curve located 18–20 cm from the anus, can require manipulative techniques such as *torquing* (rotating the sigmoidoscope on its axis), *tip deflection* (using the steering nobs to bend the tip), *dithering* (back and forth movement of the sigmoidoscope shaft), *slide-by* (advancement without full view of the lumen but with the view of mucosa sliding by the tip of the scope), and the use of air insufflation, suction, and irrigation to achieve better visualization.

Colonic spasm, poor bowel preparation, and patient discomfort may limit the completeness of the examination. Techniques to limit patient discomfort, mucosal trauma, and the risk of perforation include maintaining visualization of the lumen, stopping advancement when *redout* (loss of view due to impaction of the tip against the mucosa) or coiling of the endoscope occurs, and limiting insufflation. As the sigmoidoscope is withdrawn, the examiner uses torquing and manipulation of the steering wheels to obtain a careful 360° view of the surrounding mucosa. The position of lesions is noted in terms of their distance in centimeters from the anus. Suspicious lesions are biopsied using forceps inserted through the sigmoidoscope shaft, and their appearance and location is documented for future reference.

Standard Counseling

The patient should be advised of potential symptoms that may be experienced following the procedure (e.g., flatus, cramps). The patient should be reminded to obtain repeat screening (including FOBT) at the recommended interval and to contact the physician if blood is noted in the stool. The patient may also be advised of the possible benefits of lowering dietary fat intake and/or increasing dietary fiber intake in preventing colon cancer.

Definition of Abnormal Results

Large or adenomatous polyps, masses, diverticula, and areas of inflammation or bleeding are considered abnormal.

What to Do with Abnormal Results

See Table 17.5.

Potential Adverse Effects

A serious complication of sigmoidoscopy is perforation, which occurs in about one out of 1,000–10,000 examinations, and bleeding from biopsy sites or mucosal injuries. Transmission of infectious diseases is also possible. Sigmoidoscopy may be inappropriate or need reconsideration in patients with severe anal strictures or fissures, inadequate bowel preparation, recent pelvic or bowel surgery, severe inflammatory bowel disease, toxic megacolon, acute diverticulitis, or immune deficiency, but many of these conditions are unlikely in asymptomatic patients undergoing screening. Falsely positive results are uncommon with sigmoidoscopy, but detected polyps, even if adenomatous, may not be destined to progress to cancer. Patients can incur costs, inconvenience, discomfort, and complications for the removal of these growths and for subsequent surveillance. Falsely negative results can occur if polyps or cancers are difficult to see or are located beyond the reach of the sigmoidoscope.

Accuracy and Reliability as Screening Test

The sensitivity of sigmoidoscopy depends on the length of the instrument. The rigid sigmoidoscope, which has an average depth of insertion of 20 cm, can detect only about 25–30% of cancers and is rarely used for screening. The 35 cm flexible sigmoidoscope can visualize about 50–55% of the sigmoid colon. The 60 cm and 65 cm flexible sigmoidoscopes can reach the splenic flexure in 80% of examinations and thus can detect 40–65% of colorectal cancers. The specificity of sigmoidoscopy in detecting polyps approaches 100%, but many of these will be benign. Although adenomatous polyps are considered premalignant lesions, only a small subset of these actually progress to cancer.

Office and Clinic Organization for Routine Screening

Offices and clinics that perform sigmoidoscopy require examination rooms outfitted with a padded and adjustable examination table, a bathroom, good lighting, and certain utilities (e.g., water and suction lines). The office should also be stocked with bowel preparation kits (or standard prescriptions for the regimen), protective clothing to maintain universal precautions, an anoscope, and lubricants. Systems should be established and staff should be fully trained for proper maintenance and cleaning of the sigmoidoscope. Reminder and referral systems should also be in place to ensure that patients with abnormal results receive appropriate follow-up (e.g., colonoscopy, barium enema) and that patients return for repeat screening at recommended intervals.

Medical Record Documentation

The date and results of the sigmoidoscopy examination should be placed in the medical record, preferably on a health maintenance flow sheet. The appearance and location of polyps, diverticula, areas of inflammation, or other abnormalities should be carefully described. If equipment is available, a videotape recording of abnormal findings should be prepared. The medical record should also indicate the type and length of the sigmoidoscope, the type and adequacy of the bowel preparation and medications, depth of insertion, difficulties in advancement or visualization, reason for stopping, and discomfort or complications experienced by the patient. The record should specify whether biopsies were obtained and the plans for follow-up and repeat testing.

Mammography

Introduction

Mammography is a principal screening test for breast cancer, which accounted for an estimated 46,200 deaths in the United States in 1995 (11). A series of randomized controlled trials over the past three decades has shown that women age 50–69 who receive mammography screening every 1–2 years have a 20–50% (average of about one-third) lower risk of death from breast cancer than unscreened women (13). The effectiveness of mammography screening in women age 40–49 is less clear, since no clinical trials have demonstrated a statistically significant benefit for women in this age group. A national survey in 1990 indicated that only 40–60% of women over age 50 reported having had a mammogram within the last 3 years and that over 50% of poor women in this age group had never had a mammogram.

Official Guidelines. The American College of Physicians, American Academy of Family Physicians, U.S. Preventive Services Task Force, and Canadian Task Force on the Periodic Health Examination recommend annual mammography beginning at age 50 (the interval recommended by the U.S. Preventive Services Task Force is every 1–2 years). Some of these groups suggest earlier screening for women at increased risk of breast cancer (e.g., first-degree relative with breast cancer), although supporting evidence is lacking. The American Cancer Society, American Medical Association, American College of Radiology, American College of Obstetricians and Gynecologists, and eight other organizations recommend that all women age 40–49 receive mammography every 1–2 years, followed by annual screening at age 50 and thereafter. In 1993, the National Cancer Institute concluded that there was insufficient evidence that screening mammography reduced mortality in women age 40–49 but did not issue a practice guideline on the subject.

Technique

Radiographic methods for performing mammography are the domain of the radiologist and are not discussed here. The role of the primary care clinician in providing mammographic screening is to identify women who are due for screening, provide a proper requisition, refer patients to accredited mammographic facilities, verify that the patient obtains the study, and ensure proper interpretation and follow-up of results. In placing the requisition, the referring physician should realize that a screening mammogram typically includes only oblique and craniocaudal views. Magnification views, spot compression films, and other special imaging techniques may be needed to evaluate abnormal screening studies and for women with palpable masses, a previous history of breast cancer, or breast augmentation. Patients should only be referred to facilities that use dedicated mammography equipment. Facilities certified by the American College of Radiology are evaluated in terms of facility operations, personnel, equipment, and radiation exposure. To find a certified mammogram facility, call 800-4-CANCER. Interpretation of results is the specialty of the radiologist, but the primary care physician should also look for malignant radiographic features and consider factors that can produce false-negative results (e.g., high breast density in young women, breast implants) when interpreting the mammogram report.

Standard Counseling

Patients should be reminded to wear two-piece clothing and to not apply topical agents (e.g., deodorants) to the breasts on the day of the study. See

Chapter 20 regarding breast self-examination. The patient should be advised to contact the physician if she detects a breast lump, tenderness, or another abnormality, even if her mammogram is negative. The importance of regular breast cancer screening should be emphasized, and the patient should receive specific instructions about when to return for the next mammogram.

Definition of Abnormal Results

Radiographic features associated with malignancy include irregular margins, spiculations, and clustered microcalcifications. Indirect radiographic signs can include localized distortion of breast architecture, developing neodensities, asymmetric breast tissue, and single dilated ducts.

What to Do with Abnormal Results

See Table 17.4.

Potential Adverse Effects

Patients can experience discomfort from breast compression during imaging, and it is therefore preferable that they not obtain the study during menstruation. Risks from radiation exposure are minimal when modern, dedicated equipment is used. Average radiation exposure to each breast for two views is 0.1–0.5 rad (chest, abdominal, and lumbar spine radiographs typically deliver a dose of about 0.01–0.03, 0.5, and 0.8–1.0 rad, respectively). Falsely positive results can generate significant anxiety and may require the discomfort and anxiety of tissue biopsy to confirm the error. Costs and inconvenience are also incurred to undergo these procedures. Falsely negative results may allow women with breast cancer to escape detection.

Accuracy and Reliability as Screening Test

The reported sensitivity and specificity of mammography are 70–85% and 83–99%, respectively. Sensitivity in women age 40–49 is about 10–15% lower, and image quality is even poorer in women under age 40 due to increased tissue density. Breast implants may obscure portions of the breast and alter surrounding tissue architecture. Finally, the accuracy and reliability of the test depend greatly on the quality of the equipment, radiology technicians, views taken, and the interpretative skills of the radiologist.

Office and Clinic Organization for Routine Screening

The office or clinic should maintain a complete list of accredited mammographic facilities in the community, including high-quality facilities that will accept low-income or uninsured patients or that provide low-cost mammograms. Reminder systems should be in place to ensure that women return for repeat screening at recommended intervals and that women with abnormal results receive appropriate follow-up and treatment.

Medical Record Documentation

The date and results of the mammogram should be placed in the medical record, preferably on a health maintenance flow sheet. Abnormal results should be fully described, along with plans for follow-up and repeat testing.

Electrocardiography

Introduction

Over 19 million resting electrocardiograms are ordered or provided in doctors' offices each year in the United States (1). Electrocardiography can detect cardiac, pulmonary, and pericardial diseases, but the probability of clinically meaningful abnormal results is extremely low in asymptomatic persons. Asymptomatic cardiac ischemia is an electrocardiographically detectable condition for which early detection might be of theoretical benefit, but resting electrocardiography is a poor screening test for this condition. The false-positive rate, which is high in asymptomatic persons, may be reduced by performing stress or ambulatory electrocardiography, thallium scintigraphy, or echocardiography, but these modalities are too expensive to be considered for routine screening of asymptomatic persons. Moreover, there is currently little direct evidence that early detection of asymptomatic coronary artery disease results in improved outcome.

Official Guidelines. The U.S. Preventive Services Task Force and American College of Physicians recommend against performing routine resting electrocardiograms on asymptomatic patients. The U.S. Preventive Services Task Force indicated that it may be clinically prudent to perform screening electrocardiograms in patients at increased risk of coronary artery disease, and similar recommendations have been issued by the American Academy of Family Physicians. The American Heart Association and American College of Cardiology concluded that routine electrocardiography is of little or no usefulness in asymptomatic persons less than age 40 and with no risk factors but that a baseline tracing is useful in asymptomatic persons over age 40 and persons in special occupations that require high cardiovascular performance or that affect public safety. They recommend follow-up electrocardiograms (at unspecified intervals) for asymptomatic persons over age 40.

Technique

Methods for performing and interpreting electrocardiography are beyond the scope of this chapter. In brief, a 12-lead electrocardiogram is obtained by recording the tracing through six axial leads (I, II, III, aVR, aVL, aVF) and six precordial leads (V_{1-6}). As noted earlier, the screening electrocardiogram can detect arrhythmias, chamber enlargement, and a variety of other conditions. Asymptomatic coronary artery disease, the condition for which screening electrocardiograms are generally recommended, is often reflected in ST-segment and T-wave abnormalities and evidence of old, previously unrecognized myocardial infarctions. Other electrocardiographic findings (e.g., left ventricular hypertrophy, ectopy, conduction disorders) can also reflect coronary artery disease. In asymptomatic persons, the vast majority of these abnormalities reflect no pathology and are falsely positive. Exercise stress testing and radionuclide imaging, which have higher PPV, are often performed to evaluate resting electrocardiograms (or medical histories) suggestive of coronary artery disease, but they are inappropriate for routine screening.

Standard Counseling

Patients should be advised to reduce cardiac risk factors by stopping smoking (see Chapter 6), exercising regularly (see Chapter 7), reducing dietary intake of fat and cholesterol (see Chapter 8), and maintaining a healthy weight (see Chapter 9).

What to Do with Abnormal Results

See Table 17.3.

Potential Adverse Effects

There is no risk from electrocardiography itself, but falsely positive results may generate significant anxiety and follow-up tests, some of which are potentially harmful (e.g., coronary angiography). Costs and inconvenience are also incurred for appointments to obtain these tests.

Accuracy and Reliability as Screening Test

Over a 30-year follow-up period, studies have shown that coronary artery disease develops in only 3–15% of persons with resting electrocardiographic abnormalities. Moreover, between one-third and one-half of persons with angiographically normal coronary arteries have Q-waves, T-wave inversion, or ST-segment changes on resting electrocardiograms. Exercise electrocardiograms are more sensitive than resting electrocardiograms but they also have suboptimal performance as screening tests. In asymptomatic middle-aged men with abnormal exercise stress testing, the probability of significant stenosis on coronary angiography is 30–43%.

Office and Clinic Organization for Routine Screening

The office should be equipped with well-maintained electrocardiogram recorders. Staff who perform electrocardiograms should be properly trained in lead placement and operation of the machine. Reminder systems should be in place to ensure that patients with abnormal results receive appropriate follow-up and treatment.

Medical Record Documentation

A copy of the electrocardiogram should be dated and placed with its interpretation in the medical record. The results should be noted on a health maintenance flow sheet.

Audiometry and Newborn Hearing Screening

Introduction

Audiometry is used to detect hearing impairment, primarily in children, who are unlikely to complain of this problem and who may suffer from secondary language disorders and poor school performance. About 0.1–0.6% of newborns and nearly one million children and adolescents are believed to be hearing impaired (14). No studies have shown conclusively that routine hearing screening improves language development or school performance or that screening newborns before hospital discharge can detect most of these cases, but many hearing specialists believe that detection and treatment of hearing impairment before the age of 6 months can reduce the probability of speech and language disorders. Hearing screening of infants cannot be performed by audiometry and typically requires measurement of brainstem auditory evoked responses or otoacoustic emissions. Audiometry screening is also performed on adults to detect presbycusis. It is also used to detect noise-induced hearing loss in occupational settings, but occupational screening is not discussed in this chapter. An estimated 10 million persons in the United States suffer from noise-induced hearing loss.

Official Guidelines. In 1991, the American Speech-Language-Hearing Association, American Academy of Pediatrics, American Academy of Otolaryngology–Head and Neck Surgery, and Council for Education of the Deaf recommended that screening be performed on newborns, preferably before hospital discharge but no later than 3 months of age, if they have risk factors for hearing impairment (Table 4.6). The recommendations of the American Academy of Family Physicians are currently under review. The U.S. Preventive Services Task Force found insufficient evidence to recommend for or against newborn hearing screening. The Canadian Task Force on the Periodic Health Examination found insufficient evidence that measuring either otoacoustic emission or auditory evoked re-

Table 4.6
Risk Factors for Hearing Impairment in Newborns

Family history of hereditary childhood sensorineural hearing loss
Birth weight less than 1500 g
Stigmata or other findings associated with syndromes that can include hearing loss
Craniofacial anomalies
Congenital infection with toxoplasmosis, syphilis, rubella, cytomegalovirus, or herpes
Bacterial meningitis
Hyperbilirubinemia requiring exchange transfusion
Ototoxic medications (e.g., aminoglycosides), used in multiple courses or in combination
with loop diuretics
Apgar scores of 0–4 at 1 minute or 0–6 at 5 minutes
Mechanical ventilation lasting 5 days or longer

Adapted from Joint Committee on Infant Hearing. Joint Committee on Infant Hearing 1994 position statement. Pediatrics 1995;95:152–156.

sponses is more effective than parental questioning or the clap test. In 1993, a National Institutes of Health consensus development conference recommended universal screening of all newborns and infants within the first 3 months of life. In 1994, the Joint Committee on Infant Hearing, which includes the American Speech-Language-Hearing Association, American Academy of Pediatrics, American Academy of Otolaryngology–Head and Neck Surgery, and American Academy of Audiology endorsed "the goal of universal detection of infants with hearing loss" but stopped short of recommending universal screening or specifying which tests should be used. It recommended that certain high-risk children undergo repeat screening every 6 months until age 3, even if newborn screening is normal.

The American Speech-Language-Hearing Association recommends that pure-tone audiometry be performed annually on all children functioning at a developmental level of age 3 to grade 3 and on all high-risk children, including those above grade 3. The American Academy of Pediatrics recommends objective hearing testing by a "standard testing method" at ages 4, 5, 12, and 18 years. The Canadian Task Force on the Periodic Health Examination found poor evidence to include or exclude pure-tone audiometry in the preschool examination. The U.S. Preventive Services Task Force issued similar recommendations. The U.S. Preventive Services Task Force and the American Academy of Family Physicians recommend hearing screening of adolescents and adults with occupational or recreational exposure to excessive noise. The Canadian Task Force on the Periodic Health Examination recommends hearing screening in older adults. The American Speech-Language-Hearing Association recommends audiometry as an option in screening older adults.

Technique

Pure-tone audiometry involves the measurement of thresholds (minimum level in decibels at which the tone is detected) for each ear at different frequencies, typically ranging from 250 Hz to 8000 Hz, which are delivered for about 1 second through calibrated earphones. (Alternatively, hand-held audioscopes can be used for pure-tone testing.) Normal hearing sensitivity at each frequency is about -10 to $+20$ decibels (dB). As the examiner increases the intensity of the signal, the patient indicates when the tone becomes audible. Some of the frequencies commonly used in screening protocols are 500 Hz, 1000 Hz, 2000 Hz, and 4000 Hz, usually delivered at 25 dB, 40 dB, and 60 dB.

Infants and young children (e.g., below age 3) generally cannot cooperate with audiometry. Objective auditory screening of infants is often performed by measuring brainstem auditory evoked responses or otoacoustic emissions. The brainstem auditory evoked response test uses electroencephalographic electrodes to evaluate the integrity of the peripheral auditory system in response to an auditory stimulus delivered through an earphone. Otoacoustic emissions refer to the audiofrequency energy in the ear canal that is generated by the cochlear traveling wave that follows an auditory stimulus. A probe placed in the ear canal and containing a transmitter and sensitive microphone are used to measure the response of the cochlear hair cells to a click sound. In a two-stage screening approach, infants who fail the otoacoustic emissions test undergo repeat testing or brainstem auditory evoked response testing before being referred for further evaluation. Behavioral auditory screening tests, such as the Crib-O-Gram (in which a transducer under the crib mattress measures the infant's movement in response to auditory stimuli), have been used with decreasing frequency since the 1970s and are considered inaccurate and unreliable as screening tests for newborns.

Standard Counseling

Patients and parents should be urged to contact the clinician if evidence of hearing impairment or abnormal speech is noted.

Definition of Abnormal Results

The thresholds for abnormal hearing are 20–40 dB for mild hearing loss, 40–55 dB for moderate hearing loss, 55–70 dB for moderately severe hearing loss, 70–90 dB for severe hearing loss, and greater than 90 dB for profound hearing loss. Newborn hearing screening seeks to identify hearing loss of 30 dB or greater. Figure 4.2 illustrates the type of high-frequency hearing loss associated with presbycusis.

What to Do with Abnormal Results

See Table 17.22.

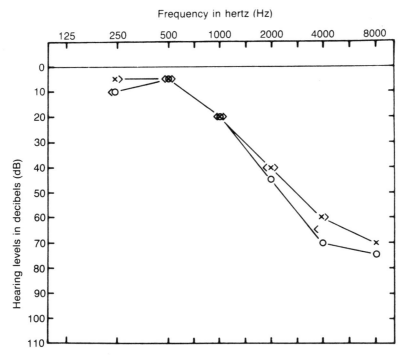

Figure 4.2. Audiometric findings in high-frequency hearing loss. (Reprinted with permission from Lass NJ, McReynolds LV, Northern JL, Yoder DE. Handbook of speech-language pathology and audiology. Toronto/Philadelphia: BC Decker, 1988:1101.

Potential Adverse Effects

There is no risk associated with hearing testing, but falsely positive results may generate unnecessary anxiety, especially among parents, and further testing. Patients, and parents of young patients, can incur costs and inconvenience for office visits and testing to rule out a hearing disorder. Abnormal results may unduly affect job and insurance eligibility. False-negative results may allow hearing impaired persons to escape detection.

Accuracy and Reliability as Screening Test

Standard air conduction audiometers can be calibrated within 2 dB of indicated levels with less than 2–3% variation from indicated frequencies. Pure-tone audiometry has a sensitivity and specificity of 90–95% in detecting sensorineural impairment. Sensitivity is thought to be lower in children, especially if the test is affected by background noise or poor cooperation. When subsequently confirmed hearing impairment (using pure-tone audiometry at a later age) is used as the reference standard, auditory brainstem responses have a reported sensitivity and specificity of 90–100%. Testing of otoacoustic emissions appears to have a lower sensitivity and specificity. When compared with subsequently confirmed mild or severe hearing impairment, the reported sensitivity and specificity are about 55% and 78–90%, respectively; with auditory brainstem responses as the reference standard, the reported sensitivity and specificity are 52–93% and 50–84%, respectively. Recent studies have demonstrated the utility of otoacoustic emissions as a first-line screen followed by auditory evoked response testing if the test is abnormal. The reported sensitivity and specificity of the Crib-O-Gram are 60–91% and 64–77%, respectively.

Office and Clinic Organization for Routine Screening

Offices and clinics that perform audiometry or measurement of otoacoustic emissions should perform the tests in a quiet room with minimal background noise from neighboring rooms or hallways. The devices should be well-maintained, calibrated regularly, and operated by staff with proper training. Offices and clinics that see infants and young children should maintain a list of local audiologic facilities that test auditory brainstem responses or otoacoustic emissions. Reminder systems should be in place to ensure that patients with abnormal results receive appropriate referral and follow-up for audiologic evaluation.

Medical Record Documentation

The date, type of hearing test, and results for each ear should be placed in the medical record, preferably on a health maintenance flow sheet. If audiometry is performed, a copy of the audiogram should be placed in the record. In the case of newborn screening, the infant's risk factors for hearing impairment should be described.

Tuberculin Skin Testing

Introduction

An estimated 10–15 million persons in the United States have latent infection with tuberculosis (15). Tuberculin skin testing of asymptomatic persons is performed to detect persons who have been infected with tuberculosis but who have not yet developed symptoms. Studies have shown that treatment of such patients with at least 6 months of antibiotics (e.g., isoniazid) can significantly reduce progression to active tuberculosis. Tuberculin skin testing can be performed by the multiple-puncture tine test, in which an uncontrolled amount of purified protein derivative (PPD) or old tuberculin is injected, but this is a less accurate screening test than the Mantoux test, in which a known quantity of PPD is injected intradermally.

Official Guidelines. The U.S. Centers for Disease Control and Prevention, U.S. Preventive Services Task Force, Canadian Task Force on the Periodic Health Examination, American Academy of Family Physicians, and American Academy of Pediatrics recommend tuberculin skin testing of persons with risk factors for acquiring tuberculosis. The risk factors identified by the U.S. Centers for Disease Control and Prevention include persons infected with HIV, close contacts of persons known or suspected of having tuberculosis, persons with medical conditions that increase the risk of infection, persons with a chest radiograph suggestive of old healed tuberculosis, immigrants from countries with a high prevalence of tuberculosis, medically underserved low-income populations (including high-risk racial or ethnic groups), alcoholics and intravenous drug users, residents of long-term institutions (e.g., nursing homes, prisons), and persons who work in health care facilities. The American Academy of Pediatrics also recommends periodic tuberculin skin testing of children without risk factors who live in high-prevalence areas or whose history for risk factors is incomplete or unreliable. It recommends against routine screening in low-prevalence areas.

Technique

In the Mantoux test, a tuberculin syringe is used to inject 0.1 ml of 5 TU (tuberculin units) of PPD intradermally on the volar surface of the forearm. The injection should produce a skin weal measuring 6–10 mm. If the patient may be anergic, control sites of mumps, *Candida,* or tetanus should be placed on the opposite arm. A circle should be placed around the injection site(s). The patient should return to the office or clinic in 48–72 hours, at which time the site is inspected for induration. (Erythema alone is an insignificant finding.) If induration is palpated, pen marks placed at the margins of induration can be helpful in measuring the diameter.

Infected persons can have false-negative tuberculin skin tests because of anergy, but anergy is disproved if the control sites are indurated. Infected persons may also have negative tuberculin skin tests if immunity has waned over time. In what is known as the "booster effect," such persons may subsequently have a positive skin test if a PPD is placed a second time. In health care and other institutional settings (e.g., nursing homes), "two-step testing," in which persons with negative tuberculin skin tests are retested in 1–2 weeks, is commonly advised to distinguish persons with booster reactions related to old infections from persons who are new converters.

Definition of Abnormal Results

According to the U.S. Centers for Disease Control and Prevention Advisory Committee for Elimination of Tuberculosis, an induration greater than 5, 10, or 15 mm is abnormal, depending on the risk category of the patient (Table 4.7). In general, induration should not be attributed to prior Bacille bilié de Calmette-Guérin (BCG) vaccination.

Table 4.7
Criteria for Abnormal PPD Induration and Chemoprophylaxis

Category	Age of patient (years)	
	<35	≥35
Patients with risk factors:		
HIV infection/suspected immunocompromised state	≥5 mm	
Close contact of person with active TB	≥5 mm	
Fibrotic lesions on chest x-ray	≥5 mm	
Illnesses that increase risk of tuberculosis (e.g., chronic renal failure, diabetes mellitus, leukemia, Hodgkin's disease, prolonged therapy with corticosteroids, immunosuppressive therapy)	≥10 mm	
Intravenous drug use	≥10 mm	
Recent converter	≥10 mm increase (within a 2-year period)	≥15 mm increase (within a 2-year period)
Patients in other risk groups: Foreign-born persons from high-prevalence countries (countries in Latin America, Asia, Africa); medically underserved, low-income populations and high-risk minorities (e.g., African Americans, Hispanics, Native Americans); residents of long-term care facilities (e.g., nursing homes, mental institutions, correctional institutions); children less than 4 years of age (and those exposed to adults who are HIV-infected, homeless persons, users of intravenous or street drugs, poor and medically indigent urban residents, residents of nursing homes, institutionalized persons, or migrant farm workers)	≥10 mm	Do not treat
Patients without risk factors	≥15 mm	Do not treat

Adapted from U.S. Centers for Disease Control and Prevention. Screening for tuberculosis in high-risk populations: recommendations of the Advisory Committee for Elimination of Tuberculosis. MMWR 1990; 39:RR-8:1-7 and American Academy of Pediatrics, Committee on Infectious Diseases. Screening for tuberculosis in infants and children. Pediatrics 1994;93:131–134.

What to Do with Abnormal Results

See Table 17.21.

Potential Adverse Effects

There is a small amount of discomfort and local erythema associated with PPD injection. Rarely, patients experience hypersensitivity reactions, ulcerated or vesicular eruptions, lymphadenopathy, or fever. Patients with falsely positive results may receive unnecessary antibiotic therapy, with potentially serious adverse effects (e.g., hepatotoxicity), and restrictions on job and insurance eligibility. They may also undergo unnecessary diagnostic procedures (e.g., chest radiography). Falsely negative results may cause patients with tuberculosis to escape detection.

Accuracy and Reliability as Screening Test

For persons who have not contacted an active case, the reported probability of infection is about 5% for 5–9 mm induration, 25% for 10–13 mm induration, 50–80% for 14–21 mm induration, and 100% for more than 21 mm induration, but the validity of these estimates depends heavily on the geographic area, local prevalence of atypical mycobacteria, and type of population being tested. Falsely positive results can be caused by improper measurement of induration (e.g., measuring erythema), cross-reactivity with atypical mycobacteria, hypersensitivity to PPD constituents, and Arthus reactions. Falsely negative results occur in 5–10% of patients due to testing in the early stages of infection, anergy, or improper technique.

Office and Clinic Organization for Routine Screening

Offices and clinics that perform tuberculin testing should maintain a fresh supply of PPD and at least two controls (e.g., mumps, *Candida,* tetanus), tuberculin syringes, and a ruler that measures millimeters. A body diagram that can be inserted in the medical record may be helpful in marking the location of the injections. Reminder systems should be in place to ensure that patients return in 48–72 hours to have the site(s) read and that patients with abnormal results receive appropriate follow-up and chemoprophylaxis for themselves and potential contacts. The health department should be notified of confirmed cases.

Medical Record Documentation

The patient's risk factors for tuberculosis should be described. The date, type of tuberculin test (tine, Mantoux), location of testing, and, if positive, the diameter of induration should appear in the medical record. It is often helpful to use a diagram to mark the location of the tuberculin and control injections. Plans for follow-up treatment of new converters should be described.

CONCLUSION

Many of the recommendations in this chapter presume that patients will be compliant in undergoing testing and in attending follow-up visits for abnormal results. In actual practice, many patients do not follow recommendations and are especially reluctant to undergo uncomfortable or distasteful screening procedures (e.g., sigmoidoscopy, FOBT, Papanicolaou smears). The clinician's chief responsibility in these settings is to ensure that the patient understands the potential benefits and harms of both undergoing and foregoing screening. Concerns about screening that are based on misconceptions, logistical problems, or other issues should be addressed by providing accurate information and proposing potential solutions to the patient's problems. Once the clinician is convinced that the patient is fully informed, however, the patient's choice to forego screening should be respected. At future visits, the decision to undergo screening can be revisited.

The latter point emphasizes the importance of continuity in the provision of quality preventive care. Primary care providers who have a longterm relationship with patients, in which the performance of screening and follow-up of results can be monitored longitudinally, are in a better position to provide comprehensive preventive care than specialists who see patients for single or time-limited visits or who concern themselves primarily with specific categorical health problems.

See Chapter 17 for information regarding the management of patients with abnormal screening test results.

RESOURCES—PATIENT EDUCATION MATERIALS

Hemoglobin and Hematocrit

American Academy of Family Physicians
8880 Ward Parkway
Kansas City, MO 64114-2797
800-944-0000
"Anemia: When Low Blood Iron Is the Cause" (brochure 1562).

Hemoglobin Electrophoresis

Agency for Health Care Policy and Research
Publications Clearinghouse
P.O. Box 8547
Silver Spring, MD 20907
800-358-9295
"Sickle Cell Disease in Newborns and Infants" (brochure 93-0564).

March of Dimes Birth Defects Foundation
P.O. Box 1657
Wilkes-Barre, PA 18703
800-367-6630
    "Sickle Cell Disease" and "Thalassemia" (information sheets).

Blood Glucose and Chemistry Profiles

American Academy of Family Physicians
8880 Ward Parkway
Kansas City, MO 64114-2797
800-944-0000
    "What is Diabetes?" (brochure 731).

Total Cholesterol and Lipid Profiles

American Heart Association
7320 Greenville Avenue
Dallas, TX 75231
214-373-6300
    "Cholesterol and Your Heart." (brochure 50-1059).

National Heart, Lung, and Blood Institute Information Center
P.O. Box 30105
Bethesda, MD 20824-0105
301-251-1222
    "Facts About Blood Cholesterol" (brochure 94-2696).

Serologic Tests for Human Immunodeficiency Virus and Syphilis

U.S. Centers for Disease Control and Prevention
AIDS and HIV Hotline
800-342-2437
800-344-7432 (Spanish)
800-243-7889 (TTY)
    To learn more about HIV and where to get the test.

American Academy of Family Physicians
8880 Ward Parkway
Kansas City, MO 64114-2797
800-944-0000
    "STDs: Signs of Common STDs and Tips on Prevention" (brochure 1565); "AIDS: How
To Reduce Your Risk of Catching It" (brochure 1507).

American Red Cross
General Supply Division
7401 Lockport Place
Lorton, VA 22079
800-969-8890
    "Testing for HIV Infection" (brochure 329547).

American Social Health Association
P.O. Box 13827
Research Triangle Park, NC 27709
919-361-8400
  "HIV Negative: When Are You Free from HIV?" (brochure).

National Institute of Allergy and Infectious Diseases
Office of Communications
Building 31, Room 7A50
9000 Rockville Pike
Bethesda, MD 20892
301-496-5717
  "Taking the HIV (AIDS) Test: How To Help Yourself" (brochure, NIH Publication No.
  93-3322).

Thyroid Function Tests

March of Dimes Birth Defects Foundation
P.O. Box 1657
Wilkes-Barre, PA 18703
800-367-6630
  "Newborn Screening Tests" (information sheet).

Phenylketonuria Screening

March of Dimes Birth Defects Foundation
P.O. Box 1657
Wilkes-Barre, PA 18703
800-367-6630
  "Newborn Screening Tests" and "PKU: Phenylketonuria" (information sheets).

Lead and Erythrocyte Protoporphyrin

U.S. Centers for Disease Control and Prevention
1600 Clifton Road, NE
Atlanta, GA 30333
  "Important Facts About Childhood Lead Poisoning Prevention" (brochure).

National Institute of Environmental Health Sciences
Office of Communications
P.O. Box 12233
Research Triangle Park, NC 27709
919-541-3345
  "Lead and Your Health" (booklet NIH Pub No. 92-3465).

Papanicolaou Smears

American Academy of Family Physicians
8880 Ward Parkway
Kansas City, MO 64114-2797
800-944-0000
  "Pap Smears: What They Are and What the Results Mean" (brochure 1539).

Office of Cancer Communications
National Cancer Institute
Building 31, Room 10A24
Bethesda, MD 20892
800-4-CANCER

> "The Pap Test: It Can Save Your Life!" (brochure, NIH Publication No. 94-3213); "Having a Pelvic Exam and Pap Test" (brochure, NIH Publication No. 93-3416); "Cancer Tests You Should Know About: A Guide for People 65 and Over" (brochure, NIH Publication No. 93-3256).

Endocervical and Urethral Screening for Gonorrhea and Chlamydia

American Academy of Family Physicians
8880 Ward Parkway
Kansas City, MO 64114-2797
800-944-0000

> "STDs: Signs of Common STDs and Tips on Prevention" (brochure 1565).

American Social Health Association
P.O. Box 13827
Research Triangle Park, NC 27709
919-361-8400

> "Stopping Gonorrhea, The Clap" (brochure); "Some Questions and Answers About Chlamydia" (brochure).

Fecal Occult Blood Test

American Cancer Society
1599 Clifton Road, NE
Atlanta, GA 30329
404-320-3333, 800-227-2345

> "Facts on Colorectal Cancer" (brochure, English 2004; Spanish 2703).

American Institute for Cancer Research
1759 R Street, NW
Washington, DC 20069
800-843-8114, 202-328-7744

> "Reducing Your Risk of Colon Cancer" (brochure E2B-BHC).

Krames Communications
1100 Grundy Lane
San Bruno, CA 94066-3030
800-333-3032

> "Colorectal Health" (brochure, English 1226; Spanish 1435).

Office of Cancer Communications
National Cancer Institute
Building 31, Room 10A24
Bethesda, MD 20892
800-4-CANCER

> "Cancer Tests You Should Know About: A Guide for People 65 and Over" (brochure, NIH Publication No. 93-3256).

SmithKline Diagnostics, Inc.
225 Baypointe Parkway
San Jose, CA 95134-1622
800-877-6242, 408-435-2660
    "There Is an Early Warning Signal for Colorectal Cancer" (brochure and instructions
    for FOBT).

Sigmoidoscopy

American Cancer Society
1599 Clifton Road, NE
Atlanta, GA 30329
404-320-3333, 800-227-2345
    "Facts on Colorectal Cancer" (brochure, English 2004; Spanish 2703).

American Institute for Cancer Research
1759 R Street, NW
Washington, DC 20069
800-843-8114, 202-328-7744
    "Reducing Your Risk of Colon Cancer" (brochure E2B-BHC).

Chek Med Systems, Inc.
1027 Mumma Road
Wormleysburg, PA 17043-9933
800-451-5797
    "Flexible Sigmoidoscopy" (brochure, English MGI-23; Spanish MSGI-23).

Krames Communications
1100 Grundy Lane
San Bruno, CA 94066-3030
800-333-3032
    "Colorectal Health" (brochure, English 1226; Spanish 1435).

Office of Cancer Communications
National Cancer Institute
Building 31, Room 10A24
Bethesda, MD 20892
800-4-CANCER
    "Cancer Tests You Should Know About: A Guide for People 65 and Over" (brochure,
    NIH Publication No. 93-3256).

Mammography

Agency for Health Care Policy and Research
Publications Clearinghouse
P.O. Box 8547
Silver Spring, MD 20907
800-358-9295
    "Things to Know About Quality Mammograms" (brochure, AHCPR Pub. No. 95-0634).

American Cancer Society
1599 Clifton Road, NE
Atlanta, GA 30329
404-320-3333, 800-227-2345
    "The Older You Get, the More You Need A Mammogram." (brochure 5020).

Office of Cancer Communications
National Cancer Institute
Building 31, Room 10A24
Bethesda, MD 20892
800-4-CANCER
"Understanding Mammography." (brochure, NIH Publication No. 94-3836); "Are You Age 50 or Over? A Mammogram Could Save Your Life." (brochure, NIH Publication No. 94-3418); "Questions and Answers About Choosing a Mammogram Facility" (brochure, NIH Publication No. 94-3228).

Electrocardiography

Channing L. Bete Co., Inc.
200 State Road
South Deerfield, MA 01373-0200
800-628-7733
"What You Should Know About ECGs" (brochure T12344A).

Chek Med Systems, Inc.
1027 Mumma Road
Wormleysburg, PA 17043-9933
800-451-5797
"The EKG and Echocardiogram" (brochure, English MC-09; Spanish MSC-09).

Audiometry and Newborn Hearing Screening

American-Speech-Language-Hearing Association
10801 Rockville Pike
Rockville, MD 20852
800-638-8255, 301-897-8682
"Can We Talk? A Guide to Your Child's Speech and Hearing" (pull-out information card); "How Does Your Child Hear and Talk? (English, Spanish brochures); "Your Guide to Preventing Hearing Loss" (pull-out information card).

National Institute on Deafness and Other Communication Disorders Information Clearinghouse
1 Communications Avenue
Bethesda, MD 20892-3456
800-241-1044, 800-241-1055 (TTY)
"Hearing and Hearing Loss" (Information packet DC-103); "Hearing and Older People" (fact sheet DC-24).

Tuberculin Skin Testing

American Lung Association
1740 Broadway
New York, NY 10019
212-315-8700, 800-586-4872
"Facts About Tuberculosis" (brochure 1091).

American Thoracic Society
1740 Broadway
New York, NY 10019-4374

Krames Communications
1100 Grundy Lane
San Bruno, CA 94066-3030, 800-333-3032
"Understanding Tuberculosis" (brochure, English 9863; Spanish 9864).

RESOURCES—PROFESSIONAL EDUCATION MATERIALS

Office of Medical Applications of Research
National Institutes of Health
Federal Building, Room 618
Bethesda, MD 20892
"NIH Consensus Statement: Early Identification of Hearing Impairment in Infants and Young Children".

U.S. Centers for Disease Control and Prevention
National Center for Prevention Services
Division of Tuberculosis Elimination
Atlanta, GA 30333

SUGGESTED READINGS

Agency for Health Care Policy and Research. Clinical practice guideline for sickle cell disease: screening, diagnosis, management, and counseling in newborns and infants (AHCPR Publication No. 93-0562). Silver Spring, MD: Agency for Health Care Policy and Research, 1993.

Agency for Health Care Policy and Research. Quality determinants of mammography (AHCPR Pub No. 95-0632). Silver Spring, MD: Agency for Health Care Policy and Research, 1995.

American Academy of Family Physicians. Commission on Public Health and Scientific Affairs. Age charts for periodic health examination. Product No. 972. Kansas City, MO: American Academy of Family Physicians, 1994.

American Academy on Pediatrics, Committee on Adolescence. Sexually transmitted diseases. Pediatrics 1994;94:568–572.

American Academy of Pediatrics, Committee on Genetics. Issues in newborn screening. Pediatrics 1992;89:345–349.

American Academy of Pediatrics, Committee on Practice and Ambulatory Medicine. Recommendations for preventive pediatric care (RE9224). Elk Grove Village, IL: American Academy of Pediatrics, 1991.

American Academy of Pediatrics, Section on Endocrinology and Committee on Genetics, and American Thyroid Association Committee on Public Health. Newborn screening for congenital hypothyroidism: recommended guidelines. Pediatrics 1993;91:1203–1209.

American Academy of Pediatrics Committee on Environmental Health. Lead poisoning: from screening to primary prevention. Pediatrics 1993;92:176–183.

American Academy of Pediatrics Committee on Infectious Diseases. Screening for tuberculosis in infants and children. Pediatrics 1994;93:131–134.

American Cancer Society. Summary of American Cancer Society recommendations for the early detection of cancer in asymptomatic people. CA 1993;43:42–46.

American College of Obstetricians and Gynecologists. Routine cancer screening (ACOG Committee Opinion No. 128). Washington, DC: American College of Obstetricians and Gynecologists, 1993.

American College of Physicians. Common screening tests. Philadelphia: American College of Physicians, 1991.

American Diabetes Association. Screening for diabetes. Diabetes Care 1993;16(Suppl. 2):7–9.

American Speech-Language-Hearing Association, Ad Hoc Committee on Hearing Screening in Adults. Considerations in screening adults/older persons for handicapping hearing impairment. ASHA 1992;34:81–85.

Bess FH, Paradise J. Universal screening for infant hearing impairment. Pediatrics 1994;93:330–334.

Canadian Task Force on the Periodic Health Examination. The Canadian guide to clinical preventive health care. Ottawa: Canada Communication Group, 1994.

Dutta SK, Kowalewski EJ, eds. Flexible sigmoidoscopy for primary care physicians. New York: Alan R Liss, 1987.

Joint Committee on Infant Hearing. Joint Committee on Infant Hearing 1994 position statement. Pediatrics 1995;95:152–156.

Kaluzny AD, Rimer B, Harris R. The National Cancer Institute and guideline development: lessons from the breast cancer screening controversy. J Natl Cancer Inst 1994;86:901–903.

National Cholesterol Education Program. Report of the Expert Panel on Blood Cholesterol Levels in Children and Adolescents. Pediatrics 1992;89:525–584.

National Cholesterol Education Program. Summary of the second report of the National Cholesterol Education Program (NCEP) Expert Panel on Detection, Evaluation, and Treatment of High Blood Cholesterol in Adults (Adult Treatment Panel II). JAMA 1993;269:3015–3023.

Schlant RC, Adolph RJ, DiMarco JP, Dreifus LS, Dunn MI, Fisch C, Garson A Jr, Haywood LJ, Levine HJ, Murray JA, Noble RJ, Ronan JA Jr. Guidelines for electrocardiography: a report of the American College of Cardiology/American Heart Association Task Force on Assessment of Diagnostic and Therapeutic Cardiovascular Procedures (Committee on Electrocardiography). Circulation 1992;85:1221–1228.

National Institutes of Health. Consensus statement: Early identification of hearing impairment in infants and young children. Bethesda, MD: National Institutes of Health, 1993;11(1).

Rodney WM, Felmar E. Flexible sigmoidoscopy: a "how to" guide. Prim Care Cancer 1985;Aug:63–74.

Schumang JL, O'Connor DM, Covell JL, Greening SE. Pap smear collection devices: technical, clinical, diagnostic, and legal considerations associated with their use. Diagn Cytopathol 1992;8:492–503.

Shapiro MF, Greenfield S. The complete blood count and leukocyte differential count: an approach to their rational application. Ann Intern Med 1987;106:65–74.

Singer PA, Cooper DS, Levy EE, Ladenson PW, Braverman LE, Daniels E, et al. Treatment guidelines for patients with hyperthyroidism and hypothyroidism. JAMA 1995;273:808–812.

Surks MI, Chopra IJ, Mariash CN, Nicoloff JT, Solomon DH. American Thyroid Association guidelines for use of laboratory tests in thyroid disorders. JAMA 1990;263:1529–1532.

U.S. Centers for Disease Control and Prevention. Public Health Service guidelines for counseling and antibody testing to prevent HIV infection and AIDS. MMWR 1987;36:509–515.

U.S. Centers for Disease Control and Prevention. Preventing lead poisoning in young children. Atlanta: U.S. Centers for Disease Control and Prevention, 1991.

U.S. Centers for Disease Control and Prevention. Screening for tuberculosis in high-risk populations: recommendations of the Advisory Committee for Elimination of Tuberculosis. MMWR 1990;39:RR-8:1–7.

U.S. Preventive Services Task Force. Guide to clinical preventive services, 2nd ed. Baltimore: Williams & Wilkins, 1996.

U.S. Public Health Service. Clinician's handbook of preventive services. Washington, DC: Government Printing Office, 1994.

Wallach J. Interpretation of diagnostic tests, 5th ed. Boston: Little, Brown & Co, 1992.

Woolf SH, Kamerow DB. Testing for uncommon conditions: the heroic search for positive test results. Arch Intern Med 1990;150:2451–2458.

REFERENCES

1. Schappert SM. National Ambulatory Medical Care Survey: 1991 summary. DHHS Pub. No. (PHS) 94-1777. Vital and Health Statistics, Series 13, No. 116. Hyattsville, MD: National Center for Health Statistics, 1994.

2. U.S. Preventive Services Task Force. Guide to clinical preventive services, 2nd ed. Baltimore: Williams & Wilkins, 1996.

3. National Center for Health Statistics. Current estimates from the National Health Interview Survey, 1993. Vital Health Stat 1994;10(190):95.

4. Geiss LS, Herman WH, Golschmid MG, DeStefano F, et al. Surveillance for diabetes mellitus—United States, 1980–1989. MMWR 1993;42:1–20.

5. Diabetes Control and Complications Trial Research Group. The effect of intensive treatment of diabetes on the development and progression of long-term complications in insulin-dependent diabetes mellitus. N Engl J Med 1993;329:977–986.

6. U.S. Centers for Disease Control and Prevention. Update: acquired immunodeficiency syndrome—United States, 1994. MMWR 1995;44:64–67.

7. U.S. Centers for Disease Control and Prevention. Cases of selected notifiable diseases, United States, week ending December 24, 1994 and December 25, 1993 (51st week). MMWR 1995;43:965.

8. Lorey FW, Cunningham GC. Birth prevalence of primary congenital hypothyroidism by sex and ethnicity. Hum Biol 1992;64:531–538.

9. Nyhan WL. Disorders of amino acid metabolism. In: Rudolph AM, Hoffman JIE, Rudolph CD. Rudolph's pediatrics, 19th ed. East Norwalk, CT: Appleton and Lange, 1991:302.

10. U.S. Centers for Disease Control and Prevention. Blood lead levels—United States, 1988–1991. MMWR 1994;43:545–548.

11. Wingo PA, Tong T, Bolden S. Cancer statistics, 1995. CA 1995;45:8–30.

12. U.S. Centers for Disease Control and Prevention. Recommendations for the prevention and management of *Chlamydia trachomatis* infections, 1993. MMWR 1993;42(RR-12):1.

13. Fletcher SW, Black W, Harris R, Rimer BK, Shapiro S. Report of the International Workshop on Screening for Breast Cancer. J Natl Cancer Inst 1993;85:1621–1624.

14. Bess FH, Paradise J. Universal screening for hearing impairment Pediatrics 1994;93:330–334.

15. U.S. Centers for Disease Control and Prevention. National action plan to combat multidrug-resistant tuberculosis. MMWR 1992;41(RR-11):5–48.

What to Do with the Information

DESIGNING A HEALTH
MAINTENANCE PLAN TARGETED TO
PERSONAL HEALTH BEHAVIORS AND
RISK FACTORS

5. Fostering Healthy Behavior

THE PROCESS

JANE WESTBERG AND HILLIARD JASON

INTRODUCTION

In our lifetimes, the demands of health care have changed substantially. Most of us grew up professionally in settings that were designed to prepare us for being good interventionists. Working mainly with people who had some form of serious acute illness or who were in the late stages of complex diseases, our dominant tasks during our education involved arriving at accurate diagnoses so that we could start appropriate treatments, often involving the prescribing of medications.

Many of us were educated by people whose attitudes about what was needed when caring for patients were shaped by the leading causes of death in the United States at that time: tuberculosis, pneumonia, diarrhea, enteritis, bronchitis, and diphtheria. In a world dominated by infections, the arrival of antibiotics seemed truly miraculous, and medical thinking, quite understandably, became oriented toward the availability of "miracle drugs." The impact was so powerful that much of medical education continues to be influenced by the notion that our task is largely that of finding the curative answer to each patient's problems.

What a different world most of us now face! Today only a small proportion of current morbidity and premature mortality is attributable to the common infectious illnesses of the past. In the 1990s, the leading causes of disability and premature death include heart disease, cancer, stroke, injuries, bronchitis, emphysema, chronic obstructive pulmonary disease, suicide, chronic liver disease, homicide and other acts of abuse and violence, and acquired immunodeficiency syndrome. These and most other major health challenges of the late twentieth century are not primarily attributable to external scourges, such as infections, but rather to the internal reality of our behaviors. Many of the illnesses and threats to life with which we and our patients must contend are largely the consequence of accumulated, multiple indiscretions. Put another way, much morbidity and premature mortality is linked to habitual, harmful ways of living and, therefore, are preventable. Consequently, a growing challenge in health care is learning how to help people adopt and sustain healthy attitudes and habits. Not an easy task (1)!

But the plot thickens. Few of us were given adequate preparation for influencing patients' behaviors. Most of us were educated in hospitals where others took care of assuring that the orders we wrote were carried out. And there are no miracle drugs available for helping people change long-standing patterns of living. Simply telling people to stop smoking, eat less fat, have safe sex, exercise more, discontinue their abusive practices, or reduce their life stresses seldom works. In the real world of ambulatory practice, unlike hospital settings, patients often do not follow their physician's advice (2). What does work far more reliably is an approach that those of us who were trained in authoritarian, interventionist models may not be accustomed to using: actively involving patients as partners in assessing their current health status and developing and monitoring their own health maintenance plans. To function collaboratively, some of us must make changes—perhaps significant changes—in the ways we practice.

Isn't it faster and more efficient, one might ask, to simply tell people what to do than to involve them in decisions about their care? Office visits are certainly briefer if all we do is offer advice. Involving patients in discussions about their health and care takes time. Yet, as we will discuss shortly, for people to make lasting changes in their lives they must feel "ownership" of their long-term health and current condition. This sense of "ownership" is most likely to emerge when time is taken for adequate discussion. Ultimately, dialogues can prove more effective and efficient than monologues.

How can a physician add health promotion to an already overloaded schedule? Health promotion is most time and cost-efficient when done as a team effort, involving nurses, other professionals in the practice, and patients themselves. Also, carefully designed office systems and patient education resources can support health promotion efforts. See Chapter 23 for more details.

Typically, in the medical literature, patients and their problems are discussed in the third person. Please note, however, that in this chapter, we use the first person (i.e., we, us). In doing this, we are acknowledging that most of us have tried making changes in our health behaviors (and in our practice patterns) and that we can draw upon these experiences to enhance our capacity for understanding, empathizing with, and helping our patients.

PROCESS OF CHANGE

Steps in Successful Change

When making changes in the ways we care for ourselves, we and our patients typically—consciously or subconsciously—take several steps. The first and often most difficult step is (*a*) *acknowledging that something is not right in our lives.* Because of our human inclination toward denial, it can take months or years to admit fully that we have a serious problem: that we are eating too much, exercising too little, using alcohol in hurtful ways, or whatever. The next critical step is (*b*) *deciding that we want to make a change in our lives.* Even if we admit we want to make a change, it can be difficult to commit to actually making that change. Subsequent steps include: (*c*) *setting a goal or goals* (e.g., losing 10 pounds in 6 weeks); (*d*) *exploring options for achieving our goal* (e.g., various diets, exercise); and (*e*) *deciding upon and trying to implement a particular plan* (e.g., eating low-fat foods on a regular basis and exercising for at least 20 minutes four times a week).

While implementing our plan, we also need to (*f*) *assess our progress* (e.g., by weighing ourselves). Quite commonly, our goals and/or plan need to be modified (e.g., extend the number of weeks for achieving our target weight). Even after we have achieved our goal, we typically need to (*g*) *guard against backsliding.* As most of us know from painful experiences, it is easy and common to regain excess weight or stop exercising or resume smoking. Most people seeking to alter established habits find that they backslide several times and must make multiple fresh starts on their way to ultimate success.

A line graph depicting the typical change process looks more like a roller coaster than a straight uphill line. For most people the process can be arduous and slow. Making changes requires patience. Impatience often causes discouragement, which can sabotage the whole process.

Why People (We and Our Patients) Tend to Resist Change

Deeply ingrained habits, even harmful ones, can be difficult to change. Most people have difficulty making even minor changes. Some health behavior changes require giving up pleasure. For example, many of us consider high-fat foods, such as ice cream, to be more appealing than their low-fat substitutes. Some changes require actions that are unpleasant (e.g., taking medications, doing certain exercises). Other changes, particularly discontinuing addictive substances, can be overtly painful. Some new behaviors, at least initially, can be stressful. For example, people who use alcohol to relieve their discomfort in social situations can experience anxiety, even panic, when facing social situations without the assistance of alcohol.

Some people are afraid that certain behavior changes will jeopardize their social relationships. For example, adolescents may feel they will be ostracized if they do not join their peers in having unprotected sex, driving without seat belts, smoking, or experimenting with drugs. To complicate the issue, adolescents and young adults in particular feel they are invulnerable to the consequences of their risk-taking behavior—witness the high injury death rate in young men. Some people, especially some older people who have engaged in certain behaviors for a long time, feel that there is no longer any point in making changes. Finally, change that requires us to alter the way we view ourselves can be especially discomforting. A person, for example, who has long defined himself as a nonstop, hard-working executive can have great difficulty introducing play and relaxation into his life. In fact, pressure to do so may initially compound his sense of being under stress.

In sum, abandoning long-standing habits and attitudes, even hurtful ones, is not natural or easy for most people.

What It Takes to Make Meaningful, Lasting Changes

As we indicated above, making and sustaining changes in health behavior usually requires *acknowledging the need for change.* Curry and colleagues (3) reported that smokers who endorsed internal reasons for wanting to quit (had "ownership" of the goal) were more successful in doing so than smokers who had external reasons, such as, "other people are nagging me to quit."

To move from simply acknowledging that they should make a change to actually taking steps toward that change, most people need to *feel that there is more to gain than to lose.* The pleasure, comfort, or other gains that people receive from overeating, smoking, and many other undesirable behaviors need to be outweighed by gains that the person values and believes are attainable.

Some people engage in self-destructive behaviors as a consequence of their lack of self-esteem. For them to muster the considerable energy needed for making significant changes, they need to move toward a greater *sense of self-worth.*

As already mentioned, to change behaviors successfully, people need to *feel "ownership" of the need for change.* When assessing participants' reasons for entering an alcohol treatment program, Plant (4) found that their internal motivation for undergoing treatment was significantly predictive of their remaining in treatment for the duration of the program. Health professionals are most likely to be successful in helping patients to feel ownership of a health improvement and maintenance plan if their approach is collaborative rather than authoritarian (5). Health professionals who use an authoritarian approach tend to do things to and for patients; they tell patients what to do and how to do it. Although some patients do follow the orders given by health professionals who use this approach, others rebel. Still others follow orders initially but revert to their old ways of doing things when they are not being monitored. In contrast, collaborative health professionals involve patients as much as possible in making decisions about their care. Patients of these health professionals are likely to feel ownership of a plan for their health improvement and maintenance and be committed to carrying it out because they participated in its formulation. The plan is their plan, not their clinician's.

Successful change is usually facilitated by *realistic goals* and *workable plans*. If people's goals are beyond their current capabilities or levels of readiness, they are unlikely to achieve them and are likely to become discouraged. If health maintenance plans are not tailored to their resources and life demands, they are likely to ignore or disregard them. Too many plans are ineffective because they focus on what the person should *stop* doing (e.g., smoking or eating high-fat diets) but fail to address what the person should *start* doing. Effective plans move people from risky or harmful behaviors toward healthy behaviors. They usually also call for gradual changes, not quick fixes. People who jump into intensive exercise programs rather than gradually increasing their level of challenge can injure themselves. Crash diets seldom have a lasting effect and can be harmful.

Changing behavior is usually made easier if there is *positive reinforcement* for the desired behavior. Rewards can be external (e.g., a gift the person receives after achieving certain goals) or internal (the sense of satisfaction associated with reaching a cherished goal). Whenever possible, internal rewards should be identified and cultivated. The most effective external rewards tend to be those that are selected and valued by the person involved and are linked to the change itself. For example, a man who successfully completes a weight loss and exercise program rewards himself with a new suit. Also, the change process is typically facilitated if the person making the change has the *support of others*: health professionals, family members, friends, and colleagues.

People are most likely to follow through with their plan for change if there is a *strategy for timely monitoring of their progress* and *for making needed changes in their plan*. The person's *self-assessments* together with *constructive feedback* from others are critical components of the process of monitoring and evaluating their progress. Initial plans are not always optimal or even workable, and can cause people to become discouraged by their lack of progress. Flawed or unworkable plans are a common reason for discontinuing efforts to make needed changes. Having a mechanism for detecting and addressing problems early and regularly can help reduce such causes of discouragement and failure.

A *mechanism for follow-up*, even after people have achieved their goals, is crucial, particularly when people are at risk for significant backsliding. Just knowing that they will be having follow-up conversations with their doctor or nurse about their current status can help some people sustain their dedication to their goals.

Patience and *practice* are especially important ingredients in the change process. Most significant change takes time. New behaviors have to be practiced repeatedly until they are integrated into people's habitual ways of functioning. Patients need to know that some backsliding is common and acceptable.

ADAPTING YOUR PRACTICE FOR HEALTH PROMOTION

Many health professionals find that they can be far more successful in attending to issues of prevention with their patients if they make systemic changes in their practice that support such an approach (6, 7). The following steps are based on a team approach to prevention and health promotion that includes systems for supporting your efforts and those of your team and patients. Similar models are discussed in more detail in Chapter 23.

Formulate Goals and Set Priorities for Your Practice

Typically, it is not practical or effective to make significant changes in a practice all at once. Rather, if you want to have more of a health promotion focus in your practice, it may be best to identify your overall goals and then determine your highest priorities, especially in terms of the needs of your patient population and those areas likely to provide the most payoff.

Decide on Your Approach to Patients

One of the key decisions that you and your colleagues can make is how you will work with patients. We recommend the collaborative, systematic approach discussed below. If several members of your practice are working with the same patient, ensure that all of you are consistent in what you say and do.

Decide How to Function as a Team

The ways in which you and your colleagues function as a team depend on the kinds of professionals on your team as well as their capabilities and interests. For example, physicians and nurses can discuss how they can support and complement each other's efforts. One member can play a key role in counseling patients about health promotion and disease prevention. Another member can update each patient's prevention flow sheet and highlight issues that need attention at each visit.

Have Visible Signs of the Emphasis on Health Promotion

You can convey your commitment to health promotion by creating a patient care environment that provides indirect and direct messages about your concerns. For example, in some offices, comfortable furniture, healthy plants, quiet music, and the absence of ashtrays help convey a sense of the healthy environment that is valued. Pamphlets, books, and video and computer programs provide more direct messages, while pre-vention-oriented posters in examination rooms remind patients and prac-titioners to attend to prevention issues.

Select and Use Systems and Resources that Support Your Efforts and Those of Your Team

Patient questionnaires, health risk assessments, reminder notices, chart stickers and alerts, and *patient education materials* are among the resources that can help you and your colleagues attend to health promotion consistently. You can ask patients to fill out a questionnaire that elicits information (e.g., about relevant risk factors, behaviors they want to change, and their level of readiness for making changes) that can help you and your colleagues indi-vidualize your approach to each person. These questionnaires can also in-clude space for patients to indicate their requests for health information. As discussed in Chapter 23, the questionnaires should be placed in the chart so that you and other team members can review them with the patient.

Health risk assessment techniques can efficiently identify health risk factors for individuals patients, even factors that otherwise might be over-looked. The Office of Disease Prevention and Health Promotion of the U.S. Department of Health and Human Services has published an exten-sive list of available health risk assessment instruments with information on how to order them. See Chapter 1 for further details.

Reminder notices that were generated at earlier visits can prompt you and/or your colleagues to address pertinent issues with each patient. Some reminder notices are computer-generated and also serve to update the computer data base. Other systems simply involve having staff make entries in paper-based record systems. See Chapter 26 for further details.

Stickers and alerts can be put in appropriate places on the chart and kept there as long as they are needed. Examples include: "Did you talk to the patient about smoking?" and "This patient has agreed to the following quit date: _____."

In addition to the patient education materials available in waiting areas, you can give patients preproduced or customized materials that are pertinent to their health maintenance needs. These materials can rein-force what you say. A listing of relevant patient education materials, and the address and telephone number for ordering them, is provided in the "Resources" section in most chapters of this book.

Select and Use Systems and Resources for Supporting Your Patients' Efforts

When patients fill out *history* and *risk factor questionnaires,* they are prompted to think about their health-related behaviors. Many *health risk as-sessment tools* provide patients with helpful personalized feedback and recommend actions to deal with aspects of lifestyle and risk exposure. These tools can also help legitimize attention to lifestyle issues. *Appropriate patient education* materials enable patients to review new information at their own pace and in their own way. *Patient reminders* typically take the form of mailed reminders or telephone calls. Sometimes both strategies are used. Reminders that convey a message about the importance of carrying out the suggested activities can help to increase adherence. *Patient-held records* (see Fig. 22.6) that are designed for recording pertinent health information as well as future needed services can assist patients or their caregivers in seeking appropriate services in a timely way. Such records can give patients some understanding of and sense of control over their health care. Patients can use *health diaries* for keeping track of more detailed information, such as the food they eat during a given period of time. See Chapter 23 for more details.

Have a Member of the Team Coordinate Special Efforts

When you and your colleagues want to introduce or give special attention to a particular health issue, such as smoking cessation, consider having one member of the health team coordinate and assume overall responsibility for the effort. For example, a nurse who is responsible for smoking cessation might check to ensure that smoking is included in the patient questionnaire, that smoking cessation posters and pamphlets are in the waiting and examination rooms, that smoking-related chart stickers are on appropriate patient charts, that all members of the health team are aware of the practice's smoking cessation resources, and that regular follow-up calls are made to designated patients.

ADDRESSING HEALTH BEHAVIOR ISSUES WITH PATIENTS

During most visits (even those that are not scheduled primarily for focusing on health behavior or other aspects of prevention), prevention issues can be addressed at least briefly. When patients seek care for a health behavior-related condition (e.g., chronic bronchitis), they can be more receptive than otherwise to talking about changes in their life that will reduce their symptoms and/or prevent them from having a recurrence. (This includes talking with patients about prevention during a hospital stay.) First visits can be a good time for patients (by themselves or with someone's help) to fill out questionnaires that deal with their risk factors, pertinent history, current health status, and their interest in receiving more information about some health issues. You can review their responses when meeting with them. Addressing prevention in the first visit emphasizes the importance you attach to this issue.

Prevention is an obvious component of some routine checkups (e.g., well-baby visits, examinations for school and work, obstetrical visits). Time can also be allowed for prevention issues during other follow-up visits. Understandably, time may not be available for prevention if the patient's visit is related to an acute or complicated condition requiring their and your full attention.

Sometimes your focus can be on helping people identify and understand their risk factors, or on helping them set goals and develop a plan for achieving those goals. If patients are already in the midst of trying to make a life change, you can use the visit to inquire about their progress and support their efforts. Depending on what you learn, you can empathize with their struggles, help them revise their plan, or congratulate them on their success. Sometimes you might simply reinforce prevention work that the patient is doing with one of your colleagues. You can often make a meaningful contribution in less than two minutes.

When addressing health behavior issues with patients, the following are some steps to consider taking.

Ensure that Patients Understand Your Reasons for Addressing Health Behavior

Although an increasing number of people expect and want health professionals to talk with them about prevention, some people (particularly those whose stated agenda is for you to treat a specific problem), might not understand why you want to talk about how they are conducting their lives. Also, some people do not appreciate the linkages between behavior and health. Before talking with them about their behavior, be diagnostic about this issue. Explore their level of understanding, and if necessary help them comprehend the relationship between behavior and health.

Discuss the Ways You Can Work as Partners in Addressing Your Patient's Health Issues

As we have indicated, patients are most likely to make lasting changes in their behavior if they are active collaborators in their care. Ultimately, they have to change themselves. No outsider can cause lasting changes in another person. External forces tend to lose their impact once they are removed. For most people, we are most helpful when we facilitate and encourage their process of change and serve as consultants. If we tell them what to do or try to exert pressure on them, we may appear to have temporary success, but in the long run this strategy usually backfires or simply fails.

Again, be diagnostic. Find out how your patients expect and/or want to relate to you. If they currently prefer being dependent and are more comfortable in an authoritarian relationship, try to help them understand the benefits of a partnership approach. But start where they are. Gradually urge them to take more responsibility for their health. If appropriate, even help them understand that unwillingness or inability to take appropriate responsibility for their own care can itself be a risk factor that needs to be addressed.

Help Patients Explore Their Health-Related Behaviors and Identify Their Risk Factors

Whether on a particular visit it is best to look broadly at a patient's health status and risk factors or to focus on particular risk factors depends on the purpose of the patient's visit, the amount of time you have together, and the patient's readiness to dwell on particular issues (e.g., behaviors related to the condition for which he or she is seeking help). Asking patients to complete a health risk assessment questionnaire before meeting with you can facilitate the process.

As you talk with patients about their behavior, especially about potentially sensitive issues, relate to them in ways that will enable them to be open and honest with you. For example, many people are more likely to acknowledge certain behaviors if they feel they are not the only ones who engage in such behavior and that you will not be shocked by what they say. You can help put them at ease by providing "normative permission," using statements and questions that indicate your comfort and expectations. For instance, in trying to determine if a patient's sexual activity puts him at risk for sexually transmitted diseases, you could say (as neutrally as possible), *"Many people find it a bother to use condoms or other forms of protection when having sex. How about you?"*

In general, you can help patients talk openly about their behavior by being nonjudgmental. For example, use neutral language when approaching sensitive topics (e.g., use the word "partner" rather than "husband," "wife," or "lover," if you are not certain of your patient's situation).

Listen carefully to the vocabulary and constructions your patients use so that when you ask questions and provide information, you can choose language that they are likely to understand. Adapt what you say and how you say it to each patient's readiness and level of understanding. After you ask a question, give patients time to respond, even if that requires providing a period of silence before they speak.

Explore Patients' Attitudes Toward Key Risk Factors

Be aware that not all patients share your understanding of and values around certain risk factors. For example, a patient who you feel is worrisomely underweight or overweight may value her current weight. In addition, her friends and family may support her condition. Clearly, before proceeding further, you have to help this patient understand the possible health-related consequences of her behavior.

Explore Patients' Experiences with Trying to Address Key Risk Factors

Most people are their own caregivers most of the time. Many of your patients are probably already aware of changes they need to make in their lives and have tried—successfully or unsuccessfully—to make some needed changes. By asking them about their health care practices and acknowledging, even congratulating them on, the efforts they have already made, you can reinforce the positive steps they have taken, empathize with any problems they have had, and help them build on what they have already done and learned. All of these steps help you to be perceived as an ally, not a judge. Your subsequent advice is likely to be taken more seriously.

Again, use strategies to facilitate communication between you and your patients. For example, open-ended questions (e.g., *"How would you describe what you currently do to try to take care of yourself?" "What steps if any have you taken to lower your cholesterol?"* and *"What was it like for you when you tried to restrict your drinking?"*) permit patients to talk with you in their own way, in their own words. Typically their responses to such questions provide you with clues about their situation that aren't as likely to surface in response to focused, short-answer questions.

Convey your empathy and compassion nonverbally and with such statements as, *"It sounds like you're going through a very tough time!"* If appropriate, demonstrate your appreciation of their situation by sharing your own experience: *"I know how hard it can be. I used to be a smoker. It took me two years of hard work before I gave up completely."* Such observations enhance your credibility and, hence, your likely impact.

Let patients know you are listening by doing such things as maintaining natural eye contact and sitting in a relaxed, open (but attentive) posture. Ask for clarification when necessary. Reflect back the key messages you have heard: *"It sounds like you don't want to stop smoking because it's one of the few things in your life that you enjoy."* To ensure you have heard correctly, after trying to paraphrase or summarize what the patient said, invite the patient's feedback: *"Did I get that right?"* or *"Is that what you meant?"*

Help Patients Explore Factors That Can Potentially Support and Obstruct Their Efforts to Change

Invite patients to think through the factors that are likely to support and block their efforts. Even use a piece of paper: divide it in half, putting supporting factors on one side of the page and barriers on the other. Include in the discussion what patients feel they are likely to gain and lose by making changes.

If before embarking on making a change, you and your patients are aware of potential barriers to their intended efforts, you and they can try to devise strategies for reducing or overcoming these barriers. For example, a patient may feel it will be difficult to give up fat in his diet. His wife does all the cooking and she has a cultural tradition of high-fat cooking. You might then suggest having her join him at the next visit so that you can try enlisting her support. Knowing about potential resources can also help patients' efforts. For example, the patient who needs to reduce fat in his diet might be helped by learning about some tasty low-fat foods.

If appropriate, also explore what the patient is getting from the behavior that needs to be changed. Quite commonly people use behaviors such as overeating, overdrinking, and smoking to compensate for unmet needs and to deal with painful problems or issues in their lives. See, for example, the discussion of self-esteem in Chapter 16. If patients attempt to change their behavior without at least being aware of their underlying problem, they can be unsuccessful in their attempt to change, or they may give up one hurtful behavior and replace it with another.

Try to Facilitate Your Patients' Commitments to Making Positive Changes

The preceding steps can all facilitate patients' readiness to commit to making changes. Explicitly voicing this commitment, however, is so key to the change process that we emphasize its importance here.

Do not be discouraged if patients are unwilling to commit to making a change the first or second time you discuss their risk-linked behavior. When patients are faced with tackling well-ingrained behaviors that are giving them pleasure and/or satisfying a need in their life, it can take months or years before they are fully prepared to take this major step. Use appropriate chart reminders so that during subsequent visits you can again raise such questions as *"Have you given any more thought to cutting back on your drinking?"*

Help Patients Establish Realistic Goals

People are most likely to be successful making changes in their lives if they try making only one change at a time. This is particularly true if they are trying to make significant changes. If patients have identified several behaviors they would like to address, you may need to help them set priorities before they start formulating goals. Factors that can contribute to the ranking and staging of priorities include the patient's perceived needs and preferences and your estimation of the level of the patient's current risks and needs.

When formulating goals, urge patients to be as specific as possible. Vague goals, such as *"I want to lose weight"* usually are not helpful. More specific goals, such as *"I want to lose 10 pounds so I can fit into my size 12 clothes again"* give patients direction and provide a tangible target, as well as a basis for feeling a sense of accomplishment when reached. For some behavior changes, it also helps for patients to give themselves a time limit (e.g., lose 10 pounds in eight weeks).

When making significant changes, it can be helpful for patients to set a reasonable long-term goal along with some short-term goals that can provide a more immediate sense of progress and success. For example, a patient may have a goal of losing 40 pounds, but decide to allow himself six months in which to do it. He can be helped by setting some short-term goals (e.g., losing 10 pounds for each of the first two months) and then maintaining his new weight for a month before continuing to lose more weight.

Help Patients Develop Workable Plans for Achieving Their Goals

Some patients have ideas about steps they might take or want you to take in helping them achieve their goals. Be sure you are aware of your patient's ideas. Also present other options you think would be useful. Consider individual counseling, group classes, written materials, audiovisual aids, and community resources.

Each patient has unique life circumstances. A plan that is effective for one person might be useless for another. As you explore plans with patients, invite them to think aloud about the advantages and disadvantages of each plan. Also, add your own thoughts about what you anticipate might be advantages and disadvantages of the various plans.

When developing plans, keep the following in mind. Major life changes (e.g., quitting smoking) are usually best accomplished in stages. Plans that include multiple strategies tend to be more effective than those that rely on a single strategy. In some cases, changes should be linked to and be congruent with people's normal activities (e.g., taking medications along with meals) so they can easily remember what they need to do. On the other hand, people who are trying to recover from addictive behaviors can be better off altering their daily activities so they can break the link between their addictive behavior and certain routine daily activities. Plans should be as simple as possible (e.g., taking a medication once a day rather than several times a day, if feasible). And, as we indicated earlier, rewards for accomplishments can help some people make changes.

Family members and others can interfere with people's attempts to change. A man who is trying to quit smoking might find it difficult to do so if his wife continues smoking. On the other hand, a woman who is trying to manage her adult-onset diabetes mellitus on diet alone can be helped in doing so if her husband, who does most of the cooking, agrees to prepare appropriate meals. If the support of family members, friends, or others is important in helping your patient make a behavior change, you might want to meet jointly with the patient and the significant people in the patient's life. Some steps to consider taking when working with family members or friends include assuring that these people understand the patient's situation and what he needs to do, gaining their commitment to support the patient, and identifying particular ways in which they can provide support.

Many people are helped to make changes if they make contracts, particularly written ones, which include their goal(s), their plan for achieving their goal(s), their responsibilities, the responsibilities of others (e.g., their physician), and a time schedule (8). Contracts can stimulate a planned approach to health maintenance, provide a clear definition of the responsibilities of the patient and other parties, and foster accountability. At the very least, we recommend recording the goal and plan in the patient's medical record. (For a sample contract, see Figure 5.1.)

Work with Patients in Monitoring Their Progress

When patients know that their progress will be reviewed, their chances of successfully accomplishing their goals increase (9, 10). Also, as we have mentioned, a mechanism for monitoring their progress can help you and your patients identify problems with their plan, enabling you and them to revise it if necessary.

Patients can report on their progress by telephone. You or other members of the practice can phone or write to patients. Patients also can come in for follow-up visits. A scheduled telephone call or visit can be linked to a short-term goal (e.g., cutting back to six cigarettes a day by the time of the next contact).

Telephone calls and visits can be scheduled to coincide with key points in the change process. For example, a visit with you or another member of the health team soon after patients have stopped smoking can provide valuable reinforcement and can help them remain nonsmokers (11, 12).

During visits or phone calls, you or your colleagues can find out what parts of a patient's plan are working and identify current or anticipated problems. If patients are making progress, you can congratulate them and help them anticipate their next steps. You can also remind them of any changes that are already taking place because of their efforts (e.g., if a patient has not smoked for two weeks, you can determine if her morning cough has diminished and, if so, emphasize that this is a sign that she is already beginning to heal). If patients are frustrated and not making progress, you can help them rethink their plans, if necessary. You might also offer additional ideas and suggestions. If it is appropriate, you and the patient can schedule further calls and visits (with you or another member of the health team) to provide further support and help. (In general, when helping patients monitor their progress, you can be most effective if

Patient's name: John Smith   Date: 6/14/95

My health goal: By October 1, 1995, I will give up all smoking

Steps I will take toward achieving my goal: By 7/1/95 I will reduce

my 2 pack/day smoking to 1 pack/day, and will then go on

patches and stop all smoking. I will strictly follow in-

tion using the nicotine patches.

Steps my family/friend have agreed to take to help me: They will not

in my presence at any time during the next 6 months, and

will give me every encouragement they can to help me stick

with my plan.

Steps my doctor (other caregiver) has agreed to take to help me: 1. Give

me all the directions and encouragement I need; 2. Be avail-

to answer my questions & concerns; 3. Provide prescriptions

need; 4. Be patient with me if I backslide; 5. Put gentle,

consistent pressure on me to stick with my plan.

If I don't achieve my goal, in addition to the negative health consequences, I

recognize that: It will be up to me to admit the difficulties I

having and to make every effort to try again.

My REWARD _____

Signed:_____   Date: _____
                        (Patient)

_____   Date: _____
               (Family member/friend)

_____   Date: _____
                    (Caregiver)

Figure 5.1.   Sample, simple health contract.

you can sustain their hope and reduce their discouragement.) As appropriate, transfer increasing responsibility for care to the patient.

Follow-up with Patients after They Achieve Goals, Especially Those That Are Difficult to Sustain

Particularly if patients have made a change that people commonly have difficulty sustaining, consider continuing regularly scheduled follow-ups, even after they have achieved their goal. Knowing that you will be communicating with them can help some patients maintain their new behavior. It is also important to know if patients have relapsed or regressed so that you can offer help promptly.

Often patients who have relapsed or regressed regard themselves as personal failures, are discouraged about trying again, and may be reluctant to admit what happened. You may need to remind them that most difficult changes do not occur in a straight line and that relapses and backsliding are common parts of the change process. You can help patients identify what went wrong and, if necessary, assist them in altering their plan or in developing a new one. Emphasize what they have achieved and encourage them to keep trying. Remind them that having achieved their goal once confirms that they can do it. Assure them of your continuing support.

CONCLUSION

Here is a summary of some key steps to take when adapting your practice for health promotion and addressing health issues with patients.

Adapting Your Practice for Health Promotion

- Formulate goals for your practice.
- Decide on your approach to patients.
- Decide how you and your colleagues can function as a team.
- Have visible signs of the emphasis on health promotion.
- Select and use systems and resources that support your team's health promotion efforts.
- Select and use systems and resources that support your patients' health promotion efforts.
- Have a member of the team coordinate special health promotion efforts.

Addressing Health Behavior Issues with Patients

You are unlikely to take all these steps at a single visit; change is an ongoing process, and several of you may need to join in taking these steps. Do try, however, to attend to prevention issues during most or all patient visits.

- Ensure that patients understand the reasons for addressing health behavior.
- Discuss the ways you can work as partners in addressing their health issues.
- Help patients explore their health-related behaviors and identify their risk factors.
- Explore patients' attitudes towards key risk factors.
- Explore patients' experiences with trying to address key risk factors.
- Help patients explore factors that can potentially support and obstruct their efforts to change.
- Try to facilitate patients' commitment to making positive changes.
- Help patients establish realistic goals.
- Help patients develop workable plans for achieving their goals.
- Work with patients in monitoring their progress.
- Schedule follow-ups with patients after they achieve their goals, especially those that are difficult to sustain.
- *Above all, be patient with your own and with your patients' efforts to make significant changes!*

SUGGESTED READINGS

Green LW. How physicians can improve patients' participation and maintenance in self-care. West J Med 1987;147:346–349.
Haynes RB, Taylor DW, Sackett DL, eds. Compliance in health care. Baltimore: Johns Hopkins University Press, 1979.
Janz NK, Becker MH. The health belief model: a decade later. Health Educ Q 1984;11:1–47.
Mullen PD, Green LW. Educating and counseling for prevention: from theory and research to principles. In: Goldbloom RB, Lawrence RS, eds. Preventing disease: beyond the rhetoric. New York: Springer-Verlag, 1990:474–479.
Roter DL, Hall JA. Doctors talking with patients/Patients talking with doctors: improving communications in medical visits. Westport, CT: Auburn House, 1992.
Waitzkin H. Information giving in medical care. J Health Soc Behav 1985;26:81–101.

REFERENCES

1. Jason H. Influencing health behavior: physicians as agents of change. Cleveland Clinic J of Med 1994;61:147–152.
2. Sackett DL, Haynes RB, Tugwell P. Clinical epidemiology: A basic science for clinical medicine. Boston: Little, Brown & Co., 1985.
3. Curry S, Wagner EH, Grothaus LC. Intrinsic and extrinsic motivation for smoking cessation. J Consult Clin Psychol 1990;58:310–316.
4. Plant RW. Motivation, expectation, and psychiatric severity in predicting early dropout from outpatient alcoholism treatment. Dissertation Abstracts International 1991;SI:3579-B.

5. Westberg J, Jason H. Collaborative clinical education: the foundation of effective patient care. New York: Springer-Verlag, 1993.
6. Cohen S, Halverson HW, Gosselink CA. Changing physician behavior to improve disease prevention. Prev Med 1994;23:284–291.
7. Pommerenke FA, Dietrich A. Improving and maintaining preventive services; Part 1: Applying the patient model. J Fam Prac 1992;34:86–97.
8. Woldum KM, Ryan-Morrell V, Towson MC, Bower KA, Zander K. Patient education: foundations of practice, Rockville, MD: Aspen Systems, 1985.
9. Fagerstrom KO. Effects of nicotine chewing gum and follow-up appointments in physician-based smoking cessation. Prev Med 1984;13:517–527.
10. Russell MA, Wilson C, Taylor C, Backer CD. Effect of general practitioners' advice against smoking. Br Med J 1979;2:231–235.
11. Kottke TE, Battista RN, DeFriese GH, Brekke ML. Attributes of successful smoking cessation interventions in medical practice. A meta-analysis of 39 controlled trials. JAMA 1988;259:2883–2889.
12. U.S. Preventive Services Task Force. Guide to clinical preventive services. Baltimore: Williams & Wilkins, 1996.

6. Tobacco Use

COUNSELING AND ADJUNCTIVE TREATMENT

MARC MANLEY

INTRODUCTION

In a landmark report to the American people, the U.S. Surgeon General concluded in 1988 that cigarettes and other forms of tobacco are addicting. Cigarettes are the leading cause of preventable death in the United States today and kill more than 400,000 people each year. This is more deaths than the number caused by alcohol, illegal drugs, car crashes, homicides, suicides, and acquired immunodeficiency syndrome, combined. Smoking is a known cause of cancer of the lung, larynx, oral cavity, and esophagus; coronary heart disease; atherosclerotic peripheral vascular disease; chronic obstructive pulmonary disease; intrauterine growth retardation; and low birth weight. Smokeless tobacco use causes oral cancer and other oral lesions. Environmental tobacco smoke, a known human carcinogen, causes lung cancer in nonsmoking adults and respiratory illness in children.

In 1991, 46.3 million Americans, or 25.7% of the adult population, smoked cigarettes; 28.1% of men smoked compared with 23.5% of women. Among whites, 25.5% smoked compared with 26.2% of blacks. The highest levels of smoking were among people age 25 to 44 (30.4%); American Indians and Alaska Natives (31.4%); people with less than a high school education (32%); and people living below poverty level (33.1%)(1).

This chapter provides physicians, nurses, other health care providers, and their associates with the necessary information to institute effective smoking cessation techniques in their practices. Although this chapter emphasizes smoking cessation, these interventions may also be used to help smokeless tobacco users stop. The interventions described are simple and brief, taking as little as 3 minutes. They are based on large clinical trials carried out by the National Cancer Institute (NCI) that clearly indicate that physicians and other health care professionals can significantly reduce the prevalence of smoking if they provide smoking cessation interventions.

BACKGROUND

Many clinicians recognize that smoking is a major threat to a patient's health but typically do not feel skilled enough to intervene effectively. Most clinicians have not experienced what they would consider success in helping patients to stop smoking. Most have treated patients with significant smoking-related disease who have been unable to stop despite multiple attempts. Repeated failures to help patients to stop smoking frequently cause clinicians to become discouraged and reinforce the belief that nothing can be done about smoking. Another barrier preventing physicians from trying to help patients quit smoking includes a lack of formal training in tested cessation techniques. Perhaps most important, many office practices are not organized to support the delivery of smoking cessation interventions.

The methods outlined here demonstrate how to recognize and overcome these barriers and how best to use the limited time available to effectively assist patients to stop smoking.

Many patients will not choose to stop smoking the first time they receive medical advice to quit. Furthermore, many patients will not stop smoking permanently after their first attempt to quit but will require several serious attempts. This chapter recommends how clinicians can incorporate smoking cessation techniques into a variety of encounters with a smoking patient until cessation is successful.

METHODS

The NCI's recommendations for promoting smoking cessation among clinic patients are detailed in *How To Help Your Patients Stop Smoking: A National Cancer Institute Manual for Physicians* (2). A summary of the recommendations is provided here. These recommendations are consistent with those of the U.S. Preventive Services Task Force. Counseling patients to stop smoking or using smokeless tobacco is also recommended by the American Academy of Family Physicians, American College of Physicians, American Academy of Pediatrics, Canadian Task Force on the Periodic Health Examination, and dozens of other medical and public health organizations and government agencies.

Clinician Intervention

The clinician intervention consists of four activities, each beginning with the letter "A":

- *Ask* all patients about smoking;
- *Advise* smokers to stop;

- *Assist* their efforts with self-help materials, a quit date, and possibly nicotine gum or the transdermal patch; and

- *Arrange* follow-up.

This intervention plan (often referred to as the "4 As") describes a general approach to smoking patients and can be used in almost any outpatient encounter, whether 30 seconds or 30 minutes is available to the clinician. Each element of the intervention is described below.

Ask about Smoking at Every Opportunity

A nurse or other staff member should routinely ask patients *"Do you smoke?"* or *"Are you still smoking?"* at each visit, usually while measuring vital signs. Once it is known that a person smokes (or previously smoked), an identifier should be placed prominently on the patient's chart to remind the physician and staff to discuss smoking at each visit. (See Chapter 23 for further information about chart alert stickers and other clinician reminder systems.) Patients who have never smoked or who formerly smoked should be briefly congratulated for their decision.

Advise All Smokers to Stop

A clear statement of advice (e.g., *"As your physician, I must advise you to stop smoking now."*) is essential. Many patients do not recall receiving this advice from their physician; therefore, the statement must be easy to understand and memorable. Personalization of the message by referring to the patient's clinical condition, social roles, personal interests, or family history may add to the effectiveness of the advice. Motivations to stop smoking vary greatly from patient to patient. A list of reasons different people might give for stopping is provided in Table 6.1 (3). While almost any clinical encounter provides an opportunity to discuss smoking, timing of the advice is still important. The so-called "teachable moment" is that time when a patient's circumstances make him or her more receptive to advice. Teachable moments occur when patients suffer from diseases caused by smoking, but they may also occur following auscultation, pulmonary function tests, or when a friend or relative is ill.

Assist the Patient in Stopping

A patient's level of interest in stopping smoking usually is evident in discussions with the clinician. If it is not, ask patients if they want to stop. For those patients who do not want to stop, nagging rarely helps. Clinicians must accept the patient's decision, make sure the patient is making an informed choice, and attempt to maintain the patient's trust and confidence so that smoking can be discussed at future visits.

Table 6.1
Good Reasons to Stop Smoking

For teenagers	Ten times the risk of lung cancer
Bad breath	5- to 8-year shorter lifespan
Stained teeth	Cost of cigarettes
Cost	Cost of sick time
Lack of independence—controlled	Bad breath
by cigarettes	Less convenient and socially unacceptable
Sore throat	Wrinkles
Cough	**For symptomatic adults**
Dyspnea (might affect sports)	Upper respiratory infection
Frequent respiratory infections	Cough
For pregnant women	Sore throat
Increased rate of spontaneous	Gum disease
abortion and fetal death	Dyspnea
Increased risk of low birth weight	Ulcers
For parents	Angina
Increased coughing and	Claudication
respiratory infections among	Osteoporosis
children of smokers	Esophagitis
Poor role model for child	**For any smoker**
For new smokers	Money saved by stopping
Easier to stop now	Feel better
For asymptomatic adults	Improved ability to exercise
Twice the risk of heart disease	May live long enough to enjoy retirement,
Six times the risk of emphysema	grandchildren, etc.

Adapted from Glynn T, Manley M. How to help your patients stop smoking: a National Cancer Institute manual for physicians. Bethesda, MD: National Institutes of Health, 1989.

For those patients who express a sincere desire to stop smoking, the clinician should help them set a specific date. There is evidence that patients who set a "quit date" are more likely to make a serious attempt to stop (4). This date should be soon (generally within 4 weeks), but not immediate, giving the patient the necessary time to prepare to stop.

Once a patient has selected a specific date to stop, information must be provided so that he or she can prepare for that date. For patients who can read, this is easily accomplished by providing them with a self-help brochure. Effective brochures provide the patient with necessary information about smoking cessation (e.g., symptoms and time course of withdrawal, tips about stopping, good reasons for stopping, answers to common questions). A list of brochures and other resources is provided later in the "Resources" section of this chapter. Patients who cannot read need to acquire this information from other sources, such as audiotapes, or from a clinician.

Arrange Follow-up Visits

When patients know their progress will be reviewed, their chances of successfully stopping improve. This monitoring may include a letter or telephone call from the office staff just before the quit date, reinforcing the decision to stop. Most relapses occur in the first weeks after cessation, and a person who comes to the office after being a nonsmoker for 1–2 weeks has a much improved chance of remaining abstinent (5). For this reason, it is critical that patients be contacted during their first 2 weeks of abstinence to reinforce their decision to stop. Follow-up office visits may be conducted by nurses or other clinicians and consist of an assessment of the patient's progress, discussion of any problems encountered or anticipated, and discussion of nicotine gum or patch use, if prescribed.

While follow-up visits are critical during the first 2 weeks after cessation, it is also important to offer patients a second follow-up visit with the physician or staff member in 1–2 months. For patients who decline this follow-up visit, contact by telephone or by mail may be helpful. Many patients can benefit from the social support and information offered through group smoking cessation programs. These are available in many communities through the American Cancer Society and the American Lung Association. However, clinicians should realize that very few patients referred to such programs will actually attend them (6). Therefore, such referrals should be given to augment, not replace, a clinician's care.

Patients may also express interest in techniques such as hypnosis and acupuncture. These have not been proven to be effective through randomized, controlled trials, but probably are not harmful. There is no reason to discourage their use by informed patients who wish to try these techniques.

Pharmacological Agents

Physicians should consider prescribing nicotine replacement therapy, especially for highly addicted patients—those who smoke more than a pack a day or who smoke within 30 minutes of waking. In clinical trials, nicotine gum and the nicotine transdermal patch generally have proven to be most helpful in the more addicted smoker when combined with advice and information from a physician or other health professional. Highly dependent smokers are often defined as patients who have experienced strong withdrawal symptoms during previous quit attempts, who smoke more than one pack of cigarettes per day, and who smoke their first cigarette within 30 minutes of waking.

The transdermal nicotine patch delivers nicotine through the skin. It is relatively easy for patients to use, placing minimal demands on their need for compliance, and often provides a higher level of nicotine replacement than nicotine gum. Several studies suggest that the patch reduces craving for cigarettes, a principal cause of smoking relapse (7). Randomized, controlled trials of nicotine patches have demonstrated long-term successful smoking cessation rates ranging from 22% to 42% among active patch users, compared with 5–28% among placebo patch users. It is important to recognize that these trials have been conducted using volunteer patients who are motivated to stop smoking. However, increased cessation rates among active patch users is a consistent finding across these trials. All trials published to date have used nicotine patches in combination with behavioral interventions.

Four brands of patches have been approved by the Food and Drug Administration for clinical use. Three brands are designed for 24-hour use (Prostep, Nicoderm, and Habitrol). The fourth brand (Nicotrol) is used for 16 hours each day, during the patient's waking hours. A lower nicotine dose during sleeping hours is thought to reduce vivid dreams and other mild sleep disorders that may be caused by higher levels of nicotine.

Patients should be provided with an information sheet on the patch and instructed in its proper use. If the patient does not stop smoking, treatment with the patch should be terminated. All four brands recommend that the patch be applied once every 24 hours, usually in the morning, to a nonhairy, clean, dry skin site on the upper torso or arm. Skin sites should be changed daily, and the same site not reused for at least 1 week. All brands of patch recommend a higher initial dose of nicotine (21–22 mg for the 24-hour patches, 15 mg for the 16-hour patch) for the first few weeks of treatment. Patients can then be given a lower dose patch for subsequent weeks. All brands except Prostep have a third and lowest dose patch for the final weaning period. A total of 6–8 weeks of treatment is recommended by the manufacturers, but shorter durations have also been used. Patients weighing less than 100 pounds and patients with cardiovascular disease may begin treatment with the lower dose patch.

The most common side effect of the nicotine patch is mild, transient itching or burning after application. Erythema, sometimes accompanied by edema, also occurs frequently at the patch site. Mild to moderate insomnia has also been reported as a side effect of the nicotine patch, but in some cases this may be caused by low nicotine levels associated with smoking cessation and not by the use of the patch. The nicotine patch is contraindicated for patients who have hypersensitivity or an allergy to nicotine, are pregnant, have serious arrhythmias or severe or worsening angina, or have had a recent myocardial infarction.

The cost of nicotine patches is a barrier to its use by some patients. However, the cost of this treatment may be less than the patient would spend on cigarettes during the same period. Physicians and pharmacists may assist patients with lower incomes by prescribing and selling patches for 1 or 2 weeks' use rather than making patients purchase the entire supply of patches at one time.

Nicotine polacrilex gum should not be chewed like chewing gum but instead chewed intermittently and then held in contact with the oral mucosa, where the nicotine is absorbed (8). Patients need careful instruction in the use of this unusual drug delivery system, or they will derive no benefit from it. The office staff can review its use with the patient. When the gum is used appropriately, withdrawal symptoms are reduced.

Using this gum for 3 months is recommended; a gradual tapering should follow. Use for more than 6 months is not recommended. However, using the gum for longer than 6 months is not rare among patients who successfully stop smoking. Physicians should warn patients of their intent to taper the dose of gum after 3 months.

Although a variety of other drugs have been used experimentally in smoking cessation, no others have been proven effective. Direct comparisons of nicotine polacrilex gum with nicotine patches have not been made; however, many patients prefer the patch because it is easy to use.

Office or Clinic Organization

Smoking cessation interventions will not be delivered to patients routinely and systematically, unless the office organization supports them. Some simple changes in office procedures will significantly increase the clinician's effectiveness in treating patients who smoke. The goal is to ensure that all patients who smoke are routinely identified, monitored, and appropriately treated. Office organizational procedures include selecting an office coordinator, making the office tobacco-free, systematically identifying and monitoring smokers, and involving staff members with the intervention and follow-up.

To act as a coordinated team, all members of the office staff need to understand that smoking cessation is an important task for the practice and they must know their roles. The team approach is facilitated by naming a smoking cessation coordinator, usually a nurse, who will incorporate the intervention into the day-to-day activities of the practice with the help of the other staff members, maintain the staff members' commitment to the program, and ensure that the system is operating smoothly (see Chapter 23). It is necessary to conduct periodic review of these activities and the performance of staff in their roles.

The team approach emphasizes staff identification of all patients who smoke. When patients are identified as smokers, their charts should be marked in a prominent manner. The typical identifier is a brightly colored permanent sticker or stamp, but this can be a removable sticker that is put on the chart at each visit. The regular use of these chart reminders has been shown to significantly increase cessation rates in office practices (9).

Staff members also should attach a progress card or flow sheet to the chart, thereby providing an easy way for the entire team to keep informed about the patient's current smoking status and allowing for brief cessation advice to become a routine part of every office visit for this patient. It is important that all staff members understand and implement this kind of charting system. See Chapter 23 for further details.

A staff member often will schedule the follow-up visits, make the contact just prior to the "quit date," and also may be the person who conducts some or all follow-up visits. Staff members also can review with patients their self-help materials and instructions for use of nicotine polacrilex gum or transdermal patches, if prescribed.

Steps for making an office or clinic tobacco-free include posting no smoking signs, removing ashtrays, displaying tobacco cessation and prevention information prominently, and eliminating tobacco advertising from the office, either by subscribing to magazines that do not carry this advertising or by crossing out the tobacco advertisements with bright markers. (A free list of publications that do not contain tobacco advertising can be obtained from the American Academy of Family Physicians by calling 800-274-2237, ext. 5542.)

COMMON PROBLEMS AND POSSIBLE SOLUTIONS

Weight Gain

The issue of weight gain is important to many patients who try to stop smoking. Some patients cite weight gain as the reason for relapse after previous attempts to stop. The average amount of weight gained after cessation is approximately 5 pounds. Some patients gain no weight after cessation, but a small proportion of people gain large amounts of weight.

Advice to a patient who is concerned about preventing weight gain can include two tactics. First, high-calorie foods should be avoided. Carrot and cinnamon sticks are time-honored, low-calorie foods that patients should have available whenever the urge to eat occurs. Attention to caloric intake may be recommended to patients to avoid weight gain (see Chapter 9). Second, recommend to weight-conscious smokers that they exercise more. This tactic may help prevent weight gain and provide the patient with activity that is usually incompatible with smoking, thus supporting smoke-free behavior (see Chapter 7).

Multiple Relapses

Many smoking patients, especially adults older than age 40, have made several serious attempts to stop but have always relapsed. These patients frequently have tried various stop-smoking products and programs, all without success. Such patients often are discouraged by their failed attempts to stop and, therefore, are less willing to try again.

These patients (and their health care providers) need to be aware that relapse is a typical part of cessation. Even in a relatively short clinic visit, a clinician can help a patient benefit from past relapses rather than view them as a personal failure and a reason to avoid future cessation attempts. During the visit, the clinician can help the patient to identify the circumstances that led to past relapses and to develop strategies for use in either avoiding those circumstances or responding to them in a different manner.

A simple question from the clinician, such as *"When you resumed smoking, where did your first cigarette come from?,"* will start the discussion of the reason for relapse. There are several common reasons offered for relapse, including withdrawal symptoms, weight gain, "stress" at work or home, alcohol intoxication, or social pressure. Once the patient has described the circumstances of the relapse, the clinician can ask, *"How would you deal with that situation if it happened again?"* or *"How could you avoid that situation in the future?"* The clinician can offer advice about some situations and help with withdrawal symptoms (see Table 6.2), but the patient must develop a specific plan for responding to circumstances that have caused past relapses.

Patients commonly say they relapsed because of stress, either at their job or at home. Marital difficulties, problems with other family members, loss of a job, or increased work responsibilities are often given as reasons for relapse. Patients, with the help of their physician, need to anticipate

Table 6.2
Responses to Patients' Common Questions and Concerns

1. I'm gaining weight.
Not every person who stops smoking gains weight.
Average weight gains are small for people who do gain (5–10 lbs).
Don't try to lose weight now—there will be time after you are an established nonsmoker.
Exercise is an effective technique to cope with withdrawal and to avoid weight gain.
Avoid high-calorie snacks. Vegetables (such as carrot sticks) and fruits are good snacks.
The risks to health from smoking are far greater than the risks to health from a small weight gain.
A small increase in weight may not hurt your appearance. Smoking is unattractive, causing yellow teeth, bad breath, stale clothing odors, and, possibly, wrinkled skin.
2. Now that I've stopped, can I smoke a cigarette occasionally?
No. Nicotine addiction seems to be retriggered quickly in most former smokers. Don't risk getting hooked again.
3. What should I do when I get an urge to smoke?
Some people relieve cravings by chewing gum, sucking on a cinnamon stick, or eating a carrot stick.
Cravings for cigarettes are a normal part of withdrawal.
Most cravings last for only a few minutes and then subside.
Cravings become rare after a few weeks.
Use nicotine gum, if prescribed.
4. When I don't smoke, I feel restless, and I can't concentrate.
These are normal symptoms of nicotine withdrawal.
These symptoms are most acute in the first 3 days after stopping.
These symptoms will disappear after a few weeks.
5. What other withdrawal symptoms will I have?
Some smokers have few or no withdrawal symptoms.
Other common symptoms include anxiety, irritability, insomnia, mild headache, and gastrointestinal symptoms such as constipation.
Few smokers experience all these symptoms.
Like other symptoms, they are only temporary.

difficult times while they are quitting and be prepared with a response other than smoking. Simple responses, such as chewing gum, taking a walk, or engaging in relaxation exercises, may be all that a patient needs to cope with a difficult personal situation. But having a concrete plan for these stressful situations is critical.

Lack of Social Support for Stopping

Social factors are frequently given as a reason for relapse, particularly when the patient is confronted by situations and friends who provide strong cues or prompts for smoking. Parties and other social gatherings are common sites of relapses, especially among patients who consume alcohol at these events.

During the time available in a brief office visit, major changes in the social skills and support of a patient cannot be expected. However, all patients should be encouraged to tell their family, friends, and coworkers of their decision to stop smoking and to seek their support and encouragement (6). Patients with little support for stopping can be referred to group cessation programs, if they are willing to attend. Referral to a counselor or other health professional also may be useful.

It is often difficult for a smoking patient to stop if his or her spouse also smokes and is unwilling to stop. The unwilling spouse should be encouraged to join in the quit attempt. If this is unsuccessful, the smoking spouse should at least be encouraged to smoke only outside the home.

SPECIAL POPULATIONS

As discussed earlier, the advice and assistance a clinician provides should reflect an understanding of the patient's medical, social, and cultural background. By asking the patient about anticipated problems with smoking cessation and potential solutions to these problems, the clinician can help the patient construct solutions that are relevant to his or her social and cultural setting. But clinicians should be prepared to provide factual medical information to any patient. For example, clinicians should be prepared to inform the older smoker who believes it is too late to stop that quitting can increase both the length and quality of life. Clinicians also need to recognize that smoking and tobacco use are viewed in different ways by different cultural groups, and that these views may influence how and why a patient stops. For example, some African Americans may be motivated to stop in order to free themselves from an addiction that is encouraged by large tobacco companies. Some Hispanic Americans may choose to stop because of concern about their family's health. An understanding of the patient's cultural norms will greatly aid any clinician in this work. Self-help materials designed for special population groups are becoming more widely available. These materials address both the cultural and language issues faced by patients, and are frequently available from local units of the American Cancer Society, American Lung Association, and local health departments.

Young people are another group who can benefit from the advice and assistance of clinicians. Because most smokers become addicted during childhood and adolescence, advice from clinicians during these periods is critical. Although any adolescent is a potential smoker, those at highest risk of becoming addicted have low self-esteem, poor academic performance, and engage in other risky behaviors such as alcohol and drug use. It is challenging but essential to provide these young people with anticipatory guidance that is appropriate for their age and developmental stage. Some clinicians have used cigarette advertisements to initiate discussions with adolescents, showing them the deceptive nature of the ads. When rapport with a young person is established, a clinicians can provide reasons for avoiding tobacco use that are relevant to an adolescent and can also help the patient practice refusal skills. Adolescents who are already regular smokers should be advised and assisted like an adult. However, adolescents are often much more concerned with the immediate effects of smoking, such as odors and poor athletic performance, and often are not influenced by risks of cancer and other diseases, which may not appear for many years.

Finally, children of any age should be protected from exposure to environmental tobacco smoke. Parents who smoke should be advised to stop and to keep their children in smoke-free environments, both at home and at day care and other settings. Some clinicians systematically identify passive smokers (including children) in their practices and routinely provide recommendations to reduce their exposure.

CONCLUSION

There is an enormous potential public health impact to be derived from clinical intervention with smoking patients. Even with very modest expectations of cessation rates, 100,000 physicians using effective intervention can enlist more than three million new ex-smokers each year. This, in conjunction with other tobacco-control efforts in communities, will result in a marked reduction in the morbidity and mortality caused by smoking and control of, according to former U.S. Surgeon General C. Everett Koop, M.D., "the most important public health issue of our time."

RESOURCES–PATIENT EDUCATION MATERIALS

American Academy of Family Physicians
8880 Ward Parkway

Kansas City, MO 64114-2797
800-944-0000

"Smoking: Steps to Help You Break the Habit" (brochure 1509); "When You're Ready to Stop" (brochure 902); "How Much Do You Know about Cigarette Smoking (brochure 903); "Stopping for Good" (brochure 904); "AAFP Stop Smoking Kit" (published in 1987: Provides instructions/materials necessary for establishing office-based smoking cessation program: physician's handbook, patient self-help materials, audiotapes for physicians and patients, sample charts, reminders, and motivating materials.

American Academy of Pediatrics
Publications Department
141 Northwest Point Blvd.
P.O. Box 927
Elk Grove Village, IL 60009-0927
800-433-9016

"Smoking: Straight Talk for Teens" (brochure HE0088).

American Cancer Society
1599 Clifton Road, NE
Atlanta, GA 30329
800-227-2345, 404-320-3333

"The Most Often Asked Questions about Smoking, Tobacco, and Health, and . . . the Answers" (brochure 2023.00); "Smokeless Tobacco: A Medical Perspective" (brochure 2090.00); "Tobacco-Free Young America: A Kit for Busy Practitioners" (published in 1989: Materials for physicians and office staff include National Cancer Institute/American Cancer Society booklet "Quit for Good: A Practitioner's Stop-Smoking Guide," "Tobacco-Free Young America: Questions and Answers," American Cancer Society resource list, samples of booklets, professional brochure on smokeless tobacco, patient chart stickers, nonsmoking contract, and legislator's cards. The American Cancer Society also has a slide/tape program for health professionals.)

American Dental Association
Division of Communications
211 East Chicago Avenue
Chicago, IL 60611

"Think Before You Chew" (brochure).

American Heart Association
7320 Greenville Avenue
Dallas, TX 75231
214-373-6300

"Calling It Quits" (packet 51-050A); "Smoking and Heart Disease" (brochure 51-1047, available in English and Spanish); "Children and Smoking: A Message to Parents" (brochure 51-033B, available in English and Spanish); "Weight Control Guidance in Smoking Cessation" (brochure 51-026A).

American Lung Association
1740 Broadway
New York, NY 10019
212-315-8700, 800-586-4872

"Freedom from Smoking" (self-help smoking cessation program); "Stop Smoking, Stay Trim: Gain Your Freedom, Control Your Weight" (brochure 2102); "A Healthy Beginning Counseling Kit" (published in 1989: Kit for pediatricians and family physicians, including guidebook on counseling about passive smoking, waiting room poster, tent card, and sample parent's packet).

National Cancer Institute
Office of Cancer Communication
Building 31, Room 10A16
9000 Rockville Pike
Rockville, MD 20892
800-4-CANCER

"Clearing the Air: How to Quit Smoking . . . And Quit for Keeps" (booklet 94-1647); "Smoking: Facts and Tips for Quitting" (booklet 93-3405); "Why Do You Smoke?" (quiz for selecting cessation techniques, 93-1822); "Smoking: Facts and Quitting Tips for Hispanics" (Spanish brochure 92-3405); "Smoking: Facts and Quitting Tips for Black Americans" (brochure 92-3405S); "Beat the Smokeless Habit" (booklet 92-3270); "How To Help Your Patients Stop Smoking: A National Cancer Institute Manual for Physicians" (Describes a brief physician intervention and simple office procedures that promote smoking intervention at every office visit.)

National Institute on Aging
NIA Information Center
P.O. Box 8057
Gaithersburg, MD 20898-8057
800-222-2225

"Smoking—It's Never Too Late to Stop."

REFERENCES

1. U.S. Department of Health and Human Services. Morbidity and mortality weekly report. Atlanta, GA: Centers for Disease Control and Prevention, 1993:1.
2. Glynn T, Manley M. How to help your patients stop smoking: a National Cancer Institute manual for physicians. National Cancer Institute. NIH Publication No. 89-3064. Bethesda, MD: National Institutes of Health, 1989.
3. Manley M, Epps RP, Glynn T. The clinician's role in promoting smoking cessation among clinic patients. Med Clin North Am 1992;76(2):477–494.
4. Cummings SR, Coates TJ, Richard RJ, et al. Training physicians in counseling about smoking cessation. A randomized trial of the Quit for Life program. Ann Intern Med 1989;110(8):640–647.
5. Kenford SL, Fiore MC, Jorenby DE, Smith SS, Wetter D, Baker TB. Predicting smoking cessation: who will quit with and without the nicotine patch. JAMA 1993;278(8):589–594.
6. Hollis JF, Lichtenstein E, Mount K, Vogt TM, Stevens VJ. Nurse-assisted smoking counseling in medical settings: minimizing demands on physicians. Prev Med 1991;20 (4):497–507.
7. Fiore MC, Jorenby DE, Baker TB, Kenford SL. Tobacco dependence and the nicotine patch. Clinical guidelines for effective use. JAMA 1992;268(19):2687–2694.
8. U.S. Department of Health and Human Services. The health consequences of smoking: nicotine addiction. A report of the Surgeon General. DHHS Publication No. (CDC) 88-8406. Washington, DC: U.S. Government Printing Office, 1988.
9. Cohen SJ, Stookey GK, Katz BP, Drook CA, Smith DM. Encouraging primary care physicians to help smokers quit. A randomized, controlled trial. Ann Intern Med 1989;110(8):648–652.

7. Exercise

STEVEN JONAS

INTRODUCTION

Definitions

The following definitions apply to the commonly used term *exercise*:

> *Physical activity* is "any bodily movement produced by skeletal muscles and resulting in energy expenditure." *Leisure activity* is "physical activity that a person or a group chooses to undertake during their discretionary time." *Exercise* is leisure time physical activity, while *training* is "repetitive bouts of exercise, conducted over periods of weeks or months, with the intention of developing physical and/or physiological fitness." (1)

In this chapter the term *regular exercise* refers to the combination of "exercise" and "training." In this chapter "regular exercise" also implies "sessions" or "workouts" or "going to the gym," rather than the more threatening-sounding "bouts."

Focus of Chapter

The U.S. Preventive Services Task Force recommends that "clinicians should counsel all patients to engage in a program of regular physical activity tailored to their health status and personal lifestyle" (2). Other groups have also encouraged physicians to counsel patients about exercise, including the American Academy of Family Physicians, the American College of Cardiology, the American Heart Association, the American College of Obstetricians and Gynecologists, and the U.S. Department of Health and Human Services.

This chapter focuses on the otherwise healthy patient: the sedentary person who wants to exercise; the sedentary person who needs to exercise for risk factor modification; and the exerciser who is looking for advice because of injury, burnout, or a need for consultation and reinforcement. This chapter specifically does not cover the role of regular exercise in either the treatment or management of disease or pathological conditions (such as hypertension), or rehabilitation (although many of the basic principles for helping any patient to become a regular exerciser happen to be the same).

BASIC CONCEPTS IN EXERCISE

Epidemiology of Exercise

Epidemiological data show that regular exercise promotes general health, while its lack, known variously as "physical inactivity" or "sedentary lifestyle," increases the risk of various diseases and negative health conditions (1–6). Less than 20% of adults in the United States exercise with sufficient frequency and intensity to improve cardiopulmonary fitness. The epidemiology of exercise and health/disease is discussed more fully in other sources (2, 7).

Exercise: Aerobic and Nonaerobic

Based on level of intensity, there are two types of regular exercise: "aerobic" and "nonaerobic." When intense enough to lead to a significant increase in muscle oxygen uptake, exercise is defined as "aerobic." Nonaerobic exercise is any physical activity above the normal resting state involving one or more major muscle groups that is sustained but not so intense as to cause a significant increase in muscle oxygen uptake. (Anaerobic exercise is intense physical activity, necessarily of very short duration, fueled by energy sources within the contracting muscles, without the use of inhaled oxygen.)

A simple measure of whether or not an episode of exercise is aerobic is the heart rate. If the pulse reaches or exceeds a level of 60% of the theoretical maximum normal, age-adjusted heart rate (220 minus the person's age), or $0.6(220 - \text{age})$, the exercise is considered aerobic. (It should be noted that this often-used formula only roughly approximates the true degree of increased oxygen uptake by the muscles (8) and is more accurate for measuring the intensity of exercise in beginners than in conditioned athletes.)

Qualitatively, one can assume that he or she is exercising aerobically if one is breathing deeply and sweating in mild to cold temperatures. Most regular exercisers do not routinely measure their heart rate during their workouts, relying instead on such subjective measures to know when they are "in the zone." Taking one's pulse, however, is definitely useful with extreme tachycardia. To assure that exercise intensity remains at a safe level, the pulse rate should remain below 85% of the person's theoretical maximum rate $(220 - \text{age})$.

While the evidence to date shows that for exercise to be beneficial in reducing long-term risk for coronary artery disease it must be aerobic, exercise at *any* level above the sedentary state is helpful for weight loss. And even modest levels of regular exercise (1 or 2 hours per week at nonaerobic intensity) probably reduce all-cause mortality. Moderate-intensity physical activity may also be beneficial.

Objectives for Regular Exercise

Given the known benefits of regular exercise and the harmful consequences of a sedentary lifestyle, the objectives for the activity can be set out
in a fairly straightforward manner. Among the "Priorities for Health Promotion and Disease Prevention" established by the U.S. Public Health Service's *Healthy People 2000* (9), "Physical Activity and Fitness" is listed first.
As the Healthy People Objectives note:

> Regular physical activity increases life expectancy, can help older adults main-
> tain functional independence, and enhances quality of life at each stage of
> life. The beneficial impact of physical activity touches widely on various dis-
> eases and conditions. (p. 55)

Most important for the clinician to know, however, is that regardless of the
accumulated data about the long-term health benefits of regular exercise,
most people who exercise regularly do so because it makes them feel good
and feel good about themselves *now*. When counseling patients about regular exercise, it is very important to bear this in mind. Further, not only do
most regular exercisers not engage in the activity to achieve future risk reduction, few nonexercisers will start for that reason (unless a negative
health event such as a first heart attack shocks them into appropriate action, or they are exercising to promote weight loss, which has both present
and future benefits).

When patients ask about the benefits of regular exercise, the clinician
should stress near-term gains: feeling good, improving personal appearance, increasing self-esteem. The clinician should stress that, while not
everyone will experience those benefits, most previously sedentary people
who become regular exercisers do.

Risks of Regular Exercise in the Otherwise Healthy Patient

Regular exercise carries with it a few risks as well as many benefits. Virtually all of the risks are preventable or modifiable. Most common is the risk
of injury. There are three types: intrinsic, extrinsic, and overuse. Intrinsic
injury is that caused by the nature of the activity or sport, e.g., shin splints
in running. Extrinsic injury is that caused by an external factor, e.g., a cy-
clist is hit by an automobile. Overuse injury results from trying to go too
far, too fast, too frequently. (The latter is the most common cause of injury
in most of the activities and sports used for regular exercise, such as running, fast walking, cycling, and swimming.)

Intrinsic injury can be ameliorated or prevented by the use of proper
equipment and correct technique. The risk of extrinsic injury can be significantly diminished by taking certain, mainly common sense, safety precautions, such as always wearing a helmet and not wearing a radio headset

while riding a bicycle (see Chapter 10). Overuse injury can be prevented by choosing a suitable sport and workout schedule, and by maintaining moderation in distance, intensity, and speed.

Intense exercise increases the risk of sudden death from myocardial infarction, but in the otherwise healthy person, these events occur primarily in previously sedentary individuals who suddenly engage in intense exercise, or in regular exercisers who suddenly begin working out at a much higher level of intensity. Thus moderation is, as always, good counsel.

GETTING UNDERWAY

"Recommendation" versus "Prescription"

Many clinicians use the term "exercise prescription" when discussing regular exercise with patients. The term hails from the disease and medical models and appeals to many clinicians, especially those new to using the intervention. "Prescription," however, means telling someone to do something, usually for a limited period of time. But regular exercise is by its very nature voluntary. No one can be forced to do it.

Furthermore, to make many other positive lifestyle changes, such as healthy eating, weight loss, smoking cessation, and substance abuse control, a regular part of patients' lives, they need to spend additional time only on a temporary basis. (For example, all people spend time food shopping and cooking. Healthy eating requires only that the time be spent differently.) In contrast, regular exercise is not only voluntary, but requires a permanent commitment of time. Clinicians should recognize this reality to be most effective in helping patients who want to become regular exercisers.

Thus, because of its special nature, exercise cannot be prescribed like a drug. Rather, the clinician is *recommending* an effort to become a regular exerciser. The aim should be to enter into a respectful partnership with patients, supporting their own decisions through advice and assistance rather than trying to tell them what to do. A primary need is to spend some time with patients just talking, communicating, recognizing obstacles to success, and equipping patients with the tools to overcome them.

Risk Assessment

Before recommending that any individual patient embark on a regular exercise program, the clinician should do a medical assessment. According to the U.S. Preventive Services Task Force, neither a resting electrocardiogram nor an exercise stress test provides information helpful in reducing the risk of an adverse outcome from regular exercise among asymptomatic persons; however, for a male over age 40 with two or more risk factors for coronary artery disease other than sedentary lifestyle (such as elevated serum cholesterol, a history of cigarette smoking, hypertension, diabetes mellitus, or a family history of early-onset coronary artery disease), a resting electrocardiogram or stress test may be indicated.

Further, the clinician should conduct a thorough evaluation (see Chapters 2 and 3) of patients for whom regular exercise presents a *definite* risk, before advising these patients to start exercising. These patients may have a history of one or more of the following diseases or conditions:

- Previous myocardial infarction;

- Exertional chest pain or pressure, or severe shortness of breath;

- Pulmonary disease, especially chronic obstructive pulmonary disease; and/or

- Bone, joint, or other musculoskeletal diseases or other limitations.

Patients for whom regular exercise presents a *possible* risk have a positive history of one or more of the following diseases or conditions:

- Hypertension;

- Cigarette smoking;

- High blood cholesterol;

- Prescription medication used on a regular basis;

- Abuse of drugs or alcohol; and/or

- Any other chronic illness, such as diabetes mellitus.

Regular exercise is very useful in the management of a number of these diseases and conditions; however, in such patients it must be embarked upon with care, especially stressing a slow, gradual, and careful start of whatever regimen is undertaken, and halting to consult with the clinician should any untoward symptoms be experienced.

COUNSELING

Getting Started

Goal-Setting

In most cases, the first subject to discuss with patients is goal setting: why is the patient even thinking about regular exercise? It may be because the patient's clinician suggested it, but virtually no one will become and remain a regular exerciser simply because he or she was told to do so. To succeed, the patient must mobilize internal motivation (see Chapter 5).

What goals does the patient want to accomplish, and why? Specifically, does the patient want to become fit, lose weight, look better and feel better, reduce future risk of various diseases and conditions, join a family member in a race? In both starting and staying with a regular exercise program it will be very helpful if patients have a good grasp of just why they are doing it in the first place.

Realism

The clinician should counsel patients to set realistic goals. A good formulation of this concept is to "explore your limits and recognize your limitations." Consider the example of endurance versus speed. After some reasonable period of training, say 3–4 months, most people can improve endurance, going quite a bit further or longer in their chosen activity without stopping than they could when they started training. They might not be able to go much faster, however. Going fast is the product of speed-specific training plus natural ability. Many people will be able to train fairly easily for endurance, which for most people is not simply the product of natural ability. But, because natural ability is such an important element in speed, not many will be able to go especially fast, no matter how hard they try. To help the patient avoid frustration, injury, and quitting, that fact should be addressed in counseling.

Inner Motivation

As noted in Chapter 5, the literature clearly shows that the only kind of motivation that works in the long run for positive lifestyle and behavior change comes from within. The patient says *"I want to do this for me, because I want to look better, feel better, feel better about myself, not for anyone else."* Purely external motivation (e.g., *"I'm doing this to make my (spouse, boy/girl friend, children/parents, employer/coworkers) feel better, but I don't anticipate getting much out of it for me"*) almost invariably leads to guilt, anxiety, anger, frustration, and, usually, injury and/or quitting.

Taking Control

"Taking control" is an important concept to stress with patients. In this formulation, patients decide to engage in physical activity on a regular basis, perhaps to do something with their bodies they have never done before or even contemplated doing. Many people find that "taking control" is an important motivator, both in starting a regular exercise program and sticking with it.

Gradual Change

"Gradual change leads to permanent change" is another basic element leading to success in becoming a regular exerciser, losing weight (see Chapter 9), and making other lifestyle changes. Thus, the previously sedentary person should start with ordinary walking, at a normal pace, for 10 minutes or so, three times a week. After a couple of weeks, the individual can increase the length of each session. Then he or she can increase the frequency of sessions, and after several more weeks, the speed with which the exercise is performed.

The hardier soul may move through this program more quickly, but all should be counseled against going out for an hour, at full tilt, on the first day, or even on the fifth or tenth. "Too much, too soon" is bound to lead to muscle pain, perhaps injury, and an increased likelihood of early quitting. Once again, a *gradual* increase in time spent, distance covered, and speed is the proven formula for adherence.

Getting Started: "It's the Regular, Not the Exercise"

Finally, the clinician should recognize that, for most people, the first challenge of becoming a regular exerciser is the "regular," not the "exercise." Most people are aware that they should exercise, that it is "good for them," even that they will feel better. But most people are busy and have schedules and other demands that cannot accommodate exercise on a regular basis.

Thus, the correct first step for many is not to learn a particular sport or activity, but rather to discover that they can indeed find the time for exercise in their lives, if they are motivated to do so. By first addressing the challenge of making the time, as suggested by the very modest training program in Table 7.1, they can actually reinforce their motivation. Making the time, rather than learning a sport or athletic activity, should be the focus of the first 2–4 weeks of an exercise program. Thus, most persons can begin with ordinary walking. This approach shows patients that the clinician understands their reality.

Duration and Frequency

The original regular exercise recommendation of the American College of Sports Medicine was that, to benefit health, it should be performed contin-

Table 7.1
The PaceWalking Plan (Phase I: Introductory Program)

Week	Day	M	T	W	Th	F	S	S	Total	Comments
				(Times in Minutes)						
1		Off	10	Off	10	Off	Off	10	30	Ordinary
2		Off	10	Off	10	Off	Off	10	30	walking
3		Off	20	Off	20	Off	Off	20	60	Ordinary
4		Off	20	Off	20	Off	Off	20	60	walking
5		Off	20	Off	20	Off	Off	20	60	Fast
6		Off	20	Off	20	Off	Off	20	60	walking
7		Off	20	Off	20	Off	Off	30	70	Fast
8		Off	20	Off	20	Off	Off	30	70	walking
9		Off	20	Off	20	Off	Off	20	60	Pace
10		Off	20	Off	20	Off	Off	30	70	Walking
11		Off	20	Off	30	Off	Off	30	80	Pace
12		Off	20	Off	30	Off	Off	30	80	Walking
13		Off	30	Off	30	Off	Off	30	90	Pace Walking

uously for a minimum of 20–60 minutes at least three times per week (7). This recommendation assumed that the exercise would be done at the aerobic level of intensity. In the tables for regular exercise schedules presented in this chapter (Tables 7.1–7.4), the recommended duration and periodicity are also based on the assumption that the exercise will be done at the aerobic level of intensity.

However, recent research and analysis have shown that physical activity, even at a moderate level of intensity, can also be beneficial to health (7). Thus, in 1995, the U.S. Centers for Disease Control and Prevention and the American College of Sports Medicine jointly recommended that, for persons not engaging in regular aerobic exercise at the original American

Table 7.2
The PaceWalking Plan (Phase II: Developmental Program)

Week	Day	M	T	W	Th	F	S	S	Total
				(Times in Minutes)					
1		Off	Off	Off	Off	Off	Off	Off	Off
2		Off	20	Off	20	Off	Off	20	60
3		Off	20	Off	20	Off	20	20	80
4		Off	20	Off	20	Off	20	30	90
5		Off	20	Off	30	Off	20	30	100
6		Off	20	Off	30	Off	20	40	110
7		Off	30	Off	30	Off	30	30	120
8		Off	30	Off	30	Off	30	40	130
9		Off	30	Off	40	Off	30	40	140
10		Off	30	Off	40	Off	30	50	150
11		Off	40	Off	30	Off	30	60	160
12		Off	40	Off	30	Off	40	60	170
13		Off	30	Off	40	Off	50	60	180

Table 7.3
The PaceWalking Plan (Phase III A: Maintenance—Two Hours per Week)

Week	Day	M	T	W	Th	F	S	S	Total
				(Times in Minutes)					
1		Off	Off	Off	Off	Off	Off	Off	Off
2		Off	30	Off	30	Off	40	Off	100
3		30	Off	40	Off	20	Off	40	130
4		Off	40	Off	30	Off	40	Off	110
5		30	Off	40	Off	20	Off	40	130
6		Off	40	Off	30	Off	60	Off	130
7		20	Off	30	Off	30	Off	40	120
8		Off	40	Off	30	Off	50	Off	120
9		20	Off	40	Off	20	Off	60	140
10		Off	30	Off	30	Off	40	Off	100
11		20	Off	30	Off	20	Off	40	110
12		Off	40	Off	30	Off	60	Off	130
13		20	Off	30	Off	30	Off	40	120

Table 7.4
The PaceWalking Plan (Phase III B: Maintenance Plus—Three Hours per Week)

Week	Day	M	T	W	Th	F	S	S	Total
				(Times in Minutes)					
1		Off	Off	Off	Off	Off	Off	Off	Off
2		Off	30	Off	40	Off	30	50	150
3		Off	30	Off	50	Off	40	60	180
4		Off	40	Off	40	Off	50	80	210
5		Off	30	Off	50	Off	40	60	180
6		Off	50	Off	30	Off	50	70	200
7		Off	40	Off	30	Off	30	60	160
8		Off	30	Off	50	Off	40	60	180
9		Off	30	Off	40	Off	30	50	150
10		Off	30	Off	50	Off	40	50	170
11		Off	40	Off	30	Off	50	70	190
12		Off	40	Off	40	Off	50	80	210
13		Off	30	Off	50	Off	40	60	180

College of Sports Medicine standard, an accumulated 30 minutes daily of moderate-intensity physical activity should be performed on as many days of the week as possible (7).

Choosing the Activity or Sport

Once the patient has begun dealing with the problem of "regular," and has learned that it is soluble, he or she will most likely want to get on to doing one or more specific sports or activities. (At the end of this chapter there is a list of suggested readings covering a variety of sports.) The first point the clinician should stress is that regular exercise is not limited to running or aerobic dance. There is a wide range of activities or sports that can be used for regular exercise, whether aerobic or nonaerobic.

There are the tried and true sports to which most people have access: running or jogging, fast walking, bicycling, and aerobic dance and its many variants, done at home, usually to the accompaniment of a videotape or television show. Less common, but suitable for home use, are such activities as rope-jumping and jogging in place on a small trampoline.

Less widely available to many are activities that usually require an athletic facility, such as swimming, stairclimbing on a machine, and group aerobic dance and its variants. Those sports listed in the preceding paragraph that are usually done outdoors of course can be performed indoors in a health club or gym if a track, treadmill, or stationary bicycle is available. A treadmill, stairclimber, or stationary bicycle can be purchased for home use as well. (For cycling, there are also devices called "indoor trainers" on which road bicycles can be mounted for riding in place.)

There are more esoteric sports with limited access for most people, like cross-country skiing and rowing in a scull or similar vessel. Machines are available on which people can do similar exercises indoors, either at home or at a health club.

Certain skill sports, both individual and team, can be done aerobically and are useful for regular exercise. These include singles tennis, squash, racquetball, handball, and full-court basketball. They require an athletic facility with courts and at least one partner. Weight training, whether with free weights or a machine, whether at home or in the gym, also can be done aerobically. As contrasted with weight training for strength and bulk, aerobic routines stress lighter resistance, more repetitions and sets of each program component, and less time between sets to keep the heart rate in the training range.

Some health clubs feature "circuit training," provided by a set of machines and stations offering different resistance. Aerobic exercises are performed by participants in series, following a timed schedule established by a prerecorded set of instructions broadcast in the circuit training area by loudspeaker.

The choice of potential sports and activities for regular exercise is therefore very broad. No one sport is "better" than any other sport for regular exercise. The heart and muscles do not "know" which sport the person is doing. If the activity increases heart rate and muscle oxygen uptake to a given level, the benefit will be the same, regardless of the sport. Thus, for example, "PaceWalking," fast walking with a strong armswing, is as "good" as running, if each is done to the same level of intensity. (With a strong armswing, PaceWalking at a rate of 11–12 minutes per mile is usually as demanding on the cardiovascular system as running 8–9 minutes per mile.)

After dealing with the problem of the "regular" by engaging in ordinary walking, it is most important that the patient choose a sport that he or she will enjoy. In fact, the chances of adhering to regular exercise will be increased if the patient chooses two different sports or activities (e.g., going down to the health club once or twice a week for low-impact aerobic dance, and PaceWalking once or twice a week). To decrease the chances of getting bored, once getting into the routine, the activities can be varied over the course of the year.

Making Exercise "Fun"

When contemplating regular exercise, many patients will say, *"Well, I know I should exercise, but I know it just isn't going to be fun."* In fact, some people find to their surprise that "just doing it" is fun, in itself. For others, unfortunately, regular exercise will never be fun. For them it would be wise to limit the total weekly exercise time (e.g., no more than 1–2 hours per week). For the third, middle group, there are some techniques for making exercise more enjoyable. (Over the long run, these techniques can also help those in the first group to maintain the fun level.)

- Let it be fun: positive anticipation is very important.

- Set appropriate goals, and avoid doing too much, too soon, as discussed previously.

- For the distance sports, train by minutes, not miles (see later in this chapter).

- Recognize that, in many distance sports in which concentration on technique is not required, time spent is uniquely private, thinking time. (For safety considerations, road bicycling should not be viewed this way.)

- Listen to music, the news, or radio talk shows through a headset. (Appropriate safety measures must be taken, however. Outdoor use of in-the-ear headphones can block out the sounds of traffic, animals, and other individuals approaching. Rather, sponge phones mounted on the temple in front of the auditory canal should be used.)

- Set nonexercise-related goals, like getting an errand or two completed in the course of a workout.

- Periodically reward oneself, with a new piece of clothing, or a long-denied snack treat.

- Many regular exercisers find that occasional racing, not for speed but for participation and personal achievement in terms of distance covered or time spent, is a very useful way to stay on a program and enjoy it.

Generic Training Program

Tables 7.1 to 7.4 present a generic training program from the beginning phase through regular maintenance, at all levels up to the training level required for racing on a regular basis. Note that the workouts are measured in minutes, not miles. Therefore, they can be used for any sport or activity the patient decides to undertake. Furthermore, by measuring workouts in minutes the mental and physical stressor of speed is removed for the distance sports. Psychologically, it is much easier to PaceWalk regularly for 40 minutes at a stretch than it is to cover 3 or 4 miles. If the person is feeling good and the weather is nice, he or she will go faster and cover more ground. A bit of stiffness on a given day will lead to a slower workout. But with minutes rather than miles defining the workout, what counts is the duration, not the speed. Also, as previously noted, the minutes formula allows the person to easily mix and match sports or activities in a single program.

The periodicity and duration of the sessions comprising the program recommended in these tables are based on the assumption that the person will be engaging in a *regular exercise* program, at a level of intensity eventually reaching at least to the lower end of the aerobic range. Of course, if the patient cannot or does not want to do this, it will be useful to suggest the new minimum recommendations of accumulating 30 minutes per day of *physical activity* at a moderate level of intensity, over the course of the day, on most days of the week (7). Physical activities that can produce a moderate level of intensity (4–7 kcal/minute) include walking briskly (3–4 mph), cycling for pleasure or transportation (≤10 mph), swimming with moderate effort, conditioning exercises and general calisthenics, table tennis, golf (without the use of a motorized cart), fishing (standing, casting), leisurely canoeing (2.0–3.9 mph), home care and repairs, general cleaning, mowing the lawn with a power mower, and painting (7).

The Introductory Program (Table 7.1) starts with ordinary walking and concludes with PaceWalking (see next section for a brief description of the technique). At the end, the person will be working out for 1.5 hours per week. The Developmental Program (Table 7.2) takes the exerciser up to 3 hours per week.

There are two Maintenance Programs. The one in Table 7.3 provides an average of 2 hours per week over a 13-week period, while that in Table 7.4 provides an average of 3 hours per week. The latter is the equivalent of 15–20 miles per week of running, all that is required to gain the maximum health benefits from regular exercise. (Musculoskeletal fitness increases with exercise intensity, time, and distance, up to about 75 miles of running per week.)

Note that, once a four-day-per-week level is reached, in either Phase II or Phase IIIB, more than half of the total workout time is scheduled for the weekends, making the program more convenient for most people. (Phase IIIA is an every-other-day program, requiring only two hours per week, on the average.) Some stretching before each workout is recommended. There are books devoted entirely to stretching (see "Resources" later in this chapter), and most sport-specific books also have a section on stretching.

Following these programs will allow virtually anyone who so desires to become a regular exerciser—slowly, gradually, and without the need to make an overwhelming time commitment.

Technique

The clinician need not be a technical expert in the sports or activities suitable for regular exercise. There are many good books written for the layman on the subject (see "Resources" later in the chapter for some examples). If exercise counseling becomes a regular part of the practice, the clinician may benefit from periodic visits to local bookshops to see what books are available.

The technique for the recommended starting sport, PaceWalking, is very simple. Here are sample instructions for the patient:

> Walk fast with a purposeful stride of medium length. With each step, land on your heel, then roll forward along the outside of the foot, and push off with the toes. Try to keep your feet pointed straight ahead, walking on an imagi-

nary white line. This will help your balance and rhythm, and will allow you to increase your speed.

The back should be comfortably straight, but not rigidly so. The shoulders should be dropped and relaxed, the head up. Swing the arms forward and back, strongly, with the elbows comfortably bent. (The elbow bend prevents the accumulation of fluid in the hands, which will happen if you swing the arms strongly while keeping them straight.) At the end of the back swing, you should feel a tug in your shoulder. On the foreswing, the hand should come up no further than midchest level. To stay in balance and maintain a smooth forward motion from the hips down, concentrate on the back swing, not the foreswing. And that's all there is to it.

For most people, it is the strong armswing that makes PaceWalking aerobic. If a person has been completely sedentary for some time, with the initiation of regular exercise, just walking quickly will most likely raise the heart rate into the aerobic range. But after he or she has been working out more regularly, fast walking alone will be insufficient. If the goal of walking is to exercise aerobically, a second major muscle group must be brought into play (i.e., swinging the arms strongly).

Equipment

As with technique, details on equipment can be found in various sport-specific books. Common to most regular exercise sports or activities is the need for properly fitting shoes (to achieve success and avoid injury). Proper fit means that the shoe should be shaped like one's foot; it should touch one's foot in as many places as possible, except over the toes; it should be flexible under the ball of the foot; and it should have a firm heel counter to keep the heel down in the shoe.

The shoe's sole design should be suited to the sport for which it will be used, i.e., shoes for PaceWalking or running should facilitate forward motion, shoes for tennis or aerobic dance should facilitate lateral motion. (If a patient has particular lower extremity weakness, say in the ankles, or a known foot deformity such as hallux valgus, consider a referral to a sports medicine orthopaedist or podiatrist for evaluation for orthotic inserts or special shoes.)

In general, a person should buy equipment in a "pro shop" rather than in a department store. A pro shop is a store dedicated to sports equipment. In general, the more sports-specific the store's focus, the more likely the buyer will come away with suitable equipment. In a pro shop, the buyer is more likely to find salespeople who are knowledgeable about the sport for which they are selling equipment and more likely to actually engage in the sport themselves.

The cost of equipment for the regular exerciser can range from nothing (the person decides to PaceWalk or jog, and their wardrobe already includes an adequate pair of shoes and the necessary clothing), to hundreds or even several thousand dollars for a health club membership, high-performance athletic shoes, or a top-of-the-line bicycle. The best recommendation for beginners is to spend as little as possible, except on buying good shoes if they lack a pair, until they are convinced they are going to stay with the sport.

OFFICE AND CLINIC ORGANIZATION

These principles must be reduced to a counseling package that can be used successfully in clinical practice. First, of course, the clinician must decide whether exercise counseling is important for some or all patients. To do that, the clinician should follow the same goal-setting process that the potential exerciser undertakes as his or her first step. See the questions posed in the section on "Setting Reasonable Limits and Priorities in Risk Assessment" in Chapter 1. It will also be necessary to decide the following:

- Is the primary clinician in the office going to offer individual counseling directly?

- Will counseling be provided by someone else in the practice or office who is qualified (or can be trained)?

- Alternatively, will exercise counseling be offered to groups of patients, rather than on an individual basis?

- Will this be done during regular office hours and/or in the evening? (There have been reports by practitioners of success with groups, meeting one evening a week, for a modest fee per person.)

As noted above, a list of patient education resources is provided at the end of this chapter. Community resources can also be used, either in place of or in addition to what is being done in the office, e.g., health clubs, sports clubs, gyms, pools, tracks, bicycle routes, walking or running trails, courts, and pro shops.

If it is decided to incorporate exercise promotion into routine clinical practice, it is worth spending time to learn about and evaluate the various community resources. Doing so saves time and provides substantive assistance to patients. The clinician can consider setting up a formal referral relationship with particularly good community facilities.

However exercise counseling is done, the clinician should make it a regular part of the practice and keep proper notes in the patient's medical record.

Finally, while not essential, clinicians who regularly exercise themselves can set examples for patients and can talk from the experience (knowing both the benefits and the difficulties) of being a regular exerciser.

RESOURCES–PATIENT EDUCATION MATERIALS

General

American Academy of Family Physicians
8880 Ward Parkway
Kansas City, MO 64114-2797
800-944-0000
   "Exercise: A Healthy Habit to Start and Keep" (brochure 1564).

American Heart Association
7320 Greenville Avenue
Dallas, TX 75231
214-373-6300
   "'E' is for Exercise" (brochure 51-1039, in English and Spanish); "About Your Heart and
   Exercise" (brochure 51-1038); "Why Exercise?" (reduced reading level brochure 64-
   1020); "Exercise Diary" (51-1016).

National Heart, Lung, Blood Institute Information Center
P.O. Box 30105
Bethesda, MD 20824-0105
301-951-3260
   "Exercise and Your Heart: A Guide to Physical Activity" (brochure 93-1677).

National Institute on Aging
NIA Information Center
P.O. Box 8057
Gaithersburg, MD 20898-8057
800-222-2225
   "Don't Take It Easy—Exercise!"

Running

Brown RL, Henderson J. Fitness running. Champaign, IL: Human Kinetics Publishers, 1994.
Cooper KH. Running without fear. New York: M. Evans and Co., 1985.
Fixx J. The complete book of running. New York: Random House, 1977.
Galloway J. Galloway's book on running. Bolinas, CA: Shelter Publications, 1984.
Glover B, Schuder P. The competitive runner's handbook. New York: Viking Penguin, 1988.
Glover B, Shepherd J. The runner's handbook. New York: Viking Penguin, 1985.
Hanc J. The essential runner. New York: Lyons and Burford, 1993.
Lebow F, Averbuch G. Friends, The New York Road Runners Club complete book of
   running. New York: NYRRC, 1992.

Bicycling

Carmichael C, Burke ER. Fitness cycling. Champaign, IL: Human Kinetics Publishers, 1994.
LeMond G, Gordis K. Greg LeMond's complete book of bicycling. New York:
   Perigee/Putnam, 1990.
Lieb T. Everybody's book of bicycle riding. Emmaus, PA: Rodale Press, 1981.

Swimming and Water Exercise

Katz J. Swimming for total fitness, updated. Garden City, NY: Doubleday/Main St. Press,
   1993.
Katz J. The W.E.T. workout. New York: Facts on File Publications, 1985.
Thomas, DG. Swimming: steps to success. Champaign, IL: Human Kinetics Press, 1989.

Walking

Balboa D, Balboa D. Walk for life. New York: Perigee Books/Putnum, 1990.
Rockport's fitness walking for women. Perigee/Putnam, 1987.
Meyers C. Walking: A complete guide to the complete exercise. New York: Random House, 1992.
Yanker G. Walking medicine: the lifetime guide to the complete exercise. New York: Random House, 1992.

Aerobics

Fox M, Broide D. Molly Fox's step on it. New York: Avon Books, 1991.
Lance K. Low-Impact aerobics. New York: Crown Publishers, 1988.
Rosas D, Rosas C, Martin K. Non-impact aerobics. New York: Villard, 1987.

Weight Training

Baechle TR, Groves BR. Weight training: steps to success. Champaign, IL: Leisure Press, 1992.
Schwarzenegger A. Arnold's bodybuilding for men. New York: Fireside/Simon and Schuster, 1981.
Vedral J. Now or never. New York: Time Warner, 1986.

Stretching

Anderson B, Anderson J. Stretching. New York: Random House, 1980.

Triathloning

Jonas S. Triathloning for ordinary mortals. New York: WW Norton, 1986.
Jonas S. The essential triathelete. New York: Lyons and Burford, in press.
Tinley S. Scott Tinley's winning triathlon, New York: Contemporary Books, 1986.

Periodicals

Runners' World, Rodale Press, Emmaus, PA.
Bicycling, Rodale Press, Emmaus, PA.
The Walking Magazine, Walking, Inc., Boston, MA.
Inside Triathlon, Boulder, CO.
Triathlete, San Francisco, CA.

SUGGESTED READINGS

American Heart Association. Statement on exercise. Dallas, TX: American Heart Association, 1992.
American Academy of Orthopaedic Surgeons. Athletic training and sports medicine, 2nd ed. Park Ridge, IL: American Academy of Orthopaedic Surgeons, 1991.
Jonas S. Regular exercise: a handbook for clinical practice. New York: Springer-Verlag, in press.
Long B, et al. Project PACE: physician-based assessment and counseling for exercise. Atlanta, GA: U.S. Centers for Disease Control and Prevention, 1992.

REFERENCES

1. Bouchard C, Shephard RJ, Stephens T, et al., eds. Exercise, fitness, and health: A consensus of current knowledge. Champaign, IL: Human Kinetics Books, 1990:6.
2. U.S. Preventive Services Task Force. Guide to clinical preventive services. Baltimore: Williams & Wilkins, 1989:297.

3. Blair SN, Kohl HW, Paffenbarger RS, et al. Physical fitness and all-cause mortality. JAMA 1989;262:2395–2401.

4. Harris SS, Caspersen CJ, De Friese GH, et al. Physical activity counseling for healthy adults. JAMA 1989;261:3590–3598.

5. Paffenbarger RS, Hyde RT, Wing AL, et al. The association of changes in physical-activity level and other lifestyle characteristics with mortality among men. N Engl J Med 1993;328:538–45.

6. Sandvik L, Erikssen J, Thaulow E, et al. Physical fitness as a predictor of mortality among healthy, middle-aged Norwegian men. N Engl J Med 1993;328:533–537.

7. Pate RR, Pratt, M, Blair SN, Haskell WL, Macera CA, Bouchard C, et al. Physical activity and public health: a recommendation from the Centers for Disease Control and Prevention and the American College of Sports Medicine. JAMA 1995;273:402–407.

8. Wier LT, Jackson AS. Exercise intensity: Misleading measurements. Running and FitNews 1993; 11(2):1.

9. U.S. Department of Health and Human Services, Public Health Service. Healthy People 2000: National Health Promotion and Disease Prevention Objectives. DHHS Pub. No. (PHS) 91-50213. Washington, DC: Government Printing Office, 1991.

8. Nutrition

MARION NESTLE

INTRODUCTION

Optimal diets should provide energy and the full complement of essential nutrients in proportions that maximize health and longevity, prevent nutritional deficiencies as well as conditions related to nutritional excesses and imbalances, and be obtained from foods that are available, palatable, acceptable, and affordable. Throughout human history, societies have developed a great variety of dietary patterns and practices that fulfill these requirements.

With improvements in economic status, dietary patterns throughout the world have tended to shift from a dependence on plant foods as sources of energy and nutrients to an increasing reliance on animal foods that are higher in fat, saturated fat, and cholesterol. This shift has been accompanied by a decline in the prevalence of health problems related to undernutrition, and an increase in the prevalence of diet-related chronic diseases.

Since the 1940s, chronic diseases such as coronary heart disease, certain cancers, diabetes, and stroke have replaced infectious diseases and conditions related to undernutrition as leading causes of death among adults in the United States. The role of diet in chronic disease prevention is well established (1–3). Substantial evidence indicates that the typical American diet—high in energy, fat, saturated fat, cholesterol, salt, sugar, and alcohol, but low in starch and fiber—contributes to chronic disease incidence and severity. Some estimates suggest that as much as one-third of coronary heart disease and cancer incidence can be attributed to dietary factors. An estimated 60 million adults have high blood cholesterol levels, 60 million have high blood pressure, and 30 million are obese; many of these individuals could benefit from improved dietary intake. Diet and physical inactivity account for an estimated 300,000 deaths each year in the United States (4).

Recommendations for clinicians to counsel patients about healthy nutritional habits have been issued by the American Academy of Family Physicians, American College of Physicians, American College of Obstetricians and Gynecologists, U.S. Preventive Services Task Force, Canadian Task Force on the Periodic Health Examination, American Heart Association, and American Dietetic Association. This chapter focuses on ways to help patients reduce dietary risk factors for the leading chronic diseases.

Dietary Recommendations

Quantitative Dietary Goals

Since the early 1960s, health associations and government agencies have issued dietary recommendations for chronic disease prevention. These recommendations have remained remarkably consistent over time, and are universal in that they apply equally well to prevention of the full range of diet-related chronic conditions (1, 2). They include:

- Energy: balance intake and expenditure to maintain desirable body weight.
- Fat: < 30% of total kcal.
- Saturated fat: < 10% of total kcal.
- Cholesterol: < 300 mg per day.
- Sodium: 1.1–3.3 g/day (average 2.4).
- Fiber: 25–30 g/day.

Dietary Guidelines

To help the public translate these recommendations into diets that provide sufficient energy and nutrients yet minimize dietary risks for chronic disease, federal agencies periodically issue dietary guidelines for Americans. The 1990 Guidelines state:

- Eat a variety of foods.
- Maintain healthy weight.
- Choose a diet low in fat, saturated fat, and cholesterol.
- Choose a diet with plenty of vegetables, fruits, and grain products.
- Use sugars only in moderation.
- Use salt and sodium only in moderation.
- If you drink alcoholic beverages, do so in moderation.

The next revision of the Guidelines is expected in 1995.

Food Guide Pyramid

The most recent food guide, illustrated in Figure 8.1, is designed to help individuals translate these recommendations into appropriate food choices. The Pyramid recommends that the daily diet contain 6–11 portions of cereal foods, 2–4 of fruits, 3–5 of vegetables, 2–3 of meats or meat substitutes, and 2–3 of dairy foods. Few Americans eat this way, however, leaving much room for positive dietary advice. The National Cancer Institute's "5-A-Day" campaign to encourage the public to consume five fruits

Food Guide Pyramid
A Guide to Daily Food Choices

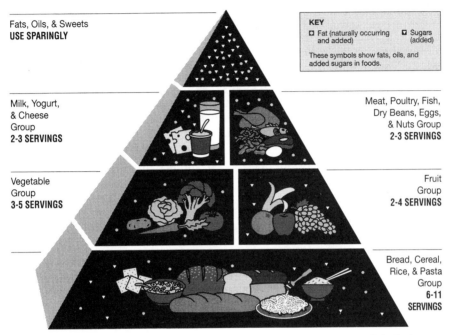

Fats, Oils, & Sweets
USE SPARINGLY

KEY
☐ Fat (naturally occurring and added)   ☑ Sugars (added)

These symbols show fats, oils, and added sugars in foods.

Milk, Yogurt, & Cheese Group
2-3 SERVINGS

Meat, Poultry, Fish, Dry Beans, Eggs, & Nuts Group
2-3 SERVINGS

Vegetable Group
3-5 SERVINGS

Fruit Group
2-4 SERVINGS

Bread, Cereal, Rice, & Pasta Group
6-11 SERVINGS

Figure 8.1. The Food Guide Pyramid, designed by the U.S. Department of Agriculture to help individuals choose healthy diets through daily intake of specific numbers of servings of foods from various groups.

and vegetables daily promotes consumption of diets that meet the Pyramid guidelines.

Dietary Counseling

Need

Surveys indicate that the American public is increasingly aware of relationships between diet and disease, and has made some improvements such as substitution of low-fat for full-fat dairy products. The proportion of energy consumed as fat remains much higher than is recommended, however, and less than 10 percent of the population consumes the recommended number of fruits and vegetables on any given day. Many features of modern life—dual career families, increasing consumption of meals outside the home, promotion of foods high in calories, fat, salt, and sugar—constitute barriers to translation of dietary knowledge into action. To help counteract these barriers, the Public Health Service has called for an increase in the proportion of primary care providers who offer nutrition assessment, counseling, and referral services (5). One reason for this objective is that the public considers physicians to be the most credible sources of nutrition advice. These principles underlie the approach to nutritional counseling outlined in this chapter.

Studies involving dietitians support the efficacy of counseling in improving patients' dietary knowledge, attitudes, and behavior. Although attitudes and eating behavior often resist change, the resistance can be overcome by counseling strategies that target specific eating behaviors, use multiple methods to achieve dietary change, are adjusted in response to evaluation, provide ongoing support, and allow sufficient time for changes to occur.

Many clinicians might like to provide such services, but lack the time, knowledge, skills, or confidence to take dietary histories, advise patients about food choices, or address barriers to appropriate dietary intake. This chapter, therefore, emphasizes specific ways clinicians can promote the benefits of good nutrition to patients, advise them about desirable dietary practices, and refer them to qualified nutrition professionals for more detailed dietary counseling.

General Principles

The objective of dietary counseling for chronic disease prevention should be to achieve normal weight, blood pressure, and serum cholesterol, as well as a more healthful food intake. The success of counseling efforts can be monitored by observing changes in measurable risk factors over time; favorable changes should become evident within 3–6 weeks of the onset of diet therapy.

Content. The basic principles of healthful diets apply to virtually all dietary interventions. Diets should be adequate—but not excessive—in energy, and should follow the guidelines illustrated in Figure 8.1. The serving sizes in the Food Guide Pyramid are intended to be small (e.g., 1 slice bread, 1 oz cereal, $1/2$ cup fruit or vegetable, 2–3 oz meat, 1 cup milk, 1.5 oz cheese), and patients should be able to consume the recommended numbers of servings.

These guidelines should greatly simplify nutritional counseling, as the basic principles apply to all diet-related chronic diseases:

- Eat more fruits, vegetables, and grains. Diets containing a large proportion of energy from fruits, vegetables, and grains are naturally low in calories, fat, saturated fat, cholesterol, salt, and sugar, but are high in vitamins, minerals, fiber, and protective nutrients such as antioxidants. Patients should be advised to increase the proportion of plant foods in their diets.

- Choose lean meats and low-fat dairy products. To reduce intake of fat and cholesterol, patients should be advised to choose the leaner cuts of meat, to substitute chicken and fish for beef, and to select lower-fat dairy foods.

- Avoid processed, packaged, and prepared foods containing added fat, salt, and sugar. Processed foods are the major sources of salt, sodium, and sugar in American diets. Patients should be advised to read package labels (see section "Use of Food Labels" later in this chapter).

- Limit the use of salt and sugar in cooking and at the table. Because the amounts of added salt and sugar usually are small relative to the amounts added to processed foods, this advice is likely to be most helpful to heavy users.

Table 8.1 summarizes this advice and provides more specific methods for making dietary changes and substitutions.

Table 8.1
Recommended Diet Modifications to Lower Blood Cholesterol: the Step-One Diet[a]

Food Group	Choose	Decrease
Lean Meat, Poultry, and Fish ≤5–6 oz. per day	Beef, pork, lamb—lean cuts well trimmed before cooking Poultry without skin Fish, shellfish Processed meat— prepared from lean meat, e.g., lean ham, lean frankfurters, lean meat with soy protein or carrageenan	Beef, pork, lamb—regular ground beef, fatty cuts, spare ribs, organ meats Poultry with skin, fried chicken Fried fish, fried shellfish Regular luncheon meat, e.g., bologna, salami, sausage, frankfurters
Eggs ≤4 yolks per week, Step I ≤2 yolks per week, Step II	Egg whites (two whites can be substituted for one whole egg in recipes), cholesterol-free egg substitute	Egg yolks (if more than four per week on Step I or if more than two per week on Step II); includes eggs used in cooking and baking
Low-Fat Dairy Products 2–3 servings per day	Milk—skim, 1/2%, or 1% fat (fluid, powdered, evaporated), buttermilk Yogurt—nonfat or low-fat yogurt or yogurt beverages Cheese—low-fat natural or processed cheese	Whole milk (fluid, evaporated, condensed), 2% fat milk (lowfat milk), imitation milk Whole milk yogurt, whole milk yogurt beverages Regular cheeses (American, blue, Brie, cheddar, Colby, Edam, Monterey Jack, whole-milk mozzarella, Parmesan, Swiss), cream cheese, Neufchatel cheese
	Low-fat or nonfat varieties, e.g.: cottage cheese— low-fat, nonfat, or dry curd (0 to 2% fat)	Cottage cheese (4% fat)

Table 8.1—*continued*

Food Group	Choose	Decrease
	Frozen dairy dessert—ice milk, frozen yogurt (low-fat or nonfat)	Ice cream
	Low-fat coffee creamer	Cream, half & half, whipping cream, nondairy creamer, whipped topping, sour cream
	Low fat or nonfat sour cream	
Fats and Oils ≤6–8 teaspoons per day	Unsaturated oils—safflower, sunflower, corn, soybean, cottonseed, canola, olive, peanut	Coconut oil, palm kernel oil, palm oil
	Margarine—made from unsaturated oils listed above, light or diet margarine, especially soft or liquid forms	Butter, lard, shortening, bacon fat, hard margarine
	Salad dressings—made with unsaturated oils listed above, low-fat or fat free	Dressings made with egg yolk, cheese, sour cream, whole milk
	Seeds and nuts—peanut butter, other nut butters	Coconut
	Cocoa powder	Milk chocolate
Breads and Cereals 6 or more servings per day	Breads—whole-grain bread, English muffins, bagels, buns, corn or flour tortilla	Bread in which eggs, fat, and/or butter are a major ingredient; croissants
	Cereals—oat, wheat, corn, multigrain	Most granolas
	Pasta	
	Rice	
	Dry beans and peas	
	Crackers, low-fat—animal-type, graham, soda crackers, breadsticks, melba toast	High-fat crackers
	Homemade baked goods using unsaturated oil, skim or 1% milk, and egg substitute—quick breads, biscuits, cornbread muffins, bran muffins, pancakes, waffles	Commercial baked pastries, muffins, biscuits
Soups	Reduced or low-fat and reduced-sodium varieties, e.g., chicken or beef noodle, minestrone, tomato, vegetable, potato, reduced-fat soups made with skim milk	Soup containing whole milk, cream, meat fat, poultry fat, or poultry skin

Table 8.1—*continued*

Food Group	Choose	Decrease
Vegetables 3–5 servings per day	Fresh, frozen, or canned, without added fat or sauce	Vegetables fried or prepared with butter, cheese, or cream sauce
Fruits 2–4 servings per day	Fruit—fresh, frozen, canned, or dried Fruit juice—fresh, frozen, or canned	Fried fruit or fruit served with butter or cream sauce
Sweets and Modified Fat Desserts	Beverages—fruit-flavored drinks, lemonade, fruit punch	
	Sweets—sugar, syrup, honey, jam, preserves, candy made without fat (candy corn, gumdrops, hard candy), fruit-flavored gelatin	Candy made with milk chocolate, coconut oil, palm kernel oil, palm oil
	Frozen desserts—low-fat and nonfat yogurt, ice milk, sherbet, sorbet, fruit ice, popsicles	Ice cream and frozen treats made with ice cream
	Cookies, cake, pie, pudding—prepared with egg whites, egg substitute, skim milk or 1% milk, and unsaturated oil or margarine; ginger snaps; fig and other fruit bar cookies, fat-free cookies; angel food cake	Commercial baked pies, cakes, doughnuts, high-fat cookies, cream pies

From National Cholesterol Education Program. Second Report of the Expert Panel on Detection, Evaluation, and Treatment of High Blood Cholesterol in Adults (Adult Treatment Panel II). NIH Publication No. 93-3095. Bethesda, MD: National Heart, Lung, and Blood Institute, 1993.

[a]Careful selection of processed foods is necessary to stay within the sodium < 2400 mg guideline.

Process. Nutritional counseling closely follows the general principles outlined in Chapter 5. As part of the history (see Chapter 2), clinicians should ask patients about their diets and take special note of information about factors that affect food intake: food and income resources, housing, employment, family and social patterns, ethnic and cultural background, cooking facilities, availability of shopping and transportation, and food preferences and dislikes.

Because dietary habits can be difficult to change, counseling is most likely to be successful when the patient is motivated to change; recommendations are consistent with the patient's cultural background, food preferences, belief systems, and economic status; suggestions are positive; and changes are made gradually and reinforced over time. These conditions may be too time-consuming for the average primary care practice. In such situations, and whenever possible, patients should be referred to trained nutrition specialists (see section on "Referral and Follow-up" later in this chapter).

METHODS

Assessment of Dietary Risk

Evaluation of the extent of dietary risk for chronic disease must consider not only the patient's daily food intake, but also the underlying food patterns and preferences, cultural and ethnic background, family history, past and present health and risk factor status, lifestyle, income, and educational level. This information should be elicited as an integral part of the prevention-focused history, physical examination, and laboratory testing described in Chapters 2–4.

Clinicians should *evaluate the dietary risks of all adult patients*. Even when no other risk factors can be identified, dietary advice is useful; cancer risks for example, cannot yet be tracked by laboratory tests. Virtually all patients are interested in nutrition and will ask questions about diet if given the opportunity. Consuming a healthful diet is a safe and desirable practice, and any patient can benefit from advice on how to do so.

To determine level of dietary risk, clinicians should *review information on the patient's height and weight, physical activity level, alcohol use, dietary intake, supplement use, blood pressure, and blood cholesterol profile.*

Risk Factor Cutpoints

Obesity. Refer to Table 3.4 to determine relative body weight:

$$\text{Current weight}/\text{Desirable weight for height} \times 100$$

If relative body weight is greater than 120%, refer to Chapter 9 for counseling instructions on weight management. If the patient is sedentary, refer to Chapter 7 for counseling instructions on exercise.

Alcohol. Current dietary recommendations state that one alcoholic drink per day for females and two drinks per day for males may decrease heart disease risk without increasing the risks for cancer or other deleterious conditions. Abstainers and individuals who drink less than these amounts need no further advice. If a patient's drinking habits exceed these guidelines or are otherwise suggestive of problem drinking, refer to Chapter 13 for counseling instructions.

High Blood Pressure or Blood Glucose. Patients with blood pressure and blood glucose levels above standard cutpoints should receive dietary counseling as part of their overall follow-up (see Chapter 17).

Blood Cholesterol. The National Cholesterol Education Program (NCEP) has established guidelines for classification, treatment, and monitoring of blood cholesterol levels based on measurement of total and HDL-cholesterol, and subsequent classification based on LDL-cholesterol (6). These guidelines are given in Tables 8.2 and 8.3; they indicate that all patients with total cholesterol measurements greater than 240 mg/dL, or with HDL-cholesterol levels less than 35 mg/dL, should receive further analysis of lipoproteins, and that those with LDL-cholesterol greater than 130 mg/dL (with two or more risk factors) or 160 mg/dL (without additional risk factors) should receive dietary therapy in two stages. If after three months, the first line diet (Step-One) has not been effective, the more stringent Step-Two Diet should be tried for another three months. If that also fails, drug treatment should be considered.

The NCEP Step-One Diet is *identical* to the basic diet for health promotion and disease prevention outlined previously under "Dietary Recommendations." To achieve the necessary reductions in intake of calories, fat, saturated fat, and cholesterol, patients should be advised to make the diet modifications suggested in Table 8.1. In many clinical situations, this diet has been effective in lowering blood cholesterol by as much as 15–20%, but in other cases it may be ineffective. The Step-Two diet restricts saturated fat intake to no more than 7% of total kcal, and cholesterol intake to no more than 200 mg/day. Although these goals may appear difficult to achieve, many authorities now believe that they are closer to ideal levels for general health promotion than the Step-One targets.

Dietary Risks

Collecting information about dietary intake can be difficult. Eating is a highly personal matter and individuals may be uncomfortable about revealing their dietary habits. They may not remember what or how much they ate. They may not know the names of the foods they ate, or the composition of mixed dishes. Consciously or unconsciously, people tend to

Table 8.2
National Cholesterol Education Program Guidelines for Classification Based on Measurement of Total Cholesterol and HDL-Cholesterol

Total Cholesterol	
<200 mg/dL	Desirable Blood Cholesterol
200–239 mg/dL	Borderline-High Blood Cholesterol
≥240 mg/dL	High Blood Cholesterol
HDL-Cholesterol	
<35 mg/dL	Low HDL-Cholesterol

From National Cholesterol Education Program. Second Report of the Expert Panel on Detection, Evaluation, and Treatment of High Blood Cholesterol in Adults (Adult Treatment Panel II). NIH Publication No. 93-3095. Bethesda, MD: National Heart, Lung, and Blood Institute, 1993.

Table 8.3
National Cholesterol Education Program Guidelines for Treatment Decisions Based on LDL-Cholesterol

Dietary Therapy	Initiation Level	LDL Goal
Without CHD and with fewer than 2 risk factors	$\geq$160 mg/dL	<160 mg/dL
Without CHD and with 2 or more risk factors	$\geq$130 mg/dL	<130 mg/dL
With CHD	>100 mg/dL	$\leq$100 mg/dL

Drug Treatment	Consideration Level	LDL Goal
Without CHD and with fewer than 2 risk factors	$\geq$190 mg/dL[a]	<160 mg/dL
Without CHD and with 2 or more risk factors	$\geq$160 mg/dL	<130 mg/dL
With CHD	$\geq$130 mg/dL[b]	$\leq$100 mg/dL

From National Cholesterol Education Program. Second Report of the Expert Panel on Detection, Evaluation, and Treatment of High Blood Cholesterol in Adults (Adult Treatment Panel II). NIH Publication No. 93-3095. Bethesda, MD: National Heart, Lung, and Blood Institute, 1993.

[a]In men under 35 years of age and premenopausal women with LDL-cholesterol levels 190–219 mg/dL, drug therapy should be delayed except in high-risk patients such as those with diabetes mellitus.

[b]In CHD patients with LDL-cholesterol levels 100–129 mg/dL, the physician should exercise clinical judgment in deciding whether to initiate drug treatment.

overreport food items they know are good for them, and underreport less healthful items. Therefore, clinicians should make some effort to assess the accuracy of the information provided in the diet history. In doing so, they should avoid making any assumptions about patients' eating patterns (e.g., eating breakfast, taking regular meals, or drinking milk or orange juice), should remain aware that patients' food habits and preferences may vary significantly from their own, and should avoid indicating any kind of judgment as to what patients should or should not be eating. Whenever possible, clinicians should provide substantial positive reinforcement for current dietary practices.

Ask patients:

- *"Does this day's diet seem about the same as the one you eat pretty much every day? How is it different? Good."*

- *"What is the first food you usually eat in the day?"*

- *"Where do you eat during the day? What do you usually have when you eat there? Good."*

- *"What are your favorite foods? How often do you eat them?"*

Qualitative Diet Screening

For a rapid screen of dietary intake, *count the number of portions of foods consumed from each group and compare to the recommended numbers from Figure 8.1.* Table 8.4 provides a format for this screening.

Table 8.4
Rapid Screen for Dietary Intake

| | Portions Consumed | |
	By Patient	Recommended
Grains, cereals, bread group	————	6–11
Fruit group	————	2–4
Vegetable group	————	3–5
Meat and meat substitute group	————	2–3
Dairy group	————	2–3
Sugars, fats, snack foods	————	—
Soft drinks	————	—
Alcoholic beverages	————	<2

Note variety (some foods in each group), balance (the number of foods in each group), and the proportion of snack foods high in fat and calories. Patterns similar to the one recommended can be considered low-risk. High-risk patterns deviate significantly from the standard; contain many foods high in calories, fat, saturated fat, cholesterol, salt, sugar, and alcohol; and are low in fiber.

Quantitative Diet Screening

More detailed information can be obtained from a 24-hour dietary history that includes questions on food portion sizes. Use of computer programs containing data on food composition requires data entry but permits rapid calculation of total amounts of energy, nutrients, fatty acids, cholesterol, and fiber consumed; such programs also permit comparison of intake levels to Recommended Dietary Allowances (RDAs), national standards for nutrient intakes adequate to prevent deficiencies in most healthy people (7), and computation of the percent of total kcal from fat, fatty acids, protein, and carbohydrate.

Compare the patient's energy and nutrient intake to RDAs and current dietary recommendations for health promotion and disease prevention (Table 8.5).

Patients whose dietary intakes are substantially above levels recom-

Table 8.5
Rapid Screen for Dietary Adequacy

	Patient	Standard
Energy, kcal	———	———
Fat, %kcal	———	<30%
Saturated fat, %kcal	———	<10%
Cholesterol, mg/d	———	<300
Sodium, g/d	———	2.4
Fiber, g/d	———	25–30

mended for fat, saturated fat, cholesterol, and sodium, but below the level recommended for fiber, should receive dietary counseling.

Basic Dietary Counseling (The NCEP Step-One Diet)

In each session, the clinician should explain the problem, negotiate the behavior change, support the change, and reinforce any previous changes that the patient has made.

Begin by telling the patient something positive: "*A good diet is important for your health. It can help you maintain a healthy weight and prevent diseases such as cancer and heart disease.*"

Refer to the diet history, and say: "*I'm glad to see that your diet contains a good balance of . . .*"

Assess the patient's motivation: "*I'm a bit concerned that your diet may be making it hard for you to (lose weight, lower your cholesterol . . .). Do you think you could be ready to make some changes in your diet? What changes do you think you might be able to make right now? Good. Let's start with . . .*"

Assess the patient's support system for dietary change: "*Who in your household shops for food, plans meals, cooks? Is there someone in your household who can help you make this change?*"

Suggest eating more of something the patient likes: "*Your diet could be improved easily if you ate more fruits and vegetables every day. What are your favorite fruits? Vegetables? Do you think you could eat them more often? How about . . . Do you think you could manage that?*"

Then go on to the foods that need substitutions or replacements (see Figure 8.1). Try to limit suggestions to one or two key options for change that will be acceptable to the patient: "*I see that you like to drink milk. Good. Have you ever tried low-fat milk? Do you think you could try low-fat or skim milk at least part of the time? Could you try skim milk with your cereal?*"

"*I see that you fry foods a lot. Have you ever tried baking or broiling these foods? Do you think you could sometimes try to bake or broil instead of frying?*"

Quantitative Dietary Counseling (The NCEP Step-Two Diet)

Patients with risk factors that require more stringent dietary modifications will need to monitor their dietary intake more carefully. Such patients must keep daily dietary records, note portion sizes, and determine the nutrient and energy composition of the diet. They also must monitor the amount of fat allowed in a given day's diet. To determine this allowance, the provider (or dietitian) will need to estimate the patient's energy needs.

To estimate energy requirements: Basal energy needs are about 25 kcal/kg/day. A sedentary person requires about 30 kcal/kg. A moderately active person requires 35 kcal/kg, and an extremely active person requires 40 kcal/kg.

To estimate fat allowance: Fat contains 9 kcal/g. Protein and carbohydrate each contain 4 kcal/g.

Example: A 70 kg sedentary man requires 2100 kcal/day (70 kg × 30 kcal/kg). No more than 30% should come from fat: 0.30 × 2100 = 630 kcal. The daily fat allowance is 630/9 = 70 g.

The provider, a nutritionist, or the patient would then need to consult food tables or a computer program to determine the number of grams of fat present in the diet and in recommended foods. As a general rule, high-fat foods are meats, dairy products, and cooking and table fats and oils. Fats that are hard at room temperature are more saturated than those that remain liquid. Much food fat is hidden; processed foods, crackers, and snack foods may be very high in fat.

Use of Food Labels

Patients on more stringent diets, and those interested in monitoring their own dietary intake, will need to be taught how to read package labels. The new food label is illustrated in Figure 8.2. It is divided by horizontal bars into three main sections. The uppermost section gives the serving size and number of servings per container. The middle section gives the number of total calories and those from fat. From this information, the percent of calories from fat can be calculated: in this example, $120/260 \times 100 = 46\%$. This section also contains information on the content of saturated fat, cholesterol, sodium, carbohydrate, fiber, sugars, and protein.

The label compares these amounts to a rather arbitrary standard called a "Daily Value." The Daily Value is based on quantitative dietary goals (given in the section "Dietary Recommendations" above) applied to a diet that contains 2000 kcal. The goal for fat, for example, is 30% of kcal. Therefore, the fat "allowance" for 2000 kcal is: 0.30 × 2000 kcal = 600 kcal. The Daily Value for fat is 600 kcal/9 kcal/g = 67 g, which is rounded off to 65 g in the label. Other Daily Values are calculated in a similar manner.

The lower section of the label provides percentages of Daily Values for vitamin A, vitamin C, calcium, and iron, and Daily Values for diets containing 2000 and 2500 kcal.

It is difficult to estimate how easily this label will be understood by patients. At a minimum, its use requires familiarity with the concept of percent; more sophisticated use requires knowledge of daily caloric intake, and the ability to use a calculator. Because higher percentages are desirable for fiber, but undesirable for fat, saturated fat, cholesterol, and sodium, the Daily Values may prove confusing. One strategy might be to advise patients to examine labels for the single dietary factor most in need of restriction, and to avoid purchasing products that contain more than 10–25% of the Daily Value for that factor.

The New Food Label at a Glance

The new food label will carry an up-to-date, easier-to-use nutrition information guide, to be required on almost all packaged foods (compared to about 60 percent of products up till now). The guide will serve as a key to help in planning a healthy diet.*

Serving sizes are now more consistent across product lines, are stated in both household and metric measures, and reflect the amounts people actually eat.

The **list of nutrients** covers those most important to the health of today's consumers, most of whom need to worry about getting <u>too much</u> of certain nutrients (fat, for example), rather than too few vitamins or minerals, as in the past.

The label of larger packages may now tell the number of calories per gram of fat, carbohydrate, and protein.

New title signals that the label contains the newly required information.

Calories from fat are now shown on the label to help consumers meet dietary guidelines that recommend people get no more than 30 percent of the calories in their overall diet from fat.

% Daily Value shows how a food fits into the overall daily diet.

Daily Values are also something new. Some are maximums, as with fat (65 grams <u>or less</u>); others are minimums, as with carbohydrate (300 grams <u>or more</u>). The daily values for a 2,000- and 2,500-calorie diet must be listed on the label of larger packages.

Nutrition Facts

Serving Size 1 cup (228g)
Servings Per Container 2

Amount Per Serving

Calories 260 Calories from Fat 120

	% Daily Value*
Total Fat 13g	**20**%
Saturated Fat 5g	**25**%
Cholesterol 30mg	**10**%
Sodium 660mg	**28**%
Total Carbohydrate 31g	**10**%
Dietary Fiber 0g	**0**%
Sugars 5g	
Protein 5g	

Vitamin A 4%	•	Vitamin C 2%
Calcium 15%	•	Iron 4%

* Percent Daily Values are based on a 2,000 calorie diet. Your daily values may be higher or lower depending on your calorie needs:

	Calories:	2,000	2,500
Total Fat	Less than	65g	80g
Sat Fat	Less than	20g	25g
Cholesterol	Less than	300mg	300mg
Sodium	Less than	2,400mg	2,400mg
Total Carbohydrate		300g	375g
Dietary Fiber		25g	30g

Calories per gram:
Fat 9 • Carbohydrate 4 • Protein 4

* This label is only a sample. Exact specifications are in the final rules.
Source: Food and Drug Administration, 1994

Figure 8.2. The new food label, required for most food products since May 1994. The Daily Value is the amount of a specific nutrient recommended in a diet containing 2000 or 2500 kcal.

Referral and Follow-up

Referral to Nutrition Specialists

Tasks such as advising patients about the information in Table 8.1 or about reading food labels are often best assigned to a dietitian or nutritionist. Registered Dietitians (with at least entry-level professional credentials certified by the American Dietetic Association) and nutritionists (who should have master's or doctoral degrees) have been trained to take diet histories, calculate nutrient intake levels, assess nutritional status, develop diet plans, and counsel patients on dietary practices. Some nurses have also received nutrition training. Clinicians can refer patients to these professionals, and should work closely with them to support and monitor patients' progress.

Follow-up Visits

Patients who require dietary intervention should be followed at regular intervals. NCEP guidelines, for example, suggest that clinicians assess patients' responses to the diet plan after three months and, if the results are not satisfactory, provide more intensive counseling, often by nutrition specialists; patients on the Step-Two diet should be seen four times during the first year and two times during subsequent years (6). The clinician or office staff members should ask:

- *"Were you able to meet with the dietitian to get some help with your diet?"*
- *"What did the two of you decide would work for you? Good."*
- *"Have you had any trouble following the plan that the nurse worked out with you?"*
- *"Do you have any questions about the diet?"*

Specific Dietary Factors and Practices

Although following the principles in Figure 8.1 and Table 8.1 should reduce dietary risk factors, some patients may require more detailed information about specific dietary factors. The techniques reviewed in the previous section "Basic Dietary Counseling" also apply to strategies designed to alter dietary proportions of specific nutrients and food components. In these situations as well, clinicians should explain the problem, negotiate the behavior change, support the change, and reinforce any previous changes that the patient has made. This section provides detailed counseling suggestions for reducing dietary fat and cholesterol. Similar suggestions apply to the additional dietary factors discussed.

Fat

Explain the Problem. *"You know, fat contains twice as many calories as either protein or starch. I'm concerned that the amount and kind of fatty foods you are eating may be making it hard for you to lose weight."*

"More than half of the hard (saturated) fat in the diet comes from meat and dairy foods. Hard fats raise your blood cholesterol level and increase your risk of developing heart disease."

Negotiate the Behavior Change. *"You can reduce the hard fat in your diet by choosing leaner cuts of meat, removing the skin from chicken, and choosing lower fat dairy items such as milk, cottage cheese, and yogurt. Do you think you might be able to substitute some of these foods for the ones you are now eating? Which substitution do you think would work best for you?"* (see Table 8.1)

Support the Behavior Change. *"I think that this change in your diet will make a big difference in your blood cholesterol. I'd like to see you again in six weeks to see how you are doing. In the meantime, I am going to [give you some information about the fat content of foods to take home and read, refer you to the dietitian who will help you plan your meals, etc.]."*

Cholesterol

Explain the Problem. *"Too much cholesterol in your foods will make your blood cholesterol go up and may make you more susceptible to having a heart attack. To get your blood cholesterol down, you need to eat less animal fat and eat less cholesterol. Cholesterol is found only in animal foods—meats, dairy products, and eggs. You can reduce your intake of both cholesterol and saturated fat by eating fewer meat and dairy foods, and by avoiding egg yolks (which are the most concentrated source of dietary cholesterol)."*

Negotiate the Behavior Change. *"Do you think you could eat less of some meats and dairy foods? Fewer eggs? What do you think you could change?"*

Support the Behavior Change. *"I think what you have decided to do will work very well. I'd like you to return in six weeks to see how you are doing. In the meantime. . . ."*

Fiber

Fiber refers to a variety of plant food components that cannot be digested. Studies associate fiber with normal digestion; control of blood glucose, pressure, and cholesterol levels; and protection against cancer and heart disease. Surveys indicate that average intakes of fiber in the United States are less than half the amounts recommended. Because the sources of fiber are fruits, vegetables, and grains, increasing the proportion of such foods in the diet to those recommended in Figure 8.1 should result in higher and more appropriate intake levels. As a first step, patients should be asked to indicate their favorite fruits, vegetables, and cereals, and encouraged to eat more of them. They should also be asked whether they might be willing to try to include any others on a regular basis.

Iron

The dietary plan illustrated in Figure 8.1 should provide adequate amounts of iron, and routine iron supplementation should not be necessary for most people. Iron supplementation may be indicated for some infants and young children at increased risk of iron deficiency. The relatively high prevalence of hemochromatosis, a relatively rare condition that is exacerbated by iron intake, and the lack of evidence of clinical benefit may argue against routine supplementation. Rates of iron-deficiency anemia are declining in the United States, and iron is plentiful in the food supply (it is used to fortify flour, for example). To enhance absorption, recommend taking iron supplements between meals with water or juice. If hemoglobin or hematocrit levels do not improve within one month, other causes of anemia should be considered (in certain clinical settings, diagnostic studies to determine the etiology of the anemia are indicated immediately). Patients should be asked about the use of supplements containing iron; those taking supplements should be asked whether they notice any associated changes in how they are feeling.

Calcium

Preliminary evidence suggests that higher-than-average intakes of calcium might help prevent osteoporosis, hypertension, and colon cancer. Although calcium is widely distributed in foods, average intakes are below recommended levels. One hypothesis for this discrepancy is that greater amounts of calcium are needed to maintain bone mineral balance when the diet is high in protein. Adult patients should be advised to follow the diet illustrated in Figure 8.1. Fruits, vegetables, and grains contain calcium, and they also contain adequate, but not excessive, protein. Advise patients who need to increase calcium intake to consume extra amounts of low-fat dairy products, small fish (with bones), tofu, and dark green leafy vegetables. If necessary, advise (or prescribe) calcium carbonate supplements, especially to young women whose bone mass has not yet reached peak levels, and to high-risk perimenopausal and postmenopausal women. Evidence that calcium supplements affect bone loss in postmenopausal women is currently equivocal.

Sodium

Average sodium intake in the United States is much higher than needed. The amount naturally present in foods is more than sufficient to meet the requirements of all but the most physically active individuals. At least 40% of the sodium in the American diet derives from that added to processed and packaged foods (cucumbers and wheat, for example, are low in salt; pickles and packaged cereals are not). The remaining dietary sodium is divided about equally between the amount in natural foods and that added at the table.

Many hypertensive patients can achieve normal blood pressure with sodium restriction alone. Restricting sodium also enhances the action of diuretics. The taste for salt is acquired; the more sodium consumed, the more people prefer its taste. Salt restriction, therefore, requires a period of adjustment; in early stages, food may not taste as good. Patients should be given advice on how to read package labels (see previous section on "Use of Food Labels") and on ways to make foods taste better without salt and with the potential use of potassium salts. They should be reassured that foods will start to taste better in a few weeks once they have adjusted.

Supplements

Increasing evidence suggests the value of adequate intake of vitamins and minerals, particularly nutrients with antioxidant functions, in chronic disease prevention. Diets that follow the precepts indicated in Figure 8.1 should provide more than adequate amounts of essential nutrients. Nevertheless, many patients take supplements or herbal products for a wide variety of reasons that may be sound or unsound. The diet history (Chapter 2) should elicit the type and amount of supplements consumed. Most supplements are harmless; excessive amounts of only a few (e.g., fat-soluble vitamins, selenium, amino acids) have been demonstrably toxic. Clinicians should determine the reasons why patients are taking supplements and should provide advice about supplements within that frame of reference. Patients should be advised against supplements known or suspected to be harmful or those taken in excessive amounts. Multinutrient supplements containing recommended amounts of key vitamins and minerals (RDA levels) are safe. If there are young children in the household, remind patients that supplements—like any other medication—should be kept out of their reach (see "Poisoning" in Chapter 10).

Unconventional Diets

Few individuals select diets for reasons of health. Instead, diets are determined by availability of foods, and by a great variety of cultural, economic, environmental, and behavioral factors. Although dietary counseling is aimed at improving nutritional status, few patients will follow advice that is inconsistent with their food beliefs and preferences. In evaluating a diet that appears unconventional or extreme, follow the principles outlined in the section on "Assessment of Dietary Risk." If the diet deviates significantly from accepted standards, be sure to ask why the patient has chosen that particular dietary pattern. Reinforce the healthful aspects of that pattern, and recommend additional food sources of energy and nutrients that are acceptable to the patient. Patients who have adopted unhealthy diets to achieve rapid or dramatic weight loss should be encouraged to instead follow the weight management principles of Chapter 9.

Vegetarian Diets. Increasing numbers of people in the United States are declaring themselves as vegetarians. Vegetarianism includes a heterogeneous group of dietary practices that share a partial or complete reliance on plant foods as principal sources of energy. The single common feature is avoidance of red meat, but practices may range from occasional waiver of this restriction to total reliance on fruits and nuts or cereals. The nutritional quality of vegetarian diets depends on the quantity and variety of foods consumed. Vegetarian diets that are adequate in energy and varied in food intake meet dietary standards and are associated with reduced chronic disease risks. A risk of undernutrition occurs when diets are limited in energy or dependent on restricted numbers of foods. Such risks are greatest in children, adolescents, and pregnant and lactating women.

Assess the diets of vegetarians in the usual manner, paying particular attention to the dietary rationale, to energy adequacy and food variety, and to the use of supplements and health foods. Advise strict vegetarians who consume no animal foods that their diets may be inadequate in vitamin B_{12} (which is obtained only from animal foods, bacteria, and certain blue-green algae), and that they should supplement their diets with an acceptable—and reliable—source of this nutrient. If necessary, also advise an increase in consumption of food sources of energy and nutrients that are consistent with the patient's belief system.

Specific Life Stages

Infancy and Early Childhood

Research on infants and young children is limited by their extreme vulnerability to nutritional deprivation as well as by ethical considerations. Thus, although many authorities believe that early precursors of chronic disease begin in childhood, it has been difficult to obtain convincing evidence for the superiority of one or another feeding practice in reducing chronic disease risk factors later in life.

Virtually all authorities recommend breastfeeding as the method of choice for infants and advise clinicians to encourage mothers to breastfeed infants whenever possible (8). Breast milk contains nutrients, immunologic factors, and other factors that cannot be duplicated in formulas. The fact that breastfeeding permits the baby to regulate caloric intake has suggested that breastfed infants will have lower rates of obesity as adults. This association remains under investigation.

Because young children are growing rapidly and require concentrated sources of energy, dietary recommendations for chronic disease prevention specifically exclude application to children under the age of two years. Children below that age should not be fed diets restricted in energy or fat. There is no need to add salt or sugar to their foods, but they should be given fluoride supplements if the local water supply has not been fluoridated. (See Chapter 15 for further information about fluoride supplementation and other feeding practices to reduce the risk of caries.) Iron supplements may also be needed for infants and children at increased risk of iron deficiency.

Childhood and Adolescence

Prospective studies of children and adolescents have demonstrated strong correlations between diet, risk factors such as blood cholesterol, blood pressure, and obesity, and early signs of atherosclerosis. Some studies also have suggested tracking of these risk factors into early adulthood. This evidence suggests that early intervention might help prevent later disease. The dietary principles of Figure 8.1 are appropriate for these age groups. Regular physical activity should also be strongly recommended. Because their bones are still growing, adolescents and young adults should be advised to consume adequate calcium through regular intake of vegetables, grains, legumes, and dairy foods. Adolescents capable of becoming pregnant should especially be advised to consume at least five fruits and vegetables daily in order to achieve an intake of at least 0.4 mg folate as a means to reduce the risk of having a child with a neural tube defect. Public health authorities have recommended that all women of childbearing age consume 0.4 mg folate per day, obtained through diet or supplements (9).

Pregnancy and Lactation

All women capable of becoming pregnant should be advised to emphasize fruits and vegetables in their daily diets as a means to increase folate intake and protect against having an infant with a neural tube defect. Healthful diets during pregnancy and lactation follow basic dietary principles, and the same counseling principles also apply. At every visit, encourage healthful dietary practices, discourage use of potentially harmful substances (e.g., alcohol, cigarettes), and address the patient's questions and concerns. Because iron deficiency is the most common cause of anemia during pregnancy, oral iron supplements (30 mg elemental iron/day) are prescribed routinely during the second and third trimesters, with higher doses prescribed for anemic women. There is little direct evidence, however, that this practice reduces the risk of adverse outcomes for the mother, fetus, or newborn (10).

Support from the clinician is an important factor in a mother's decision to breastfeed. Inform pregnant women about the benefits of breast feeding, and encourage them to breastfeed their infants. Once the baby is delivered, support the mother's efforts to breastfeed and refer her to additional sources of support (11).

Older Ages

Although few clinical trials have directly examined the benefits of dietary counseling in older adults, many experts recommend doing so; chronic disease risk factors increase with age, and dietary improvements at any age have been shown to reduce risk factors, improve functional ability, reduce the need for drug treatment, and lower health care costs. The basic dietary patterns of Figure 8.1 are prudent recommendations for individuals of any age. More intensive suggestions such as those of the Step-Two diet may not be advisable or may be too difficult for many older adults to follow. Decisions to counsel older patients about diet should be decided case by case, and should be based on reliable information about elderly patients' dietary intake (see Chapter 2), assessment of patients' or caregivers' interest in dietary improvements, ability to understand the diet, access to food, and physical or economic impairments that might limit food shopping and preparation (see "Functional Status" in Chapter 16).

Several recent studies of older adults indicate beneficial effects of multinutrient supplements on cognitive and immune functions, and of mild-to-moderate exercise on overall quality of life. These can be recommended whenever appropriate. Whether extra calcium will prevent bone loss in postmenopausal women is as yet uncertain, but older as well as younger adults should receive regular sun exposure to activate vitamin D, following the recommendations in Chapter 14, or should receive supplements of vitamin D.

OTHER ISSUES

Potential Adverse Effects

Since the diets recommended for reduction of chronic disease risk factors are the same as those recommended for general health promotion, no adverse effects should be expected from following them. Patients may be concerned that dietary restrictions will decrease their enjoyment of food. In such cases, they should be reassured that healthy foods also taste good, and should be given guidance on more interesting food preparation methods. Referrals to nutrition specialists and to the cookbooks and patient education materials in Chapter 9 may be helpful in these situations.

In some cases, patients may take dietary recommendations to an extreme and, for example, attempt to eliminate all fat from their diets. The diet history should elicit information about such practices, and patients should be counseled about the need for adequate energy and variety in food intake. These needs are most pronounced in infants and children; they should not be placed on restrictive diets. As noted earlier, counseling about restrictive practices should be conducted within the patient's frame of reference.

Costs

Dietary counseling is best referred to nutrition professionals (see "Community Resources" later in this chapter). Although many large insurance carriers will reimburse clinicians for such services, reimbursement policies are not uniform; they vary widely according to state, specific carrier, diagnosis, and setting. Services are more likely to be reimbursed when clinicians can document the effectiveness of the intervention in reducing disease risks, and can assign the counseling intervention to a specific insurance code (see Chapter 25).

The costs of referrals also vary widely, depending on geographic location and type of practice. In 1993, consulting nutritionists charged $40–100 for an initial counseling session, and about half that amount for subsequent visits. To successfully reinforce dietary intervention, patients typically receive follow-up counseling two to four times per year.

Office and Clinic Organization

The receptionist or nurse can administer the diet history while the patient is waiting in the reception area. The reception area is also an appropriate site for distribution of patient questionnaires and education materials, display of posters, and viewing of videos related to diet and health. Receptionists or nurses can direct patients to these materials, with indications that they will be happy to answer any questions that are elicited. Sources of such materials are listed under "Patient Education Materials" below.

Medical Record Documentation

Dietary prescriptions and counseling suggestions should be entered in the medical record in the usual manner.

RESOURCES–PATIENT EDUCATION MATERIALS

American Heart Association
7272 Greenville Avenue
Dallas, TX 75231-4596
214-373-6300, 800-242-8721
    Especially recommended are the publications "The American Heart Association Diet:
    An Eating Plan for Healthy Americans" and "How to Read the New Food Label
    (brochure 51-1075)."

National Cancer Institute
Office of Cancer Communications
Building 31, Room 10A16
9000 Rockville Pike

Bethesda, MD 20892
800-4-CANCER
    "Eat More Fruits and Vegetables: 5 A Day for Better Health" (brochure 92-3248); "Diet, Nutrition and Cancer Prevention" (NIH Pub. No. 87-2878).

Other patient education materials can be obtained from these resources:

American Dietetic Association
216 W. Jackson Blvd.
Chicago, IL 60606-6995

Center for Science in the Public Interest
1875 Connecticut Ave, NW Suite 300
Washington, DC 20009

National Heart, Lung and Blood Institute
Communications and Public Information Branch
National Institutes of Health, Building 31
Bethesda, MD 20892
301-951-3260

Society for Nutrition Education
2001 Killebrew Drive, Suite 340
Minneapolis, MN 55425-1882

Materials can also be obtained through local chapters of the American Heart Association, American Cancer Society, and American Diabetes Association.

SUGGESTED READINGS

U.S. Department of Agriculture. The Food guide pyramid. Home and Garden Bull. No. 252. Hyattsville, MD: Human Nutrition Information Service, 1992. Order from Food and Drug Administration (product FDA93-2259), Information and Outreach Staff, HFE-88, Room 16-63, 5600 Fishers Lane, Rockville, MD 29857, 301-443-3170.

U.S. Department of Agriculture and U.S. Department of Health and Human Services. Nutrition and your health: Dietary guidelines for Americans. Home and Garden Bull. No. 232, U.S. GPO 1990-273-930. Washington, DC: Government Printing Office, 1990. Order from Food and Drug Administration (product FDA90-3170), Information and Outreach Staff, HFE-88, Room 16-63, 5600 Fishers Lane, Rockville, MD 29857, 301-443-3170.

REFERENCES

1. U.S. Department of Health and Human Services. The surgeon general's report on nutrition and health. Publication no. DHHS (PHS) 88-50210. Washington, DC: Government Printing Office, 1988.
2. National Research Council, Food and Nutrition Board. Diet and health: implications for reducing chronic disease. Washington, DC: National Academy Press, 1989.
3. U.S. Preventive Services Task Force. Guide to clinical preventive services. Baltimore: Williams & Wilkins, 1989:305–314.
4. McGinnis JM, Foege WH. Actual causes of death in the United States. JAMA 1993;270:2207–2212.

5. U.S. Department of Health and Human Services. Healthy people 2000: national health promotion and disease prevention objectives. Conference edition. Washington, DC: Government Printing Office, 1990:131–132.

6. National Cholesterol Education Program. Second Report of the Expert Panel on Detection, Evaluation, and Treatment of High Blood Cholesterol in Adults (Adult Treatment Panel II). NIH Publication No. 93-3095. Bethesda, MD: National Heart, Lung, and Blood Institute, 1993.

7. National Research Council, Food and Nutrition Board. Recommended dietary allowances, 10th edition. Washington, DC: National Academy Press, 1989.

8. Pediatric nutrition handbook, 3rd edition. Elk Grove, IL: American Academy of Pediatrics, 1993.

9. U.S. Centers for Disease Control and Prevention. Recommendations for the use of folic acid to reduce the number of cases of spina bifida and other neural tube defects. MMWR 1992;41:1–7.

11. Institute of Medicine. Nutrition during pregnancy and lactation: an implementation guide. Washington, DC: National Academy Press, 1992.

9. Weight Management

STEVEN JONAS

INTRODUCTION

Overweight and Obesity

The term *overweight* means more than simply "too heavy," according to some generally accepted parameters for normal height and weight (e.g., see Table 3.4). In the more complex health sense, *overweight* means excess weight of a particular type; that is, too much weight, in the form of excess body fat, for a given height, by age and sex. The "normal" weight and body fat proportions to which overweight in the health sense refers are defined by the distributions in the population of three physical parameters (height, weight, body fat) by two demographic parameters (age, sex). Thus, excess body fat is the primary concern, not simply excess weight. Excess body fat is potentially harmful, even if the person is not overweight.

The term *obesity* (carrying excess body fat, whether overweight or not) actually describes more accurately the condition with which health promotion/disease prevention is concerned than does the term *overweight*. In the health care context, the terms *obesity management* and *obesity loss* are more scientifically accurate than are *weight management* and *weight loss*: for people who are overweight due to excess fat, the only desirable weight loss is of fat, not excess muscle. Since weight management and weight loss are the commonly used terms, however, and since for most people the word *obese* is more pejorative than the word *overweight*, weight management and loss are the terms used in this chapter.

In terms of potential health risk, the overweight type of obesity can be divided into four categories: 0 to 19% above the upper limit of normal weight by age and height, for which there is no significant elevation of risk (not considered obese); 20–40% above (mild obesity); 41–100% above (moderate obesity); and above 100% (severe or morbid obesity) (1). While obesity can also be defined in terms of body fat percentages, the

The theory and practice presented in this chapter were originally developed for the book: Jonas S, the Editors of Consumer Reports Books. Taking control of your weight. Yonkers, NY: Consumer Reports Book, 1993.

overfat but not overweight type has no common descriptors. For a discussion of the health risks associated with different levels of obesity, see "Health Significance of Obesity" below.

Overweight and Obesity as Social Constructs

Regardless of the various medically-defined categories, most people think of obesity as a matter of self-perception as well as of weight and body fat: how one looks, feels, and thinks about one's body image. American society stresses thinness for women (2). Thus, a 5'7" tall woman weighing 125 pounds, even if described by most observers as "attractive" may *think* of herself as "fat" if she carries some excess adipose tissue on the lateral aspects of her thighs. In evaluating a patient for obesity, it is important to bear in mind not only what the tables have to say about the subject, but also what the patient has to say about it.

Given societal norms, certain patients will set their goals for weight loss not on the basis of health or other physical needs, but rather on the basis of perceived societal or other interpersonal demands. The clinician should recognize that patients who find it difficult if not impossible to lose weight for metabolic reasons may well experience serious conflict created by societally determined weight/fat *desiderata* (3). Therefore, in weight management for certain patients, the clinician should focus not on weight loss but rather on self-acceptance, healthy eating for its own sake, and regular exercise for its own sake (4).

EPIDEMIOLOGY OF OBESITY

Health Significance of Obesity

About 32 million American adults (aged 25–74) are obese [body weight more than 20% above the upper limit of normal by sex, age, and height]. The prevalence of obesity among children is uncertain, but it is estimated to be between 5% and 25%. . . .

Increased mortality in adults has been clearly documented as a result of morbid obesity, weight that is at least twice (or 100 pounds over) the desirable weight. In the case of moderate obesity, however, experts differ on whether the observed decrease in longevity [sic] is due to the effect of obesity alone or to the effect of closely related variables such as smoking, concurrent diseases, physical inactivity, socioeconomic status, or diet. It is known, however, that the overweight are more likely to have diabetes, hypertension and risk factors for other diseases, . . . [and] hypercholesterolemia. . . . [Obesity is] a possible independent [risk factor for] coronary artery disease . . . [and] may influence the risk of cancer of the colon, rectum, prostate, gallbladder, biliary tract, breast, cervix, endometrium and ovary. Finally, obesity affects the quality of life through social discrimination and by limiting mobility, physical endurance, and other functional measures. (5)

Further, obesity increases the risk of developing a number of the possible complications of pregnancy, and is associated with gout and osteoarthritis (the latter through simple excess mechanical wear on the joints).

Being overweight has few benefits. One benefit is the reason the characteristic developed in the first place: protection against famine (see "Mechanisms for Saving Energy" later in this chapter). It may also be associated with slightly decreased risk of osteoporosis.

Benefits and Risks of Weight/Fat Loss

In health terms, the benefit of weight/fat loss is the reduction or elimination of risks associated with obesity. Beyond that, the overweight person who manages to lose weight will often feel better physically and psychologically, will look better to self and others, will be more able to engage in regular physical activity, and will have dealt with the personal social negatives of being obese.

But weight/fat loss carries certain risks as well, primarily fear of failure and fear of success. Fear of failure often inhibits the initiation of weight loss, especially for persons who have experienced yo-yo dieting (see "Starvation Response and 'Yo-Yo' Dieting" later in this chapter). In addition, the difficulty inherent in successfully losing weight is well-known, especially in organized weight loss programs. The clinician should address this fear of failure and should point out to patients that, if they are ready to try weight/fat loss on their own, their chance of success may be significantly greater than for persons using organized programs (6, 7) (see "Is Weight/Fat Loss Possible?" later in this chapter).

Weight-loss therapists report that, for some patients, a major risk of success in weight loss concerns sexuality and relationships with the opposite sex. Many persons with adult-onset obesity report that their sex life has diminished or disappeared entirely. Weight loss may bring increased anxiety over the prospect of becoming sexually active once again. It may be possible to deal with these fears early on in the assessment and goal-setting steps of the weight loss program. If the clinician senses that the fear is deep-seated and could be a significant barrier to success (and the risk associated with the obesity is substantial), a referral for psychotherapy might be in order. For some people, however, accepting overweight and its health risks may be preferred over the psychosocial risks of once again being thin.

METABOLISM OF WEIGHT GAIN AND LOSS

Mechanisms for Saving Energy

When individuals consume food energy (calories) beyond their immediate needs, the body stores much of the excess as body fat. Body fat, other than that which plays a protective, cushioning function, serves mainly to store potential energy. For many people, the storage capacity is quite high, leading to obesity. Given the place that obesity occupies in our culture, it is important to share with patients the concept that excess body fat is nothing more than stored potential energy.

Social Constructs versus Metabolism

Although our culture often uses moralistic terms to refer to overeating/overweight (e.g., "I was *bad*; I ate too much," "I feel *guilty* for eating that hot fudge sundae"), obesity is obviously *not* caused by wickedness. Neither overeating nor underexercising is a sin or a failure of will (8). While the fact that overweight has nothing to do with immorality may seem obvious to the clinician, prevailing social attitudes towards overweight may make the distinction less obvious to patients. For these patients, it is useful to review the metabolic origins of excess body fat.

Food Fat Is Calorie Rich

Patients should also be given two other relevant facts about fat metabolism. First, a gram of food fat contains about 9 calories of potential energy, whereas a gram of protein or carbohydrate contains only about four. (This is one reason why low-fat eating is helpful for both weight loss and weight loss maintenance.) Second, because of the energy requirements for internal carbohydrate and protein conversion to fat, excess calories presented to the body in the form of food fat are stored as body fat with much less extra energy expenditure than are excess carbohydrate or protein calories: about 3% of food fat calories are metabolized in the conversion to body fat; about 33% of carbohydrate or protein calories are metabolized to convert them to body fat (9).

Starvation Response and "Yo-Yo" Dieting

Finally, a critical metabolic factor in weight gain, especially relevant to our weight reduction, diet-conscious culture, is a phenomenon called the Starvation Response. Like the fat energy storage system, it is a mechanism to enhance the survival of the individual and species (10). If a person experiences a sudden decrease in caloric intake, the resting metabolic rate (RMR, the measure of energy required to maintain organ system function) will start to decrease, probably within 24–36 hours. This process is designed to conserve energy. The RMR, which normally is about 75 calories per hour, can drop to 60 calories per hour. A second exposure to sudden caloric deficit can lower RMR further to about 50 calories per hour. In some people, the RMR may drop as low as 35–40 calories per hour.

The Starvation Response can be elicited by sudden calorie restriction dieting. Unfortunately, the body's metabolic system responds the same way to intentional caloric deficit as it does to externally induced deficits. The body's metabolic system cannot recognize that the immediate caloric deficit in this instance does *not* indicate that food might be in short supply for quite some time. Thus, when the person concludes the diet and returns to a normal eating pattern (as often happens), there is no available built-in "second signal" to stimulate an immediate return to normal RMR.

Usually, the sudden calorie restriction diets described in the lay literature contain little information about permanent healthy eating. Many dieters using these methods lose some weight and then return to their normal eating pattern. If a person with a lowered RMR resumes normal eating without increasing energy expenditure, calories in excess of metabolic need will be consumed. Most of the excess calories will be stored as body fat, and body weight will increase again. That outcome may well induce the person to try losing weight once more.

If the same sudden calorie-restriction dieting approach is followed, the RMR may be further depressed. And again, even if some weight is lost on subsequent tries, unless the person has managed to change his or her regular eating patterns, the diet often produces immediate, sometimes significant, weight loss, followed by slow, but steady weight regain. This dieting-induced pattern is called "yo-yo" dieting (3). (After a number of such cycles, the RMR may be depressed to the point that the next episode of calorie restriction dieting has no effect on body weight at all, as well as having no further effect on a greatly depressed RMR.)

There is one known mechanism by which a depressed RMR can be raised, however: engaging in regular exercise (11). Muscle requires more energy for maintenance of its basal functions than does fat. Regular exercise raises the RMR by gradually creating new muscle mass. For patients averse to regular exercise, this will be a "good news/bad news" message, but they should be encouraged to use this method to raise their RMR.

Pathways to Overweight

It was formerly thought that body weight/fat proportion was simply the result of the interplay of caloric intake and caloric expenditure. According to this model, weight loss was simply a matter of taking in fewer calories than were required to satisfy a person's energy needs. It is now known that the process is not quite so simple as the old "calories in/calories out" formula. The Starvation Response demonstrates that body weight/fat proportion is the product of the interplay among caloric intake, physical activity, *and* metabolic rate. Because this interplay exists, it is now apparent that there is more than a single pathway, overeating, to overweight/obesity. In addition to the relatively rare organic disease causes of overweight such as hypothyroidism, four principal dietary/metabolic pathways to overweight have been theorized (12):

1. Adult-onset overeating: High-calorie overweight.

2. Childhood-onset overeating, arising from familial eating patterns (which may result in a high or normal caloric intake in adult life): Familial overweight.

3. Dieting-induced, lowered RMR, with low caloric intake: Dieting-induced low calorie overweight (DI-LCO).

4. Genetically-determined, lowered RMR, with low caloric intake: Genetic predisposition low calorie overweight (similar in outcome to DI-LCO).

While observational data support this theoretical construct, the epidemiology of the pathways to overweight, other than the genetically determined one, has not been studied with any rigor. Thus, in the overweight population, the distribution of the causes of overweight/obesity among the postulated four pathways is not known. Nevertheless, assuming that the pathways construct is correct, one of the first steps in helping patients find a successful long-term weight reduction plan is to determine which pathway led to overweight in the first place (see "Program Development" later in this chapter).

Achieving Success in Weight Loss

Weight loss success is measured not just by how much weight and body fat decrease, but by the extent to which one remains at or near the target weight/body fat level. Further, success is determined by whether that goal can be achieved without permanently "going on a diet." One of the keys to success is for the patient to understand that permanent weight loss is usually achieved not just by reducing caloric intake for a finite period of time, but also by changing one's *whole way of eating*, and, often, how energy is expended. As noted by F. Xavier Pi-Sunyer:

> Exercise is extraordinarily important, not so much for the number of calories it expends but because it seems to keep a person focused. Physical activity keeps an individual motivated to maintain the dietary discipline that's required in weight control. Persons who exercise are much more likely to successfully manage their weight than those who don't. (13)

To achieve *permanent* weight loss, a program must help the person to make *permanent* changes in eating habits and activity patterns. It must make *nor-*

mal, healthy eating part of the person's life *from the beginning of the program,* not something added on in a maintenance program after the weight is lost. (See Chapter 8 for the principles of healthy eating.) Carefully defining "success" (in a manner that fits the patient) can help the patient deal with both the fear of failure and the fear of success.

PROGRAM DEVELOPMENT

Is Weight/Fat Loss Possible?

Before discussing with the patient the details of a program for weight loss, it is often necessary to deal with the question, is weight loss possible? In contrast with the situation faced, for example, when counseling patients about regular exercise, few patients need to be convinced of the benefits of weight loss or that they ought to try to lose weight if they are overweight or overfat. In fact, of the approximately 20% of the population who are overweight, at any one time an estimated 50% are trying to lose weight.

It is well-known that organized weight loss programs have long-term success rates of only 5–20%. Less well-recognized are the results of at least two studies of self-directed weight loss regimens that showed a success rate of 60–75% (6, 7). It stands to reason that self-directed regimens might work best.

At the same time that the possibility of success is being considered, it should also be recognized that a variety of physiological, metabolic, and psychological factors make it difficult for every overweight person to lose weight (3). It is important for these people to strive for self-acceptance (and for society to increase its tolerance of overweight people) (2). Furthermore, for some patients for whom weight reduction to the "normal" range is not possible, partial weight reduction is a worthwhile goal (14). Such goals should be considered with the patient, including a determination of whether achieving them will provide self-acceptance.

"Four Pathways Up/Three Pathways Down" Model

According to the pathways theory, depending upon which pathway led to weight gain, the patient will have to accomplish one or more of the following to lose weight: reduce total caloric intake; lower the amount of dietary fat (both for metabolic conversion purposes and to lower caloric intake); and engage in regular exercise (both to consume excess calories stored in body fat and to raise the RMR).

Three possible pathways to weight reduction can also be postulated (12):

1. for high-calorie overweight, reducing caloric intake is obligatory and regular exercise is desirable;

2. for normal calorie overweight (as in stabilized familial), caloric intake reduction and regular exercise are both equally important;

3. for diet-induced or genetically predisposed LCO, regular exercise is obligatory and low-fat eating is desirable (not only to lower caloric intake but also to maintain lean body mass as weight is lost and to establish a lifelong pattern of healthy eating).

Assessment

To choose the correct pathway to weight loss, it helps to know how the patient became overweight. The following questions will help make the correct determination, as well as provide the basis for making general eating habit recommendations.

General questions on weight and eating history include: What is the patient's weight? According to Table 3.4, given the range and allowances for body frame size, is the patient overweight? By how much? For how long? Is the excess weight composed primarily of fat? Was the patient's weight ever in the normal range? What has the patient's adult weight range been? Is the patient really overweight, in the physical sense, or only by self-perception? Is body image adjustment possibly more appropriate than weight loss?

See Chapter 8 for information on how to assess eating habits. If the patient eats large amounts frequently and consumes food high in fats and simple sugars, high calorie overweight is the probable etiology. If, on the other hand, the patient can truly say, "I don't eat, but I can't lose weight," either diet-induced or genetically-predisposed LCO is likely.

In taking the history of overweight/obesity, the following questions may help distinguish between family-induced and genetically predisposed overweight: Is there a parental history of overweight? For all or part of their lives? Were the grandparents overweight? Are any siblings overweight? Was the patient overweight as a child? What were the childhood eating patterns? Were any other relatives morbidly obese? Is there an identifiable, perhaps cultural, attitude toward body size/shape, eating, and weight gain in the family? Was weight loss dieting common in the family during childhood?

In general, negative answers to these questions make either genetically predisposed or family-induced overweight unlikely. Positive answers generally indicate one of the two, but it can be difficult to distinguish between them, unless the patient has LCO. Genetic predisposition does not require the appearance of overweight in childhood. *If* the patient was overweight as a child, *and* the parents (and likely siblings as well) were overweight, *and* food and eating were a major center of family life, *and* the patient is presently eating a high or normal calorie diet, then the chances are good that the familial pathway is responsible for the obesity (unless adult-onset, dieting-induced LCO is superimposed on the familial overweight of childhood origin).

If one or both parents were overweight (and possibly siblings as well), *and* food was not ample on the table during childhood, *and* weight loss dieting was common in the family, *and* the patient has had a great deal of difficulty losing weight as an adult, *and* has been eating a low-calorie diet for an extended period without seeing significant weight loss, then genetically predisposed LCO is the probable etiology.

To elicit the presence of diet-induced LCO, the following questions may be helpful. If the answer to more than half of them is yes, this is the likely pathway. Was the patient of normal weight until a particular point in adulthood, such as having her first child? Did the patient then become a chronic dieter? Was an attempt made to lose weight on a fad diet (such as a fruit only, grain only, or high protein diet)?

Has the patient tried without success to lose weight on a very low-calorie diet (under 1000 calories per day), liquid or otherwise? Does the patient remain overweight despite regularly consuming less than 1000 calories per day? On a crash diet, have 10 pounds or more been lost in a short time, say 2–3 weeks, only to be regained within 2–3 months of completing the diet? Have major weight fluctuations been experienced more than twice? Is each diet thought of as a short-term, but nevertheless "final," solution?

Once the patient and clinician have agreed on the pathway that led to the patient's obesity and together have identified the correct pathway to weight reduction, program design can begin. (If regular exercise is to be part of the program, please refer to Chapter 7 for guidance in developing that component.)

Basic Approach

The basic approach for engaging in behavior change to achieve weight loss is the same as for becoming a regular exerciser or for engaging in most forms of behavior change (see also Chapter 5), and will be reviewed only briefly here.

The first step is *goal-setting*: establishing what the patient wants to do and why. The patient should take some time to think about this undertaking. *Realism* is essential. What is feasible, achievable, and desirable, given the identified pathway to overweight? As noted in Chapters 5 and 7, *inner motivation* is required for long-term results. External motivation, *"I'm doing this for my spouse (or boy/girl friend, children/parents, em-*

ployer/coworkers)," almost invariably leads to guilt, anxiety, anger, frustration, and quitting.

It is important to stress with patients the concept of *taking control* (6, 12). They are deciding what they want to do with their bodies. Many people find that "taking control" is an important element both in starting a weight management program and in sticking with it. *Gradual change*, as in "gradual change leads to permanent change," applies as much to weight loss as it does to any other behavior change endeavor. Rejecting both *perfectionism* and the *"fat is sinful"* concept is also very helpful, as is dealing with the *fears of failure and success*. Some persons find it helpful to deal with the loss of *immediate physical gratification* by replacing it with the immediate mental gratification that comes from taking control.

Approaches to Eating

The key to successful weight loss is learning a pattern of generally healthy eating that can be maintained for life. The eating plan to be adopted for weight loss should be tailored to the patient's type of obesity. One constant, however, is that lowering the fat content of the diet is essential to success. Low-fat eating achieves caloric restriction, if that is required. For the person with LCO, low-fat eating is beneficial for several reasons. It will encourage the body to use fat to meet energy needs, thereby avoiding muscle loss; as caloric intake needs increase secondary to the addition of muscle mass, low-fat eating will help prevent excess calorie consumption; and low-fat intake will reduce serum cholesterol and low-density lipoprotein levels.

Because people select *types* of food and generally do not count calories or fat grams on a regular, ongoing basis, the plan should aim to achieve change qualitatively (by helping the patient to choose different *types* of foods), rather than quantitatively (by counting fat grams and/or calories). In addition to types of foods, the plan will likely have to address the amount of food, the optimal frequency of eating, and daily/weekly eating patterns.

Lowering Fat

The best way to lower fat in the diet is by food-substitution on a gradual basis. The person learns to identify the high-fat foods in his or her regular diet, chooses which foods to gradually remove, and chooses which low or lower fat foods to substitute for them. In this approach, it is important for the patient to understand that healthy eating begins in the supermarket and continues in the food preparation process. Healthy shopping and healthy cooking, the precursors to healthy eating, are essential to successful weight loss.

Absolutism is not required, and in fact may be counterproductive. Once gradual change is learned, the patient will come to see healthy eating and managing weight as a lifelong process. Occasional consumption of high-fat food is normal. As eating habits change, tolerance for fatty foods often declines.

PLAN IMPLEMENTATION

Healthy Eating

The first step in developing a healthy eating plan is to find out what the patient is eating now (see Chapter 8). The next step is to identify low-fat foods that might be substituted for current foods. These choices, which can appear fairly complicated at first, can be reduced to some fairly simple food choices (see also Chapter 8, especially Table 8.1).

Low-Fat Food Choices Simplified

- The patient should substitute lower fat for higher fat milk, aiming towards 1% fat or skim milk. Low or nonfat yogurt is a very useful substitute for butter, margarine, or sour cream on baked potatoes; as a base for a vegetable spread; or with fresh fruit for a pleasing dessert.

- Red meat should be eaten sparingly (although it does not have to be eliminated from the diet completely), and it helps to choose lower fat cuts such as flank steak, pork tenderloin, or loin lamb chops, with visible fat trimmed off, and to limit portion size to about 3 ounces. (Not all food descriptions have the same meaning. About 60% of the calories in both "extra lean" and "lean" hamburger come from fat.) Sausages, hot dogs, and luncheon meats should be avoided (unless they are made from poultry and the label shows that they are low in fat. Not all poultry luncheon meats are low in fat.) Poultry cuts should be chosen carefully. White meat is much lower in fat content than dark meat, and the skin should be removed. Ground turkey is usually high in fat.

- Prepared carbohydrates can be very tasty. Patients can consider beans, rice, potatoes, pasta, whole grain cereals, bread and bread products (such as bagels), green and orange vegetables, and fruit. High-fat toppings for these foods should be avoided.

- The lower fat varieties of fish, such as cod, haddock, northern pike, flounder, grouper, halibut, red snapper, Dover sole, bass, bluefish, swordfish, and tuna are preferred. Higher fat varieties include coho salmon, mackerel, pompano, and sardines.

- Frozen "lite" meals (after checking the labels to make sure that they really are low in fat) can be recommended for easy dinner preparation.

- Frozen low or nonfat yogurt, ice milk, sherbet, fruit sorbets, and frozen fruit bars can be substituted for ice cream.

Food Substitution and Gradual Change

The goal of food substitution is to achieve *qualitative* change in eating. The recommended food substitution pattern is to take one small, dietary fat lowering step at a time. The person does not have to stop eating chocolate, ice cream, red meat, cheese, and butter all at once, or eliminate them entirely. As Dr. Pi-Sunyer has noted:

> High-fat foods aren't prohibited, but people should understand that if they eat extra fat one day, they should eat less the next. No food is forbidden, but some foods only can be eaten on occasion for successful weight maintenance. (13)

If the patient eats red meat five times a week, he can try reducing it to four times per week for the first 2 weeks of a new weight loss program. If that goes well, he can try reducing it to three times per week for the next 2 weeks. If the patient feels that ultimately he cannot do without red meat less than two times a week, that number should be set as the goal, achieved by substituting lower fat foods of the patient's own choice. The patient should repeat this process for all the identified major high-fat foods.

Healthy Eating Patterns

In addition to lowering fat in the diet, the patient can consider other aids to developing a healthy eating pattern. The old saw "eat three square meals a day" is especially valuable for weight loss. Many people think that skipping breakfast, and the calories and fat it might contain, is a good way to lose weight. There is evidence that both eating breakfast and eating at regular intervals are elements of successful weight loss that can be as important as the content of the meals.

Behavioral Interventions

Behavior modification is commonly recommended as a weight loss tool. By itself, however, it is not a method for weight loss but rather a means to an end. While behavior modification techniques can be useful in helping the patient to implement a plan, developing the plan must come first. Useful behavioral techniques include keeping an eating log, controlling "mindless eating" (eating for reasons other than to satisfy hunger), not continuing to eat after feeling full, avoiding distractions and interruptions while eating, not eating too fast (taking smaller bites, chewing completely, putting the fork down between bites, etc.), and reducing portion size.

Healthy Shopping

Unless the patient is one of the relatively rare persons who can eat the same meals over and over again, he or she is not going to maintain a healthy eating pattern unless the menu is varied and appetizing. The patient's family members will also be unlikely to maintain healthy eating patterns, especially if they do not have a weight problem. There are many low-fat cookbooks on the market (some of which are presented in the "Resources" section), and there are plenty of recipes, ranging from the simple to the complex, for healthy and tasty low-fat dishes.

Low-fat eating begins in the supermarket. Among the keys to health-conscious food-shopping are these: not shopping when hungry; shopping with a list for the ingredients of planned low-fat dishes and for other low-fat foods; making sure that high-fat foods are not bought on impulse; learning the layout of one's supermarket, so that the high-fat food aisles can be avoided; and learning to read and use the new FDA-mandated food labels (see Chapter 8).

Healthy Cooking

The preparation of low-fat foods can vary greatly. Chinese cuisine, for example, can take the same ingredients of chicken and vegetables and vary the seasonings, combinations, coatings, sauces, slicing, and mode of cooking to make vastly different dishes. Healthy foods can be prepared in so many different ways that in a month of dinners made from the same basic ingredients the same taste and texture need not be experienced twice. For example, a low-fat eating plan could include chicken (primarily white meat) three times a week, and as long as a little time is taken in its preparation, the meals will never become boring. The initial step is to make low-fat meals so satisfying that the customary high-fat foods are not missed.

Vegetables form the centerpiece of any low-fat diet. Paying attention to cooking time (the less the better) and using imaginative recipes can overcome the reputation vegetables sometimes receive as being tasteless, soft, and overcooked.

Chicken is a staple of many low-fat diets. Found in virtually every major cuisine around the world, it can be prepared in many different ways. It is easy to prepare and cook. Fish is very important to the low-fat eater too, but it should be prepared with a low-fat method such as broiling or grilling. Meat can be included if low-fat varieties and cuts are chosen, all visible fat is trimmed off, and it is prepared in such a way as to remove as much of its intrinsic fat as possible.

Salads are, of course, an important part of any low-fat diet, as long as fat is not added in the form of meat, cheese, mayonnaise, or oily or creamy dressings. Many tasty low-fat dessert ideas can be found in low-fat cookbooks.

A variety of food preparation and cooking equipment can make low-fat cooking easier and can also help to produce the best flavor, texture, and appearance. Useful equipment include a steamer for cooking vegetables; a greaseless frying pan; a greaseless/waterless cookware system; a microwave oven; an oriental wok; an automatic bread making machine; a food processor or blender (for making dressings, dips, toppings, and drinks from stock or nonfat yogurt); a bulb baster for removing fat from gravies and sauces; a gravy separator; and sharp knives and poultry shears (helpful for trimming visible fat from meat and removing poultry skin before cooking).

Several cooking ingredients can facilitate tasty low-fat cooking: herbs and spices used creatively; low-fat lubricants such as vegetable oil; a low-fat nonstick spray; wine; lemon juice; wine or herb vinegar; a low-fat broth; cooking soy sauce (low-salt, if preferred); marinades for lower fat cuts of meat; and olive oil, used sparingly, for pan-frying.

CONCLUSION

Weight loss can be a complex, difficult, and frustrating process for both patient and clinician. Success can be achieved, however, especially if these principles are followed: both clinician and patient must understand overweight in general and the patient's type of overweight in particular; goal-setting is essential and should be realistic; inner motivation is the only kind that works; feeling good *now* should be the emphasis in motivation; doing it oneself while taking control is the guide, and gradual change is the route.

OFFICE AND CLINIC ORGANIZATION

Clinicians must decide if emphasis on weight management is important, for some or all patients, in clinical practice. It may help the clinician to answer the same goal-setting questions that the patient asks as his or her first step in deciding whether and how to change behavior (see "Setting Reasonable Limits and Priorities in Risk Assessment" section of Chapter 1).

It is also necessary to decide the following:

- Is the primary clinician in the office going to offer individual counseling directly?

- Will counseling be provided by someone else in the practice who is qualified?

- Will weight loss counseling be offered to groups of patients or on an individual basis?

- When will counseling be offered, during regular office hours or in the evening? (For example, some practitioners have reported success with groups, meeting one evening a week, for a modest fee per person.)

Finally, while not essential, clinicians engaging in weight loss counseling should consider their own weight. They will set an example for their patients by demonstrating healthy weight management. Clinicians who have dealt with weight loss can also talk from experience, knowing both the benefits and the difficulties of the process.

RESOURCES

Patient Education Materials

American Academy of Family Physicians
8880 Ward Parkway
Kansas City, MO 64114-2796
800-944-0000
"Weight Control: Losing Weight and Keeping It Off" (brochure 1522).

American Heart Association
7272 Greenville Avenue
Dallas, TX 75231-4596
800-242-8721
"A Guide to Losing Weight" (brochure 50-1035, available in English and Spanish); "Taking It Off" (brochure 50-079A).

Cookbooks

American Heart Association. Cookbook, 5th ed. New York: Times Books/Random House, 1991.
American Heart Association. Low-fat, low-cholesterol cookbook. New York: Times Books/Random House, 1990.
Cutler C, the Editors of Consumer Reports Books. Catch of the day. Yonkers, NY: Consumer Reports Books, 1990.
Jonas, S, the Editors of Consumer Reports Books. Take control of your weight. Yonkers, NY: Consumer Reports Books, 1993.
Kaufman PC, the Editors of Consumer Reports Books. Good eating, good health cookbook. Yonkers, NY: Consumer Reports Books, 1990.
Kreitzman S, the Editors of Consumer Reports Books. Slim cuisine. Yonkers, NY: Consumer Reports Books, 1991.
Kreitzman S, the Editors of Consumer Reports Books. Indulgent desserts. Yonkers, NY: Consumer Reports Books, 1993.
Light and easy cooking collection. Birmingham, AL: Oxmoor House, 1990.
Piscatella JC. Controlling your fat tooth. New York: Workman Publishing, 1991.
Scott ML, Scott JD, the Editors of Consumer Reports Books. Bean, pea and lentil cookbook. Yonkers, NY: Consumer Reports Books, 1991.
Spear R. Low fat and loving it. New York: Warner Books, 1991.
Weight Watchers. Fast fabulous cookbook. New York: New American Library, 1983.

Professional Education Materials

American Heart Association. Guidelines for weight management for healthy adults. Dallas: American Heart Association, 1994.
Lissner L, et al. Variability of body weight and health outcomes in the Framingham population. N Engl J Med 1991;324:1839.
U.S. Department of Health and Human Services, Public Health Service. Healthy people 2000. National health promotion and disease prevention objectives (PHS Pub. No. 91-50213). Washington, DC: Government Printing Office, 1991.

REFERENCES

1. Stunkard AJ. The current status of treatment for obesity in adults. In: Stunkard AJ, Stellar E, eds. Eating and its disorders. New York: Raven, 1983;157–173.
2. Brownell KD. Dieting and the search for the perfect body: where physiology and culture collide. Behavior Therapy 1991;22:1–12.
3. Garner DM, Wooley SC. Confronting the failure of behavioral and dietary treatments for obesity. Clinical Psychology Review 1991;11:729–780.
4. Lyons P, Burgard D. Great shape. Palo Alto, CA: Bull Publishing Co., 1990.
5. U.S. Preventive Services Task Force. Guide to clinical preventive services. Baltimore: Williams & Wilkins, 1989:111–114.
6. Kayman S, Bruvold W, Stern JS. Maintenance and relapse after weight loss in women: behavioral aspects. Am J Clin Nutr 1990;52:800–807.
7. Schachter S. Recidivism and self-cure of smoking and obesity. Am Psychol 1982;37:436.
8. Brownell KD. Personal responsibility and control over our bodies: when expectation exceeds reality. Health Psychol 1991;10:303–310.
9. Flatt JP. The biochemistry of energy expenditure. In: Bjorntorp P, Brodoff BN, ed. Obesity. New York: JB Lippincott, 1988.
10. Jonas S, Aronson V. The "I don't eat (but I can't lose)" weight loss program. New York: Rawson Associates, 1989.
11. Mole PA, et al. Exercise reverses depressed metabolic rate produced by severe caloric restriction. Med Sci Sports Exerc 1989;21:29.
12. Jonas S, Editors of Consumer Reports Books. Take control of your weight. Yonkers, NY: Consumer Reports Books, 1993.
13. An interview with F. Xavier Pi-Sunyer: obesity trends. Food Insight 1994;March/April:2.
14. Brownell KD, Wadden TA. The heterogeneity of obesity: fitting treatments to individuals. Behavior Therapy 1991 22:153–177.

10. Injury Prevention

STEVEN H. WOOLF

INTRODUCTION

All patients should be counseled about injury prevention. Injuries threaten the well-being and safety of all individuals, regardless of their health status or age. As the fourth leading cause of death in the United States, intentional and unintentional injuries together account for about 150,000 deaths each year (1). Persons under 45 years of age are more likely to die from injuries than from any other cause (2). It is therefore not surprising that injuries are the leading cause of years of potential life lost before age 65 (3). The lifetime costs of injuries sustained in the United States during a single year exceed an estimated one trillion dollars (4).

Injuries can be defined as unintentional or intentional events that cause physical or psychological harm. Unintentional injuries account for about 90,000 deaths annually in the United States. In 1990, the most common causes of unintentional injury deaths were motor vehicle crashes (45,827 deaths), falls (12,313 deaths), poisoning (5,803 deaths), fires and burns (4,175 deaths), and drowning (3,979 deaths) (1). Intentional injuries include psychological, sexual, and physical abuse; homicide; and suicide. Homicide and suicide account for about 55,000 deaths each year in the United States. About one to two million children and about one million older adults are abused or neglected each year in the United States (5).

Despite this enormous burden of morbidity and mortality, both clinicians and patients often view injuries as outside the domain of ambulatory medical practice. For many years, the public and the profession regarded injuries as a social policy problem to be addressed by legislators, engineers, product manufacturers, and employers. Their medical outcomes were seen solely as the province of the emergency department and hospital. Their relevance to ambulatory practice was overlooked, as was the clinician's ability to help prevent injuries. The belief that injuries are unrelated to clinical practice was clearly inaccurate. Injuries are the second most common cause of patient visits to physicians, accounting for 114 million physician contacts annually. Injuries generate one out of four visits to emergency departments and 2.8 million hospital admissions; they are the leading cause of hospital admissions for persons under age 45 (4).

Another common misconception is that patients are less endangered by injuries than by serious medical problems that clinicians are more accustomed to addressing, such as prostate cancer, leukemia, and acquired immunodeficiency syndrome (AIDS). Based on mortality data alone, these assumptions are clearly inaccurate. More persons die each year in the United States from motor vehicle injuries (about 50,000 deaths) than from prostate cancer (40,000), AIDS (38,500) or leukemia (20,000) (1–2, 6). In fact, among persons 1–34 years of age, unintentional and intentional injuries account for more deaths each year than all other causes combined (1). The public health significance of AIDS and its high death toll among young persons are widely recognized. Yet its total impact on years of potential life lost (YPLL) before age 65 (0.8 million YPLL) is far less than that of injuries (3.6 million YPLL) (2).

In light of these facts, clinicians cannot afford to ignore the effect of injuries upon the health of their patients. This often requires a reorientation of the history and physical examination to reflect the true risks faced by the patient rather than what the clinician considers "normal" clinical concerns. For example, most physicians examining an 18-year-old male would be reluctant to omit cardiac auscultation or testicular palpation for fear of missing congenital heart disease or testicular cancer. Time spent performing these procedures, however, often comes at the expense of discussing how the patient gets home from parties after drinking alcohol or whether he understands the importance of seat belts. These medical attitudes need to be reconciled with the facts. Motor vehicle injuries, the leading cause of death for persons under age 35 (4), are more likely to kill the patient than any single other cause (1). The chances that this patient will die in a car crash (45:100,000) are about 150 times greater than his risk of death from genital neoplasms (0.3:100,000) (2).

It is therefore not surprising that several physician organizations have recommended routine injury prevention counseling. The American Academy of Pediatrics (7), American Academy of Family Physicians (8), and U.S. Preventive Services Task Force (9) have recommended that clinicians counsel adult patients and the parents of pediatric patients about these and other injury prevention measures: motor vehicle safety; smoke detectors; barriers to keep children away from the hazards of windows, stairways, and swimming pools; bicycle safety helmets; syrup of ipecac; water heater temperature; and smoking near bedding or upholstery.

This chapter reviews the essential counseling that should be provided for the most common unintentional and intentional injuries. It also discusses the physician's role in reducing medical causes of injuries. The most effective injury prevention measures, however, are not performed in the doctor's office but result from population-wide or community-based interventions, such as design changes, safety regulations, and other public policies. These broader activities that fall outside the clinical domain are

Table 10.1
Leading Causes of Injury-Related Deaths, By Age (Death Rates per 100,000)

Rank	0–1	1–4	5–9	10–14	15–19	20–24	25–29	30–34	35–44	45–54	55–64	65–74	75–84
						Age (Years)							
1	Hom (8)	MV (6)	MV (5)	MV (6)	MV (33)	MV (34)	MV (26)	MV (21)	MV (17)	MV (15)	Sui (16)	MV (18)	Falls (34)
2	MV (5)	Drow (4)	Drow (1)	Hom (2)	Hom (17)	Hom (23)	Hom (20)	Hom (16)	Sui (15)	Sui (15)	MV (16)	Sui (18)	MV (29)
3	Suff (5)	F/B (4)	F/B (1)	Sui (2)	Sui (11)	Sui (15)	Sui (15)	Sui (15)	Hom (12)	Hom (8)	Hom (5)	Falls (9)	Sui (25)
4	F/B (3)	Hom (3)	Hom (1)	Drow (1)	Drow (2)	Drow (2)	Pois (3)	Pois (3)	Pois (5)	Falls (2)	Falls (4)	Hom (4)	F/B (5)
5	Asp (3)	Suff (0.2)	UF (0.3)	UF (1)	UF (2)	Pois (2)	Drow (2)	Drow (2)	Drow (1)	F/B (1)	F/B (2)	F/B (3)	Hom (4)

Adapted from National Center for Health Statistics. Vital Statistics of the United States, 1990, vol. II, mortality, part A. Washington, DC: Public Health Service, 1994. *Legend: Asp* = Aspiration (food); *Drow* = Drowning; *F/B* = Fires and burns; *Hom* = Homicide; *MV* = Motor vehicle injuries; *Pois* = Poisoning (solids and liquids); *Suff* = Suffocation; *Sui* = Suicide; *UF* = Unintentional firearm injuries.

not discussed here. Although work site injuries are extremely common, they are also not discussed here: the complexity and extensive regulations associated with the prevention of occupational injuries are beyond the scope of a single chapter. Clinicians practicing in an area where many patients work in a hazardous setting (e.g., mining, foundry, lead smelting, farming) should become familiar with appropriate counseling interventions for that industry. Although incidents in which injuries are sustained are often referred to in this chapter as "accidents," the injury prevention community tries to avoid this term because such events are considered predictable, preventable, and therefore not true accidents (10).

Although this chapter addresses nine injury topics, most clinicians lack the time to discuss each of them in a single visit. Instead, counseling should be tailored to the most likely injury risks facing the individual patient. Table 10.1 reviews the leading causes of injury deaths for patients in different age groups. This information can be used by the clinician to determine which topics to emphasize when counseling individual patients or parents. For example, counseling of adolescents should emphasize alcohol and seat belt use in motor vehicles, whereas counseling of older adults should devote more time to the prevention of falls.

UNINTENTIONAL INJURIES

Motor Vehicle Injuries

Almost 50,000 persons die each year in the United States from motor vehicle injuries (2). Each year, motor vehicle injuries account for about 5 million injuries requiring treatment in emergency departments, about

500,000 hospital admissions, 57% of head injury deaths, 44% of brain injuries (about 180,000 injuries), 56% of acute spinal cord injuries (about 6,800 injuries), 20% of facial injuries treated in emergency departments (about 630,000 injuries), and an estimated 50 billion dollars in direct and indirect costs. About 670,000 office visits to physicians are for motor vehicle injuries (11). Motor vehicle crashes account for 40% of all deaths among teenagers. Although fatal and severe nonfatal motor vehicle injuries are most common among young persons (ages 15–24), the elderly are most likely to die from motor vehicle injuries (4).

Essentials of Counseling

All persons who drive or ride in motor vehicles should be urged to use seat belts, even if the planned trip is short. At least 48 states and the District of Columbia currently require this by law. The clinician can help motivate the patient to follow this advice by describing the risks of injury and death for unbelted passengers, contrasting the risk of motor vehicle injuries with diseases that the patient assumes, incorrectly, pose a greater threat to their health, clarifying that short trips may be the most likely setting for injurious accidents, and emphasizing the proven efficacy of seat belts in reducing the risk of death and nonfatal injuries by 50%. Although patients should be encouraged to purchase vehicles with passive restraint and injury protection systems (e.g., air bags, automatic seat belts, energy-absorbing structures), they should understand that these features do not replace the need for using seat belts. Patients should also understand that the risk of fatal motor vehicle injuries is about 20–30% higher when driving speeds increase from 55 to 65 miles per hour (4).

Parents should be counseled regularly (e.g., during well-child visits) about the importance of properly securing their children in safety seats or seat belts. Infants and small children should be secured in a rearward-facing position and restrained in appropriate safety seats for their weight: *infant seats* for babies weighing up to 20 pounds, *convertible seats* for babies or toddlers weighing up to 40 pounds, *vests and integral seats* for toddlers weighing more than 20 pounds, and *booster seats* for children weighing 40–70 pounds who have outgrown convertible/toddler seats but cannot use a regular harness. Only seats meeting Federal Motor Vehicle Safety Standard 213 should be used, and the manufacturer's instructions should be followed. Parents should be reminded that failure to restrain children in safety seats is illegal in all states. Many communities have programs that provide child safety seats to parents who cannot afford to purchase them at retail stores. Parents should be encouraged to teach children to fasten seat belts on their own whenever riding in a motor vehicle. Grandparents, babysitters, and others who regularly transport children should receive similar counseling about the use of safety seats and belts for children.

Driving while intoxicated by alcohol or other drugs increases the risk of being involved in motor vehicle accidents, dying in the accident, and suffering nonfatal injuries. About 40% of fatal motor vehicle crashes (18,000 deaths) involve drivers with blood alcohol concentrations of 0.10 or greater (4). About 25% of males ages 18–29 years admit in surveys to having driven at least once in the past year after drinking excessively (12). Clinicians should warn all patients who drive, especially those who use alcohol or other drugs, that it is extremely dangerous to drive while intoxicated. Since alcohol impairs driving skills before one becomes intoxicated, patients should be informed that driving after drinking as few as one or two drinks may be dangerous (13). The likelihood of a fatal crash doubles for every 0.02% increase in blood alcohol concentration; a driver with a blood alcohol concentration of 0.15 is 300–600 times more likely to have an accident than one who is sober (4). The value of identifying a "designated driver" when attending social functions where alcohol is used should be emphasized.

Patients who ride motorcycles should be urged to wear safety helmets, as required by law in many states. About 7% of traffic deaths involve motorcyclists, whose risk of being killed per mile driven is 35 times greater than that for automobile drivers (4). Head injuries account for about 85% of these deaths. Patients may be motivated to wear helmets if the clinician describes the lethal and disabling nature of high-impact head injuries and the efficacy of safety helmets (about 30% reduction in mortality and 75% reduction in head injuries) (4, 14). Since about 80% of motorcyclists killed in accidents are intoxicated by alcohol, patients who ride motorcycles should also be counseled against drinking and driving. Safety helmets are also recommended for persons who ride all-terrain vehicles. Use of safety helmets when riding bicycles is discussed later under "Falls."

Adolescents and young adults are at increased risk of being involved in a motor vehicle accident, driving without seat belts, and driving while intoxicated. This age group, however, which has a tendency to minimize risk and to ignore the advice of authority figures, is less likely to be persuaded by traditional motor vehicle counseling. Parents of adolescents should receive special counseling about the need to teach children about responsible options when they attend parties or other social functions at which alcohol or other drugs are used or when they are considering riding in a vehicle operated by an intoxicated driver. The clinician should counsel the adolescent to avoid using alcohol or other drugs when driving is anticipated and to discuss with their families transportation alternatives for teen parties or other functions at which alcohol and other drugs are used.

Older adults and patients suffering from neuromuscular and other disorders may also be at increased risk of motor vehicle injuries. Such individuals should receive special counseling about the importance of both regular prevention strategies (e.g., seat belts, avoiding driving while intoxicated) and special measures to compensate for their impairment (e.g., corrective lenses, hearing aids). Patients with impairment from certain endocrine, neurological, psychiatric, cardiac, pulmonary, and musculoskeletal disorders should be discouraged from obtaining a driver's license (15). The questions listed in Table 10.2 can help determine whether driving should be restricted.

Falls

Falls are the most common cause of injuries, the leading cause of hospital admissions for trauma, and the second leading cause of injury-related deaths (about 12,000 annually). An estimated one of out 20 persons receives emergency room care for injuries sustained in falls; the total lifetime cost of falls approaches 40 billion dollars annually (4). Fall injuries can affect all age groups. Small children who fall from furniture or buildings (e.g., by climbing out of opened windows) and older children who fall from bicycles can sustain head trauma and other serious injuries. An estimated one out of ten children ages 1–3 years are treated in emergency rooms for fall injuries. Most fatal falls among children are from buildings or other elevated structures (4). One out of six children (ages 5–14) killed in motor vehicle accidents are riding bicycles. Adolescents and adults who ride bicycles are also at risk for serious injuries from head trauma.

Older adults are more likely to fall during normal household activities due to postural instability and decreased proprioception, muscle strength, and vision. Due to decreased bone density and other factors, the elderly are also more likely to sustain serious injuries when they fall (e.g., hip fractures, subdural hemorrhages). Falls cause nearly 90% of all fractures among older adults. Hip fractures account for about 250,000 hospital admissions annually and are associated with a 15–20% reduction in survival in the first year following the fracture. Among persons over 85 years of

Table 10.2
Assessment of Driving Impairment

1. How reliable is the patient in describing their driving skills?
2. Does the patient have the physical and mental characteristics to drive safely?
3. Does the patient have a medical problem or multiple problems that might affect driving safety?
4. Would prescription medications affect driving skills?
5. What is the patient's driving history?
6. Is there a history of previous crashes or moving violations?
7. Is there evidence of episodic impairment due to substance abuse?
8. What is the prognosis for the patient during the period of licensing?
9. Does the person have a driving occupation that would put other persons at risk?
10. Should a driving test be recommended?

Adapted from Doege TC, Engelberg AL, eds. Medical conditions affecting drivers. Chicago: American Medical Association, 1986.

age, the risk of dying from a fall is three times greater than an adolescent's risk of dying in a motor vehicle crash (4).

Essentials of Counseling

Parents of infants and small children should be counseled about the risks of falls. They should be reminded about the ease with which children can fall from changing tables, beds, and other surfaces on which they may be left unattended. Once small children begin crawling and walking, they are at risk of falling down stairs. This risk can be lowered by installing protective gates or other devices to block access to the top and bottom of dangerous stairways. Parents who live in high-rise buildings should be encouraged to install window guards or locks on windows not designed as emergency fire exits. Similar advice should be given to grandparents and other persons who care for small children.

Parents of children who ride bicycles or tricycles should be urged to purchase child safety helmets and to ensure that their children wear properly fitted helmets whenever the bicycle or tricycle is used. Many communities have programs that provide safety helmets to parents who cannot afford to purchase them at retail stores. Only helmets approved by the American National Standards Institute, the Snell Memorial Foundation, American Society for Testing and Materials, or Consumer Product Safety Commission should be used. The same advice should be given to adolescents and adults who ride bicycles or engage in other forms of cycling, rollerblading, and high-speed sports.

Fall prevention among older adults involves home improvements and the reduction of medical risk factors. Home improvements that can reduce the risk of falls include installing good lighting, visual cues, hand railings, and nonstick traction strips on floor surfaces; the removal of loose rugs, electrical cords, and other items that promote tripping; and the removal or padding of sharply cornered furniture. The clinician should encourage the patient and family members to inspect the home for these problems. Stable footwear should replace slippers, loose slip-on shoes, and high heels. Since about 1400 fatal falls occur in nursing homes and other residential institutions (4), physicians who work with nursing homes should urge administrators to correct building conditions or practices that precipitate falls. The physician should also address medical factors that increase the risk of falls. Patients with impaired vision or hearing should be counseled to obtain correct prescription lenses and hearing aids, respectively (see Chapters 3 and 4). Older adults should be encouraged to perform exercises or undergo physical therapy to improve gait and balance, strengthen muscles, and increase bone density (see Chapter 7). Patients with neuromuscular conditions that impair balance should be prescribed appropriate walkers, canes, or wheelchairs. Whenever possible, physicians should either discontinue medications that increase the risk of falls or prescribe safer substitutes. Older adults who use alcohol should receive appropriate counseling (see Chapter 13).

Poisoning

The third leading cause of unintentional injuries are poisonings, which account for about 6000 deaths each year in the United States (4). Poison control centers receive about 1.4 million reports of exposures each year, 60% involving children under the age of five. The most common agents known to cause poisoning deaths in adults are motor vehicle exhaust (25%), cocaine and heroin (11%), antidepressants and tranquilizers (10%), and barbiturates (2%). Of the approximately 850,000 childhood poisonings reported each year to poison control centers, most of which are nonlethal, the most common agents are unspecified substances (61%), cleaning or polishing agents (10%), plants (10%), and pesticides and fertilizers (3%) (16). The most common lethal agents ingested by children are antidepressants, anticonvulsants, and cardiovascular drugs. Most poisonings occur when unattended small children enter medicine cabinets, kitchen cabinets, or other areas in which potentially toxic chemicals are stored. Among small children, death rates from drug poisoning have fallen by 75% since 1970, a trend widely attributed to childproof packaging of medications. Absorption of some poisons can be minimized by inducing vomiting with an emetic (e.g., ipecac) as soon as possible after ingestion.

Essentials of Counseling

Parents of infants and small children should be counseled about the use of ipecac and urged to purchase a 1 ounce bottle of ipecac syrup and place it in a quickly accessible location in the home. The clinician should provide parents with the telephone number of the local poison control center, suggest that they post the number near their telephone, and instruct them to call the number immediately in the event of an exposure. They should be reminded not to administer syrup of ipecac without instructions from a physician or poison control center. Parents should be advised to install door catches to prevent small children from opening cabinets that contain harmful chemicals. Potentially harmful medicines or chemicals should be transferred from areas to which access cannot be restricted to high cabinets or other locations out of the reach of children. Grandparents or other individuals who care for small children in the home should receive similar advice.

Burns and Fires

Burns and fires account for 1.4 million injuries, 54,000 hospital admissions, and about 4,000 deaths each year in the United States, making it the fourth leading cause of unintentional injury deaths. About 75% of these deaths occur in house fires, which are usually caused by cigarettes or heating equipment. Elevated blood alcohol levels are found in about half of adults who die in fires. Unintentional burn injuries are usually the result of fires or hot water scalds. An estimated 3,500 persons with scald burns from showers or bathtubs receive emergency treatment each year, and about one-quarter require hospitalization (4).

Essentials of Counseling

Patients who are homeowners (including landlords, hotel managers, etc.) should be advised to install and test periodically smoke detectors. Periodic testing should be emphasized; although five out of six homes in the United States have smoke detectors, studies suggest that at least one-third are not functional because of dead batteries (4). Smoke detectors should be installed in locations that are near potential sources of smoke, are easily audible in all rooms, and provide occupants with sufficient warning to escape in safety. Patients with questions about fire safety should contact their local fire department, many of which will conduct free fire safety inspections of the home and will help design an appropriate escape plan. The plan should pay special attention to young children or older adults, who are more likely to die in house fires due to difficulty in escaping the building.

Parents and other homeowners with small children or impaired adults should be reminded that hot water accidents can result in severe burn injuries. The temperature of hot water heaters should be kept below 120° Fahrenheit, or antiscald tap water devices should be installed. Parents should also be reminded to purchase fire-retardant clothing for their children, to store matches and lighters in child-resistant containers, and to place plastic covers over accessible electrical wall outlets. Patients who smoke cigarettes, in addition to being counseled to stop smoking (see Chapter 6), should be warned against smoking in bed or while intoxicated, both of which are common causes of household fires.

Drowning

Approximately 4000 persons in the United States die each year from drowning, making it the fifth most common cause of unintentional injury deaths (2). About 20% of drownings are related to boating accidents. Although many drownings result from unexpected and poorly preventable circumstances (e.g., motor vehicle immersion, flash floods, marine accidents), some drownings are preventable. For example, about 230 children under age five die annually in swimming pools, and about 350 drownings occur each year in bathtubs (4). For every fatal case of pediatric drowning, there are an estimated four hospitalizations and 15 emergency department visits for pediatric drowning. Adolescents and adults often drown because of swimming or boating while intoxicated by alcohol or other drugs. High blood alcohol concentrations are reported in 40–50% of adult drownings (4).

Essentials of Counseling

Patients who participate in water sports should be counseled about the importance of water safety (e.g., learning how to swim, boating skills, wearing life vests) and should be warned against swimming or boating while intoxicated by alcohol or other drugs. Such counseling is most timely during the summer months, when patients are more likely to participate in water sports or attend activities near water. Parents of infants and small children should be reminded to watch children closely when they are near swimming pools, rivers, lakes, or bathtubs. Parents of small children who own swimming pools should be encouraged to install a 4.5–5 foot "childproof" protective fence around the pool and to keep the entrance gate securely closed. Because a large number of swimming pool drowning deaths could be prevented by immediate cardiopulmonary resuscitation, owners of swimming pools should be encouraged to obtain basic resuscitation training.

Sports Injuries

Although sports activities account for a relatively small proportion of injury deaths in the United States, they are a major cause of nonfatal injuries. Studies suggest that sports injuries may be the leading cause of hospital admissions and emergency department visits for children and adolescents. About one-third of hospital admissions for eye trauma are due to sports-related injuries. An estimated two-thirds of sports injuries result from contact sports. In 1980, emergency rooms treated about 1.5 million injuries from football, baseball, basketball, soccer, and racquet sports (4). Surveys suggest that about 10% of persons who exercise at fitness clubs seek medical attention for exercise-induced musculoskeletal injuries (17).

Essentials of Counseling

Clinicians should discourage patients from participating in especially dangerous sports, such as boxing, or using dangerous sports equipment, such as trampolines and all-terrain vehicles. For other sports, patients should be encouraged to obtain proper training to reduce injuries (e.g., ski lessons), to perform recommended preparatory activities (e.g., stretching), to avoid beginning sports at a strenuous intensity, and to wear appropriate protective equipment (e.g., eye protection devices during racquet sports (18), helmets and face masks during football and horseback riding). See Chapter 7 for further details. Patients should be reminded to avoid playing sports when intoxicated by alcohol or other drugs.

INTENTIONAL INJURIES

Abuse and Neglect

Abuse refers to intentional acts that harm or threaten an individual's physical or mental well-being. *Neglect* refers to the failure to provide for an individual's basic needs (e.g., food, clothing, shelter, hygiene). Abuse can be physical (e.g., kicking, hitting, burning), sexual (fondling, intercourse, or other sexual acts without consent), or emotional (verbal or behavioral attacks on self-worth). Child sexual abuse also includes sexual activities for which the child is developmentally unprepared. Patients at increased risk of abuse and neglect include children, older adults, and other persons who are vulnerable due to physical or mental limitations. Spouses are common victims of physical and sexual abuse, with about one million American women receiving emergency treatment each year for battering (19). Epidemiologic studies suggest that pregnant women are more likely than other women to be victims of violence (20).

Screening and Reporting

There is insufficient evidence of effectiveness to support the routine use of screening instruments to detect abuse or neglect (21). Recommendations to this effect have been issued by the U.S. Preventive Services Task Force and the Canadian Task Force on the Periodic Health Examination. As discussed in Chapters 2 and 3, clinicians should watch for signs of abuse when talking with and examining patients, especially children, older adults, pregnant women, or other vulnerable patients. During the physical examination, they should be alert for abnormal bruises, scars, or orthopedic injuries that rarely result from routine accidents or that do not correspond with the description of events. Clinicians who consider themselves unqualified to conduct this examination should refer the patient to a qualified colleague.

Two common approaches are used when questioning patients or caretakers about the possibility of abuse. One is to link the question to information that the patient has already provided in the encounter. *"You said that one bad thing about your marriage is the frequent arguments. Does your husband ever hurt you during these arguments?" "These bruises on Johnny's back are somewhat unusual. Can you tell me what happened?"* Another approach is to normalize the problem. *"Many of my patients have told me that their husbands hit them—they complain of being abused. How is it for you?"* *"Many parents have difficulty dealing with the stress of a baby's constant crying. How do you handle it?"* Questions can also be directed at children. Using age-appropriate language, the clinician may wish to ask children directly about feelings of sadness or an unpleasant home situation if an abnormal affect, behavior, or family dynamic is noted in the clinical encounter that might suggest depression, abuse, or neglect.

The physical findings of child abuse are often subtle or nonspecific: children who are not abused commonly have abrasions and lacerations from normal play activities; abused children are often manipulated into secrecy; and some injuries are difficult to detect. A good example of the latter is shaken baby syndrome, in which the child may sustain severe brain injuries (e.g., subdural hemorrhage) with no external signs of trauma (22). Other physical findings and behaviors seen in physically or sexually abused children are listed in Table 10.3. Clinicians who suspect child abuse or neglect are required by law in all states to report their concerns to the local child protective services agency. This reporting requirement is not satisfied by informing colleagues, a hospital social worker, or other individuals outside the official agency.

The signs of elder abuse can also be subtle or nonspecific, since injuries from falls are common among older adults. Moreover, patients suffering from dementia and other forms of cognitive impairment may be unable to report abuse or may issue false claims of abuse against caretakers as a result of delusional thinking. Elder neglect includes withholding of necessary food, clothing, hygiene, medical care, or social contact. Clinicians who discover evidence of abuse or neglect (e.g., malnutrition, pressure ulcers, misuse of personal finances) should report their concerns to the local adult protective services agency. Table 10.4 lists the telephone number to report elder abuse in each state (23).

Essentials of Counseling

The clinician's responsibilities when abuse or neglect are suspected extend beyond the legal requirement to contact a protective services agency. The clinician should also document physical findings (using either a body diagram or photographs to describe the size, location, and appearance of injuries) and pertinent laboratory data. This information should be placed in the patient's chart. In cases of suspected sexual abuse, a pelvic examination is often necessary to check for abrasions or bruises of the vagina and external genitalia; in children and adolescents, in particular, the physician should check for distortion of the hymen, alterations in rectal tone, sexually transmitted diseases, or signs of pregnancy. If a recent sexual assault is

Table 10.3
Common Behaviors and Physical Findings Among Abused Children

Behaviors

Extremes of activity (hyperactivity or withdrawal)
Poor self-esteem
Poor peer relationships
General feelings of shame and guilt
Distortion of body image (distorted drawings)
Regressive behavior
Enuresis/encopresis
Fear, phobia directed toward adults
Pseudomature behavior
Poor academic performance
Eating disorder
Sexual promiscuity or provocative behavior
Compulsive masturbation
Sexual abuse of sibling, friend, or younger child
Early pregnancy
Running away from home
Attempted suicide

Physical Findings

Burns or bruises in patterns that resemble hands, belts, cords, and other weapons
Wounds in locations of corporal punishment (e.g., buttocks, lower back, upper thighs, face)
Multiple traumatic injuries without a plausible explanation

Adapted from American Medical Association. Diagnostic and treatment guidelines on child sexual abuse. Arch Fam Med 1993;2:19–27.

suspected, clothing and samples of blood, hair, urine, and saliva may be useful for laboratory and forensic analysis.

The next concern is the patient's safety. Although protective service agencies will take responsibility for removing patients from dangerous living situations, the clinician should take the additional step of making the patient aware of community resources that can provide immediate help in the event of future abuse. For example, women who are victims of spouse abuse or parents who worry that their partner may injure the children should be given information about local battered women's shelters and crisis centers that can provide safe housing, psychological support, and other services (e.g., legal advice). The clinician and patient can reach agreement on a safety plan should a future crisis arise. These extra efforts by the clinician provide a safety net in case the investigating agency reaches incorrect conclusions about the risk of abuse or provides inadequate help for victims at risk.

The clinician should next address relevant psychosocial issues. Patients or parents who report abuse to the clinician often suffer from guilt and fear of reprisals from the abuser. The act of informing the clinician and acknowledging the abuse can shatter the denial that previously masked the problem, thereby releasing powerful emotions. The clinician

Table 10.4
Telephone Contacts for Elder Abuse

Alabama	800-458-7214
Alaska	907-465-2145
Arizona	602-542-4446
Arkansas	800-482-8049, 800-922-5330
California	916-657-2186
Colorado	303-866-5910
Connecticut	203-566-3117
Delaware	302-421-6791
District of Columbia	202-727-0113
Florida	800-96-ABUSE
Georgia	404-894-4440
Hawaii	808-548-5902
Idaho	208-334-5531
Illinois	800-252-8966
Indiana	800-992-6978
Iowa	800-362-2178
Kansas	800-432-3535
Kentucky	502-564-7043
Louisiana	504-342-9931
Maine	207-624-5335
Maryland	410-333-0161
Massachusetts	800-922-2275
Michigan	517-373-2869
Minnesota	800-652-9747
Mississippi	800-354-6347
Missouri	800-392-0210
Montana	406-444-5900
Nebraska	800-652-1999
Nevada	702-687-4588
New Hampshire	800-852-3345
New Jersey	800-792-8820
New Mexico	800-432-6217
New York	518-432-2980
North Carolina	800-662-7030
North Dakota	701-224-2577
Ohio	800-686-1581
Oklahoma	800-522-3511
Oregon	800-232-3020
Pennsylvania	800-992-2433
Rhode Island	800-322-2880
South Carolina	800-734-5670
South Dakota	605-773-3656
Tennessee	615-741-5926
Texas	800-252-5400
Utah	801-538-3910
Vermont	800-564-1612
Virginia	804-662-9241
Washington	206-753-5227
West Virginia	800-352-6513
Wisconsin	608-266-2536
Wyoming	800-528-3396

Adapted from: Aravanis SC, Adelman RD, Breckman R, Fulmer TT, Holder E, Lachs M, O'Brien JG, Sanders AB. Diagnostic and treatment guidelines on elder abuse and neglect. Arch Fam Med 1993;2:371–388.

should be prepared to provide emotional support, to recommend that the patient return for future visits, and to provide information about appropriate community resources (e.g., therapist, clergy, women's centers) for further counseling.

A more difficult psychosocial problem is faced by clinicians who, based on their own findings, suspect abuse that is unmentioned or denied by the parents or caregivers. The law requires clinicians to report their concerns to the local protective services agency, but doing so may jeopardize their relationship with the parents or caregivers. Although most agencies do not disclose the identity of the person who reported the case, it is a common and healthy practice for clinicians to tell parents or caregivers that they need to report the case; even if they do not reveal their intentions, the clinician is often suspected anyway. Anger directed at the clinician for violating confidentiality and for initiating a potentially embarrassing and threatening investigation may cause patients to terminate their relationship with the clinician. Although this can sometimes be avoided through empathy and the clinician's genuine concern for the patient, the relationship with the clinician may not survive the anger and mistrust generated by the incident.

Finally, the clinician can play a role in getting help for the abuser, especially if the abuser is a patient. Many abusers were themselves victims of abuse and are suffering from environmental stress, social isolation, poor impulse control, substance abuse, or personal crises. Fundamental issues related to self-esteem may have a causal role (see Chapter 16). The clinician should encourage the abuser to obtain counseling from a qualified mental health professional and should be prepared to recommend therapists in the community with special expertise in this area. In some cases, neglect of children or older adults is due to economic or other personal circumstances rather than psychological factors. In these cases, the clinician should direct the caregiver to appropriate social services agencies that can help remedy the problem or provide better care for the patient. Elder neglect can occur when children incapable of providing appropriate care are reluctant to acknowledge their limitations and pursue other options (e.g., nursing home) because of denial or guilt. The clinician can help them to overcome their denial and to separate their feelings from the needs of the patient. Finally, abuse is sometimes related to alcohol or other drug abuse. In such cases, the clinician can arrange appropriate substance abuse counseling and rehabilitation services (see Chapter 13).

Homicide

About 25,000 persons are murdered each year in the United States. Homicide is the second leading cause of death among adolescents and young adults (age 15–24) and the third leading cause of death among children

ages 5–14 (1). In 1993, the homicide rate for African American males between 15 and 24 years of age was 10 times that for white males of the same
age (1). In fact, firearms are the leading cause of death among African
American males age 15–34. About 55% of homicide victims are killed by
family members or acquaintances (4). Two-thirds of homicides are committed with firearms (about 34,000 Americans are killed each year by
firearms), making shootings the second most common cause of fatal injuries (24). In the last 30 years, homicide rates for children and adolescents have doubled.

Essentials of Counseling

Complex societal and personal factors lead individuals to commit murder,
and thus the capacity of the clinician to help prevent homicide is quite
limited. Several potential interventions are possible, however. First, patients or families that have difficulty with conflict resolution can be referred for individual or group counseling to learn nonviolent options for
dealing with disagreement. Arguments are a precipitating factor in almost
half of all homicides (4). Second, since many homicides are related to alcohol or other drug use, substance abuse counseling and rehabilitation may be
helpful (see Chapter 13). Third, clinicians who become aware of an individual's intent to harm or kill another individual should report this information to the local police department. The threat of harm to other individuals
permits violation of the confidentiality of the clinician-patient relationship.

Another intervention that can prevent both intentional and accidental
homicide is the removal of firearms from the home. Persons engaged in
domestic violence or other angry conflicts may be more likely to shoot and
kill another individual if there is easy access to firearms (25). Removal of
firearms from the home is especially important if children live in or visit
the home. Approximately 32% of accidental firearm-related deaths occur
among children and adolescents (26). If firearms are kept in the home,
they should be unloaded, the bullets should be stored separately, and both
the weapon and ammunition should be locked in a compartment that children cannot open.

Evidence that these measures are effective in decreasing violent injuries
is limited. The U.S. Preventive Services Task Force concluded that there was
insufficient evidence to recommend for or against counseling to prevent violent injuries. See Chapter 28 regarding promotion by health professionals of
local and national policies to control the availability of firearms.

Suicide

Over 30,000 persons in the United States commit suicide each year, making it the eighth leading cause of death in the general population. Among

persons under age 35, who account for about 12,000 suicides each year, it is the third leading cause of death (2). The most common means of committing suicide are firearms (59%), hanging (15%), poison ingestion (10%), carbon monoxide inhalation (8%), drowning (2%), and cutting with a sharp instrument (1%). In unsuccessful suicide attempts, drug ingestion (70%) and wrist cutting (15%) are the most common methods (4). The incidence of successful suicide is highest among elderly males, whereas the highest incidence of attempted suicide is among adolescents and young adults below age 25 (4). Risk factors for suicide include previous suicide attempts, depression, substance abuse, divorce or separation, and availability of firearms (4). In the last 30 years, suicide rates for children and adolescents have tripled.

Essentials of Counseling

A large proportion of suicides result from depression, and thus some suicides may be prevented by the early diagnosis and treatment of depression (see Chapter 16). Similarly, suicide is often related to alcohol and other drug use, and thus the treatment of substance abuse may have a preventive role (see Chapter 13). As noted in Chapters 2 and 16, clinicians should ask patients who are depressed whether they have ever thought of hurting themselves. This can be done in a nonjudgmental manner by saying, *"When people feel the way that you do, they often think of hurting themselves. Have you ever considered killing yourself?"* If the patient has considered suicide, the clinician should ask about the frequency of such thoughts and the most recent suicidal ideation, preparatory actions (e.g., obtaining a weapon, preparing a plan, giving away prized possessions), and prior suicide gestures or attempts. If this information and the patient's mood generate suspicion that the patient may commit suicide in the near future, the patient should generally be admitted to the hospital for inpatient psychiatric care. Otherwise, arrangements should be made for outpatient counseling and the prescription of antidepressant medication. The patient should also be given the telephone number of local mental health agencies and suicide hotlines to contact during future crises.

Routine screening for suicide risk has been recommended by some authorities. For example, the American Academy of Pediatrics (27) recommends asking all adolescents about suicidal thoughts during the routine medical history. Current evidence suggests, however, that answers to such questions have poor sensitivity and specificity in predicting subsequent suicidal behavior. Furthermore, there is no available evidence that early detection of suicidal intent is an effective means of reducing suicide rates. Accordingly, the Canadian Task Force on the Periodic Health Examination recommends that clinicians routinely evaluate suicidal risk factors only in high-risk patients (28), and the U.S. Preventive Services Task Force recommends against routine screening to detect suicide risk (9).

OFFICE AND CLINIC ORGANIZATION FOR INJURY PREVENTION COUNSELING

The office or clinic with excellence in injury prevention counseling should have immediate access to the telephone number and address of the local poison control center; agencies or private organizations providing child safety seats, safety helmets, and smoke detectors for disadvantaged families; crisis centers, shelters, and hotlines for abuse victims and persons considering suicide; therapists with special skills in domestic violence, child physical or sexual abuse, and conflict resolution; protective services agencies for children, older adults, and other abused persons; and other social service agencies for economically deprived caregivers. If other services are available in the community (e.g., fire department home safety inspections, cardiopulmonary resuscitation training), the appropriate telephone number should be available in the office for interested patients or parents. Patient education brochures on timely injury prevention topics (e.g., "water safety" during summer months) should be placed in the waiting room, and selected copies should be available in the examining room so that clinicians can hand them directly to patients or parents to reinforce counseling messages. Examples of such brochures are listed under "Resources— Patient Education Materials."

MEDICAL RECORD DOCUMENTATION

Clinicians should make brief notations in the medical record whenever injury prevention counseling is provided. Physical findings or other evidence suggestive of abuse or neglect (including photographs or body diagrams) should also be placed in the chart, as well as documentation that the appropriate protective services agency was notified. A flow sheet should summarize all medications being taken by patients, especially older adults, to help determine whether the risk of falls or other adverse effects can be minimized.

RESOURCES—PROFESSIONAL EDUCATION MATERIALS

Injury Prevention

American Academy of Pediatrics
Publications Department
141 Northwest Point Boulevard
P.O. Box 927
Elk Grove Village, IL 60009-0927
800-433-9016

"Injury Control for Children and Youth." (300-page manual MA0024); "A Guide to Safety Counseling in Office Practice." (56-page manual HE0042); "TIPP—The Injury Prevention Program" (a comprehensive childhood injury prevention packet for professionals that includes questionnaires to be completed by parents and children and eight age-specific safety sheets HE0013).

National Maternal and Child Health Clearinghouse
8201 Greensboro Drive, Suite 600
McLean, VA 22102-3843
703-821-8955, ext. 254
Several professional publications on childhood injury prevention are available.

Motor Vehicle Injury Prevention

American Academy of Family Physicians
8880 Ward Parkway
Kansas City, MO
800-944-0000
"Take 40 Seconds" (brochure for physicians on counseling patients regarding seat belts). The Academy also offers a free subscription to "Safe Ride News," a quarterly newsletter on childhood occupant protection, recalls, and product updates.

American Academy of Pediatrics
Publications Department
141 Northwest Point Boulevard
P.O. Box 927
Elk Grove Village, IL 60009-0927
800-433-9016
"Physician's Resource Guide for Bicycle Safety Education." (26-page manual, HE0084).

National Highway Traffic Safety Administration
Auto Safety Hotline
800-424-9393
Information and notices about car safety and child safety seats.

Family Violence and Child Abuse

Clearinghouse on Family Violence Information
P.O. Box 1182
Washington, DC 20013
703-385-7565, 800-FYI-3366
Services include publications, databases, posters, and other materials.

National Maternal and Child Health Clearinghouse
8201 Greensboro Drive, Suite 600
McLean, VA 22102-3843
703-821-8955, ext. 254
Numerous professional publications on child abuse are available.

Violence Prevention Project
1010 Massachusetts Avenue, 2nd Floor
Boston, MA 02118
617-534-5196
"Identification and Prevention of Acquaintance Violence Among Young Patients: A Protocol for Health Providers" (training tool for counseling adolescents about violence, firearms, and safety issues).

RESOURCES—PATIENT EDUCATION MATERIALS

Motor Vehicle Injury

American Academy of Family Physicians
8880 Ward Parkway
Kansas City, MO
800-944-0000
"Take 3 Seconds" (patient education brochure and door hanger reminder to buckle seat belts).

American Academy of Pediatrics
Safe Ride Program
141 Northwest Point Boulevard
P.O. Box 927
Elk Grove Village, IL 60009-0927
800-433-9016
"Family Shopping Guide to Car Seats" (brochure ER6006); "Teens Who Drink and Drive: Reducing the Death Toll" (brochure HE0026); "Caring for Your Adolescent: Ages 12 to 21" (book); "Are You Using Your Car Seat Correctly?" (brochure ER6004).

Channing L. Bete Co., Inc.
200 State Road
South Deerfield, MA 01373
800-628-7733
"Protect Your Kids With Safety Seats" (Item No. 40840A-8-93); "About Drugs and Driving" (booklet).

Florida Alcohol and Drug Abuse Association Resource Organization
1030 East Lafayette, Suite 100
Tallahassee, FL 32301-4559
904-878-2196
"Just the Facts . . . Driving Under the Influence" (fact sheet).

Mothers Against Drunk Driving
920 North Valley Mills Drive
Waco, TX 76710
"Your Loved One Drinks and Drives" (booklet).

National Clearinghouse for Alcohol and Drug Information
P.O. Box 2345
Rockville, MD 20847-2345
800-729-6686
"Helping Your Child Say 'No': A Parent's Guide" (PH 283).

National Highway Traffic Safety Administration
U.S. Department of Transportation
400 Seventh Street, SW
Washington, DC 20590
800-424-9393
    "Seat Belts: They Only Work When You Wear Them" (brochure 1Z0005); "Sudden Impact: An Occupant Protection Fact Book" (booklet DOTHS 807-743); "Shopping Guide to Child Safety Seats" (annually updated fact sheet 1P0306); "Motorcycle Helmets" (brochure DOTHS 807-603); "Choosing a Helmet" (DOTHS 808-098).

National SAFE KIDS Campaign
111 Michigan Avenue, SW
Washington, DC 20010-2970
202-884-4993
    "Safe Kids Buckle Up" (brochure) and "Traffic Safety Magazine for Kids."

Syndistar, Inc.
125 Mallard Street, Suite A
St. Rose, LA 70087-9471
504-468-1100
    "A Parent's Guide to Drinking, Driving, and Drugs" (brochure).

Burns and Fires

American Academy of Pediatrics
Publications Department
141 Northwest Point Boulevard
P.O. Box 927
Elk Grove Village, IL 60009-0927
800-433-9016
    "Protect Your Home Against Fire . . . Planning Saves Lives" (brochure HE0039).

Channing L. Bete Co., Inc.
200 State Road
South Deerfield, MA 01373-0200
800-628-7733
    "Housekeeping for Fire Prevention" (brochure T43109A).

National SAFE KIDS Campaign
111 Michigan Avenue, SW
Washington, DC 20010-2970
202-884-4993
    "How Fire Safe is Your Home?" and "A Fire Safety Booklet for Kids."

Drowning

American Academy of Pediatrics
Publications Department
141 Northwest Point Boulevard
P.O. Box 927
Elk Grove Village, IL 60009-0927
800-433-9016
    "Home Water Hazards for Infants and Toddlers" (brochure HE0131); "Pool Safety for Toddlers" (brochure HE0132); "Water Safety for Your School-Aged Child" (brochure HE0129); "Swim Lessons for Kids" (videotape).

Michigan Substance Abuse and Traffic Safety Information Center
2409 East Michigan Avenue
Lansing, MI 48912-4019
517-482-9902
> "Just When You Thought It Was Safe" (brochure, poster).

U.S. Coast Guard Boating Safety Hotline
800-368-5647

Poisoning

American Academy of Pediatrics
Publications Department
141 Northwest Point Boulevard
P.O. Box 927
Elk Grove Village, IL 60009-0927
800-433-9016
> "Protect Your Child: Prevent Poisoning." (brochure HE0033); "Choking Prevention and First Aid for Infants and Children" (brochure HE0066).

Falls

American Academy of Pediatrics
Publications Department
141 Northwest Point Boulevard
P.O. Box 927
Elk Grove Village, IL 60009-0927
800-433-9016
> "Infant Furniture" (brochure HE0030); "About Bicycle Helmets" (brochure HE0075); "Bicycle Safety: Myths and Facts" (brochure HE0076); "Tips for Getting Your Kids to Wear Helmets" (brochure HE0079).

Channing L. Bete Co., Inc.
200 State Road
South Deerfield, MA 01373-0200
800-628-7733
> "Accident Prevention and Older People" (brochure T13490A).

Massachusetts Department of Public Health
150 Tremont Street
Boston, MA 02111
> "Elder Home Safety Checklist."

National Highway Traffic Safety Administration
U.S. Department of Transportation
400 Seventh Street, SW
Washington, DC 20590
800-424-9393
> "Prevent Bicycle Accidents" (fact sheet 6P0019); "10 Smart Routes to Bicycle Safety" (brochure 6P0046).

National Institute on Aging
NIA Information Center
P.O. Box 8057

Gaithersburg, MD 20898-8057
800-222-2225
    "Preventing Falls and Fractures" (brochure).

Intentional Injuries

American Academy of Family Physicians
8880 Ward Parkway
Kansas City, MO 64114-2797
800-944-0000
    "Black-on-Black Violence" (brochure 733).

American Academy of Pediatrics
Publications Department
141 Northwest Point Boulevard
P.O. Box 927
Elk Grove Village, IL 60009-0927
800-433-9016
    "Child Sexual Abuse: What It Is and How To Prevent It" (brochure HE0029); "Surviving: Coping With Adolescent Depression and Suicide" (brochure HE0046); "Keep Your Family Safe from Firearm Injury" (brochure, English HE0163; Spanish HE0164).

Center to Prevent Handgun Violence
1225 Eye Street, NW
Suite 1100
Washington, DC 20005
202-475-6714
    Numerous free brochures for preventing firearm injuries.

Channing L. Bete Co., Inc.
200 State Road
South Deerfield, MA 01373-0200
800-628-7733
    "What Everyone Should Know About Family Violence" (brochure, English T16741A; Spanish T18713A); "Elder Abuse" (brochure T16956A); "About Suicide" (brochure T16550A).

ETR Associates
Attention: Pamphlet Samples
P.O. Box 1830
Santa Cruz, CA 95061-1830
800-321-4407
    Free samples of pamphlets for adolescents regarding injury prevention, suicide, conflict resolution, and rape.

Monterey County Health Department
Violence and Injury Prevention Program
1200 Aguajito Road
Monterey, CA
408-755-4583
    "Store Guns Properly" (English/Spanish).

National Child Abuse Hotline
800-422-4453

National Clearinghouse on Child Abuse and Neglect and Family Violence Information
800-394-3366

Rise High Projects, Inc.
3712 North Broadway
Box 329
Chicago, IL 60613-4105
312-528-4320
   "Stop the Violence" posters (e.g., "Real men don't play with guns," "Let pride be your weapon," "Carry your peace").

SUGGESTED READINGS

Injury Prevention

Bass JL, et al. Childhood injury prevention counseling in primary care settings: a critical review of the literature. Pediatrics 1993;92:544–550.
Smith GS. The physician's role in injury prevention: beyond the U.S. Preventive Services Task Force report. J Gen Intern Med 1990;5(5 Suppl..):S67–S73.

Falls

U.S. Centers for Disease Control and Prevention. Injury-control recommendations: bicycle helmets. MMWR 1995;44(RR-1):1–17.
Cutson TM. Falls in the elderly. Am Fam Physician 1994;49:149–156.
Tinetti ME. Performance-oriented assessment of mobility problems in elderly patients. J Am Geriatr Soc 1986;34:119–126.

Family Violence and Child Abuse

American Medical Association. Diagnostic and treatment guidelines on domestic violence. Arch Fam Med 1992;1:39–47.

Suicide

American Academy of Pediatrics, Committee on Adolescence. Suicide and suicide attempts in adolescents and young adults. Pediatrics 1988;81:322–324.

REFERENCES

1. National Center for Health Statistics. Annual summary of births, marriages, divorces, and deaths: United States, 1993. Monthly vital statistics report, vol 42, no. 13. Hyattsville, MD: Public Health Service, 1994.
2. National Center for Health Statistics. Vital statistics of the United States, 1990, vol. II, mortality, part A. Washington, DC: Public Health Service, 1994.
3. U.S. Centers for Disease Control and Prevention. Years of potential life lost before age 65—United States, 1990 and 1991. MMWR 1993;42:251–253.
4. Baker SP, O'Neill B, Ginsburg MJ, Li G. The Injury fact book, 2nd ed. New York: Oxford University Press, 1992.
5. Novello AC. From the Surgeon General: A medical response to violence. JAMA 1992;267:3007.
6. Wingo PA, Tong T, Bolden S. Cancer statistics, 1995. CA 1995;45:8–30.
7. American Academy of Pediatrics, Committee on Injury and Poison Prevention. Office-based counseling for injury prevention. Pediatrics 1994;94:566–567.
8. American Academy of Family Physicians. Age charts for the periodic health examination. Reprint No. 510. Kansas City, MO: American Academy of Family Physicians, 1991.

9. U.S. Preventive Services Task Force. Guide to clinical preventive services, 2nd ed. Baltimore: Williams & Wilkins, 1996.

10. Smith R, Pless IB. Preventing injuries in childhood. Br Med J 1994;308:1312–1313.

11. Schappert SM. National Ambulatory Medical Care Survey, 1991 Summary. National Center for Health Statistics. Vital Health Stat 1994;13:22.

12. Piani A, Schoenborn C. Health promotion and disease prevention: United States, 1990. National Center for Health Statistics. Vital Health Stat 1993;10:52.

13. Council on Scientific Affairs. Alcohol and the driver. JAMA 1986;255:522–527.

14. Sosin DM, Sacks JJ. Motorcycle helmet-use laws and head injury prevention. JAMA 1992;267:1649–1651.

15. Doege TC, Engelberg AL, eds. Medical conditions affecting drivers. Chicago: American Medical Association, 1986.

16. Litovitz TL, Schmitz BF, Holm KC. 1988 annual report of the American Association of Poison Control Centers National Data Collection System. Am J Emerg Med 1989;7:495–545.

17. Requa K, DeAvilla LN, Garrick JG. Injuries in recreational adult fitness activities. Am J Sports Med 1993;21:461–467.

18. Stock JG, Cornell FM. Prevention of sports-related eye injury. Am Fam Physician 1991;44:515–520.

19. National Committee for Injury Prevention and Control. Injury prevention: Meeting the challenge. Am J Prev Med 1989;5(Suppl.):1–303.

20. Newberger EH, Barkan SE, Lieberman ES, McCormick MC, Yllo K, Gary LT, Schechter S. Abuse of pregnant women and adverse birth outcome: current knowledge and implications for practice. JAMA 1992;267:2370–2372.

21. MacMillan HL, MacMillan JH, Offord DR, and the Canadian Task Force on the Periodic Health Examination. Periodic health examination, 1993 update: I. Primary prevention of child maltreatment. Can Med Assoc J 1993;148:151–163.

22. Spaide RF, Swengel RM, Scharre DW, Mein CE. Shaken baby syndrome. Am Fam Phys 1990;41:1145–1152.

23. Aravanis SC, Adelman RD, Breckman R, Fulmer TT, Holder E, Lachs M, O'Brien JG, Sanders AB. Diagnostic and treatment guidelines on elder abuse and neglect. Arch Fam Med 1993;2:371–388.

24. Mercy JA. The public health impact of firearm injuries. Am J Prev Med 1993;9(Suppl. 1):8–11.

25. Saltzman LE, Mercy JA, O'Carroll PW, Rosenberg ML, Rhodes PH. Weapon involvement and injury outcomes in family and intimate assaults. JAMA 1992;267:3043–3047.

26. U.S. Centers for Disease Control and Prevention. Unintentional firearm-related fatalities among children, teenagers—United States, 1982–1988. MMWR 1992;268:451–452.

27. American Academy of Pediatrics, Committee on Adolescence. Suicide and suicide attempts in adolescents and young adults. Pediatrics 1988;81:322–324.

28. Canadian Task Force on the Periodic Health Examination. The Canadian guide to clinical preventive health care. Ottawa: Canada Communication Group, 1994.

11. Family Planning through Reversible Contraception

DAVID A. GRIMES

INTRODUCTION

Family planning, like immunization, is a prototype for health promotion and disease prevention (1). The health benefits for women and their children of spacing pregnancies are well established. Moreover, the health benefits of some methods of family planning, such as barrier methods, extend to prevention of sexually transmitted diseases (see Chapter 12) and possibly cervical cancer.

Family planning methods include lactation, reversible contraception, sterilization, and induced abortion. While an important method of fertility control, abortion is secondary rather than primary prevention. Lactational amenorrhea plays an important role in postponing the return of fertility after childbirth, especially in developing countries. Since breast-feeding requires little medical intervention, it will not be discussed here (see Chapter 8). Sterilization is covered in gynecology and urology texts. This chapter reviews reversible methods of contraception.

In 1988 approximately 60% of women of reproductive age in the United States were using some form of family planning (2). Surgical sterilization was the most common method (28%), followed by oral contraceptives (19%), condoms (9%), diaphragms (4%), periodic abstinence (1%), intrauterine devices (1%), and other methods. Overall, about 90% of women at risk of unintended pregnancy were using a method of family planning in 1988 (Fig. 11.1). Regrettably, hundreds of thousands of American women at risk of accidental pregnancy are not using contraception because of erroneous information about the safety and efficacy of available methods and because of barriers to access to family planning services.

Health care providers have a key role to play in dispelling these fears. This chapter examines the principal forms of reversible contraception and the basic information that patients should receive about available options. Estimates of contraceptive efficacy and the likelihood of adverse effects are based on studies that are too numerous to cite individually because of space limitations. The interested reader should consult the "References"

258

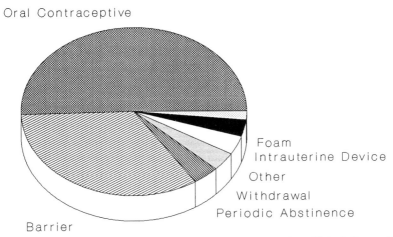

Figure 11.1.   Distribution of reversible methods of contraception, United States, 1988. (From Mosher WD, Pratt WF. Contraceptive use in the United States, 1973–88. Hyattsville, MD: National Center for Health Statistics. Advance Data No. 182, 1990, p. 1–7.)

and "Resources—Professional Education Materials" sections at the end of the chapter.

METHODS

In general, the best contraceptive for a couple is the method that they prefer to use. A partially effective method used faithfully is better than a package of oral contraceptives left in a dresser drawer. A "cafeteria" approach to contraception is customary: the clinician describes the array of contraceptives available; discusses the efficacy, risks, and benefits; and advises the patient about potential contraindications. The decision should take into account risk factors identified through the history, physical examination, and laboratory testing (see Chapters 2–4).

Counseling is important. Contraceptive effectiveness is the product of method efficacy and continuation rate. Appropriate counseling can dramatically improve compliance and continuation rates and, hence, may be more important than inherent differences in the efficacy of the contraceptives (3). In addition to information, counseling should include a discussion of the patient's sexual circumstances, her experience with and understanding of contraception, and her concerns. Counseling often is done better by nurses, counselors, and health educators than by physicians; these individuals may develop better rapport and take more time in counseling than do most physicians.

Counseling is especially important for adolescents (4). About one million teenage pregnancies occur each year in the United States, with about half of adolescents using no contraception during the first episode of sexual intercourse. In 1985 and 1993, Gallup polls revealed that most U.S. women are grossly misinformed about the safety and efficacy of contraceptives; teenagers tend to be more confused than are older women. For example, unfounded fears about weight gain and acne frequently scuttle interest in oral contraception.

All contraceptive counseling for teenagers should be done in private. Teens must be assured that all discussions are strictly confidential and that no information will be shared with parents (or anyone else) without the explicit consent of the patient. Young patients need to know that all states allow physicians to prescribe contraception for minors without parental consent. If an adolescent seems hesitant to talk, the clinician may start by discussing issues commonly raised by other women of similar age or by inquiring about what the patient has heard about various contraceptives from her friends. Although the important advantages of abstinence merit discussion, clinicians must not be judgmental with sexually active teens.

Finally, all teens should be advised not to make any unilateral decisions about contraception. Specifically, before stopping a method, the patient should make an office visit or call to discuss her concerns. Problems looming large in the life of a teenager, such as breakthrough bleeding while on oral contraceptives, may be both innocuous and transient. Compliance among adolescents can be encouraged by explaining how contraceptives work, reviewing anticipated side effects, discussing necessary tests, giving oral and written instructions, and providing samples at the initial visit. Other strategies include arranging regular follow-up visits (e.g., every 8–12 weeks) and emphasizing the importance of attending, designating a contact person for questions or problems, offering positive reinforcement for keeping appointments and complying with instructions, and telephoning patients who miss appointments.

COMPLIANCE-INDEPENDENT METHODS

Subdermal Levonorgestrel Implants

Subdermal implants are a new approach to chronic administration of systemic progestin for contraception. Levonorgestrel is released from six subdermal rods over a period of five years' use. The system becomes effective for contraception the day after implantation, and fertility returns promptly upon removal.

The pregnancy rate with subdermal implants is very low (Table 11.1). Although early studies noted higher failure rates in women weighing over 70 kg than in lighter women, this problem does not relate to the currently marketed rods, which are more permeable to the steroid.

Counseling of patients requesting progestin-only methods is crucial to

Table 11.1
Typical Failure Rates during the First Year of Use of a Method, United States

Method	Percent of Women Experiencing an Accidental Pregnancy
Chance	85
Spermicides	21
Periodic abstinence	20
Withdrawal	19
Cervical cap	18 (nulliparous)
Sponge	18 (nulliparous) 36 (parous)
Diaphragm	18
Male condom	12
Female condom	21
Copper T380A	0.8
Pill	3
Depo-medroxyprogesterone acetate injections	0.3
Levonorgestrel implants	0.09

From Hatcher RA, Trussel J, Stewart GK, Kowal D, Guest F, et al. Contraceptive technology, 16th revised ed. New York: Irvington Publishers, 1994:652.

successful use, since erratic bleeding is very common, especially in the early months of use. Women should be advised to expect unpredictable bleeding patterns, although these tend to resolve with time. While the total number of days of bleeding usually increases with subdermal implants, the total volume of menstrual blood loss in general decreases, leading to increases in hematocrit. Women who find irregular bleeding unacceptable should not use progestin only contraceptives. About 10% of women request removal in the first year because of irregular menses. Complications associated with insertion and removal of the rods have recently received attention in the professional literature and lay media (5), and therefore patients should receive adequate counseling about what to expect.

Subdermal implants are inserted under local anesthesia in an office setting. Nurses, nurse practitioners, and other midlevel practitioners can be taught to perform insertions and removals as skillfully as physicians.

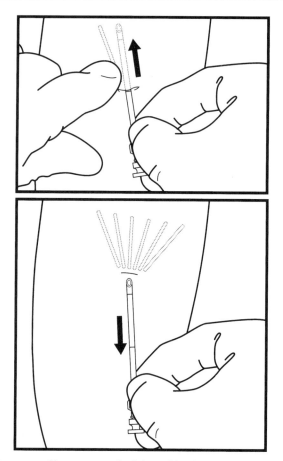

Figure 11.2.   Placement of levonorgestrel subdermal implants. Insertion of trocar for second rod (*top*). Removal of trocar from skin only after insertion of all six rods (*bottom*). (Reproduced with permission from Speroff L, Darney PD. A clinical guide for contraception. Baltimore: Williams & Wilkins, 1992.)

The six rods are placed in the inner aspect of the arm in a fan-shaped pattern using a special trocar and obturator provided with the device (Fig. 11.2). Superficial placement is important to facilitate future removal. Removal is also performed with local anesthesia. After a small (4 mm) incision is made, the first rod is maneuvered into the incision by the clinician's fingers. After a fibrous sheath is dissected from the tip of the rod, the clinician slides the rod out with a small clamp. This process continues until all the rods have been removed. Another set of rods can be inserted at this time if desired. The skin is closed with skin tapes; no sutures are required.

One and two-rod implants are currently being evaluated for possible use if the woman desires a shorter period of contraception.

Injectable Progestin

In 1992, the Food and Drug Administration approved a long-acting injectable progestin (depo-medroxyprogesterone acetate, DMPA) for contraception. The dose for contraception is 150 mg intramuscularly every 3 months. The efficacy of this method rivals or surpasses that of surgical sterilization, yet it is reversible. It reduces to four the number of days a year a woman needs to think about contraception. The mechanism of action is suppression of ovulation, perhaps supplemented by changes in cervical mucus and other effects.

As with other progestin only methods, DMPA causes irregular bleeding; however, the likelihood of amenorrhea increases with time. After a year's use, the majority of women have no menstrual bleeding, which many patients find very appealing. Another disadvantage of this method is that it is not immediately reversible. Because of the depot administration in muscle, months may be required before fertility returns. The mean duration is about 9 months, but it may be as long as 18 months for some. Hence, this method should not be used by women who plan to conceive in the near future.

Intrauterine Devices

Two safe and effective intrauterine devices (IUDs) are currently marketed in the United States. The progesterone T device releases synthetic progesterone from its vertical stem into the endometrial cavity over the course of a year, after which it must be removed and, if desired, replaced. Its failure rate is higher than that associated with the copper IUD (Table 11.1). In contrast to other IUDs, the progesterone device reduces menstrual blood loss and decreases dysmenorrhea. The newer device on the market is the copper T380A. This IUD has annual failure rates of less than 1%. It is marketed for up to 10 years' use.

Previously, the mechanism of action of IUDs was thought to be prevention of implantation of zygotes. More recent evidence indicates that IUDs may work much earlier in the reproductive process. The IUD appears to be a spermicide, preventing sperm from reaching the fallopian tubes. It is important for women to understand that the IUD is not an abortifacient.

Candidates for IUD use are those women who are at low risk of sexually transmitted diseases. Unlike several other methods of contraception, the IUD use does not protect a woman from sexually transmitted diseases.

The insertion process for both devices involves a withdrawal technique. After washing the vagina with antiseptic, the clinician applies a

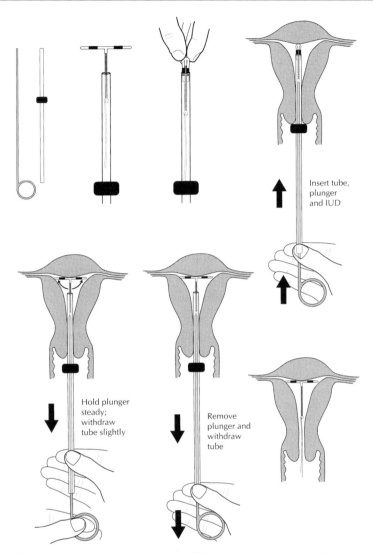

Figure 11.3. Insertion technique for copper T380A intrauterine device. High fundal placement is achieved by using a withdrawal technique. (Reproduced with permission from Speroff L, Darney PD. A clinical guide for contraception. Baltimore: Williams & Wilkins, 1992.)

tenaculum to the cervix for traction and determines the depth and direction of the uterine cavity with a sound. The lateral arms of the device are folded back (with an arm cocker provided with the progesterone device or by hand with the copper device) and the IUD is placed at the superior aspect of the endometrial cavity; the insertion instruments are then withdrawn, leaving the IUD at the apex of the uterus (Fig. 11.3).

COMPLIANCE-DEPENDENT METHODS

Oral Contraceptives

Oral contraceptives remain the most popular reversible method of contraception in the United States. Two general types are available: combination estrogen and progestin formulations and progestin only pills. The former work principally by preventing ovulation and the latter by making the cervical mucus impenetrable. Among combination pills, several varieties are sold: fixed-dosed monophasic pills and multiphasic pills, in which the dose of estrogen, progestin, or both varies over the cycle. In addition, 21 and 28-day preparations are available, with 7 days of placebo pills in the latter.

There is no scientific basis for choosing between monophasic and multiphasic pills. Randomized controlled trials have not established the superiority of the newer multiphasic pills. Hence, the general approach is to use a low-dose pill, defined as less than 35 µg of estrogen and ≤1 mg of norethindrone (or its biological equivalent). Among the multiphasic pills, randomized controlled trials have found better bleeding patterns with those containing the progestin levonorgestrel.

A recent change in oral contraceptives has been the introduction of formulations containing new progestins, such as norgestimate and desogestrel. These are alleged to have purer progestational activity with less undesirable androgen activity than do earlier generation progestins. Nevertheless, large comparative trials will be required to demonstrate the purported superiority of the new progestin pills over the older progestin preparations.

Condoms

Condoms remain a popular method of contraception, and interest in them for prevention of disease transmission, including human immunodeficiency virus infection, has grown over the past decade. Two general types are marketed: latex rubber and natural membrane condoms made from animal intestine. Because the latter have larger pore sizes that may allow passage of viruses, they are not recommended for prophylaxis against disease. In addition, the natural membrane condoms are more expensive.

Latex condoms are available with and without lubricant or spermicide. While the addition of spermicide has theoretical appeal, studies comparing them to plain condoms are lacking. In addition, some condoms have a nipple tip to serve as a reservoir for ejaculate. Condoms should be applied to the erect penis before any vaginal contact and removed promptly after ejaculation to prevent spill of semen during detumescence. As discussed in Chapter 12, patients often need to be reminded to hold the condom at the base of the penis during withdrawal, to use a new condom with each act of intercourse, and to avoid using petroleum or oil-based lubricants (e.g., Vaseline) that can weaken latex condoms.

Female Barriers

Diaphragm

The diaphragm has been a mainstay of contraception for decades. It consists of a dome of latex rubber over a flexible ring. After a spermicide is placed in the center of the dome, the diaphragm is inserted into the vagina so as to cover the cervix, with the spermicide held against the cervix. The ring lodges beneath the pubis and in the posterior fornix of the vagina. Several different types of diaphragm rings are available; some bend in only one plane, while others bend in all directions. No comparative studies have been done. Although recommendations call for leaving the device in place for 6 hours after coitus, the minimum time required for contraceptive effectiveness is unknown. If coitus is repeated, additional spermicide is usually advised, but the diaphragm should remain in place.

Diaphragms come in a variety of sizes, in 5 mm diameter increments. This method can be considered a vehicle to hold a spermicide close to the cervical os. To fit a diaphragm, the clinician should try several sizes to determine the largest that will fit without the patient sensing its presence. The patient should be allowed to practice insertion and removal (a finger can hook the ring beneath the pubis and pull it out) before leaving the office or clinic (Fig. 11.4). If vaginal dimensions may change (e.g., after birth or marked weight change) another fitting may be advisable.

Cervical Cap

Cervical caps can be considered a miniature diaphragm covering only the cervix. These thimble-shaped cups must be fit to the cervix by a clinician. After spermicide is placed in the cap, the device is applied to the cervix, where it may remain in place for several days. Failure rates with the cap approximate those of the diaphragm, and the insertion and removal process requires more skill than that for the diaphragm. Use of caps in the United States is limited.

Female Condom

The female condom was approved by the Food and Drug Administration in 1993. It is a lubricated polyurethane sheath with a flexible ring on each end; one ring covers the cervix and the other ring is on the vulva. This method has the advantage of being controlled by the woman and providing theoretical protection against both unintended pregnancy and sexually transmitted diseases. Preliminary trials revealed high contraceptive failure rates, raising questions about compliance with the method. Patient instructions for proper use of the female condom are provided in Table 12.1.

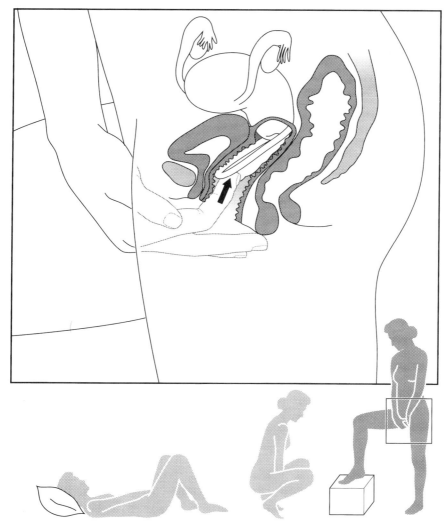

Figure 11.4.   Insertion of the diaphragm. Proximal edge fits in posterior fornix and distal edge behind symphysis. (Reproduced with permission from Speroff L, Darney PD. A clinical guide for contraception. Baltimore: Williams & Wilkins, 1992.)

Spermicides

Spermicides have been used for millennia. The most popular spermicide is nonoxynol-9, an alcoholic detergent. Toxic to both sperm and bacteria, spermicides have been shown *in vitro* and *in vivo* to confer some protection against sexually transmitted diseases.

Several delivery systems for spermicides are available: suppositories, jellies, film sheets that dissolve in the vagina, and foams. Cans of foam should be thoroughly shaken before dispensing into the applicator to disperse the nonoxynol-9 throughout the foam. The contraceptive sponge, which contains 1 g of nonoxynol-9, was designed to be left in place for up to 24 hours and to be used for multiple acts of intercourse without adding more spermicide. Production was discontinued by the manufacturer in 1995, however, for financial reasons.

Periodic Abstinence

Periodic abstinence methods (rhythm method) are designed to avoid coitus during perceived fertile days of the menstrual cycle. All hinge on assumptions about poorly understood and variable biologic events. Examples of periodic abstinence methods include the calendar method (which estimates fertile days based on cycle length), the temperature method (which relies on basal body temperature to detect ovulation), and the sympto-thermal method, which uses temperature and cervical mucus changes. Advantages of periodic abstinence methods include their lack of expense and negligible medical risk; disadvantages include long training periods, unreliability in predicting fertility, poor compliance and continuation rates, and resulting high failure rates.

Emergency Contraception

Emergency contraception is used to avoid pregnancy after unprotected coitus or failure of a barrier (e.g., a damaged condom) has occurred (6). Hence, emergency contraception, also known as "postcoital contraception," is ad hoc prevention of pregnancy. The precise mechanism of action is unknown, but it probably involves prevention of ovulation, impairment of ovum transport, or prevention of implantation.

The most popular method of emergency contraception is a regimen of two oral contraceptive tablets containing ethinyl estradiol 50 μg and levonorgestrel 150 μg taken as soon as possible but no later than 72 hours after intercourse. Another two tablets are taken 12 hours later. The failure rate is about 2%. Although there are no known contraindications to this protocol, about half of women who use this regimen will have nausea. Serious complications have not been reported. Administration of danazol for emergency contraception appears to have a higher failure rate than that with oral contraceptives used for this purpose.

Another form of emergency contraception is insertion of a copper IUD within 5 days of unprotected coitus. Here the failure rate is less than 1%, and the woman also benefits from ongoing contraception. The same contraindications for IUDs apply here as in other clinical settings.

ADVERSE EFFECTS

Modern contraceptives infrequently have serious adverse effects; many of these can be avoided by appropriate screening of potential users (7). Modern, low-dose oral contraceptives appear to be associated with either no risk or a slightly increased risk of either myocardial infarction or cerebrovascular accidents in healthy women who do not smoke (7). While an increased risk of thromboembolic disease has been reported among users of oral contraceptives, this may reflect detection bias rather than a causal association. No population-based data on the incidence of this rare complication exist for contemporary low-dose pills. Breakthrough bleeding tends to be self-limited, and absence of withdrawal bleeding can often be managed with hormones if treatment is desired.

Contemporary IUDs appear to be associated with a small increase in the likelihood of upper genital tract infection related to the insertion process in some women at risk. In the largest United States study, the risk was about four times baseline in the first month after insertion and returned to baseline by 5 months. The increased risk of infection was not statistically significant among low-risk women. International trials have indicated that the risk is limited to the first 20 days and is less than 1% during that time. Limited data from randomized controlled trials support use of a single 200 mg oral dose of doxycycline at the time of insertion to reduce the risk of subsequent upper genital tract infection.

Mechanical problems, such as perforation of the uterus and embedding in the uterus, are infrequent. Recent series indicate a perforation rate of less than 1:1000. Spontaneous expulsion of the device, should it occur, often happens within the first few cycles after insertion. Hence, many clinicians have patients return for a checkup after the first menstrual period following insertion. About 10% of women will request removal of an IUD because of pain or bleeding.

Progestin only contraception (minipill, subdermal implant, and depomedroxyprogesterone acetate) is associated with irregular, unpredictable bleeding that improves with time. The latter two methods are associated with weight gain as well. Subdermal implants have a low rate of surgical complications; infection of the insertion site occurs in less than 1% of patients.

Barrier contraceptives have few serious side effects. Limited evidence points to an association between use of the diaphragm and toxic shock syndrome. Should an association exist, its public health impact is probably negligible because of the infrequency of this condition. The risk of urinary tract infection is doubled in women who use diaphragms, perhaps due to overgrowth of pathogenic flora in the vagina. Spermicides may cause irritation of mucous membranes in both men and women.

CONTRAINDICATIONS

Contraindications to oral contraceptives are described in detail in package labeling and mandatory patient package inserts. Prior thromboembolic disease and active liver disease are contraindications, and women who have been treated for breast cancer should probably consider nonsteroidal contraception.

Exclusion criteria for an IUD include women at high risk of sexually transmitted diseases. Although package labeling recommends these devices for parous women, nulliparity does not, in itself, appear to be a contraindication, although rates of expulsion may be higher in nulliparous women than in women with previous pregnancies. Women with uterine anomalies, e.g., distorted cavities from leiomyomata or congenital anomalies, should not use this form of contraception, because of higher failure rates.

Women with frequent urinary tract infections should probably not use diaphragms for contraception. Sensitivity to latex rubber precludes use of this method and of condoms.

OFFICE AND CLINIC ORGANIZATION

Separate rooms for group and individual counseling can improve the efficiency of patient education in an office or clinic. Extensive teaching aids are available, ranging from pamphlets and flip charts to anatomic models and videotapes. Specific examples of useful brochures are provided below under "Resources—Patient Education Materials."

MEDICAL RECORD DOCUMENTATION

Medical records should document pertinent history and physical examination findings as well as relevant laboratory tests (e.g., hematocrit). In addition, the clinician or counselor should document the discussion of appropriate methods, their risks and benefits, efficacy, and alternatives. Notation of patient education materials or patient package inserts given to the patient can be useful to subsequent treating clinicians. Informed consent documents, such as those for intrauterine devices, should be incorporated into the medical record.

RESOURCES—PATIENT EDUCATION MATERIALS

American Academy of Family Physicians
8880 Ward Parkway
Kansas City, MO 64114-2797
800-944-0000
    "Birth Control: Choosing the Method That's Right For You" (brochure 1524); "Stop Adolescent Pregnancy" (brochure 732).

American Academy of Pediatrics
Publications Department
141 Northwest Point Blvd.
P.O. Box 927
Elk Grove Village, IL 60009-0927
800-433-9016
> "Deciding to Wait: What You Need to Know" (brochure HE0128); "Making the Right Choice: Facts Young People Need To Know About Avoiding Pregnancy" (brochure HE0055).

Food and Drug Administration
Information and Outreach Staff
HFE-88, Room 16-63
5600 Fishers Lane
Rockville, MD 29857
301-443-3170
> "Choosing a Contraceptive" (brochure FDA94-1213).

National Center for Education in Maternal and Child Health
2000 15th Street North, Suite 701
Arlington, VA 22201-2617
> "Birth Control Methods" (Chinese B266; Korean B267; Vietnamese B269).

Planned Parenthood Federation of America, Inc.
810 Seventh Avenue
New York, NY 10019
800-230-PLAN
> "How To Talk With Your Teen About the Facts of Life" (brochure 1436); "Facts About Birth Control" (brochure 1800, English; 1801, Spanish); "The Condom: What It is For, How to Use It" (brochure 1550); "It Can't Happen to Me" (brochure 1689).

RESOURCES—PROFESSIONAL EDUCATION MATERIALS

American College of Obstetricians and Gynecologists
409 12th Street, SW
Washington, DC 20024-2588

American Public Health Association
1015 15th Street, NW
Washington, DC 20005

Association of Reproductive Health Professionals
2401 Pennsylvania Avenue, NW
Washington, DC 20037

SUGGESTED READINGS

Hatcher RA, Trussel J, Stewart F, Stewart GK, Kowal D, Guest F, et al. Contraceptive technology, 16th revised ed. New York: Irvington Publishers, 1994.
Speroff L, Darney PD. A clinical guide for contraception. Baltimore: Williams & Wilkins, 1992.

REFERENCES

1. Harlap S, Kost K, Forrest JD. Preventing pregnancy, protecting health. New York: Alan Guttmacher Institute, 1991.
2. Mosher WD, Pratt WF. Contraceptive use in the United States, 1973–88. Hyattsville, MD: National Center for Health Statistics. Advance Data No. 182, 1990, p. 1–7.
3. Jones EF, Forrest JD. Contraceptive failure rates based on the 1988 NSFG. Fam Plann Perspect 1992;24;12–19.
4. Ringdahl EN. The role of the family physician in preventing teenage pregnancy. Am Fam Phys 1992;45:2215–2219.
5. Thomas AG Jr, LeMelle SM. The Norplant system: where are we in 1995? J Fam Pract 1995;40:125–128.
6. IMAP statement on emergency contraception. IPPF Medical Bulletin 1994;28(6).
7. Kost K, Forrest JD, Harlap S. Comparing the health risks and benefits of contraceptive choices. Fam Plann Perspect 1991;23:54–61.

12. Sexually Transmitted Diseases

WILLIAM J. KASSLER, JUDITH N. WASSERHEIT, and WILLARD CATES, JR.

INTRODUCTION

Sexually transmitted diseases (STDs) are among the most important public health problems in the United States. More than 30 million persons in the United States are infected with genital herpes, and one million persons are infected with human immunodeficiency virus (HIV). An estimated annual incidence of four million cases of chlamydia, 1.3 million cases of gonorrhea, 500,000 cases of genital warts, and 134,000 cases of syphilis attest to the magnitude of the problem. Besides acquired immunodeficiency syndrome (AIDS), the long-term sequelae of STDs include anogenital neoplasias, tubal infertility, ectopic pregnancy, and such adverse pregnancy outcomes as prematurity, low birth weight, fetal wastage, infant morbidity, and death. The enormous morbidity and mortality associated with AIDS is well-known. Over 80,000 new cases were reported in 1994. By 1993, AIDS had become the leading cause of death among persons age 25–44 years in the United States (1).The impact of these diseases in terms of financial cost and human suffering has made STD prevention one of the country's top public health priorities.

Primary care physicians and other health care providers are in a unique position to play a central role in the prevention of STDs. Providers have the opportunity to make an early diagnosis, to treat infected persons, to provide a reliable source for patient education and counseling, and to participate in the identification and treatment of infected sex partners.

These clinical strategies to prevent the spread of STDs can be classified by the stage of illness they target. *Primary prevention* strategies are intended to prevent infection. They are implemented before the sexually transmitted infection occurs and involve reducing or eliminating risk factors. *Secondary prevention* strategies are implemented to prevent adverse health outcomes once an infection has occurred and involve early detection and treatment of patients with STDs. Because treating an infected person breaks the chain of transmission, many STD prevention strategies are directed towards the infected individual, serving both primary and secondary prevention functions.

This chapter provides information for primary care clinicians providing STD prevention services addressing (*a*) interventions that clinicians

273

should apply to all patients, such as recognizing patients who are at risk for STDs and counseling them about behavior changes; and (*b*) interventions that clinicians should apply to patients with presumptive or documented infection, such as diagnosis, treatment, counseling, and management of sex partners.

TALKING TO PATIENTS ABOUT SEX, STDS, AND HIV

Because the risk factors for STDs involve intensely personal, often taboo, and sometimes illegal behaviors, clinicians often find it difficult to talk with patients about sexual behaviors that might place patients at risk for STDs and HIV infection (2, 3). Given the large proportion of asymptomatic infected persons, proper questions must be asked in the right way to identify patients who might be infected. Furthermore, because preventing the spread of STDs requires people to change their unsafe behaviors, clinicians must elicit information about the specific practices that place patients at risk so that they can deliver appropriate prevention messages that are tailored to the individual patient's risks.

Sexual History

The sexual history, like other aspects of the medical history, should be tailored to the individual. The first step with all adult and adolescent patients is to determine whether their behaviors place them at high risk for sexually acquired infections (4). This minimal history should include the patient's sexual orientation; whether the patient is sexually active, either in an exclusive relationship or with several partners; whether the patient has recently changed sex partners or acquired a new partner; and whether the patient has a history of STDs.

Since discussing sexual behavior and drug use can be uncomfortable for both health professionals and patients, the clinician might begin with an introductory or qualifying statement to tell the patient why it is important to discuss these sensitive issues (5). *"To give you the best care I can, I need to ask some specific questions about your lifestyle and sexual behaviors."* Another introduction might include an acknowledgment that these are sensitive questions: *"I realize that a person's sexual behavior is a very personal thing, but I need to ask you some questions so we can explore whether you are at risk for certain medical conditions, such as sexually transmitted infections."* (6)

Give patients permission to discuss "taboo" topics by asking global questions about risk behaviors (3). *"Many people are worried that they might be infected with the virus that causes AIDS; have you been concerned about that?"*

Use clear, open-ended questions to encourage more complete histories. Pose questions nonjudgmentally and in words that the patient understands. Additional techniques that can be effective in developing rapport with the patient include reassuring the patient that treatment will be provided regardless of ability to pay, legal immigration status, or language spoken.

Avoid assumptions. Marriage does not guarantee that a person is either monogamous or heterosexual (7). For married persons, explicitly ask about extramarital sex partners.

Avoid labels. Instead of asking someone if he or she has engaged in prostitution, ask *"Have you ever exchanged sex for drugs or money?"* Instead of asking, *"Are you a homosexual?"* ask, *"Do you have sex with men, women, or both?"* Phrasing the question this way avoids the assumption that a patient is exclusively heterosexual or homosexual, and lets the patient know that any answer is "acceptable" (8). Many men who have sex with men do not consider themselves homosexual or bisexual. They may not perceive themselves to be at risk and may not respond affirmatively to general questions about homosexual or bisexual activities. To these men one could say, *"Some men, although they are married or have a girlfriend, occasionally have sex with another man. Have you done that?"* Another way of asking this would be to say, *"Many men have sex with other men. Have you ever had sex with another man?"*

Avoid leading questions. Patients may find it difficult to truthfully answer leading questions such as *"You do use condoms, don't you?"* A more successful technique might include the use of validation in asking questions; *"Many women find it difficult to get their men to use condoms. Has this been a problem for you?"* See Chapter 2 for further details about techniques for asking about sensitive topics in the history.

Ask about a past medical history of STDs. A recent STD is a marker for unsafe sexual behavior. In addition, ulcerative and inflammatory STDs such as syphilis, herpes, gonorrhea, chlamydia, and trichomoniasis may facilitate HIV transmission (9). Therefore, persons with a recent history of STDs are at increased risk of HIV infection.

Ask about sex partners. Does the patient have more than one sex partner? Has the patient recently changed partners or acquired a new partner? What does the patient know about the sexual or drug injection activities of his or her partner(s)? Finally, it is often helpful to know how a patient met his or her partner.

As risks are identified, more in-depth questions should focus on specific behaviors. These questions should be explicit and should refer to specific body parts and practices (8): *"Do you engage in anal sex (inserting your penis into a person's rectum or allowing someone to insert his penis into your rectum)?" "Do you engage in oral sex?"*

Depending on the patient, the clinician may also want to seek information about drug use and sexual activity under the influence of alcohol or other drugs. Drugs such as alcohol, cocaine, barbiturates, or amphetamines impair judgment, can promote unsafe sexual behaviors, and have been associated with increased risks of STDs (7, 10). See Chapter 13 for further discussion of alcohol and other drug misuse.

Prevention Counseling

Once risks have been identified, the primary care provider is in an excellent position to talk with the patient about risk reduction. The sexual history provides an opportunity for education and can lead to a discussion about risk reduction. This chapter describes two different approaches for talking to patients about risk reduction: health education and prevention counseling. *Health education* involves providing didactic information to (*a*) persons at risk of STDs so that they can avoid infection, and (*b*) persons with sexually transmitted infections so that they can avoid the complications of infection and prevent transmission of their infection to others. *Counseling* involves greater interaction with the patient. It helps patients to recognize their risk for STDs and assists them in developing a plan to reduce those risks. Techniques such as role playing and interactive discussions facilitate the counseling approach.

Prevention Message

The prevention message should be tailored to the individual patient's specific risks. The message should be delivered with the same respect, compassion, and nonjudgmental attitude as displayed while taking the sexual history; the advice should be practical, specific, and simple.

These prevention messages may include:

1. Abstaining from sex and from injecting drugs is the surest way to prevent STDs, including HIV infection.

2. A mutually monogamous relationship in which neither partner is infected with an STD nor uses injected drugs is the safest sexual relationship.

3. If abstinence or monogamy is not possible, always use condoms during sexual intercourse. Avoid sexual practices involving the exchange of body fluids, such as vaginal, anal, or oral sex without a condom.

4. Limit the number of sex partners.

5. Know the symptoms of STDs and seek care as soon as symptoms are suspected.

6. When infection is detected, take all medications as directed, and ensure that all sex partners are also examined and/or treated before resuming sexual intercourse.

A reasonable strategy for personal protection would be to decrease the number of one's sex partners, which will reduce the risk of having sex with an infected partner. Limiting anonymous or casual sex will further reduce

that risk. Patients should use condoms consistently with all new sex partners and with partners whose HIV status and risk status are unknown. The
use of such drugs as cocaine, barbiturates, and amphetamines, or the excessive use of alcohol should be limited, because they impair judgment
and therefore may lead to unsafe sex.

Patients at risk of STDs should be advised that condoms must be used
correctly and consistently to be effective. They should be instructed in the
proper use of condoms (Table 12.1). Latex condoms, if used correctly,
protect the wearer and his partner against sexually transmitted infection
by providing a mechanical barrier against semen, genital discharge, genital lesions, or infectious secretions. (Their role in preventing pregnancy is
discussed in Chapter 11.) Most condom failure is due to nonuse or to incorrect use. Condom breakage rates are low (about 1–2% among hetero-
sexuals in the United States) (11).

The female condom, as discussed in Chapter 11, has the theoretical
advantage of shifting control of the decision to use a condom from the
man to the woman. Prevention methods that are under female control are
important, because without such methods women are often unable to negotiate safer sex. Unfortunately, the female condom is more expensive
than male condoms, and there are few data to assess its effectiveness in
preventing STD transmission. Instructions for use of the female condom
are provided in Table 12.1.

Some other methods of contraception, such as the diaphragm combined with a spermicide, vaginal spermicides alone, or nonoxynol-9
sponge (no longer commercially available) provide some protection
against bacterial infections but have not been shown to protect against

Table 12.1
Proper Use of a Condom

Male Condom
  Put on condom before you have any genital contact with your partner.
  Hold condom at the base of penis during withdrawal.
  Use a new condom for each act of intercourse. Never use a condom twice.
  Never use petroleum or oil-based lubricants such as Vaseline with a latex condom because
    they can weaken latex. Use water soluble lubricants such as K-Y Jelly with a latex
    condom.
Female Condom
  Practice insertion before using during intercourse to make sure procedure is understood.
  Put on condom before you have any genital contact with your partner.
  Squeeze the inner ring and insert into the vagina, similarly to inserting a tampon without
    an applicator.
  The outer ring should be outside the vagina during sex.
  Be careful to guide the penis into the vagina to avoid misrouting the penis to the side of
    the device.
  After intercourse, twist the outer ring. Pull out gently.
  Use a new condom for each act of intercourse. Never use a condom twice.

HIV infection (12). Frequent use of high-dose spermicides may even increase the risk of HIV transmission by causing genital irritation (13). Therefore, no recommendations can be made about the use of spermicides without condoms for prevention of HIV infection (11).

HIV Counseling and Testing

U.S. Public Health Service guidelines recommend that HIV testing be accompanied by counseling. Pretest counseling takes place when the blood is drawn, and posttest counseling takes place later when the results are provided to the patient. During pretest counseling, the clinician should ask for informed consent for the HIV test. The clinician should also assess the patient's risk behaviors, help the patient recognize his or her risk, and help the patient develop a plan to reduce those risks. During posttest counseling, the clinician should review, and discuss the meaning of, test results: a positive test means that the patient is infected with HIV and is capable of infecting others; a negative test means that the patient is probably not infected but is still susceptible to infection unless he or she changes risk behaviors. In the HIV-negative patient, the posttest session is a good time for the clinician to reinforce the steps necessary for the patient to avoid becoming infected in the future. For the HIV-positive patient, the posttest session should be used to reinforce the behaviors necessary to avoid transmitting infection to others, to make appointments for medical follow-up, and to provide referral for additional services if needed, such as psychological or behavioral counseling, or social services (see Chapter 17) (14–17).

The U.S. Public Health Service recommendations were developed for use in publicly funded HIV counseling and testing centers by persons with specialized training in HIV counseling, and may not be practical for all settings in which patients are tested for HIV. In busy office-based practices, for example, the intensive, interactive counseling specified in the Public Health Service model may not be feasible. Depending on the patient's needs, the setting, the time available, and the counseling skills of the clinician, a brief, didactic health education session may be more appropriate. In such cases, patients who require intensive, interactive counseling can be referred to a trained HIV counselor. There are currently no data available to demonstrate the superiority of either approach, though it may be unrealistic to expect that one or two sessions of either health education or the standard pretest and posttest counseling will be sufficient to achieve sustained reductions in longstanding sexual risk behaviors (18).

Whichever way the clinician chooses to communicate the HIV prevention message, minimum requirements at the time of HIV testing are to ensure that patients give informed consent and that all patients are aware of how their behavior can influence the risk of transmission. These requirements constitute the same standard of care as that for testing for any other communicable disease.

Adolescents and Young Adults

Because adolescence is a time of sexual curiosity, experimentation, and risk-taking, adolescents have the highest risk of exposure to STDs. Many teenagers mistakenly believe it is not possible for them to come into contact with anyone who is infected. They view multiple sex partners as an achievement rather than a health risk. Adolescents also tend to have spontaneous rather than premeditated sex, which hinders preventive measures. Furthermore, female adolescents are at disproportionately increased risk of STDs and HIV infection due to physiological factors, such as an immature cervix that is more vulnerable to infection, and social factors, such as lack of assertiveness and the pressure to agree to sex (19).

Establishing rapport with adolescents can be difficult. Two common pitfalls are assuming the role of the surrogate parent or overcompensating by acting as the adolescent's peer. The clinician's role is more of an adult (but not a parent) who is both an advocate and an advisor. As discussed in Chapter 2, to establish rapport, it is frequently helpful to assure the teenager about the confidentiality of the discussion, to display interest and concern, to pay attention to nonverbal cues and body language, and to be sensitive to hidden agendas (the chief complaint is often unrelated to the real reason the patient is in the office). A good opening line would be to ask the patient, *"Do you have any questions or concerns about sex, sexually transmitted diseases, contraception, or pregnancy?"*

While the adolescent is the primary patient, the parents cannot be overlooked. The adolescent's need for privacy and the need to reassure the parents' concerns may conflict. One way to help is to say in advance, *"After I finish talking with you all together, I will spend a few minutes alone with your son (daughter), and then I will examine him (her). During this time we may discuss some issues that we will prefer to keep in confidence. Then I will call you back to discuss my findings and recommendations."* (20)

IMMUNIZATIONS

Hepatitis B is the only STD for which an effective vaccine exists. Vaccination is recommended for all persons known to be at high risk of sexual transmission. This includes persons who have multiple sex partners, sex partners of hepatitis B virus carriers, men who have sex with other men, persons seeking treatment for STDs, and prostitutes (21–22). Hepatitis B immune globulin combined with vaccination can prevent infection in persons exposed sexually to hepatitis B virus if administered within 14 days after exposure. Please refer to Chapter 18 for vaccination schedules, guidelines on managing those exposed to hepatitis B virus, and information about universal neonatal vaccination.

EARLY DIAGNOSIS AND TREATMENT

Diagnosis and treatment of STDs is a primary as well as secondary prevention strategy. Early antibiotic treatment of infected patients and their sex partners is an effective way to help prevent the spread of bacterial STDs within a community. Early diagnosis and treatment may also prevent serious sequelae for the individual, such as infertility, ectopic pregnancy, adverse pregnancy outcomes, and infant morbidity and mortality.

Early detection of infection can be accomplished by clinical diagnosis based on signs and symptoms, confirmatory diagnostic testing of patients where clinical suspicion exists, targeted screening of asymptomatic individuals considered to be at risk of STDs, and examination of sex partners of persons diagnosed with STDs.

The diagnosis of an STD should be based on the specific medical history, symptoms, and physical signs of each patient. This means applying a knowledge of the epidemiology of STDs in the geographic area of one's practice, and assessing the specific risk for individual patients. However, even in low-prevalence areas, patients can practice behaviors that place them at risk for STDs. A patient who has a history of an STD, a partner with an STD, or multiple sex partners should be considered at risk.

Screening

Screening, the testing of asymptomatic persons for evidence of infection, can play an important role in the early diagnosis and treatment of persons with STDs. Bacterial and parasitic STDs are high priorities for screening because the treatments are of short duration, safe, effective, and inexpensive.

Screening tests should achieve a high sensitivity because false-negative results may place the patient at risk for secondary complications and may result in further spread of disease. While achieving high specificity may not be as important from a public health perspective as achieving high sensitivity, the emotional consequences of falsely stigmatizing a patient cannot be ignored. As explained in Chapter 4, when screening tests are applied broadly to a low-prevalence population, they are likely to yield a high rate of false-positives.

Given the low prevalence of STDs in many primary care settings, screening is best directed towards individuals with known behaviors that place them at high risk for acquiring an STD. Therefore, screening for STDs should be considered for sexually active patients who have had mul-

Table 12.2
Recommended Regimens for Treating Common, Uncomplicated Sexually Transmitted Diseases

Disease	Intervention
Gonorrhea	Ceftriaxone 125 mg i.m. once *or* Cefixime 400 mg p.o. once *or* Ciprofloxacin 500 mg p.o. once[a] *or* Ofloxacin 400 mg p.o. once[a] *plus* Doxycycline 100 mg p.o. BID for 7 days (for possible co-infection with chlamydia)
Nongonococcal urethritis	Doxycycline 100 mg p.o. BID for 7 days
Mucopurulent cervicitis	Treat for gonorrhea and chlamydia in populations with high prevalence of both infections. Treat for chlamydia only if the prevalence of gonorrhea is low but the likelihood of chlamydia is substantial. Await test results if the prevalence of both infections is low and compliance with a recommendation for a return visit is likely.
Chlamydia	Doxycycline 100 mg p.o. BID for 7 days *or* Azithromycin 1 gm p.o. once
Bacterial vaginosis	Metronidazole 500 mg p.o. BID for 7 days
Trichomonas	Metronidazole 2 gm p.o. once
Syphilis	Primary, secondary, early latent: Benzathine penicillin G 2.4 million units i.m. once Nonpregnant penicillin allergic patients should be treated with doxycycline 100 mg p.o. BID for 14 days. Late-latent, latent of unknown duration, or late: Benzathine penicillin G 2.4 million units i.m., three doses at 1 week intervals
Chancroid	Azithromycin 1 gm p.o. once *or* Ceftriaxone 250 mg i.m. once *or* Erythromycin base 500 mg p.o. QID for 7 days
Genital herpes	First episode: Acyclovir 200 mg p.o. 5 times a day for 7–10 days or until lesions clear Recurrent episodes: For most patients treatment is not recommended; some may have limited benefit from therapy when treatment is instituted during the prodrome. Acyclovir 200 mg p.o. 5 times a day for 5 days Suppressive therapy: Daily suppressive therapy reduces frequency of recurrences among patients with frequent recurrences. Acyclovir 400 mg p.o. BID

Table 12.2
Recommended Regimens for Treating Common, Uncomplicated Sexually
Transmitted Diseases—Continued

Disease	Intervention
Genital warts	Treatment of genital warts is based on the preference of the patient. The goal of treatment is removal of warts and alleviation of signs and symptoms, not eradication of human papilloma virus. Treatment of external warts is not likely to have any effect on the development of cervical cancer. Expensive or toxic therapies, and therapies that result in scarring, should be avoided.
	External genital warts:
	Cryotherapy with liquid nitrogen
	or
	Podofilox 0.5% solution BID for 3 days for self-treatment (contraindicated during pregnancy)
	or
	Podophyllin 10–25% applied to warts and washed off in 1–4 hours. Repeat weekly PRN (contraindicated during pregnancy)
	or
	Trichloroacetic acid 80–90% applied to warts; powder with talc or baking soda to remove unreacted acid. Repeat weekly PRN
Ectoparasites	Pediculosis pubis:
	Lindane 1% shampoo (not recommended during pregnancy)—applied and washed off after 4 minutes
	or
	Permethrine 1% cream—applied and washed off after 10 minues
	or
	Pyrethrins with piperonyl butoxide—applied and washed off after 10 minutes.
	Scabies:
	Permethrin cream (5%) applied to all areas of the body from the neck down and washed off after 8 to 14 hours
	or
	Lindane (1%) 1 oz of lotion or 30 g cream applied to all areas of the body from the neck down and washed off thoroughly after 8 hours (contraindicated for pregnant or lactating women, or for children < age 2 years)
Pelvic inflammatory disease	Outpatient treatment:[b]
	Ofloxacin 400 mg p.o. BID *plus* either clindamycin 450 mg p.o. QID or metronidazole 500 mg p.o. BID for 14 days.
	or
	Either cefoxitin 2 g i.m. *plus* probenecid 1 gm p.o.; or ceftriaxone 250 mg i.m. or other parenteral third generation cephalosporin *plus* doxycycline 100 mg p.o. BID for 14 days.

Adapted from U.S. Centers for Disease Control and Prevention. 1993 sexually transmitted diseases treatment guidelines. MMWR 1993;42(RR-14):i–102.

[a]Contraindicated for pregnant or lactating women or for persons under age17.

[b]Many experts recommend that all patients with pelvic inflammatory disease be hospitalized so that supervised treatment with parenteral antibiotics can be initiated.

tiple sex partners, a history of STDs, a sex partner who has multiple sexual contacts or who is known or suspected to have an STD, and in health care settings that see high-risk patients, such as STD clinics.

For a more detailed discussion of screening, please refer to Chapter 4. The U.S. Centers for Disease Control and Prevention have developed specific recommendations for treating common, uncomplicated STDs in outpatient settings (Table 12.2).

Epidemiologic Treatment

In some circumstances, when a diagnosis is considered likely, antibiotics should be administered without clinical signs of infection, or before proof of infection by laboratory methods has been obtained. This presumptive therapy, called *epidemiologic treatment* because it is based on epidemiologic indications, can play an important role in STD control by interrupting the chain of transmission. Epidemiologic treatment ensures treatment of infectious individuals who have false-negative laboratory results or who are seen before their tests turn positive. Epidemiologic treatment also guarantees treatment for those who might not return when notified of positive test results.

Epidemiologic treatment is indicated for sex partners of patients with syphilis, chancroid, gonorrhea, or chlamydia, because a high proportion of such persons are likely to be infected. That same philosophy underlies the recommendation that patients with confirmed gonococcal infections receive presumptive treatment for chlamydia (23). Epidemiologic treatment is indicated when syndromes such as nongonococcal urethritis, mucopurulent cervicitis, or genital ulceration are recognized but when laboratory facilities are not readily available to confirm a microbiological diagnosis. Epidemiologic treatment is also indicated in settings such as walk-in clinics and emergency rooms, where follow-up may be uncertain.

In the original recommendations of the U.S. Preventive Services Task Force, epidemiologic treatment received the highest grade of evidence and level of recommendation.

PARTNER NOTIFICATION AND MANAGEMENT OF SEX PARTNERS

Breaking the chain of transmission is central to STD prevention at both the clinical (e.g., individual) and public health (e.g., community) level. Therefore, sex partners of patients diagnosed with an STD should be evaluated, examined, and, in circumstances in which infection is considered likely, treated in spite of the absence of clinical signs of infection, or before proof of infection by laboratory methods is available (see previous discussion of epidemiologic treatment). Sex partners of patients diagnosed with specific STDs require different management strategies (Table 12.3).

Table 12.3
Management of Sex Partners

Disease	Intervention
Gonorrhea	Partners should be referred for evaluation and treatment according to the following schedule:
	If the index patient is symptomatic, partners should be evaluated and treated for gonorrhea and chlamydia if their last sexual contact with the patient was within 30 days of onset of the patient's symptoms.
	If the index patient is asymptomatic, partners should be evaluated and treated for gonorrhea and chlamydia if their last sexual contact with the patient was within 60 days of diagnosis.
	Patients must be instructed to avoid sexual intercourse until patient and partner(s) are cured (when therapy is completed and patient and partner are without symptoms).
	The mothers of infants with gonococcal infection and their sex partners should be evaluated and treated.
Nongonococcal urethritis	If the index patient is symptomatic, partners should be evaluated and treated for gonorrhea and chlamydia if their last sexual contact with the patient was within 30 days of onset of the patient's symptoms.
	If the index patient is asymptomatic, partners should be evaluated and treated for gonorrhea and chlamydia if their last sexual contact with the patient was within 60 days of diagnosis.
	Patients must be instructed to avoid sexual intercourse until patient and partner(s) are cured (when therapy is completed and patient and partner are without symptoms).
Mucopurulent cervicitis	Partners should be managed appropriately for the specific STD (chlamydia or gonorrhea) identified in the index patient. Partners of patients treated presumptively should receive the same treatment as the patient.
Chlamydia	If the index patient is symptomatic, partners should be evaluated and treated for gonorrhea and chlamydia if their last sexual contact with the patient was within 30 days of onset of the patient's symptoms.
	If the index patient is asymptomatic, partners should be evaluated and treated for gonorrhea and chlamydia if their last sexual contact with the patient was within 60 days of diagnosis.
	Patients must be instructed to avoid sex until patient and partner(s) are cured (when therapy is completed and patient and partner are without symptoms).
	The mothers of infants with chlamydial infection and their sex partners should be evaluated and treated.
Trichomonas	Partners should be treated.
	Patients should be instructed to avoid sex until therapy is completed and patient and partner(s) are without symptoms.
Bacterial vaginosis	Routine treatment of partners is not recommended.
Syphilis	Sexual transmission occurs only when mucocutaneous syphilitic lesions are present; such manifestations are uncommon after the first year of infection.
	All partners exposed to a patient with early syphilis (primary, secondary, or latent with duration < 1 year) should be evaluated clinically and serologically.

Disease	Intervention
Syphilis (continued)	Partners exposed to a patient with early syphilis within the preceding 90 days might be infected yet seronegative; they should be treated presumptively. It may be advisable to presumptively treat persons exposed more than 90 days ago if serologic test results are not immediately available and follow-up is uncertain. Long-term sex partners of patients with late syphilis should be evaluated clinically and serologically for syphilis. The time periods usually used for identifying at-risk partners are 3 months plus duration of symptoms for primary syphilis, 6 months plus duration of symptoms for secondary syphilis, and 1 year for early latent syphilis.
Chancroid	Partners exposed to chancroid within 10 days before onset of the patient's symptoms should be examined and treated, whether symptomatic or not.
HIV infection	Sexual and needle-sharing partners of HIV infected persons must receive HIV prevention counseling (see text) and must be offered HIV testing.
Genital herpes	Symptomatic partners should be managed as would any patient with genital lesions. Asymptomatic individuals may benefit from evaluation and counseling.
Genital warts	Examination of sex partners is not necessary for management of genital warts, since the role of re-infection is probably minimal. Sex partners may have warts and desire treatment, and they also may benefit from counseling.
Hepatitis B	Susceptible partners should receive post-exposure hepatitis B immune globulin prophylaxis within 14 days of their last exposure. This should be followed by the standard three-dose immunization series with hepatitis B vaccine beginning at the time of hepatitis B immune globulin administration. (See Chapter 18 for more details.)
Ectoparasites	Partners of patients with lice or scabies within the past 30 days should be examined and treated.
Pelvic inflammatory disease	Treatment of partners of women with pelvic inflammatory disease is imperative, because of the risk of reinfection. Since diagnostic testing for *C. trachomatis* and *N. gonorrhoeae* is thought to be insensitive in asymptomatic males, all sex partners should be treated empirically with regimens effective against these infections. In clinical settings in which only women are seen, special arrangements should be made to provide care for male sex partners of women with pelvic inflammatory disease. When this is not feasible, clinicians should ensure that partners are referred for treatment.

U.S. Centers for Disease Control and Prevention. 1993 sexually transmitted diseases treatment guidelines. MMWR 1993;42(RR-14):i–102.

Partner notification is both a primary and a secondary STD prevention strategy. As a primary prevention strategy, uninfected partners can reduce the risks of acquiring infection by changing their behaviors. Infected partners can receive early medical intervention and can avoid transmitting infection to others, including reinfecting themselves. As a secondary prevention strategy, infected sex partners can receive prompt medical treatment. This is particularly important for those who have bacterial STDs such as gonorrhea or chlamydia, which can remain inapparent and, unless cured, can lead to pelvic inflammatory disease and long-term sequelae.

Patient versus Provider Referral

There are two strategies for partner notification: patient referral, where index patients themselves notify their partners, and provider referral, where named partners are notified and counseled by health department staff (24). The choice of how to notify partners must be based on the wishes of the index patient, the legal requirements of the local health department, and the resources available for the provider referral process.

If provider referral is chosen, clinicians should contact their local health department or state STD program. If patient referral is chosen, clinicians may want to assist in notifying partners, particularly if they also care for one of the partners. Because of the relationships that primary care clinicians develop with their patients, they may be in the best position to help patients disclose STD diagnoses to their partners. Helping these patients may involve not only counseling sessions, but role-playing or rehearsal techniques to coach patients in ways to inform their partners. For example, *"How will you tell your partner about this? What if he (she) gets angry or starts crying? What will you say?"* (25). In some circumstances, the clinician may want to meet with a couple or may offer to disclose the results to a partner. The follow-up evaluation of partners should then proceed.

Persons with STDs have a responsibility to protect their partners. However, some patients may be unwilling to disclose a sexually acquired infection or positive HIV test result to their partners because of anticipated unfavorable reactions (26). There are several approaches for persuading a reluctant patient to notify his or her partner(s). Men need to be informed that their female sex partners can develop severe, irreversible complications from STDs unless these infections are treated promptly. *"Won't your partner find out eventually? How do you think your partner will feel when she (he) finds out that you didn't tell her (him) right away?"* (25). If a patient with an STD refuses to notify sex partners while continuing to place them at risk, the clinician has an ethical and legal duty to inform persons that they are being exposed. (The ethical principle on which this is based is discussed in Chapter 27.) This duty to warn may be particularly applicable to primary care clinicians who often have special knowledge about a patient's social and family relationships, but it should be exercised only when all other attempts to persuade a patient to inform his or her partner have failed.

DISEASE REPORTING

Disease reporting is a critical component of the public health response to STD control, and primary care physicians have a major role to play. The data gained through disease reporting are used by researchers to understand the transmission dynamics of STDs, and by public health planners to direct STD prevention activities. Morbidity trends are used to set public health priorities, to allocate scarce resources, and to evaluate the effectiveness of STD control programs.

In addition, reporting is essential to maintaining partner notification activities. Reporting STDs may fulfill a physician's duty to warn persons who are at risk of being infected by their patients. STD reports are held in the strictest confidence; in some jurisdictions they are even protected by statute from subpoena. Before any follow-up of a positive STD test is conducted by STD program representatives, they consult with the provider to verify the diagnosis and treatment.

STD/HIV cases should be reported in accordance with local statutory requirements, and in as timely a manner as possible. Syphilis, gonorrhea, and AIDS are reportable diseases in every state. Requirements for reporting other STDs such as chancroid, chlamydia, and asymptomatic HIV infection differ from state to state; physicians should become familiar with local STD reporting requirements. Reporting may be provider-based, laboratory-based, or both. Clinicians who are unsure of local reporting requirements should seek advice from their local health department or state STD program.

OFFICE ORGANIZATION

Waiting areas should be arranged so that registration information can be obtained in a confidential manner. The office waiting room or patient examination rooms can provide a good setting to distribute health promotion materials (see "Resources" section later in this chapter). These materials should be linguistically and culturally appropriate for the patient population, and targeted to the appropriate reading level. In settings where high-risk patients are frequently seen, consider making condoms available, along with instructions for their proper use. The U.S. Centers for Disease Control and Prevention publish recommendations for the treatment and counseling of patients with STDs as well as guidelines for improving the structure and management of publicly funded STD clinics. These may also be useful in private practice settings. Free copies of either reference can be obtained by calling 404-639-8063. See also the specific guidelines for the workup and treatment of patients with HIV and other STDs listed in Chapter 17.

MEDICAL RECORDS

The medical record should contain information to identify and locate the patient if necessary. In addition to documenting the presenting symptoms, medical history, physical examination, laboratory results, diagnosis, and treatment, the record should document high-risk behaviors, counseling, and plans for follow-up. Many patients worry that sensitive behavioral information, when written in the chart, can be embarrassing if read by someone other than the physician (e.g., by nurses or insurance companies). Some clinicians recommend a coding system for this information to reassure patients about their privacy. In such a system, for example, insertive anal intercourse could be abbreviated as "IA," while receptive anal intercourse could be referred to as "RA" (6).

CONCLUSION

STDs, including HIV infection, remain among the most important public health problems in the United States. Primary care physicians and other health care providers are uniquely situated to play a major role in preventing the spread of STDs through early diagnosis and treatment of STDs, patient education and counseling, appropriate management of sex partners, targeted screening or presumptive epidemiologic treatment of high-risk individuals, and timely reporting of disease.

RESOURCES—PATIENT EDUCATION MATERIALS

National STD Hotline
800-227-8922

U.S. Centers for Disease Control and Prevention
AIDS and HIV Hotline
800-342-2437
800-344-7432 (Spanish)
800-243-7889 (TTY)
    To learn more about HIV and where to get the test.

Agency for Health Care Policy and Research
Publications Clearinghouse
P.O. Box 8547
Silver Spring, MD 20907
800-358-9295
    "Understanding HIV" (brochure 94-0574); "HIV and Your Child" (brochure 94-0576).

American Academy of Family Physicians
8880 Ward Parkway
Kansas City, MO 64114-2797
800-944-0000

"STDs: Signs of Common STDs and Tips on Prevention" (brochure 1565); "AIDS: How To Reduce Your Risk of Catching It" (brochure 1507).

American Social Health Association
P.O. Box 13827
Research Triangle Park, NC 27709
919-361-8400
"STD (VD): Questions and Answers"; "Stopping Gonorrhea, The Clap"; "Some Questions and Answers About Chlamydia"; "HIV Negative: When Are You Free from HIV?"

Channing L. Bete Co., Inc.
200 State Road
South Deerfield, MA 01373-0200
800-628-7733
"What Everyone Should Know About Syphilis and Gonorrhea" (brochure T38414A); "What Everyone Should Know About Chlamydia" (brochure T14738A).

Krames Communications
1100 Grundy Lane
San Bruno, CA 94066-3030
800-333-3032
"Sexually Transmitted Diseases" (booklet 1181); "Condoms and STDs" (booklet, English, 1422; Spanish, 1423); "Safer Sex" (booklet 1267).

National Institute of Allergy and Infectious Diseases
Office of Communications
Building 31, Room 7A50
9000 Rockville Pike
Bethesda, MD 20892
301-496-5717
"An Introduction to Sexually Transmitted Diseases" (brochure 92-909A); "Taking the HIV (AIDS) Test: How To Help Yourself" (brochure 93-3322); "Testing Positive for HIV: How to Help Yourself (booklet 93-3323); "HIV Infection and AIDS" (brochure 92-909F).

REFERENCES

1. U.S. Centers for Disease Control and Prevention. Update: acquired immunodeficiency syndrome—United States, 1994. MMWR 1995;44:64–67.
2. Lewis CE, Freeman HE. The sexual history-taking and counseling practices of primary care physicians. West J Med 1987;147:165–167.
3. Ferguson KJ, Stapleton JT, Helms CM. Physicians' effectiveness in assessing risk for human immunodeficiency virus infection. Arch Intern Med 1991;151:561–564.
4. Siwek J. Taking a sexual history: an individualized approach. Am Fam Physician 1989;40(1):83–84.
5. American Medical Association. HIV blood test counseling: physician guidelines, 2nd ed. Chicago: American Medical Association, 1993
6. Kassler WJ, Wu AW. Addressing HIV in the office practice: assessing risk, counseling, and testing. Primary Care 1992;19:19–33.
7. American Medical Association. HIV blood test counseling: AMA physician guidelines. Chicago: American Medical Association, 1988:1–14.
8. Jewell ME, Jewell GS. How to assess the risk of HIV exposure. Am Fam Physician 1989;40(1):153–161.
9. Wasserheit JN. Epidemiological synergy: interrelationships between human immunodefi-

ciency virus infection and other sexually transmitted diseases. Sex Trans Dis 1992;19(2):61–77.

10. Marx R, Aral SO, Rolfs RT, Sterk C. Crack, sex, and STD. Sex Trans Dis 1991;18(2):92–101.

11. U.S. Centers for Disease Control and Prevention. Update: barrier protection against HIV infection and other sexually transmitted diseases. MMWR 1993;42(30) Aug 6:589–591.

12. Cates W, Stone KM. Family planning, sexually transmitted diseases and contraceptive choice: a literature update—part I. Family Planning Perspectives 1992;24:75–84.

13. Stone KM, Peterson HB. Spermicides, HIV, and the vaginal sponge. JAMA 1992;268:521–523.

14. U.S. Centers for Disease Control and Prevention. Technical guidance on HIV counseling. MMWR 1993;42(RR-2):11–16.

15. Gerber AR, Valdiserri RO, Holtgrave DR, et al. Preventive services guidelines for primary care clinicians caring for adults and adolescents infected with the human immunodeficiency virus. Arch Fam Med 1993;2:969–976.

16. U.S. Centers for Disease Control and Prevention. Recommendations for HIV testing services for inpatients and outpatients in acute care hospital settings. MMWR 1993;42(RR-2):1–6.

17. El-Sadr W, Oleske JM, Agins BD, et al. Evaluation and management of early HIV infection. Clinical practice guideline No. 7 (AHCPR Publication No. 94-0572). Rockville, MD: Agency for Health Care Policy and Research, 1994.

18. Doll LS, Kennedy MB. HIV Counseling and testing: what is it and how well does it work? In: Schochetman G, George JR, eds. AIDS testing. New York: Springer-Verlag, 1994:302–319.

19. Cates W. The epidemiology and control of sexually transmitted diseases in adolescents. Adolescent Medicine 1990;1(3):409–427.

20. Neinstein LS. Adolescent health care: a practical guide, 2nd ed. Baltimore: Urban & Schwarzenberg, 1991.

21. U.S. Preventive Services Task Force. Guide to clinical preventive services. Baltimore: Williams & Wilkins, 1996.

22. U. S. Centers for Disease Control and Prevention. Protection against viral hepatitis. MMWR 1990;39(RR-2):1–26.

23. U. S. Centers for Disease Control and Prevention. 1993 sexually transmitted diseases treatment guidelines. MMWR 1993;42(RR-14):1–102.

24. U. S. Centers for Disease Control and Prevention. Partner notification for preventing human immunodeficiency virus (HIV) infection—Colorado, Idaho, South Carolina, Virginia. MMWR 1988;37(25) Jul 1:393–402.

25. Coates TJ, Lo B. Counseling patients seropositive for human immunodeficiency virus: an approach for medical practice. West J Med 1991;153:629–634.

26. Stempel A, Moulton J, Bachetti P, Moss A. Disclosure of HIV-antibody test results & reactions of sexual partners, friends, family, and health professionals. Int Conf AIDS 1989;Abstract E.729:(abstract).

13. Substance Use and Abuse: Alcohol and Other Drugs

HENRIETTA N. BARNES AND DAVID H. BOR

INTRODUCTION

The majority of patients seen by primary care providers use or have used alcohol or other psychoactive drugs. While the adverse effects of heavy drug and alcohol use are well-known, moderate or episodic alcohol or drug use may also have serious health consequences (1). The clinician's role is to assess where the patient is on the spectrum of alcohol and drug use and to provide appropriate education, counseling, or medical intervention. Although the pharmacologies of alcohol and other abused drugs lead to different clinical presentations, the common underlying problem is addiction. In this chapter we shall consider the abuse of alcohol and other drugs as different facets of the same problem.

The natural history of alcohol and drug use covers a spectrum of nonuse, use, misuse, abuse, and dependence. The use of alcohol and drugs is a learned social behavior that usually starts with youthful experimentation. Most alcohol and drug users arrive at a level of drug use that maximizes the pleasurable effects and minimizes adverse consequences. People in this category may experience occasional episodes of *misuse* which range from minor (the morning hangover) to severe (fatal automobile crash). The 15–20% of drinkers with repeated problems related to their alcohol use comprise the *abuse* category (2). An even smaller number manifest physiological dependence. This chapter will focus on the primary care clinician's responsibility toward the large number of patients who use alcohol or other drugs but do not have significant problems of abuse or dependence.

Although the devastation of inner city communities by illicit drug use and the "War on Drugs" have rightly commanded national attention, problems due to the use of ethyl alcohol account for a much larger public health burden in terms of mortality, morbidity, days of work lost, and effect on the economy (Fig. 13.1) (1, 3). Similarly, the misuse of prescribed psychoactive drugs, often in combination with alcohol, presents a significant and often unrecognized problem (4).

Through patient education, the primary care provider can help pa-

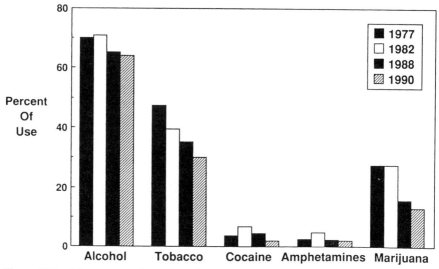

Figure 13.1. Most commonly used psychoactive drugs. (Adapted from Fleming MF, Barry KL, eds. Addictive disorders. St. Louis: Mosby Year Book, 1992. Reprinted with permission.)

tients take a more active role in assessing their alcohol and drug use and in recognizing and changing risky behaviors. Clinical research indicates that techniques of brief intervention (5) and motivational interviewing (6) are useful prevention strategies for patients with alcohol problems. Furthermore, because of the high prevalence of alcohol problems, even modest results from an intervention would have substantial impact on the nation's public health (3). The recommendations in this chapter are based on available scientific evidence about behavioral change and on the authors' clinical experience.

ASSESSMENT

Routine assessment and counseling of patients (and the parents of pediatric patients) about alcohol and other drug use is recommended by the U.S. Preventive Services Task Force, Canadian Task Force on the Periodic Health Examination, American Academy of Pediatrics, American Academy of Family Physicians, American Medical Association, and other groups. In this chapter we shall describe techniques for assessment of risk for problems related to drug and alcohol use and strategies for primary and secondary prevention—including education, anticipatory guidance, and brief therapeutic intervention. We discuss how some techniques of motivational interviewing may be useful to the practicing clinician. These assessment and counseling techniques are summarized in Table 13.1.

Table 13.1
Approach to the Patient Who Uses Alcohol or Other Drugs

I Assessment
  A. Rule out substance *abuse* or *dependence*
    1. Screening instruments
      a. ascertain quantity and frequency of use
      b. CAGE
    2. Data from medical history
      a. personal and social history
      b. family history
      c. review of systems
  B. Assess for unhealthy use, *misuse*
    1. Host factors
      a. genetic predisposition
      b. comorbid conditions (psychiatric disorders)
      c. use of other drugs
      d. positive review of systems
      e. hostile, defensive affect during interview
    2. Environmental factors
      a. family stress
      b. leisure centered around alcohol-related activities
      c. occupation
    3. Agent/Substance
      a. pharmacology
      b. illegality
  C. Counseling
    1. Share concern about effects of use or potential risk. Use *specific* data from history
    2. Educate patient about effects of alcohol or drugs
    3. Offer options and set goals for healthier behaviors
    4. Plan follow-up

In assessing a patient's use of alcohol or other drugs, the primary care clinician has two responsibilities:

1. to rule out substance abuse or dependence that requires prompt, active intervention;

2. to understand the patient's use of these substances in order to provide appropriate education about prevention.

The initial assessment determines whether a patient drinks alcohol or uses drugs and the average quantity and frequency (e.g., drinks per week). More than 12 standard drinks per week for women and 15 drinks per week for men implies a significant risk for developing problems related to alcohol (4). A standard drink contains approximately 13 grams of absolute alcohol and is equivalent to one 12-ounce can of beer, one shot of liquor, or one 6-ounce glass of wine.

Questions about quantity and frequency are *not* useful in screening for abuse or dependence, which is best performed using specific instruments such as the CAGE questionnaire (see Table 2.2) (7). In one study, two positive answers to the CAGE questionnaire provided a sensitivity and specificity of about 80–85% in detecting alcohol abuse or dependence in an ambulatory medical population (7). Lower accuracy has been reported in other studies (see Chapter 2 and Table 2.7). Clinicians have adapted the CAGE for drug use, but this has not been validated (4).

Because early problems with alcohol and drugs are primarily behavioral, rather than physiological, it is not surprising that brief questionnaires are more sensitive for screening than any combination of physical examination findings and laboratory tests (8). Groups such as the U.S. Preventive Services Task Force and the Canadian Task Force on the Periodic Health Examination specifically recommend against the use of biochemical markers or drug testing to screen routinely for these disorders (see also Chapter 21).

Whether trying to confirm the results of a positive screening test or assessing risk from alcohol or drug use, the clinician will find that a picture of the person's use of these substances will emerge from the family, social, and occupational histories. Consideration of these data in terms of the *host*, the *environment*, and the *agent* can make the information more understandable. *Host* risk factors include genetic susceptibility for alcoholism, psychiatric disorders, chronic pain, and use of psychoactive medications and other drugs, including tobacco (5). Patients with sleep disturbances, anxiety, or multiple somatic complaints may often use alcohol or drugs in an unhealthy way. Defensive, vague, or hostile responses from the patient during the interview may indicate a problematic relation to alcohol or drugs.

Elucidation of the patient's interaction with his or her *environment* may also yield useful information. Is there evidence of family stress: divorce, inadequate family resources, behavioral problems in the children, domestic violence? Do the patient's leisure activities center around the use of alcohol or drugs? Is he in an occupation with low supervision, isolation, or access to alcohol and drugs, which may increase the potential for problems? Does she engage in risky behaviors such as driving or having unprotected sex while intoxicated? A positive family history, reflecting both genetic and environmental factors, is a significant risk factor, tripling a person's chance of developing drug or alcohol problems.

The choice of *agent* may indicate risky behavior in terms of personal health and social consequences. The illicit use of drugs, whether alcohol by an adolescent or marijuana by a judge, poses legal risks, although the risks to physical health may be minimal. The intravenous use of drugs, particularly street drugs, implies a willingness to take health risks that is usually seen only in people with significant dependence. The particular pattern of drug use (drinking to intoxication every weekend, taking leftover oxycodone to help with sleep, or smoking marijuana daily before work) may suggest an unhealthy use of a psychoactive drug.

A complete medical history offers many opportunities to assess a patient's use of alcohol and drugs and the consequences of that use:

1. Health habits: *"Do you use coffee? Smoke cigarettes? Do you use alcohol or other drugs?"* If patient responds affirmatively: *"In an average week, how many drinks do you have?"* Because self-reports about quantity and frequency are frequently misleading, patients who describe drinking "a couple of glasses of wine with dinner" or "just a six-pack on the weekends" should still be screened for alcohol abuse and dependence. If the patient does not use alcohol or drugs, asking *"why not?"* may uncover a diagnosis of alcoholism in remission or a strong family history of alcohol and drug problems.

2. Driving habits: *"Do you use seat belts?" "Do you ever drive after drinking, or ride with a driver who has been drinking?"*

3. Family history: *"... any history of diabetes, cancer, heart disease, alcohol problems, drug use, psychiatric illness?"*

4. Social/personal/occupational history: *"Who are the important people in your life?" "How are things at home?" "What do you do for fun or to relax?" "How do you cope with stress?" "What kind of work do you do?"* These questions are not specific to screening for drug and alcohol problems, but they may uncover valuable information about the patient's relationship with alcohol and other drugs.

5. Review of systems: This part of the history is very valuable for uncovering minor complaints which may indicate an unhealthy use of alcohol or drugs (heartburn, insomnia, menstrual or sexual difficulties, palpitations, constipation, anxiety, rhinitis, fatigue).

COUNSELING

After assessing the severity of health risks from alcohol and drug use, the clinician should counsel the patient about prevention or treatment. This section focuses on primary prevention, including anticipatory guidance and education, and secondary prevention, including brief intervention and motivating behavioral change. Clinicians should tailor their approach to the severity of the patient's problems with alcohol or drugs. If a significant problem is uncovered, the clinician will need to make very specific recommendations about treatment. For a patient just learning to use alcohol or drugs, a discussion of "normal" use in her sociocultural milieu and of its potential risks may help facilitate responsible choices about drug use in the future.

The steps for counseling patients as described in different models for brief intervention (5, 6) provide a structure for talking to patients about alcohol and drugs. The principal components of brief intervention include:

1. Sharing concern with patients about the effects of their use of alcohol or drugs or their potential risks;

2. Educating the patient about adverse consequences related to alcohol or drug use;

3. Setting goals or discussing options for behavioral change;

4. Planning follow-up.

The first step is to *share concern* about the patient's use of alcohol or drugs. In primary prevention, the clinician helps the patient anticipate future problems:

> *"Paul, you're certainly doing well in school this year—on the honor roll and the varsity basketball team. But your friends' use of alcohol worries me; I'm very concerned about what will happen if you or one of your friends gets behind the wheel after drinking at the victory parties."*

If the clinician has concerns about the effects of current drinking behavior, she should share them before reviewing the *specific* evidence from the history that has caused concern:

> *"Mrs. Johnson, I'm concerned that your use of alcohol may be unhealthy for you. You told me that you've been having problems with anxiety and sleep since your divorce, that you frequently have several drinks in the evening to relax and then have trouble correcting the papers for your students the next morning."*

In discussing the adverse effects of drinking or other drug use, the clinician should *educate* patients about the potentially harmful effects of the drug, so that they can make more informed decisions about their use of alcohol or drugs:

> *"One or two drinks, Paul, can affect your judgment and slow your reflex time, even if you don't feel drunk, and that's just the kind of situation that can turn a minor driving problem into a lethal crash."*

> *"You're right, Mrs. Johnson, that alcohol can help you fall asleep, but your nighttime drinking is more likely to cause sleep problems than to help them. I think alcohol may be causing more harm than help."*

Once the clinician and patient have discussed the patient's use of alcohol or drugs, they need to *set goals* and *review options* for healthier behavior. As primary prevention, the clinician should make explicit recommendations as a guide to future behavior:

> *"You know I think that high school kids are dealing with too many other issues to take on the task of learning how to drink responsibly. I recommend that you not drink alcohol at all, but if you do, I'd like us to work out a plan with your folks and your friends' parents that gets you and your friends home safe after a party."*

When a problem is identified, the clinician, as a part of secondary prevention, should provide concrete advice as a plan for change:

> *"Mrs. Johnson, I think it would make sense for you to stop drinking for a while so that we can see how much of a role alcohol is playing. But I also think we need to focus on other ways to help you handle the stress you're under. You had mentioned getting back to your yoga class at the gym. A course on stress reduction techniques might be helpful too."*

Finally, the clinician should *plan follow-up*, to reassess risks from alcohol and drug use, to reinforce the patient's efforts toward healthier use, and to provide the opportunity for patients to consider again the health risks presented by their drug or alcohol use.

> *"Paul, I'm really glad you feel you can talk to your parents about this. I'd like to hear how things work out. Why don't you schedule another appointment for next month after your exams?"*

> *"Mrs. Johnson, it's clear that you and I disagree about whether your use of alcohol is causing any problems; but we both agree that helping you with the stress and trouble sleeping is very important. I'd like you to think about our discussion today and take a look at this pamphlet. Let's get together in a month to see how you're doing."*

Brief advice coupled with written materials and follow-up has resulted in a decrease in alcohol consumption among heavy drinkers (5, 9, 10). Sample patient education materials are listed later under "Resources."

The clinician's understanding of patients' willingness to change and his use of motivational interviewing techniques can assist patients to change behaviors. A model of the different stages of change developed by Prochaska and DiClemente in their work with smokers is helpful in assessing patients' readiness to change (11). The stages of precontemplation ("I don't have any problem with alcohol"), contemplation ("Maybe driving home after those drinking parties isn't such a good idea"), and determination ("I'll be sure to appoint a designated driver when I go out drinking"), followed by action, maintenance, and relapse describe the cyclical pattern of an individual trying to change behavior. Clinicians should tailor their approach to the patient's appropriate stage; e.g., a patient who denies having any problem will benefit more from a discussion of what *would* constitute a problem rather than from a referral to a treatment program. Brief interventions are likely to be more successful if the clinician is empathic and able to empower the patient's sense of self-efficacy (6).

For the patient with more serious problems, the options for further intervention depend on the patient's assessment of the problem. If the patient disagrees that a problem exists, the clinician can refer the patient to an addiction specialist for a consultation or suggest a trial of controlled drinking and reassessment in a few weeks. Recommendations for treatment depend on the severity of the patient's alcohol and drug problem. Many well-functioning alcoholic patients do well with a referral to a mutual support group or an outpatient counselor, and close follow-up by the primary care provider. The most well known of these support groups, Alcoholics Anonymous (see "Resources" later in this chapter), has meetings throughout the United States and many parts of the world. Patients with more severe addiction may require hospitalization for detoxification and a more intensive rehabilitation program. In either case, the clinician must negotiate a plan acceptable to the patient.

Special Populations

Adolescents, with their sense of personal invulnerability, pose a particular challenge. The clinician should acknowledge both the effects of peer pressure and the normalcy of teens taking risks and challenging authority. As noted earlier, such a discussion can be important for persons just learning to use alcohol or other drugs and can set the stage for a discussion of responsible options. A discussion of what the adolescent enjoys about drinking can lead to an exploration of other ways to achieve the same social benefits that may be less risky.

Family members may express concern about a child's or spouse's use of alcohol or drugs. The primary care clinician can educate them about the effects of alcohol and drugs and help them to provide guidance or set limits with their loved one's problem. A brief assessment of the family member's use of alcohol or drugs will elucidate their own risk for problems. Organizations that specifically provide support for such family members are listed later in the "Resources" section.

Assessing health risks in patients who use illicit drugs requires clinicians to separate their medical opinion from their moral or legal stance. There is no evidence to suggest that the occasional recreational use of marijuana is any more harmful medically than similar use of alcohol. Cocaine is more problematic; significant intoxication may be associated with cardiac arrhythmias, violent behavior, and risky sexual practices. The legal ramifications of illicit drug use can be significant. A discussion of the patient's perception of those risks can provide useful information regarding the patient's attitude about risky behaviors.

> *"Ms. Taylor, you've told me how excited you are to be finishing your graduate degree in criminal justice and that you've been interviewing for a government position. And yet you also tell me that you frequently enjoy smoking pot at parties. To me, there seems to be a contradiction here. Can you help me understand it?"*

After smoking and alcohol use, prescription drug abuse may be the most common drug abuse problem encountered in ambulatory medicine. The physician should include possible drug abuse in the differential diagnosis when interviewing patients with chronic pain syndromes (migraine headaches, back pain), especially those without objective signs, anxiety, insomnia, and depression. Certain patient behaviors (weekend requests for narcotics or tranquilizers, "allergies" to all analgesics except one particular brand, frequently "lost" prescriptions) should alert the physician to possible drug abuse. Opiate analgesics and benzodiazepines head the list of frequently abused prescription drugs, followed by barbiturates, stimulants, muscle relaxants, and anabolic steroids.

For patients whose addiction is in remission, the clinician can play an important role in relapse prevention. Anticipating situations when patients will be at risk for drug use and helping them develop appropriate coping strategies allow patients to exert more control over addiction.

Potential Adverse Effects of Counseling

Patients whose use of alcohol or other drugs is unhealthy may feel stigmatized by the label of "alcoholic" or "addict." Clinicians can avoid reinforcing that stigma by framing the problem as one of unhealthy behaviors that the clinician and patient need to address together. Even so, the societal stigma perceived by patients may interfere with their ability to receive care.

Many clinicians are concerned that patients will leave their practices if questions about alcohol and drug use are raised. This may reflect the clinician's personal discomfort with these issues or prior negative experiences when talking with patients about alcoholism or addiction. Although these discussions may be painful for patients struggling with drug or alcohol problems, a frank, compassionate conversation about the health risks and the options for changing behavior with the doctor's help can empower patients to take more responsibility for their alcohol and drug use.

Occasionally, such an explicit discussion will precipitate a patient's decision to leave a clinician's practice. Although the clinician may feel that she has been ineffective, many people whose alcohol or drug problems are in remission date the beginning of their recovery to such a clear statement, even if they were unable to acknowledge it at the time.

Actively intoxicated patients are unable to participate in any meaningful discussion of health behaviors. Clinicians should share their assessment with such patients, recommend detoxification, and make an appropriate referral. Patients with histories of intravenous drug use or chronic pain syndromes virtually always require an in-depth alcohol and drug history and a more intensive intervention than a brief discussion of unhealthy behaviors. See Chapters 4 and 18 for screening and immunization guidelines for patients who use intravenous drugs.

OFFICE AND CLINIC ORGANIZATION

Pamphlets on the effects of alcohol and other drugs and information on mutual help groups should be available in examining rooms for clinicians to give to patients as part of counseling. Similar pamphlets should be available in the waiting room. Educational literature describing the effects of alcohol and other drugs on individuals and their families is published by the National Clearinghouse on Alcohol and Drug Abuse Information, Alcoholics Anonymous, and other programs. (See section on "Resources" below.)

MEDICAL RECORD DOCUMENTATION

Both the assessment of alcohol and drug use and counseling should be documented in the medical record. Because problems with alcohol and drugs may be episodic and require ongoing observation, any suspicion of a drug or alcohol problem should be recorded in the problem list to remind the clinician to reassess the matter at a later visit. Under federal law any release of information pertaining to drug or alcohol abuse requires specific authorization from the patient. Clinicians need to be sensitive to issues of confidentiality, because the inadvertent release of such information without explicit authorization could affect a person's employability or insurability.

Careful prescribing practices and documentation of prescriptions in the medical record can obviate prescription drug abuse. The amount of drug, the directions, the indication, and the number of refills should be carefully recorded. Similarly, prescriptions for psychoactive drugs should have the dosage and number dispensed written numerically and in words to prevent alteration of the prescription.

RESOURCES—PROFESSIONAL EDUCATION MATERIALS

An overview of current diagnostic and treatment strategies for substance abuse is provided in "Recent Advances in Addictive Disorders," an entire issue of Psychiatric Clinics of North America 1993;16(1). See also Kitchens JM. Does this patient have an alcohol problem? JAMA 1994;272: 1782–1787, or contact the National Clearinghouse for Alcohol and Drug Information, 800-729-6686.

RESOURCES—PATIENT EDUCATION MATERIALS

Patient Education

Alcoholics Anonymous
P.O. Box 459
Grand Central Station
New York, NY 10163
212-686-1100

Local A.A. chapters are listed in most telephone directories. Publications: "A Newcomer Asks" (brochure P-24); "A.A. At a Glance" (fact sheet, English F-1, Spanish FS-75) "A Brief Guide to Alcoholics Anonymous (brochure P-42); "Is AA For You?" (brochure P-3); "A Message To Teenagers: How To Tell When Drinking is Becoming a Problem" (brochure F-9); "AA For the Native North American" (brochure P-21).

American Academy of Family Physicians
8880 Ward Parkway
Kansas City, MO 64114-2797
800-944-0000
"Alcohol: What To Do If It's A Problem For You" (brochure 1517).

American Academy of Pediatrics
Publications Department
141 Northwest Point Blvd.
P.O. Box 927
Elk Grove Village, IL 60009-0927
800-433-9016
"Alcohol: Your Child and Drugs" (brochure HE0059).

National Clearinghouse for Alcohol and Drug Information
P.O. Box 2345
Rockville, MD 20847-2345
800-729-6686
800-487-4889 TTY/TDD
Publications: "If Someone Close...Has A Problem With Alcohol or Other Drugs" (DHHS Pub. No. ADM-92-1916), "Helping Your Child Say 'No': A Parent's Guide" (PH283).

National Council on Alcoholism and Drug Dependence
12 West 21st Street, 8th Floor
New York, NY 10010
800-622-2255
212-206-6770
Offers list of agencies providing treatment for alcoholism and drug dependence, some of which also offer counseling and treatment services.

National Drug Information Treatment and Referral Hotline
800-662-HELP (4357)
800-662-9832 (Spanish)
800-228-0427 (TTY/TDD)
Offers alcohol and drug abuse-related information and/or referrals for persons seeking treatment.

Family Members

Adult Children of Alcoholics
P.O. Box 3216
Torrance, CA 90505
310-534-1815

Al-Anon/Alateen Family Groups
P.O. Box 862
Midtown Station, New York, NY 10018-0862
800-359-9996
Local chapters are listed in most telephone directories.

COCANON Family Groups
P.O. Box 64742-66
Los Angeles, CA 90064
213-859-2206

Nar-Anon Family Groups
P.O. Box 2562
Palos Verdes Peninsula, CA 90274
213-547-5800

National Association for Children of Alcoholics
11426 Rockville Pike, Suite 100
Rockville, MD 20852
301-468-0985

National Association for Native American Children of Alcoholics
P.O. Box 18736
Seattle, WA 98118
206-322-5601

REFERENCES

1. National Institute on Alcohol Abuse and Alcoholism. Eighth special report to the U. S. Congress on alcohol and health. DHSS Publication No. (ADM) 281-91-0003. Washington, DC: Public Health Service, 1993.
2. Skinner HA. Spectrum of drinkers and intervention opportunities. Can Med Assoc J 1990;143:1054–1059.
3. Institute of Medicine. Broadening the base of treatment for alcohol problems. Washington, DC: National Academy Press, 1990:511–549.
4. Fleming MF, Barry KL, eds. Addictive disorders. St. Louis: Mosby Yearbook, 1992.
5. Babor TF, Ritson B, Hodgson R. Alcohol-related problems in the primary care health setting: a review of early intervention strategies. Brit J Addict 1986;81:23–46.
6. Miller WR, Rollnick S. Motivational interviewing: preparing people to change addictive behavior. New York: Guilford Press, 1991.
7. Ewing J. Detecting alcoholism: the CAGE questionnaire. JAMA 1984;252:1905–1907.
8. Bernadt M, Taylor C, Mumford J, et al. Comparison of questionnaire and laboratory tests in the detection of excessive drinking and alcoholism. Lancet 1982;1:325–328.
9. Wallace P, Cutler S, Haines A. Randomized controlled trial of general practitioner intervention in patients with excessive alcohol consumption. Brit Med J 1988;297:663–669.
10. Anderson P, Scott E. The effect of general practitioners' advice to heavy drinking men. Brit J Addict 1992;87:891–900.
11. Prochaska J, DiClemente C. Stages of change in the modification of problem behaviors. In: Hersen M, Eisler R, Miller P, eds. Progress in behavior modification. Sycamore, IL; Sycamore Press, 1992.

14. Exposure to Ultraviolet Light and the Prevention of Skin Disease

DORIAN LIZABETH GRAVENESE and STEVEN JONAS

EPIDEMIOLOGY

Excess exposure to the ultraviolet radiation of sunlight carries a significantly increased risk of skin cancer, as well as of photoaging. The American Cancer Society estimated that approximately 34,000 cases of malignant melanoma were diagnosed in 1995 (1). The incidence of melanoma approximately doubled during the 1980s (2). Melanoma is fatal in about 21% of cases, accounting for about 7000 deaths in 1995 (1).

Basal cell and squamous cell carcinoma, the nonmelanoma skin cancers, are the most common cancers in the United States. Their combined annual incidence is approximately 600,000 (1). Basal cell carcinoma, the most common human malignancy, accounts for about 75% of cases. Although these malignancies rarely metastasize and therefore have a low mortality rate, they have a high morbidity rate, resulting primarily from the significant disfigurement often associated with their removal.

Numerous environmental and extrinsic factors contribute to the development of basal and squamous cell carcinomas, but clearly the most prominent is long-term sunlight exposure (3). Both experimental and epidemiologic evidence indicates that ultraviolet B (UV-B) solar radiation is the major cause of nonmelanoma skin cancers and appears to be a significant (although not the only) risk factor for malignant melanoma as well. This association is supported by the clinical observation that most squamous and basal cell carcinomas occur on sun-exposed areas, such as the head, neck, and hands (4).

For nonmelanoma skin cancer, any excess sunlight exposure increases risk. In contrast, however, melanomas arise frequently on areas not usually exposed to the sun, raising questions about the role of sun exposure in the development of melanoma.

Epidemiologic studies have suggested that the development of melanoma is strongly related to intermittent and intense sun exposure (5–7), rather than to long-term, mild sun exposure. Furthermore, studies have linked the occurrence of blistering sunburns in childhood with increased melanoma risk later in life (8). A definitive answer to this question

303

has not been found (9). As of 1994, the American Academy of Dermatology held that the available evidence supported the view that sunlight is an important factor in subsequent melanoma development, but agreed that many unanswered questions remain regarding the role of other risk factors (10).

Melanoma primarily affects Caucasians with one or more of the following risk factors: (*a*) Family history of melanoma in a blood relative; (*b*) significant number of nevi, especially large atypical nevi (see later) or familial atypical mole syndrome (a nevus is a benign localized overgrowth in the skin of melanin-producing cells, usually appearing early in life); (*c*) family history of atypical nevi or familial atypical mole syndrome; (*d*) history of severe sunburn; (*e*) ease of burning and inability to tan; (*f*) fair complexion (with light hair and light colored eyes); (*g*) history of previous melanoma or nonmelanoma skin cancer.

EXPOSURE FACTORS

There is no such thing as a "healthy tan" resulting from ultraviolet light exposure. Furthermore, while sunburn increases the relative risk of skin cancer, many people mistakenly assume that they are only at risk if they burn; there is no single dose-response curve for ultraviolet exposure that affects everyone in the same way.

Ultraviolet rays from solar radiation range in wavelength from below 290 nm (nanometers) (UV-C), to 290–320 nm (UV-B), and 320–400 nm (UV-A). UV-A causes photoaging and immediate darkening of the skin after sun exposure. UV-B is the most important cause of redness and sunburn. It is also the predominant cause of skin cancer, although UV-A can potentiate the effects of UV-B.

Of the three categories, UV-C rays are the most carcinogenic. Fortunately, ozone in the stratosphere blocks UV-C (and partially blocks UV-B). However, ozone depletion in the Southern Hemisphere, a topic of global concern, has been accompanied by increasing amounts of UV-B and (potentially) UV-C reaching the earth's surface, especially in Australia and New Zealand (11, 12).

TYPES OF INTERVENTION

All patients should be counseled about the dangers of exposure to sunlight. There are two useful interventions to reduce one's risk of skin cancer. First and foremost is to limit unnecessary sun exposure by avoiding outdoor activity during midday, when UV-B radiation is at its highest. Second is to wear protective clothing, such as broad-brimmed hats and densely woven clothing, and to use sunscreen at all other times. Clinicians, especially primary care providers, should educate their patients about the harmful effects of the sun's ultraviolet radiation as part of routine health promotion counseling.

HISTORY TAKING AND COUNSELING

The first step in history taking is to identify the patient's pattern of exposure to ultraviolet light. A history of severe or frequent sunburns is a risk factor for the development of both melanoma and nonmelanoma skin cancer. While it is not clear whether cumulative sun exposure is a risk factor for melanoma, it is clearly a risk factor for nonmelanoma skin cancer. There is no standard means for quantifying cumulative sun exposure (e.g., the "pack-years" measure of cigarette smoking).

In assessing overall exposure, one should ask about weekend hobbies (for example, sailing, wind surfing, long-distance running or cycling, gardening, and, of course, sunbathing), occupations requiring sun exposure (farming, telephone line repair, outdoor construction), and a history of severe or frequent sunburns.

The clinician should also inquire about family history. A significant risk factor is the familial atypical/dysplastic nevi syndrome, characterized by the presence of more than 50 atypical nevi on the body, with at least one being more than 8 mm in diameter. Some think that the risk of cancer in persons with this history approaches 100% (13, 14). Atypical/dysplastic nevi have a variegated color, irregular or ill-defined borders, and an asymmetric shape. A family history of melanoma is also a risk factor. The most significant risk factor for melanoma is a family history of melanoma in combination with the atypical mole syndrome.

It is especially important to identify young adults who have a blood relative, especially a parent, sibling, or child, who either has had malignant melanoma or has an unusual number of large nevi. These patients require more intensive counseling, warning them against excessive exposure and especially against sunburn. Significant though less marked associations with melanoma risk have also been noted for individuals with an increased number of nevi (15).

Tanning bed usage for cosmetic purposes or light box ultraviolet therapy for psoriasis increases the risk of melanoma and nonmelanoma skin cancer. Commercial tanning salons generally use tanning beds and stalls emitting primarily UV-A, but some still combine UV-A and UV-B. Thus, tanning bed use can be considered a cancer risk factor and should be explored in the history. Patients should be discouraged from using tanning salons at any time, especially to provide a "primer" tan before going on sunny vacations.

Therapeutic radiation, either alone or in combination with ultraviolet radiation, is also a risk factor for skin cancer. In the past, therapeutic radiation was offered for some benign conditions, such as acne vulgaris and scalp infections.

Lifestyle Counseling and Care: Children

It has been estimated that at least 50% of the total lifetime sun exposure is received prior to age 18. Counseling for sun protection should therefore start in infancy with parental counseling. Health care providers should recommend that parents limit the child's sun exposure as much as possible in the first few years, especially by keeping children from playing outdoors during midday (10:00 AM–2:00 PM). Infants and young children should be provided with protective clothing (i.e. broad-brimmed hats, densely woven shirts), especially at early ages when frequent application of sunscreen may be logistically difficult.

If the child tolerates them, sun protection products can be used safely on children as young as six months of age. Specific features required for children are that the cream or spray be easily applied and waterproof (in this instance, defined as active for up to 80 minutes of continuous water exposure). The product should be applied 30 minutes before exposure to the sun. It is important to teach parents that, at the beach, hats, umbrellas, and even sitting in the shade are only partially protective, because water and sand can reflect significant amounts of ultraviolet radiation. Thus, sunscreen should be used even in those situations.

Lifestyle Counseling and Care: Adolescents and Adults

As is well-known to any clinician, it is particularly difficult to persuade teenagers and young adults to change their behaviors. This is especially true for sun exposure counseling. Photoaging and skin cancer are not concerns of the average adolescent. However, while few teenagers will be persuaded by counseling about cancer risk, some will respond to advice that curtailing sun exposure will prevent or at least diminish the photoaging process. Photoaged skin typically appears leathery, blotchy, and covered with brown spots (lentigines) and deep wrinkles. It is not a "natural" skin change but rather a direct result of excess ultraviolet exposure.

This photodamage occurs on sun-exposed areas and hence can be prevented by photoprotection. The best way to illustrate this phenomenon to patients, whether young or older, is to have them compare sun-protected surfaces (e.g., breasts, buttocks) to sun-exposed surfaces (e.g., chest, face, and shoulders). The difference in color and texture may convince even the most dubious of teenagers that sunlight causes undesirable changes in the skin, which will only become worse with accumulating sun exposure.

Many teenagers and adults use suntanning as an important cosmetic device. These patients may be convinced to use self-tanning creams or bronzing gels as substitutes. Because a tan may mask acneiform lesions, some adolescents use tanning and even burning as a substitute for medical treatment of acne. These patients should be encouraged to try traditional acne therapies and/or to consult with a dermatologist.

Older adult patients should also be counseled about sun avoidance and protection. See also Chapter 8 regarding the need for calcium and vitamin D in older adults.

PHYSICAL EXAMINATION FOR SKIN CANCER

Self-Examination

The best screen for both melanoma and nonmelanoma skin cancer is visual inspection. Early detection (secondary prevention) of skin cancer relies on examining skin on a regular basis. Except for high-risk patients, who should be seen periodically by a clinician, this can often be done by self-examination. Patients should know the basic features of the three main types of skin cancer. Many organizations offer visual and written learning aids to assist this teaching (see "Resources" section at the end of this chapter).

Skin self-examination recommendations are controversial, however, with some groups (e.g., U.S. Preventive Services Task Force) not recommending the practice (see Chapter 20). According to the Skin Cancer Foundation, self-examination should be done every 3 months, regardless of risk factors. Other authorities (e.g., American Cancer Society) recommend other frequencies. The Skin Cancer Foundation recommends that patients at high risk of melanoma, e.g., those with atypical nevi syndrome, be advised to undertake a self-examination monthly and be seen yearly by a clinician.

Clinician Examination

The physical examination of the skin is described in Chapter 3. The potential benefit of periodic examinations by a physician is illustrated by the fact that, for melanoma in situ (early melanoma in which the atypical melanocytes are confined to the epithelium), the long-term disease-free survival rate is 99%, whereas survival for thicker lesions is often poor. Direct evidence that physician screening reduces morbidity or mortality is currently lacking. Although the sensitivity and specificity of periodic skin examinations vary, both by type of observer and proportion of total body area examined, many melanomas are found by primary care physicians, nurses, and paraprofessionals, as well as by dermatologists.

The American Cancer Society currently recommends a physician examination of the skin every 3 years for people between age 20 and 40 and annually for those over age 40. The U.S. Preventive Services Task Force, on the other hand, found insufficient evidence to recommend for or against screening for skin cancer. In the initial encounter, primary care physicians should determine if the patient is at high risk (see previously) and whether to examine the skin completely.

Any patient with a suspicious lesion requires further evaluation by an appropriately trained physician and possible biopsy and histological examination of the lesion. A punch or excisional biopsy removing the lesion in its entirety is considered the standard of practice. Primary care clinicians who are unqualified to perform skin biopsies or to evaluate suspicious lesions should refer such patients to a dermatologist (see Chapter 17).

Melanoma

Melanoma can appear suddenly as a dark spot, either in or around a previous nevus or on normal skin. In patients with atypical nevus syndrome, both clinicians and patients may overlook a new, potentially malignant, lesion in the background of many unusual nevi. This is an important reason for regular follow-up of patients with multiple nevi. Familiarity with an individual's pattern of nevi will make changes more noticeable to both patient and clinician.

Changes in the size, pigmentation, border, and surface of any nevus are potential warning signs of a developing melanoma. These signs are often referred to as the "ABCDs" of melanoma (Fig. 14.1). "A" refers to *asymmetry* within the dark area. "B" indicates a *border* which is irregular, ragged, or blurred. "C" represents the *color* variation within a lesion. (Lesions with more than two tones should be regarded with suspicion.) "D," a *diameter* of more than 6 mm, should also raise concern.

Many of the features seen in melanoma are shared with their potential precursor lesion, the atypical or dysplastic nevus. Patients with benign nevi (small, homogeneous in color, with regular borders) should be made aware of changes that may indicate malignant transformation into melanoma.

Clinicians should not be confused by the seborrheic keratosis, a benign pigmented lesion which can mimic an atypical mole or malignant melanoma. It is a brown or black warty growth which, because of its deep pigmentation, can alarm both self-examiner and clinician. Its "stuck on" appearance is quite typical, as is its common presentation in clusters.

Basal and Squamous Cell Carcinoma

Basal and squamous cell carcinomas usually present on sun-exposed areas. Both appear as small, shiny bumps or as red, scaly patches (Fig. 14.2). Squamous cell carcinomas that develop on the lower lip have a higher like-

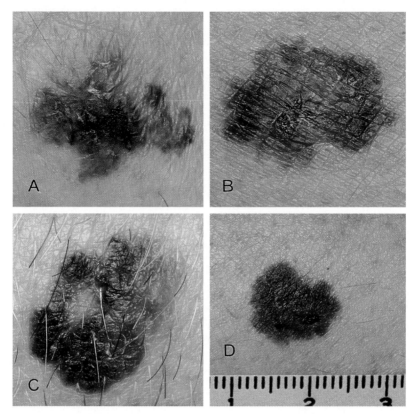

Figure 14.1. The ABCDs of melanoma: **A.** Asymmetry—one half unlike the other half. **B.** Border—irregular, scalloped, or poorly circumscribed border. **C.** Color—varied from one area to another: shades of tan and brown; black; sometimes white, red, or blue. **D.** Diameter—larger than 6 mm, the diameter of a pencil eraser. (Reprinted with permission from the American Academy of Dermatology.)

lihood of metastasis than those at other sites. Because of their frequent sun exposure, the ears, temple, and nose are also areas particularly vulnerable to the development of squamous cell carcinoma.

Another precancerous lesion, actinic keratosis, can often be detected on sun-exposed areas as well. Patients often interpret these scaly, rather innocuous appearing patches simply as dry skin. Nevertheless, they can develop into squamous cell carcinoma and require treatment. Recognition of actinic keratosis is also important to identify patients with actinic (solar) damage.

Follow-up

Patients at risk of developing skin cancer should be given relevant patient education materials (see "Resources" later in this chapter) and told what

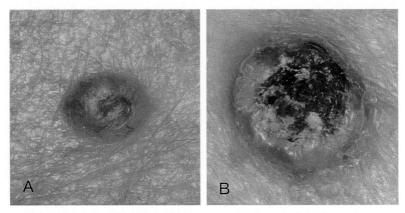

Figure 14.2. A. Basal cell carcinoma. This lesion does not metastasize but it can extend below the skin to the bone. **B.** Squamous cell carcinoma. This lesion can increase in size, developing into large masses, and it can metastasize. (Reprinted with permission from the American Academy of Dermatology.)

signs to look for when examining their skin. All patients with a prior history of malignant melanoma need close follow-up. The choice of interval is arbitrary but the recommendation of a National Institutes of Health Consensus Conference is a full skin examination every 6 months for the first 2 years, then yearly. Patients who have a history of nonmelanoma skin cancer should be followed every 6 months for the first 2 years, then yearly for 5 years to detect tumor recurrence at the treatment site or new skin cancers. See Chapter 17 for further information about follow-up.

SPECIFIC PREVENTIVE AND TREATMENT MEASURES

As already noted, it is important to minimize sun exposure (wearing tightly woven clothing and applying sunscreen) when engaging in outdoor activities. The consumer has many choices of sun protection oils and creams, with manufacturers ranging from top cosmetic houses to those supplying supermarkets. Patients can easily spend a great deal of money on sunscreens, but, if they carefully read labels for Sun Protection Factor (SPF) and substantivity ratings (concepts discussed later), they can protect their skin even if they are on a limited budget. There are two types of sunscreens: those that physically block the sun's rays from reaching the skin, and those that absorb light energy and change it to a form that is not damaging to the skin.

Physical Blocking Sunscreens

Physical blocking sunscreens (e.g., titanium dioxide, zinc oxide, red petrolatum) block and scatter up to 99% of light in both the visible and ultraviolet spectrums (290 nm–760 nm). These heavy, paste-like products are used primarily to augment the effects of light-absorbing sunscreens on especially vulnerable areas (ears, nose, lips, and shoulders). Being opaque, they are very effective as sun blocks. They are cosmetically unattractive, however, and their thickness can make them difficult to apply. However, recent developments in the production of titanium dioxide in a smaller particle size ("micronized") may in the future make physical sunscreens an effective alternative to chemical sunscreens.

Light-Absorbing Sunscreens

There are approximately 20 different light-absorbing sunscreens approved by the Food and Drug Administration. Each preparation has a characteristic absorption spectrum. The strength of a sunscreen is expressed as its SPF. The SPF is determined by exposing treated and untreated skin to ultraviolet radiation at the UV-B wavelength and measuring the length of time required to produce redness, the "minimal erythema dose." The SPF is the ratio of the time required (in minutes) for treated skin to become erythematous to the time required for untreated skin to become erythematous. If, for example, treated skin requires 100 minutes to become red and untreated skin requires 10 minutes, the SPF is 10.

Because the SPF is a ratio and not an absolute number, its value does not correlate linearly with the magnitude of its protective effect. An SPF of 15 protects against 93% of UV-B, while an SPF of 30 increases the blocking effect by only another 4%. This fact can be confusing to patients (as well as to practitioners who are unfamiliar with how SPF is calculated). The minimum protection level generally recommended by the American Academy of Dermatology and most dermatologists is an SPF of 15. Individuals with skin that burns easily and never tans may require higher SPFs.

Products with SPFs greater than 15 can be used, but the patient should be informed that they provide little additional protection. More important than a high SPF value is how well the product adheres to the skin (see later discussion). Also, SPF refers only to UV-B protection. There is no comparable scale for quantifying UV-A protection. (For "broad spectrum" sun protection products with a chemical composition that absorbs both UV-B and UV-A, the advertised SPF refers only to UV-B protection.)

Specific Protective Substances

Para-aminobenzoic acid, PABA, is one of the best known sunscreen agents. PABA compounds can cause contact dermatitis in some people—thus the focus on "PABA-free" products—and it binds well to the skin. To prevent a generalized allergic reaction, patients should be taught to test PABA-containing products on a small area of forearm skin before using them on their whole body. Taking this precaution is especially important for individuals with a history of itching or skin rash when wearing sunscreen. Cinnamates and salicylates have a range of protection similar to PABA and are often used as a substitute in PABA-free products.

Broad spectrum protection can be achieved by mixing different compounds in a sunscreen product. For example, benzophenones, commonly found in sun protection products, have a wide range of ultraviolet absorption capable of protecting against all three UV ranges. Parsol 1789 is a member of the newest class of sunscreen agents to be introduced in the United States, the dibenzoylmethane derivatives, and can block the entire UV wave band.

A third sunscreen characteristic of almost equal importance to the SPF and absorption spectrum is "substantivity," the product's ability to remain on the skin. Active individuals, for example, get little benefit from an SPF 30 product if it is not waterproof, because heavy perspiration or a wipe of a towel on sweaty skin will remove the product. Several labeling terms rate substantivity. "Water-resistant" products protect for up to 40 minutes of continuous water exposure, "waterproof" products for up to 80 minutes of continuous water exposure. These product characteristics are a function of both the chemical sunscreen itself and the vehicle base in which it is mixed.

"Self-Tanning" Substances

Self-tanning lotions and creams are generally considered a safe alternative to tanning from natural sunlight, tanning beds, or lamps. Self-tanning substances contain dihydroxyacetone (approved by the Food and Drug Administration), which binds to the epidermis and chemically produces a brown skin color resembling a sunlight-induced tan. It affects neither the melanocytes nor melanogenesis and is not dependent on ultraviolet light. Patients need to be reminded that sunless tanners do not increase melanin levels, and therefore do not provide the same UV protection as a natural tan.

Protective Clothing

Clothing may or may not be protective, depending on its characteristics. For example, the average, lightweight cotton T-shirt is only partially protective against sunlight. Densely woven clothing is sometimes suggested, because it does not allow significant ultraviolet penetration. New evidence suggests that certain tightly woven fabrics can provide exceptional protection from the sun, perhaps as much as a SPF 30 lotion. Such clothing may not be comfortable to wear on a warm summer's day, however.

MEDICAL RECORD DOCUMENTATION

Discussions with the patient regarding skin cancer prevention should be noted in the chart. Documentation of skin lesions can be done most accurately by using preprinted body diagrams that allow the clinician to specify the lesion location(s), with descriptive notations made in the margins. The size, shape, color, and texture of both suspicious and benign lesions can also be documented. See Chapter 3 for further details.

OFFICE AND CLINIC ORGANIZATION

Patient information pamphlcts and posters (such as those listed below under "Resources") can be placed in the waiting area, as well as in the examination room or nearby, so that the clinician can hand the patient literature for further reading. Such patient education material is informative, can prompt patients to ask questions about skin cancer prevention, and can help make the clinician's role in counseling interactive rather than didactic. Office and clinic organization for routine skin examinations is discussed in Chapter 3. Patient education materials for skin self-examination are listed in Chapter 20.

RESOURCES—PATIENT EDUCATION MATERIALS

American Academy of Dermatology
930 North Meacham Road
P.O. Box 4014
Schaumberg, IL 60169-4014
　　"Common Sense About Moles"; "The Sun and Your Skin"; "Sun Protection for Children: A Parent's Guide"; "Melanoma/Skin Cancer: You Can Recognize the Signs"; "Moles"; "Skin Cancer" (brochures).

American Academy of Family Physicians
8800 Ward Parkway
Kansas City, MO 64114-2797
800-944-0000
　　"Skin Cancer: Saving Your Skin from Sun Damage" (brochure 1527).

American Cancer Society
1599 Clifton Road, NE
Atlanta, GA 30329
800-227-2345, 404-320-3333
　　"Facts on Skin Cancer" (brochure 2049); "Fry Now, Pay Later" (brochure 2611); "Play it Safe . . . Beat Skin Cancer" (brochure 2675); "Why You Should Know about Melanoma" (brochure 2619).

Food and Drug Administration
Information and Outreach Staff
HFE-88, Room 16-63
5600 Fishers Lane
Rockville, MD 29857
301-443-3170
　　"The Darker Side of Indoor Tanning" (brochure FDA87-8272).

National Cancer Institute
Office of Cancer Communications
Building 31, Room 10A24
Bethesda, MD 20892
800-4-CANCER
   "What You Need to Know about Skin Cancer" (brochure 94-1563); "What You Need to
   Know about Moles and Dysplastic Nevi" (brochure 93-3133).

Skin Cancer Foundation
245 Fifth Avenue, Suite 2402
New York, NY 10016
   "ABCDs of Melanoma"; "Sunproofing Your Baby"; "Basal Cell Carcinoma: The Most
   Common Cancer"; "Squamous Cell Carcinoma: The Second Most Common Skin Can-
   cer"; "Simple Guidelines to Sun Protection" (brochures).

REFERENCES

1. Wingo PA, Tong T, Bolden S. Cancer statistics, 1995. CA 1995;45:8–30.
2. Koh HK. Cutaneous melanoma. N Engl J Med 1991;325:171–182.
3. Brash DE, Rudolph JA, Simon JA, et al. A role for sunlight in skin cancer. Proc Nat Acad
   of Sci USA 1991;88:10124–10128.
4. Miller SJ. Biology of basal cell carcinoma (Part I). J Am Acad Dermatol 1991;24:1–13.
5. Elwood JM. Melanoma and sunexposure: Contrasts between intermittent and chronic exposure. World Journal of Surgery 1992;16:157–165.
6. Anaise D, Steinitz K, BenHur N. Solar radiation: A possible etiologic factor in malignant
   melanoma in Israel. A retrospective study (1960–1972). CA 1978;42:299–304.
7. Gallagher RP, Elwood JM, Threlfall WJ, et al. Socioeconomic status sunlight exposure
   and risk of malignant melanoma. J Nat Cancer Inst 1987;79:647–652.
8. Zanetti R, Franceschi S, Rosso S, et al. Cutaneous melanoma and sunburns in childhood
   in a Southern European population. Eur J Cancer 1992;28A:1172.
9. Koh HK, Lew RA. Sunscreens and melanoma: Implications for prevention. J Nat Cancer
   Inst 1994;86:78–79.
10. American Academy of Dermatology. Sunscreens still essential to sun protection arsenal.
    Schaumberg, IL: News Release, Jan. 21, 1994.
11. Coldiron BM. Thinning of the ozone layer: Facts and consequences. J Am Acad Derma-
    tol 1992;27:653–662.
12. Environmental Protection Agency. Regulatory impact analysis: protection of stratos-
    pheric ozone. Washington, DC: Government Printing Office, 1988.
13. Rigel DS, Rivers JK, Kopf AW, et al. Dysplastic nevi: markers for increased risk for
    melanoma. CA 1989;63:386–389.
14. Albert LS, Rhodes AR, Sober AJ. Dysplastic melanocytic nevi and cutaneous melanoma:
    markers of increased melanoma risk for affected persons and blood relatives. J Am Acad
    Dermatol 1990;22:69–75.
15. Schneider JS, et al. Risk factors for melanoma incidence in prospective followup. Arch
    Dermatol 1994;130:1002–1007.

15. Oral Health

JOHN C. GREENE and ALAN R. GREENE

"If you don't have oral health, you're simply not healthy."
FORMER SURGEON GENERAL C. EVERETT KOOP, M.D. (1)

Oral health refers to the condition and adequate function of the soft and hard tissues that compose the mouth and contiguous structures. Of particular concern are the teeth, gingiva (gums), oral mucosa lining the mouth, tongue, salivary glands, oropharynx, mandible, maxilla, and temporomandibular joints. This chapter discusses risk factors and behaviors that increase the risk of abnormal development, impaired function, or pathology of these structures and what should be done about them. The interventions recommended for physicians or nurses are for the purpose of removing or mitigating these risk factors or for secondary prevention to avoid further damage. The recommendations in this chapter are generally consistent with those made by the U.S. Preventive Services Task Force and the Canadian Task Force on the Periodic Health Examination, although some preventive dentistry topics were not examined by either group.

TAKING AN ORAL HISTORY

When taking the patient's medical history, ask the patient (or the parent if the patient is a child) the following questions about oral health:

1. *"Who is your dentist?"*

2. *"When did you last visit a dentist?"* It should have been within the previous 12 months, beginning by age 2.

3. *"What did he or she do for you?"* It should have included an oral examination and treatment of any pathology, but it is important to learn whether the patient is receiving regular preventive care or only visiting episodically in response to pain or discomfort.

4. *"How often do you brush your teeth?"* Teeth should be brushed thoroughly at least daily, and preferably twice each day, with a dentifrice containing fluoride. Brushing should be accompanied by the use of dental floss to clean between the teeth.

5. *"Are you having any problems with your mouth, throat, or teeth?"* Ask appropriate follow-up questions if the answer is yes.

315

6. *"Do your gums bleed when you brush?"* Bleeding gums can indicate the presence of periodontal disease or possibly of systemic disease such as leukemia or a suppressed immune system.

7. *"Do you have trouble chewing your food?"* A properly functioning dentition is important for adequate nutrition.

8. *"Do you smoke, dip, or chew tobacco?"* Cigarette smoking can cause gingivitis and increases the risk of oral cancer, especially when combined with the use of alcohol. The use of smokeless tobacco (snuff or chew) increases the risk of oral cancer and gum recession.

9. *"Do you use sunscreen for your lips?"* Cancer of the lip is more common in persons with increased sun exposure.

10. *"Do you engage in contact sports or use skateboards?"* These activities are risk factors for traumatic injuries to the face, including the jaws and teeth.

11. *"Do you routinely use seat belts?"* Automobile accidents often result in facial and/or head injuries, especially to those who ride in the front seat without seat belts or use them improperly.

12. *"Do you have any sores or lumps in your mouth? Are you having any pain?"*

13. *"Do you engage, or have you ever engaged, in a lifestyle that might place you at risk of developing human immunodeficiency virus (HIV) infection?"* Some of the first signs of acquired immunodeficiency syndrome often appear in the mouth. HIV risk factors are discussed in more detail in Chapters 3, 4, and 12.

14. If the patient is a child, ask the parent: *"Is your child receiving fluoride supplements to prevent tooth decay? If so, how much?"*

15. *"Do you have any questions about your oral health?"*

CONDUCTING THE ORAL EXAMINATION

A good light and tongue blade are essential. Have the patient open his or her mouth. Evaluate the cleanliness of the teeth. The accumulation of soft material on the teeth (bacterial plaque) is a major risk factor for gingivitis, periodontitis, and dental caries. Look at all of the teeth and note any open carious lesions (holes in the teeth or broken fillings). Rampant tooth decay in young children may be a sign of baby bottle tooth decay (BBTD) or ad libitum breastfeeding. Early signs of BBTD or nursing caries can be detected by looking carefully for white-spot lesions along the gum line of the upper incisor teeth (Fig. 15.1). This scrutiny is critical because physicians and nurses are more likely to see infants and very young children than are dentists. Inspect the gingivae (gums) for signs of inflammation, bleeding, pus, or recession as possible signs of periodontal disease. Bad breath is often associated with periodontal disease. With advanced periodontal disease, sufficient supporting bone may have been lost to cause individual teeth to move easily when pressed with a tongue blade. Have the

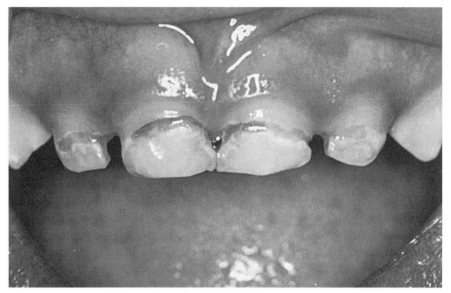

Figure 15.1. Early signs of baby bottle tooth decay or nursing caries. (Courtesy of Dr. Francisco Ramos-Gomez, San Francisco, CA.)

patient close the mouth, and with the tongue blade retract the cheek on one side and then the other. The upper and lower teeth should fit together snugly, with the maxillary teeth slightly overlapping the mandibular teeth.

As discussed in Chapter 3, the oral cavity examination should not be limited to the teeth and gums. With the mouth open, examine the mucous membrane lining the cheeks and lips, as well as the floor of the mouth and the palate. This tissue should be free from ulcers or white or red lesions. The examination should be especially thorough in patients reporting regular use of tobacco or alcohol. The dorsal, ventral, and lateral surfaces of the tongue should be inspected for ulceration, leukoplakia, or other deviations from normal.

If the patient is wearing a denture or any removable dental appliance, ask that it be removed so that the soft tissue underneath can be inspected. That tissue also should be free from inflammation, ulceration, or hypertrophy. This is especially important for edentulous persons because many do not receive an oral examination from a dentist on a regular basis.

PROFESSIONAL CARE

One of the most important components of counseling a patient regarding oral health is to encourage regular visits to a dentist. Patients can do several things to protect their own oral health, but there are additional measures that a dentist can take to prevent oral health problems and to intervene at early stages when problems do arise. *Advise patients to visit their dentist at least once every 12 months throughout life, beginning by two years of age.* The American Academy of Pediatrics recommends that the first dental visit should occur at age 3, whereas the American Academy of Pediatric Dentistry and American Dental Association recommend that infants should be seen by a dentist by at least 12 months of age (2). We recommend that the child be seen by a dentist by 24 months of age, primarily as a cost/benefit judgment. A major advantage of seeing the child before this age is for early detection of BBTD or nursing caries and for ensuring that the child is receiving proper fluoride coverage. Both of these matters, however, can be attended to by the pediatrician or family physician, who is more likely to see the patient at this early age and who can then refer to the dentist as necessary. The American Dental Association recommends that adults be examined annually. This annual schedule will need modification for persons with special risk factors, but recommending at least an annual dental visit is appropriate. The dentist will adjust the schedule to meet the patient's needs.

The patient may need prompt referral to a dentist, otolaryngologist, or oral surgeon if the oral examination reveals any of the following: inflamed or bleeding gums, white spot lesions along the gum line of the upper front teeth of young children, overtly decayed or loose teeth, ulceration of the tongue or oral mucous membranes, presence of leukoplakia or erythroplakia, lumps or swelling in the mouth, or other deviations from normal (see Chapter 17).

RISK FACTORS

Risk factors for developing oral health problems will be discussed separately for children and adolescents (persons from birth to age 18), for adults (age 19 to 65), and for older adults. Some of these risk factors are covered in other chapters, but their particular oral health implications are emphasized here.

Tobacco Use

Children

The use of smokeless tobacco (chewing tobacco and snuff) among young males in the United States has grown rapidly in the past two decades. An estimated 19% of school-aged boys (nearly 12 million) and almost 2% of school-aged girls currently use snuff (3). This practice is more common in rural than in urban settings. Some boys start using snuff by age 8 or 9. Most do so just because they want to be "one of the guys" or want to emulate the habits of a sports idol.

Physicians and nurses should remember that the use of tobacco in any form is harmful to health and should be avoided. *Advise young patients that long-term use of smokeless tobacco may lead to mouth or throat cancer—diseases with a very poor survival rate.* Several points may help reinforce this message. The U.S. Surgeon General's report estimates that the risk of mouth cancer is several times greater among smokeless tobacco users (4). Furthermore, it causes gum recession, which could lead to loss of teeth, it makes one's breath smell bad, and chewing and spitting is an unattractive habit. Moreover, the more smokeless tobacco is used and the stronger the brands, the greater the effects (5). Once a person starts the smokeless habit, it is very difficult to stop.

The use of smoking tobacco (cigarettes, cigars, pipes) also is harmful to oral health. The risk of gingivitis and periodontitis as well as of oral cancer is increased among smokers. Up to 70% of oropharyngeal cancers have been attributed to tobacco use (6).

All patients who report using tobacco in any form should be advised to quit because of the risks to oral and general health. Patients may need help in breaking the smokeless or the smoking tobacco habit. See Chapter 6 for further details.

Adults

In 1991 an estimated 5.3 million (3%) adults in the United States were current users of smokeless tobacco, including 4.8 million (6%) men and 553,000 (1%) women. For adult males, the prevalence of use was highest among those age 18 to 24 years (7).

The use of smoking or smokeless tobacco increases the risk of periodontal disease, leukoplakia, oral cancer, and other serious diseases. The longer the use, the greater the risk (see previous discussion under "Children"). Help in quitting should be given to those who desire assistance (see Chapter 6).

Older Adults

A 1991 study of smokeless tobacco use in the United States found that the prevalence rate in women was highest among those age 75 or older (7). Older adults who have used tobacco for a prolonged period have an even higher risk of experiencing the negative oral health effects of tobacco and should be urged to quit. See Chapter 6 for further discussion of cessation techniques.

Nutrition

Children

Fluoride Deficiency   The most cost-effective measure for preventing tooth decay is the use of fluoride in its various forms (8, 9). The most common natural sources of dietary fluoride are drinking water and foods. Children raised in areas with inadequate fluoride in the drinking water supply are at a greater risk of developing tooth decay.

Dental enamel that is formed without an adequate amount of fluoride is particularly susceptible to decalcification by acids produced by cariogenic bacteria. The crowns of permanent teeth in the human begin to calcify near, or just after the end of, the normal gestation period.

Fluoride that is ingested while tooth enamel is calcifying causes the enamel to develop a crystalline structure that is less susceptible to decalcification. On the other hand, too much fluoride ingested during enamel calcification can result in aesthetically undesirable dental fluorosis. Thus, as is discussed in Chapter 2, it is important to *ask the parents of newborn, pediatric, and adolescent children whether their water supply contains fluoride. Check with the local health department to verify the amount of fluoride in the drinking water in the area where patients reside.* The optimum concentration of fluoride in community drinking water is one part per million. *Ask parents if their children are ingesting other sources of fluoride, such as toothpaste, fluoride drops, or vitamins with fluoride. Fluoride supplements should be prescribed through the 14th year of age for patients who are receiving less than optimum amounts.* The proper supplemental amount will vary according to the patient's age and the amount of fluoride in the local water supply (Table 15.1) (10). Fluoride supplements, either by themselves or in combination with vitamins, should never be prescribed without confirming the fluoride content of the child's water supply. Supplemental fluoride should be in liquid form for young children and in tablet form when the child is old enough to use it.

Most dietary fluoride supplements are available as sodium fluoride (NaF) in which 2.2 mg of NaF provides 1 mg of fluoride. Fluoride supple-

Table 15.1
Supplemental Fluoride Dosage (mg/day)

Age of Child	Parts Per Million of Fluoride in Water Supply		
	Less than 0.3	0.3 to 0.6	Greater than 0.6
6 mo to 3 yr	0.25	0	0
3 to 6 yr	0.50	0.25	0
6 to 16 yr	1.0	0.50	0

Adapted from Cost effectiveness of caries prevention in dental public health. J Public Health Dentistry 1989; 49(5): Special Issue; ADA Council on Dental Therapeutics. New fluoride schedule adopted. ADA News, May 16, 1994.

ments are available in liquid form, with and without vitamins, and in chewable tablets. The liquid form of NaF is available in 0.125 mg, 0.25 mg, and 0.5 mg of fluoride per drop. Liquid preparations containing both fluoride and vitamins are available in concentrations that provide 0.25 mg/ml and 0.5 mg/ml of fluoride. Chewable fluoride tablets are available in 0.25 mg, 0.50 mg, and 1.0 mg fluoride doses. Chewable tablets should be chewed well and swished around the mouth to provide both topical and systemic effects. Scientific evidence suggests that chewable fluoride tablets or lozenges are more effective than other oral supplements (11).

The additional topical effect of fluoride in toothpaste should be introduced to the child between the ages of 2 and 3 years. Before age 6, only a pea-sized amount of fluoride toothpaste should be applied to the toothbrush each time, to avoid excessive ingestion of fluoride. Excess amounts of fluoride dentifrice should be wiped or rinsed out of the child's mouth to minimize ingestion.

Although fluoride is discussed here in regard to children's oral health, it is important for the prevention of tooth decay in persons of any age. Adults with dry mouth caused by disease or medications and those with gingival recession are particularly vulnerable to dental caries.

Improper Diet. The role of sucrose and other sugars in the colonization and metabolic activities of cariogenic bacteria in dental plaque has been well established (12). Children, whose newly erupted teeth are most vulnerable to decay, should therefore minimize their use of highly refined, sucrose-laden sweets. Noncaloric sweeteners such as saccharin, cyclamate, and aspartame are not metabolized to acid by oral microorganisms and thus are not cariogenic. From the standpoint of oral health, they are far superior to sucrose as a sweetener. The primary factors to emphasize in counseling children and their parents are the frequency of ingestion of sweets and the length of time the cariogenic substance remains in the mouth. *Advise patients to avoid between-meal snacks of candy or sugared foods, particularly those that tend to stick to the teeth.*

Infant Feeding Practices. Ad libitum breast or bottle feeding to pacify, rather than feed, the infant or frequent use of the bottle at bedtime may increase the risk of decay of primary teeth (13). Baby bottle tooth decay (BBTD) or nursing caries is a specific form of severe decay of the primary teeth in infants (Fig. 15.2). It usually affects the labial surfaces of maxillary incisor teeth, which otherwise are seldom affected by caries. The cavities first appear at the gum line as white, decalcified lesions. In advanced cases, the crowns of the four maxillary incisors may be completely destroyed, leaving decayed brownish-black stumps. The pattern of caries unique to BBTD appears to be caused by multiple factors, including the chronology of primary tooth eruption, the muscular pattern of infant sucking, vertical

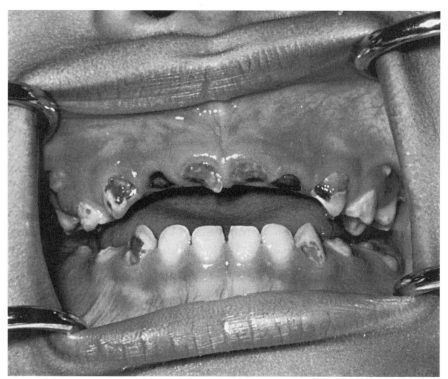

Figure 15.2. Baby bottle tooth decay or nursing caries, a specific form of severe decay of the primary teeth in infants. (Courtesy of Dr. Francisco Ramos-Gomez, San Francisco, CA.)

transmission of certain bacteria from the mother and the duration of the feeding and sucking habit. The maxillary incisors, being the first to erupt, are subjected to the cariogenic habit longest. Other teeth may become affected if the habit is continued beyond 18 months to age 2. The lower incisors, perhaps protected by the tongue during sucking and washed by saliva from the mandibular salivary glands, usually remain sound.

Given the dependence of cariogenic dental plaque on dietary sucrose levels, it is not surprising that many studies and case reports of children with BBTD found that table sugar or other cariogenic sweetening agents had been added to the nursing bottle contents. Nursing bottle liquids responsible for BBTD can include milk sweetened with sugar, sugared water, fruit juices, carbonated or noncarbonated beverages, and cow's milk. Milk-based baby formula, because of its lactose content, also is a potential promoter of BBTD. Some reports have indicated an association as well between the use of a sweetened pacifier and BBTD in preschool children.

The main strategy for preventing BBTD is to alert prospective parents and new parents about the condition and its causes. *Tell prospective parents that they can demonstrate love for their children without putting them to bed with a bottle or honey-dipped pacifier. Pay particular attention to parents who demonstrate a tendency to overindulge their children. If parents insist that a night bottle is necessary for the child to sleep, suggest that the bottle contain only water.* Baby bottle tooth decay can result from the child sleeping with a bottle containing anything but water. Weaning a child from a bedtime bottle can be an intense experience for three or four nights but, once the habit is broken, the child should be able to sleep normally. Cuddling with the child more than usual may help to ease the transition.

Adults

Just as for children and adolescents, it is important for adults to avoid highly refined carbohydrates to reduce the risk of tooth decay. Sweet foods that stick to tooth surfaces should especially be avoided. Frequent between-meal snacks containing sucrose are conducive to tooth decay. The frequency of eating sucrose-laden foods is more important than the quantity consumed. *Tell patients that, if they need frequent snacks, it is far better to eat fresh fruits or raw vegetables than processed sweets. If they do eat sweets, they should eat them with a meal and not as between-meal snacks.*

Older Adults

Frequent intake of sticky foods high in sucrose should be avoided by older adults who retain natural teeth, as well as by others. Older adults face the added risk of caries developing on root surfaces exposed by gum recession.

The exact role of diet and nutrition in other oral and dental diseases continues to be difficult to document. Malnutrition, in and of itself, does not cause gingivitis or periodontal disease; however, it can result in deterioration of host defense mechanisms, making a person more vulnerable to infections. In the well-nourished individual, mild gingivitis may remain in a chronic or static state for several years. But when the body becomes malnourished or debilitated, the infection may rapidly progress to fulminating periodontitis. HIV-infected individuals, especially those with significant immunosuppression, are susceptible to highly destructive and rapidly progressive forms of periodontal infection (14). Older adults who suffer from chronic illness, or who are receiving therapies that interfere with proper nutrition, are at increased risk of more rapid loss of tooth-supporting bone due to advancing periodontitis.

Injuries

Children

Unrestrained children involved in automobile accidents often sustain serious oral/facial injuries, and children and adolescents involved in certain sports and recreational events are at increased risk of trauma to the mouth, face, head, and neck (15). Injuries to the face can result in loss of teeth and broken jaws. The loss of teeth can be very significant. It may mean dealing with costly artificial replacements for the rest of one's life. Usually the teeth are lost in the most conspicuous location, the incisor area, which changes one's appearance. When an injury to the teeth or jaws does occur, immediate referral to or consultation with the patient's dentist is essential because the prognosis usually worsens with delay in treatment. Avulsed teeth should be kept moist in a cloth or in saliva for possible reimplantation.

Fortunately, athletic mouth protectors (mouth guards) greatly reduce the risk of dental injuries for those engaged in contact sports. They are required for organized football and should be encouraged for basketball, soccer, wrestling, skateboarding, and any sport where mouth injuries are a likely possibility. Stock mouth guards are available in sporting goods stores. Custom mouth guards that fit better can be prepared by a dentist. *Encourage and reinforce the active use of automobile seat belts, child restraints, and safety helmets to avoid head injuries.* See Chapter 10 for more details on injury prevention.

Adults

The same precautions outlined above for children and adolescents apply to adults engaged in contact sports and other activities that can produce severe head or facial injuries (e.g., driving or riding in automobiles, bicycling).

Other Oral Health Risk Factors

Children

Poor Oral Hygiene. To maintain a healthy oral environment and establish a pattern of daily oral care, oral hygiene measures should be established during the first years of life. *Tell parents they should assume primary responsibility for cleaning the newly erupted teeth of infants and toddlers until their children gain sufficient dexterity to do it on their own.* A clean washcloth may be used to wipe off the first few teeth, and a small soft bristle toothbrush should be used as soon as feasible. The preferable time is at bedtime, because salivary flow, a caries-protective mechanism, decreases at night.

By age 7, the child should begin to use dental floss, under the parent's supervision. *Parents should continue to monitor frequency and thoroughness of oral hygiene practices at least to age 12, or until the practice of brushing twice a day with fluoride toothpaste and the use of floss once a day are well established.* Numerous studies have demonstrated the beneficial effects of good oral hygiene on periodontal health (16, 17). Gingivitis, an early form of periodontal disease, is present in most children and adolescents and may be exacerbated during puberty. Periodontitis, a more advanced form of periodontal disease, is uncommon before adulthood. Some rare forms, however, can be serious during the teen years. For example, juvenile periodontitis can lead to rapid bone loss and loosening of teeth. Thus, it is very important for children and adolescents to use good home care practices to maintain healthy gingival support of their teeth into adulthood.

Occlusal Pits and Fissures. Pits and fissures on the chewing surfaces of permanent teeth are primary sites for caries in children, even in localities with optimally fluoridated drinking water. The single most effective measure for preventing pit and fissure decay is professionally applied dental sealants—plastic coatings applied to the chewing surfaces of posterior teeth to keep bacteria and food out of the pits and fissures. When correctly applied, sealants are essentially 100% effective in preventing cavities, as long as they remain intact (18). To be most effective, however, sealants must be applied early, soon after tooth eruption, and before cavities form. *Physicians and nurses can help in this regard, particularly with high-risk children—those who have grown up in areas without fluoride or who already have multiple cavities. In these cases, encourage parents to take the child to a dentist, not only for repair of diseased teeth, but also for the application of sealants to currently unaffected teeth.* The first permanent molars erupt at about age 6, and the pits and fissures of these teeth are primary targets for tooth decay. Thus, the eruption of these teeth signals the need to begin a sealant program. Sealants should be placed between the ages of 6–8 and 12–14 years (18).

Premature Tooth Loss. Loss of posterior primary teeth before the normal exfoliation time increases the risk of malocclusion or malalignment of permanent teeth at a later age. When a primary second molar is lost prematurely, the permanent first molar drifts forward into the open space, contributing to crowding later when more permanent teeth erupt. Generally speaking, the more primary teeth that are lost prematurely, the more likely that malocclusion will develop later.

Refer children with premature loss of primary teeth to a dentist for appropriate treatment. Space-maintaining appliances have proved to be very effective in preventing the drift of other teeth into spaces created by early loss of primary teeth.

Mouth Breathing. A regular, prolonged pattern of mouth breathing during periods of normal growth and development of the face may adversely affect the ultimate shape and size of the jaws, leading to dental malocclusion (19). The resulting change in facial form and occlusion is not due simply to air passing through the mouth, but to altered positioning of the tongue, jaws, lips, and other muscles of the head and neck.

When a regular pattern of mouth breathing is noted or suspected, the physician should examine the airway to determine the underlying cause and to make sure it is kept open during childhood and adolescence. In some cases it may be necessary to refer the patient to an orthodontist for facial growth monitoring.

Thumb Sucking. Estimates of the prevalence of thumb or digit sucking are wide ranging. Most children stop this behavior by age 3 to 4. Why some children adopt this habit and others do not is unclear, but it is clear that pressure habits such as sucking on a thumb or finger for several hours each day can and do move teeth. Generally, if such habits are discontinued before the permanent front teeth erupt, there is no lasting effect on their alignment. Lip pressure tends to help restore normal alignment when the habit is stopped. Therefore, thumb sucking should not be treated unless potential risks outweigh potential benefits. *Advise parents to be tolerant and not to intervene unless the habit continues after permanent teeth erupt or is associated with some other behavior problem.* Tolerance is the operative word until about age 4½ or 5; however, if the habit is continued beyond age 5 or 6, disfiguring malalignment can result. When treatment seems desirable, inform parents that there are a number of options such as special appliances fabricated by a dentist, Band-Aids, tape, or mittens. Perhaps the simplest and most effective treatment is a bitter-tasting liquid purchased at a pharmacy and applied to the thumb or finger for a few days.

Adults

Poor Oral Hygiene. There is a direct association between bacterial plaque accumulation on teeth and the presence and severity of periodontal diseases (15). The first manifestation usually appears as gingivitis, which, if not treated, usually progresses to involve tooth-supporting hard and soft tissue. The prevalence and severity of periodontal disease and tooth loss increase with age in any given population.

Advise patients that the best way to prevent development or progression of periodontal disease is with good daily oral hygiene practices and at least an annual oral prophylaxis by a dentist or dental hygienist. Thorough tooth brushing with a soft-bristled toothbrush and flossing at least once each day to remove bacterial plaque are essential for maintaining healthy tooth-supporting structures. Inevitably, however, some plaque remains undisturbed long enough to become calcified (calculus) and cannot be removed by a toothbrush or floss. For this reason it is important that teeth be cleaned professionally at least once every 12 months. Some people need to have their teeth cleaned as often as every three months because they form dental calculus so rapidly. The dentist can recommend the proper cleaning schedule for each patient.

Decreased Salivary Flow. Saliva provides natural cleansing and lubrication and assists with the body's immune and digestive functions. When it is absent or scant, patients may experience great discomfort, increased tooth decay, mucositis, difficulty in speaking and swallowing, and gingivitis. Reduced salivary flow can result from the use of a number of medications, chemotherapy, or head and neck radiation or surgery. *Advise patients scheduled to undergo any therapy that will significantly reduce salivary function to see their dentist first so that any existing problems can be treated and a plan developed to prevent problems that may occur from loss of salivary function.* Patients with xerostomia may use candies and mints to increase salivary flow. *Caution them to use sugarless products if they choose this way to increase moisture in their mouths.*

Lack of Regular Professional Care. One characteristic of oral health is that if one does not take care of it, matters only get worse. Lost bone support for teeth will not regenerate. Missing permanent teeth will not be replaced by growing another tooth. Moreover, most dental restorations deteriorate with time, and recurrent decay appears. Continued neglect often leads to increasingly complex problems with less satisfactory and more expensive solutions. *Again, encourage all patients to obtain dental care on a regular basis so that the dentist and hygienist can help prevent most of these problems.*

Older Adults

Although older adults in the United States are keeping their natural teeth longer today than in the past, many still experience oral problems. Primary and recurrent tooth decay and advancing periodontal diseases are major oral health problems of the elderly. These and other oral diseases experienced by older adults are preventable or controllable, yet many do not obtain needed care. Most people over age 60 today did not have the benefit of preventive dentistry when they were young, so getting them to appreciate its value at this stage of life is often difficult. The belief that losing one's teeth is an inevitable consequence of the aging process is still common among older adults. *Physicians and nurses can help correct this misconception by paying attention to the oral health status of older adults and encouraging them to obtain regular care from their dentists.*

Information gathered from the history and examination of the oral structures is especially important in this age group. Pay particular attention to causes of tooth loss, the ability to chew firm foods, medications being taken, and physical and emotional states that may affect the ability to carry out proper oral hygiene procedures.

Poor Oral Hygiene. Effective, frequent removal of dental plaque remains the basic and essential element of proper oral health home care for the older adult. Tooth brushing and flossing, the two primary approaches to plaque removal, require time and some dexterity, however. For older adults, they can be more difficult to perform, depending on the condition of the mouth and the degree of manual dexterity the individual retains.

For the person with gingival recession and exposed tooth root surfaces, daily plaque removal helps to prevent root caries and further gingival recession. The use of a soft toothbrush with light pressure will help to avoid abrasion or wearing away of the exposed root surface, which is much softer than dental enamel.

Dental floss is the basic method for removing plaque between the teeth where the brush cannot reach. Bacterial plaque readily forms on these surfaces, and periodontal pockets most commonly develop in these interproximal areas. Since periodontal pockets are most common in older adults, the daily use of dental floss is especially important in this age group. Usually, careful instruction and coaching by a dental hygienist or dentist are necessary to ensure proper use of the floss. Persons in this age cohort often use wooden toothpicks routinely after eating to remove food from between the teeth and around the gumline. This practice should be discouraged, as it increases the risk of trauma to the gums in those with limited dexterity. Such injuries can result in bacteremia, a condition to be avoided, especially in the elderly and the immunocompromised.

The clinician may be asked about the advisability of routine use of mouth rinses, another common practice in the elderly. If asked, the clinician should find out why the patient is using or wants to use the rinse. The practice of using rinses just to make the mouth feel better is of questionable value. The refreshing effect is short-lived, and use of the rinse may mask some serious underlying periodontal problems. There are several nonprescription fluoride mouth rinses on the market that may be useful in caries prevention. Also, there are therapeutic rinses that may be prescribed by the dentist, such as a fluoride rinse to help control root caries or a chlorhexidine rinse to control advanced periodontitis.

Personal oral hygiene practices and frequent cleanings to prevent gingival inflammation and periodontal disease are particularly important for persons with certain cardiovascular diseases or implanted joints, valves, and other body parts, because treatment of these oral problems can cause transient bacteremia that may seed heart valves and prostheses. Persons with heart murmurs and implanted prostheses and heart valves also require antibiotic prophylaxis before dental treatment of periodontal problems to prevent bacteremia and possible bacterial endocarditis (20).

The gingival tissues of patients with diabetes mellitus are unusually vulnerable to bacterial plaque. Decreased resistance to infection in combination with circulatory problems in these patients makes effective oral hygiene practices essential to maintaining oral health (21). There is evidence that indicates that oral infections are exacerbated in diabetic patients and that oral infections complicate glycemic control. Persons with diabetes mellitus often have increased gingival swelling, bleeding, and ultimately periodontal disease. Burning tongue, candidiasis, and lichen planus are also more common in diabetic patients.

Artificial Dentures. The wearing of dentures can contribute to numerous health problems of the oral soft tissues. Dentures are not intended to be worn continuously. *Patients should be instructed to remove their dentures before retiring for the night and to immerse them in a liquid to prevent drying and warping.* This allows time for relief of pressure on the soft tissue on which the denture rests. *Instruct denture wearers also to remove their dentures and clean and massage the tissues under the dentures at least once a day.* They may use a soft-bristled toothbrush for this purpose, followed by a vigorous rinsing with water. *They also need to be taught to clean their dentures at least once each day with a brush, rinse them thoroughly, and allow them to soak in a cleansing solution overnight.* The presence of plaque and calculus on dentures provides a breeding ground for bacteria and fungal organisms that can damage oral soft tissues. Also, accumulated food on dentures can cause offensive mouth odors.

Iatrogenic Factors. Of the nearly 30,000 patients each year who develop primary cancers of the head and neck and are treated with radiation, chemotherapy, or surgery, most experience serious oral complications. Chemotherapy of malignancies elsewhere in the body also can result in oral complications. These complications can be so debilitating as to severely limit the recovery process. Among them are dryness of the mouth, osteoradionecrosis of the mandible or maxilla, loss of taste, difficulty in chewing and swallowing food, severe inflammation of the oral mucosa, rampant dental caries, and severe weight loss.

Before a patient is subjected to cancer therapy, he or she should be under the care of a dentist and, preferably, all necessary dental treatment should be completed. Many of the oral complications of cancer therapies can be eliminated or greatly diminished with appropriate home and professional oral health care. Diminished salivary flow, a major risk factor for tooth decay in older adults, is also a possible side effect of many drugs. These include antihypertensives, anticonvulsants, antiparkinsonian drugs, antidepressants, and tranquilizers. *Physicians should make certain that patients undergoing prolonged use of medications that cause decreased salivary flow are under the regular care of a dentist.*

POTENTIAL ADVERSE EFFECTS

Excessive intake of fluoride by children during the tooth development years can result in unsightly aberrations in the formation and appearance of dental enamel. For this reason, it is very important to check the amount of fluoride occurring naturally in (or artificially added to) drinking water

Table 15.2
Recommendations of the American Association for World Health

Oral Health Problem	Description of Signs and Symptoms	Causes and Risk Factors	Prevention and Treatment
Abrasion/recession	• Gums receding • Root exposure • Sensitive root surfaces	• Excessive pressure when brushing • Use of stiff-bristled toothbrush	• Use soft-bristled toothbrush • Avoid excessive pressure when brushing
Congenital Anomalies	• Defects in newborns which include abnormalities of the lips, palate, face, and structure of the mouth	• Heredity (genetic) factors • Substance abuse during pregnancy (i.e., drugs and alcohol)	• Genetic counseling • Early detection by physicians at birth, for referral to teams of health care providers
Dental Caries (tooth decay) • Smooth surface caries • Occlusal (chewing) surface caries • Root surface caries • Baby-Bottle Tooth Decay	• Demineralization/remineralization of the tooth surface • White spot lesions (early stage) • Dark spot lesions (late stage) • Sensitivity to heat, cold, or pressure • Pain • Tooth loss	• Bacterial infection present • Improper eating practices • Frequent consumption of sweetened snacks and beverages • Inadequate use or access to fluorides • Reduced flow of saliva • Improper infant feeding practices	• Use fluorides • Assure community or school water fluoridation • Dental sealants • Proper personal oral hygiene • Xylitol chewing gum • Healthy dietary practices
Dry Mouth	• Decrease in saliva flow • Difficulty speaking, chewing, or swallowing • Burning mouth • Increased demineralization of tooth structure • Rampant tooth decay	• Medication • Diseases and other conditions • Cancer treatment (radiation and chemotherapy)	• Take frequent sips of water • Avoid drinks containing caffeine • Avoid tobacco and alcohol • Use toothpaste with fluoride and fluoride rinses • Ask health care provider about fluoride supplements • Ask dentist about use of pilocarpine • Use of artificial saliva

	Signs	Risk Factors	Prevention
Injuries	• Trauma to head, neck, face, mouth, gums, and teeth	• Vehicular (auto, bike, other) injuries • Sports injuries • Interpersonal violence • Occupational injuries • Unintentional injuries	• Use care seat belts • Use car child restraints • Use sports mouth guards • Use head and face protection devices • Detect and report injuries to appropriate professonals • Limit availability of guns and other weapons
Oral Cancers (mouth and pharynx)	• A mouth sore that fails to heal or bleeds easily • A lump, thickening, or soreness • Difficulty in chewing or swallowing • White, red, or dark patches • Hoarseness or sore throat that persists • Unexplained numbness or pain	• Tobacco use (smoking and spit) • Alcohol use • Unprotected exposure to sunlight (lip) • Age (especially over 40) • Occupational exposure (working with textiles, wood, leather, printing, asphalt, dyes, solvents, etc.) • Immune deficiencies • Poor nutrition	• Avoid use of tobacco products • Avoid alcohol intake • Limit recreational and occupational exposure to sunlight by wearing sunscreen and a hat • Seek regular oral cancer examinations • Self-check monthly for early warning signs
Periodontal Diseases • Disease of the soft and hard tissues around the teeth	• Bleeding, red, or swollen gums • Gums pulling away from teeth • Tenderness of gums • Pus discharge from around teeth • Bad breath or bad taste in the mouth • Loose permanent teeth	• Bacterial infection present • Other factors • Systemic diseases (diabetes) • Pregnancy • Medications • Improperly fitting fillings, bridges, and crowns • Use of cigarettes or spit tobacco • Poorly aligned teeth	• Remove plaque thoroughly by regular brushing and interdental cleaning • Seek regular dental exams/care • Avoid abrasion/recession by using soft bristle toothbrush. • Avoid excessive pressure when brushing • Self-check regularly for early warning signs • Use prescription therapeutic rinses

From Oral health for a healthy life: resource booklet for World Health Day, April 7, 1994. Washington, DC: American Association for World Health, 1994.

before prescribing fluoride supplements. As noted earlier, for the very young child who uses fluoride toothpaste, it is important to place only a very small (pea-sized) amount of the paste on the toothbrush and to make sure the child does not swallow the paste. Other adverse effects from preventive dentistry are uncommon.

CONTRAINDICATIONS

Fluoride supplementation is contraindicated in areas where the drinking water contains more than 0.6 parts per million fluoride (10, 11). Where bottled water is used, determining the need for fluoride supplementation is more complicated because bottled water contents are unregulated. These products may have little or no fluoride or they may have very high concentrations. Before prescribing fluoride supplements, find out whether bottled water is used for drinking and food preparation and then obtain a chemical assay of the water. Doing so is important to provide protection from tooth decay and, at the same time, to avoid causing unsightly dental fluorosis.

There is a growing practice among physicians in optimally fluoridated communities to prescribe fluoride supplements when parents report that their child does not drink water. *Rather than writing a prescription in such cases, urge the parent to encourage the child to drink water or juice that is reconstituted with tap water.* The use of optimally fluoridated community water, not a prescription, is the best answer.

OFFICE AND CLINIC ORGANIZATION

See Chapter 3 for details on equipment and facilities for performing routine oral cavity examinations. Educational materials about oral health can be placed in the waiting area for review by patients and parents before the examination. Brochures on specific topics (see "Resources" at the end of the chapter) should also be readily accessible to the clinician to hand to the patient or parent during counseling. A listing of local areas that lack adequate water fluoridation should be obtained from the public health department and kept readily available in the office, along with guidelines on fluoride dosing (Table 15.1). See Chapter 6 for recommendations on organizing an office or clinic to provide tobacco cessation counseling.

Certain special situations call for close collaboration and consultation with the patient's dentist. Examples are patients with such conditions as diabetes mellitus, Down's syndrome, congenital clefts of the lip and palate, ectodermal dysplasia, compromised immune system (such as acquired immunodeficiency syndrome or organ transplantation), or leukemia; patients receiving medications or radiation that decrease salivary flow; and patients presenting with acute dental problems that require prompt referral. The office should have access to the names of dental providers and clinics for patients who do not have a dentist and those who lack funds or insurance to pay for services.

MEDICAL RECORD DOCUMENTATION

The results of the history and physical examination of the oral cavity should be recorded in the medical record. When supplemental fluoride is prescribed, the details should be documented in the patient's record. Notations regarding the patient's last visit to the dentist can be monitored on a health maintenance flow sheet.

CONCLUSION

The American Association for World Health has published an oral health resource booklet that contains recommendations for prevention of oral problems (22). Their recommendations are consistent with those in this chapter, and are summarized in Table 15.2.

RESOURCES

American Dental Association
Division of Communications
211 East Chicago Avenue
Chicago, IL 60611-2678

> Brochures for patients: "Basic Brushing"; "Basic Flossing"; "Diet and Dental Health"; "Baby Bottle Tooth Decay"; "Facts About Fluoride"; "Keeping a Healthy Mouth: Tips for Older Adults." Professional materials can also be obtained from this resource.

Other community resources are the local dental or medical society and the local health department and water department. The faculty of a dental school, if conveniently located, is also an excellent resource.

REFERENCES

1. Oral Health 2000 News (vol.1, no. 1) (published by American Fund for Dental Health, Chicago).
2. Recommendations for preventive pediatric dental care. Chicago: American Academy of Pediatric Dentistry, May 1992.
3. U. S. Centers for Disease Control and Prevention. Tobacco use among high school students—United States, 1990. MMWR 1991;40:617–619.
4. The Advisory Committee to the Surgeon General on the health consequences of using smokeless tobacco: a report to the Surgeon General. NIH Publication No. 86-2874. Bethesda, MD: U.S. Department of Health and Human Services, Public Health Service, 1986.
5. Ernster VL, Grady DG, Greene JC, Walsh M, Robertson PB, Daniels T, Benowitz N, Siegel D, Gerbert B, Hauck W. Smokeless tobacco use and health effects among baseball players. JAMA 1990;264:218–224.
6. Cancers of the oral cavity and pharynx: A statistics review monograph, 1973–1987. NIH Publication No. 91-3191. Bethesda, MD: U.S. Department of Health and Human Services, 1990.

7. U.S. Centers for Disease Control and Prevention. Use of smokeless tobacco among adults—United States, 1991. MMWR 1993;42:263–266.
8. Greene JC, Louie R, Wycoff, SJ. Preventive dentistry I: dental caries. U.S. Preventive Services Task Force. JAMA 1989;262:3459–3463.
9. Cost effectiveness of caries prevention in dental public health. J Public Health Dentistry 1989;49(5): Special Issue.
10. American Dental Association Council on Dental Therapeutics. New fluoride schedule adopted. ADA News, May 16, 1994.
11. Riordan PJ. Fluoride supplements in caries prevention: a literature review and proposal for a new dosage schedule. J Public Health Dent 1993;53:174–189.
12. Newbrun E. Cariology, 22nd ed. Baltimore: Williams & Wilkins, 1993.
13. Ripa LW. Nursing caries: a comprehensive review. Pediatr Dent 1988;10:268–282.
14. Greenspan D, Greenspan J, Pindborg J, Schiot M. AIDS and the dental team. Copenhagen: Munksgaard, 1986.
15. Greene, JC, Louie R, Wycoff, SJ. Preventive dentistry II: periodontal diseases, malocclusion, trauma, and oral cancer. U.S. Preventive Services Task Force. JAMA 1990;263:421–425.
16. Horowitz AM, Suomi JD, Peterson JK, et al. Effects of supervised daily dental plaque removal by children after 3 years. Community Dent Oral Epidemiol 1980;8:171–176.
17. Lang NP, Cumming BK, Loe H. Toothbrushing frequency as it is related to plaque development and gingival health. J Periodontol 1973;44:398–405.
18. Llodra JC, Bravo M, Delgado-Rodriguez M, Baca P, Galvez R. Factors in influencing the effectiveness of sealants: a meta-analysis. Community Dent Oral Epidemiol 1993; 21:261–268.
19. Vargervik K, Harvold EP. Experiments on the interaction between orofacial function and morphology. Ear Nose Throat J 1987;66:201–208.
20. Dajani AS, Bisno AL, Chung KJ, et al. Prevention of bacterial endocarditis: recommendations by the American Heart Association. JAMA 1990;264:2919–2922.
21. Katz PP, Wirthlin MR Jr, Szpunar SM, Selby JV, Sepe SJ, Showstack JA. Epidemiology and prevention of periodontal disease in individuals with diabetes. Diabetes Care 1991;14:375–385.
22. Oral health for a healthy life: resource booklet for World Health Day, April 7, 1994. Washington, DC: American Association for World Health, 1994.

16. Functional Status and Mental Health

STEVEN H. WOOLF

INTRODUCTION

An intriguing question in health promotion is the true definition of *health*. In 1948, the World Health Organization defined health as "a state of complete physical, mental, and social well-being and not merely the absence of disease or infirmity" (1). Although this definition may appear utopian and unattainable for most people, it serves the useful purpose of emphasizing the interrelationship of social, psychological, and physical factors in determining health status. The recent trend in health policy is to return to this more holistic outlook, in which effective health interventions are defined by effects on quality of life rather than biophysical processes. Health-related quality of life is defined not only by the signs and symptoms of disease or its effects on survival, but by functional status, opportunity, and one's self-perception of relative well-being (2).

If this is true, then a comprehensive approach to disease prevention and health promotion must look beyond the prevention of organic disease (e.g., coronary artery disease, cancer) to examine broader measures for improving a patient's functional status and quality of life. Early detection and treatment of such problems as inability to maintain personal hygiene, purchase and prepare meals, or obtain satisfaction from life may accomplish more to improve a patient's overall well-being (and prevent disease) than dealing exclusively with "medical" problems. Although addressing some of these issues may be more in the realm of social workers and other mental health professionals than physicians, the effect of disease on functional status and the effect of functional status on the patient's medical care are clearly interrelated.

FUNCTIONAL STATUS

Functional status, the ability of individuals to perform age-appropriate tasks of self-care and self-fulfillment, is important at any age but is particularly critical among children, older adults, and those with medical disabilities. Impaired functional status during childhood is often associated with abnormal growth and development. Functional status among older adults and those with medical disorders can be impaired by the physical limitations related to disease and aging and by psychiatric factors (e.g., cognitive impairment). About 20% of older adults living in the community report difficulty in performing at least one of the basic activities of daily living (e.g., dressing, bathing, eating) (3). The inability of an individual to tend to hygiene and other personal needs, to manage household and financial responsibilities, and to pursue personal interests is a source of great anguish, embarrassment, frustration, and illness for many thousands of individuals in the United States. The rationale for early detection and treatment is that medical and social service interventions may prevent further deterioration in functional status and limit the duration of suffering experienced by these individuals.

Preventive interventions are possible for each of the three components of functional status: social, physical, and psychological function (1). Patients with impaired *social function* (e.g., limitations in usual roles, inadequate social contact and participation in the community, decreased intimacy and sexual function) can benefit from a broad range of social and community service programs. Patients with impaired *physical function*, such as decreased fitness or activity restrictions (e.g., decreased mobility, inadequate self-care, communication disorders), can benefit from interventions that range from traditional medical care to physical, occupational, and speech and language therapy; home health care; and assistive devices (e.g., hearing aids, wheelchairs). Patients with impaired *psychological function*, who are unable to enjoy life because of cognitive impairment (e.g., dementia) or affective disorders (e.g., depression), can benefit from a variety of services for themselves and their caregivers.

Early Detection

Although asking patients about personal living conditions is unnecessary during routine clinical interviews, it is appropriate to ask older adults and those suffering from chronic diseases whether they are able to perform the activities of daily living. The American College of Physicians and Society of General Internal Medicine recommend routine assessment of a patient's ability to perform daily tasks as part of the periodic health examination. A sample primary screening question is, *"Are you having any trouble taking care of things at home, like getting your meals or cleaning yourself?"* (see Chapter 2). If a problem is suspected, further questions about physical and social functional status should be asked. Sample questions are listed in Table 16.1, and more focused questions may be indicated depending on the patient's responses. A number of formal screening instruments are also available for assessing functional status. Examples include the Quality of Well-Being Scale, Instrumental Activities of Daily Living, Functional Activities Ques-

Table 16.1
Sample Questions for Assessing Physical and Social Functional Status

Physical Function

1. How far can you walk?
2. How many stairs can you climb?
3. Do you have difficulty standing up or sitting down?
4. Have people commented about your hearing or vision or have you noticed a change? (see Chapters 3–4)
5. Do you have difficulty getting out of bed or moving around your home?
6. Are you able to prepare and eat your meals?
7. Are you able to dress yourself?
8. Are you able to take a shower or bath, comb or brush your hair, and brush and floss your teeth?
9. Are you able to clean your home (e.g., dusting, cleaning floors, light housework)?
10. Are you able to drive a car or catch a bus, train, or taxi to run errands (e.g., shopping, banking)?

Social Function

1. Do you have a job?
2. Do you go to church or attend other social functions?
3. How often do you visit relatives or friends?
4. Do you have a telephone?
5. How often are you visited at home by family? friends? social workers?
6. Do you receive financial or other social services?
7. Have you recently retired, separated, or divorced?
8. Have there been any recent illnesses or deaths involving close friends or relatives?
9. Are you having problems with friends or relatives?
10. Have there been any other major changes in your life?

tionnaire, Nottingham Health Profile, McMaster Health Index Questionnaire, Index of Health-Related Quality of Life, and Medical Outcomes Study Framework of Health Indicators. See Chapters 2 and 17, respectively, for information about screening children for developmental delay and about what to do if a problem is suspected.

Treatment

Interventions to enhance functional status are generally directed toward the underlying problem. Physical dysfunction due to medical factors is addressed by treating the underlying disease, discontinuing medications that impair function, and providing ancillary care services. Potentially helpful services that are frequently overlooked include physical, occupational, recreational, and speech-language therapy; the prescription of walking aids; and other home health devices. Many aspects of social dysfunction can be addressed by public or private social service agencies. These services include arranging and financing home health care, food delivery services, transportation, and financial and legal assistance. Many communities offer activities and other structured programs for older adults and disabled persons. Clinicians should be prepared to provide patients with information about these services or the names and telephone numbers of appropriate contacts.

PSYCHOLOGICAL WELL-BEING

Following social and physical function, the third component of functional status is psychological well-being. Many individuals are unable to enjoy life because of mental illness or personality disorders, resulting in poor functional status for emotional or cognitive reasons. These patients can benefit from psychotherapeutic and social service interventions. Often, however, the disorders have an insidious onset and are difficult to detect until they progress to an advanced stage. Virtually every psychiatric and psychologic disorder can affect the quality of life, but this chapter focuses on four major causes of disordered psychological well-being that present commonly in the primary care setting and that may benefit from early treatment: poor self-esteem, anxiety, depression, and cognitive impairment.

In dealing with these disorders, most clinicians use an eclectic approach that incorporates different theoretical and treatment models as determined by the needs of the patient. Few clinicians outside the mental health professions are wedded to a particular treatment philosophy, such as Jungian, cognitive-behavioral, psychoanalytic, or rational-emotive therapy. They instead borrow concepts and techniques from various schools, based on the clinician's personal style and individual clinical circumstances, and rely on the recommendations of the mental health professionals whom they consult. A complete discussion of each of these approaches is beyond the scope of this chapter. The following discussion of self-esteem, which reflects one useful orientation to understanding the causes of emotional and behavioral disorders, is presented as an example and not to exclude other conceptual frameworks for understanding mental illness and emotional disorders.

Self-Esteem

Clinicians should concern themselves with a patient's self-esteem for several important reasons. First, poor self-esteem can lead to more severe psychological and emotional disorders, such as depression, substance abuse, and eating disorders. Second, poor self-esteem influences interpersonal relationships and may contribute to the patient's involvement in family dysfunction, marital discord, abuse, or other violent behavior. Third, patients with poor self-esteem and emotional distress often present with somatic complaints, such as headaches, fatigue, abdominal complaints, or chest pain. Understanding the role of emotions in producing these symptoms can avoid unnecessary diagnostic testing and help provide more appropriate treatment for the patient's problem.

Self-esteem exists naturally when individuals understand and value their true *self* (the genuine person, who exists independently of social roles and expectations) and live their lives according to their own agenda (self-actualization) rather than the agenda of others. Healthy self-esteem and the skills to live a self-actualized life are typically acquired during childhood, when the ability to understand and value one's identity is facilitated by wholesome parental nurturing and reassurance. Children who are criticized, shamed, or ignored and those who undergo physical or sexual abuse often emerge from childhood with weakened self-esteem and an overreliance on pleasing others. The mask, or *false self*, that children pull over their true identity to obtain parental and family acceptance is often reproduced in adult relationships with friends, relatives, lovers, and coworkers.

Individuals who depend on the acceptance and praise of others to gain self-worth can place inappropriate demands on spouses, other family members, and friends. Their difficulty in understanding the boundaries of the self often lie at the heart of marital conflicts, family dysfunction, and divorce. Those who depend on personal achievements and success to find self-worth may adopt a compulsive lifestyle to excel in work, body image, sex, or finances, often to the point of interfering with relationships and personal self-growth. Those who cannot acquire self-esteem through these measures or who become frustrated with the failure of others to give them self-esteem often express their anger by attacking others, sometimes through physically hostile acts or violent crime. Many turn to a false sense of emotional well-being through mind-altering experiences, such as intoxication with alcohol or other drugs, compulsive eating, or other addictive behaviors.

Growing disaffection with life can also produce somatic complaints. Traditionally, the somatic complaints of depressed persons have been viewed by physicians as manifestations of their mental state and not as true organic disease. This model, however, has been unable to explain fully certain conditions (e.g., fibromyalgia, chronic fatigue syndrome) that are common in depressed persons and are often accompanied by objective physical findings and laboratory abnormalities. Some view depression as a symptom of these chronic conditions, while other researchers are exploring whether the emotional states alter physiologic mechanisms (e.g., cellular immunity) to cause the disorders (4). The connection between mind and body, although a new concept in Western medicine, has been the centerpiece of highly effective treatment practices in China and other Eastern societies for centuries.

Some believe that poor self-esteem lies at the heart of many psychological, interpersonal, and physical complaints. It may represent the common pathway to such varied social problems as depression, family dysfunction, abuse, and violent crime. Its relevance to health promotion and disease prevention is that early recognition and treatment of poor self-esteem may reduce the patient's risk of developing or continuing to suffer from these problems. Improvements in self-esteem may also enable the patient to adopt health-promoting behaviors such as exercise, smoking cessation, or dietary fat reduction. The etiologic role of self-esteem in causing these problems is unproven, however, and no studies have demonstrated the effectiveness of early detection and treatment. Sections later in this chapter discuss how to detect and treat patients suffering from anxiety, depression, or impaired cognition. Chapters 10 and 13, respectively, discuss how to help patients who have become victims or perpetrators of abuse or who have begun to misuse alcohol or other drugs. A strategy aimed at enhancing self-esteem before these more advanced problems develop (or as a form of direct treatment once they occur) may offer a more rational and promising preventive strategy.

Early Detection

There is no scientific evidence to support routine screening for self-esteem, nor are there validated screening instruments or questions for detecting this problem. Nonetheless, because of the importance of this issue, the conscientious clinician should remain alert for signs of poor self-esteem in patients' descriptions of their lifestyle or in relation to somatic complaints. Intrapersonal clues that suggest an overreliance on the false self and a dissociation from the true self include excessive preoccupation with career, body appearance, sports, sex, personal or family prestige, or money; excessive unhappiness or anxiety about the loss of these life elements; and comments about personal inadequacy, unworthiness, or inability to identify one's true desires independent of others' expectations. Interpersonal clues include recurring complaints about the behavior of others; excessive concern about the expectations of others; frustration in not being recognized or appreciated; and a pattern of unfulfilling relationships with lovers, spouses, or friends. Somatic complaints in the absence of an obvious organic etiology may also provide important clues.

Treatment

Patients in whom poor self-esteem has been diagnosed or suspected should be encouraged to explore the underlying reasons for their diminished sense of self-worth, either through counseling or independent reading. Psychotherapy is the preferred approach, because it enables patients to clarify the diagnosis, to understand the full dimensions of the problem, and to receive encouragement and guidance as they adopt a new lifestyle aimed at self-actualization and the fulfillment of their own agenda. Taking these steps is often difficult and anxiety-provoking, and the support of the therapist is helpful in facing these fears and the resistance and anger that may be generated among family and friends as the patient's "people-pleasing" behavior is withdrawn. Excellent books on this subject, some of which are listed later in this chapter, can be helpful to both patients in counseling and those who are unable or unwilling to consider psychotherapy.

Anxiety

Like poor self-esteem, anxiety disorders are encountered commonly in the primary care setting and are often associated with somatic complaints that can distract the clinician's attention from the underlying emotional cause. The anxiety disorders include generalized anxiety disorder (excessive, habitual anxiety and worry for at least six months), panic disorder (frequent and sudden attacks of anxiety accompanied by specific physical symptoms), social phobia (persistent, irrational fear of embarrassment or humiliation), obsessive-compulsive disorder (recurrent intrusive and disabling thoughts accompanied by repetitive stereotypical behavior), and post-traumatic stress disorder (a specific behavioral syndrome that occurs following exposure to a traumatic stressor). Detailed diagnostic criteria for each of these disorders are provided in the *Diagnostic and Statistical Manual of Mental Disorders* (DSM-IV) (5). Together, these disorders occur commonly in the population, with an estimated prevalence of 15%.

Early Detection

Most persons with anxiety disorders do not identify anxiety or stress as their chief complaint but instead draw attention to somatic complaints. The typical symptoms associated with anxiety disorders include chest pain, hyperventilation, tachycardia, palpitations, abdominal pain or cramping, and diarrhea. There is little evidence to support routine screening for anxiety disorders in patients with these complaints (which, strictly speaking, falls outside the definition of screening) or the asymptomatic general population. Although diagnostic instruments, such as the Hamilton Anxiety Rating Scale (6), have been developed, none has been properly validated for routine use as a screening test. Indirect evidence suggests that treatment of stress and anxiety may be effective in improving health outcomes. For example, studies suggest that stress reduction, along with intensive cardiac risk factor modification, may decelerate or reverse the process of atherosclerosis (7). Similarly, the relationship between stress and myocardial infarction, gastrointestinal disease, panic disorder, and other conditions is being explored.

Treatment

Medications and talk therapy are the mainstays of treatment for anxiety disorders. Commonly used pharmacologic agents include benzodiazepines, tricyclic antidepressants, monoamine oxidase inhibitors, beta-blocker agents, centrally acting agents, selective serotonin reuptake inhibitors, and other agents (e.g., buspirone). Appropriate medications vary for different types of anxiety disorders. For example, some patients with panic disorder are most effectively treated with tricyclic antidepressants rather than with anxiolytic agents. Available agents also vary in terms of potential side effects and risks of dependency, and they therefore need to be selected based on the individual circumstances of each patient.

Psychotherapy to develop coping skills and insights to deal with anxiety represents an important adjunct or alternative to pharmacologic therapy, especially when patients experience, or are at risk for, side effects from medication. Typical providers include psychiatrists, psychologists, social workers, family therapists, and psychiatric nurses. Supportive, cognitive, behavioral, or combined psychotherapy are commonly useful in treating anxiety disorders. Psychotherapy has been shown in some studies to be at least as effective in treating panic disorder as pharmacologic therapy (8).

Depression

Primary mood disorders include unipolar and bipolar conditions. Unipolar conditions include major depression, dysthymia, and depression not otherwise specified (DNOS). Bipolar conditions include bipolar disorder (e.g., manic-depressive disorder) and cyclothymia. About 7–12% of men and 20–25% of women experience major depression at some time in their lives, whereas dysthymia is experienced by 2% and 4%, respectively. About 1% of the population experiences bipolar disorders. Studies suggest that about 5–9% of patients seen in ambulatory primary care settings are suffering from major depression and 8–10% are suffering from DNOS, although both problems are often overlooked. A large survey suggested that 21% of persons visiting primary care physicians are depressed, although only 1% cited depression as the reason for their visits (9). The consequences of untreated depression include severe emotional anguish, the disruption of job performance and family dynamics, the exacerbation of concurrent medical illnesses, and suicide. The risk of suicide is eight times greater in depressed persons than in the general population. Up to 15% of untreated bipolar patients or depressed persons requiring hospitalization eventually commit suicide (10).

Early Detection

Depression should be considered in all patients with a sad mood or low interest in life, but these symptoms are frequently absent, masked, or nonspecific in depressed persons. Often the only presentation is the patient's somatic complaints, such as fatigue, headache, abdominal pain, body aches, and decreased sexual performance. Other risk factors for depression include age under 40 years, prior history of depression, family history of major depressive or bipolar disorder, personal or family history of suicide, concurrent medical illness, substance abuse, and stressful life events.

Table 16.2 lists the diagnostic criteria for major depressive disorder. To meet these criteria, (*a*) the symptoms must be present during the same time period, (*b*) at least one of the first two symptoms must be present, (*c*) symptoms must be present most of the day, nearly daily, for at least two weeks, (*d*) symptoms must cause clinically significant distress or functional impairment, (*e*) symptoms must not be due to direct physiological effects of a substance or medical condition, and (*f*) symptoms must not represent a normal grief reaction (e.g., death of a loved one) or a mixed episode. Some anxiety disorders can also present with depressive symptoms. Screening questionnaires completed by the patient or clinician may help assess the likelihood of depression. Commonly used questionnaires include the General Health Questionnaire, the Center for Epidemiological Studies Depression Scale, the Beck Depression Inventory, and the Zung Self-Rating Depression Scale (see Chapter 2 and Table 2.2).

If depression is suspected or confirmed, the clinician should ask the patient about suicidal ideation and prior history of suicide attempts. If the risk of suicide appears to be significant, the patient should be referred to a mental health specialist and/or be hospitalized. Patients at increased risk have a stated desire to commit suicide, a clear plan of action, a means of

Table 16.2
Diagnostic Criteria for Major Depressive Episode

At least five of the following symptoms must be present:
• Depressed mood most of the day;
• Markedly diminished interest or pleasure in all or almost all activities;
• Significant weight loss when not dieting, weight gain (e.g., a change of more than 5% of body weight in a month), or decrease or increase in appetite;
• Insomnia or hypersomnia;
• Psychomotor agitation or retardation;
• Fatigue or loss of energy;
• Feelings of worthlessness or excessive, inappropriate guilt;
• Diminished ability to think or concentrate, or indecisiveness;
• Recurrent thoughts of death, recurrent suicidal ideation without a specific plan, a suicide attempt, or a specific plan for committing suicide.

Adapted from Diagnostic and statistical manual of mental disorders, 4th ed. Washington, DC: American Psychiatric Association, 1994.

committing suicide (e.g., owning a firearm), poor support structures, and ill-defined plans for the future. See Chapter 10 for further details about suicide.

Treatment

About 10–15% of major depressive disorders are associated with concurrent medical disorders (e.g., hypothyroidism), medications, or substance abuse. A targeted history, physical, and laboratory examination may be helpful in detecting these causes. If medical causes of depression are diagnosed, treatment of the underlying problems should be emphasized among the first steps in therapy. If the mood disorder persists, treatment with medication and/or psychotherapy should be considered. Treatment of depression usually begins with an acute phase of care (6–12 weeks), which is followed by continuation treatment (4–9 months), during which medication is continued at the full dosage and psychotherapy may be continued, followed by maintenance treatment.

Antidepressant Medication. Studies suggest that over 50% of depressed outpatients who are treated with antidepressant medication experience marked improvement in or complete remission of their depressive symptoms. Potential indications for prescribing antidepressants include incomplete response to psychotherapy, unwillingness or inability to undergo psychotherapy, severe or chronic symptoms, melancholy, prior positive response to medication, family history of depression, or psychotic features. Classes of antidepressant medications include tricyclic and heterocyclic agents, selective serotonin-reuptake inhibitors, and monoamine oxidase inhibitors. Dosages and principal side effects of commonly used agents are listed in Table 16.3. Most studies have found that primary care physicians often fail to prescribe antidepressant medication to patients who would benefit from these agents, prompting several national campaigns to educate providers about the indications for pharmacologic treatment.

Psychotherapy. Psychotherapy can be helpful in treating mild to moderate depression. Commonly used techniques include family, marital, interpersonal, cognitive, behavioral, psychodynamic, psychoanalytic, and rational-emotive therapies. Typical providers include psychiatrists, psychologists, social workers, family therapists, and psychiatric nurses. Considerations for using psychotherapy without antidepressant medication include mild depression, less chronic or disabling depression, absence of psychotic symptoms, prior response to psychotherapy, prior failure of medication, chronic psychosocial problems, and contraindications to medications. Some studies suggest that combined psychotherapy and antidepressant medications may act synergistically in controlling the symptoms of depression.

Table 16.3
Common Antidepressant Medications

Drug	Therapeutic Dosage Range (mg/day)	Average (Range) of Elimination Half-Life (Hours)	Drowsiness	Orthostatic Hypotension	Anticholinergic Effects[a]
Tricyclic Antidepressants					
Amitriptyline (Elavil, Endep)	75–300	24 (16–46)	4+[b]	4+	4+
Desipramine (Norpramin, Pertofrane)	75–300	18 (12–50)	1+	2+	1+
Doxepin (Adapin, Sinequan)	75–300	17 (10–47)	4+	2+	3+
Imipramine (Janimine, Tofranil)	75–300	22 (12–34)	3+	4+	3+
Nortriptyline (Aventyl, Pamelor)	40–200	26 (18–88)	1+	2+	1+
Protriptyline (Vivactil)	20–60	76 (54–124)	1+	2+	2+
Trimipramine (Surmontil)	75–300	12 (8–30)	4+	2+	1+
Heterocyclic Antidepressants					
Amoxapine (Asendin)	100–600	10 (8–14)	2+	2+	2+
Bupropion (Wellbutrin)	225–450	14 (8–24)	0	0	0
Maprotiline (Ludiomil)	100–225	43 (27–58)	4+	0	2+
Trazodone (Desyrel)	150–600	8 (4–14)	4+	0	0
Selective Serotonin Reuptake Inhibitors					
Fluoxetine (Prozac)	10–40	168 (72–360)	0	0	0
Paroxetine (Paxil)	20–50	24 (3–65)	0	0	0
Sertraline (Zoloft)	50–150	24 (10–30)	0	0	0
Venlafaxine (Effexor)	75–225	5–11 (3–13)	0	0	0
Monoamine Oxidase Inhibitors					
Isocarboxazid (Marplan)	30–50	Unknown	1+	2+	1+
Phenelzine (Nardil)	45–90	2 (1.5–4.0)	1+	2+	1+
Tranylcypromine (Parnate)	20–60	2 (1.5–3.0)	1+	2+	1+

From (with subsequent updating) Depression in primary care: volume II. Treatment of major depression (AHCPR Publication No. 93-0551). Rockville, MD: Agency for Health Care Policy and Research, 1993.

[a]Dry mouth, blurred vision, urinary hesitancy, constipation.

[b]0 = absent or rare, 2+ = in between, 4+ = relatively common.

Other Treatments for Depression

Other pharmaceutical agents (e.g., lithium), electroconvulsive therapy, and other interventions are indicated in some depressed persons. The use of these agents is beyond the scope of this book and should be pursued in consultation with a psychiatrist.

Recommendations of Other Groups

Routine depression screening is not recommended by the Canadian Task Force on the Periodic Health Examination or the U.S. Preventive Services Task Force. An expert panel of the Agency for Health Care Policy and Research recommended that providers maintain a high index of suspicion for depression, a recommendation that is supported by most other groups. The American Academy of Pediatrics and American Medical Association recommend routine behavioral assessment and asking about suicidal ideation throughout childhood and adolescence.

Cognitive Impairment

A common cause of poor functional status among older persons is cognitive impairment, or dementia, which occurs in 5–10% of persons over age 65. Although about one-half to two-thirds of cases are caused by Alzheimer's disease, the differential diagnosis also includes multi-infarct dementia, alcoholic dementia, Parkinson's disease, Creutzfeldt-Jakob disease, and Niemann-Pick disease. In about 8–11% of cases, the causes are potentially reversible (e.g., thyroid disorders, hypoglycemia, acid-base disturbance, electrolyte abnormalities). Alzheimer's disease is characterized by progressive memory disturbance, wandering, agitation, hallucinations, paranoia, and inability to perform the activities of daily living. With an estimated four million Americans suffering from this disease (11), its impact on patients, families, and society is enormous. The rationale for early detection and treatment is that some forms of cognitive impairment are reversible or partially treatable with supportive care and medications. Such measures may reduce the duration and severity of suffering experienced by patients and caregivers, but direct evidence of these outcomes is limited.

Early Detection

There is insufficient evidence to recommend routine screening for cognitive impairment, but clinicians should remain alert for this diagnosis in their older patients. Recommendations to this effect have been issued by the U.S. Preventive Services Task Force and the Canadian Task Force on the Periodic Health Examination. Clues are often apparent in the patient's behavior in the office or in their inability to understand instructions, but perhaps the most useful information comes from family members, friends, and caregivers, who may report increasing episodes of memory loss, confusion, wandering, agitation, or paranoia. Screening questionnaires that can be useful in this setting, such as the Mini-Mental State Exam, are discussed later in this chapter and in Chapter 2.

Table 16.4 lists the diagnostic criteria for dementia. The mainstay for making the diagnosis is a complete mental status examination. This typically includes an assessment of the patient's appearance, interpersonal interactions, orientation, appropriateness of behavior, affect, mood, language, attention and concentration, short-term and long-term memory, ability to perform calculations and abstractions, ability to reproduce geometric figures, thought content, sensory perception, social and moral judgment, and impulse control. Standardized scales for assessing cognitive impairment include the Mini-Mental State Examination (see Table 2.6), Blessed Rating Scale, Short Portable Mental Status Questionnaire, Mattis Dementia Rating Scale, Brief Cognitive Rating Scale, Alzheimer's Disease Assessment Scale, Global Deterioration Scale, Functional Dementia Scale, and Clinical Dementia Rating.

Other causes of dementia need to be excluded. Dementia caused by depression, subdural hematoma, brain tumor, and infectious causes is more likely to have an acute and/or recent onset. A metabolic or toxic etiology should be considered when delirium is present. Common metabolic causes of cognitive impairment include hypothyroidism, hypoglycemia, hypercalcemia, Cushing's disease, hyponatremia, hyperosmolar states, metabolic acidosis or alkalosis, hepatic encephalopathy, uremia, nutritional deficiencies (e.g., thiamine or vitamin B_{12} deficiency), and anemia. Drugs that can cause cognitive impairment (e.g., phenothiazines, barbiturates, benzodiazepines, insulin, sulfonylureas, diuretics) should also be considered. Simple causes such as fecal impaction should not be overlooked. The correct diagnosis is determined by a careful history and physical examination, supplemented by selected laboratory tests (e.g., complete

Table 16.4
Diagnostic Criteria for Alzheimer's Dementia

- Multiple cognitive deficits that are manifested by both memory impairment and one or more of the following cognitive disturbances: aphasia, apraxia, agnosia, disturbance in executive functioning (i.e., planning, organizing, abstracting).
- Cognitive defects that cause significant impairment in social or occupational functioning and represent a significant decline from previous level of functioning.
- Course is characterized by gradual onset and continuing decline.
- Cognitive deficits are not due to other central nervous system conditions that cause progressive deficits in memory and cognition (e.g., cerebrovascular disease, Parkinson's disease, Huntington's disease, subdural hematoma, normal pressure hydrocephalus, brain tumor), systemic conditions that cause dementia (e.g., hypothyroidism, vitamin B_{12} or folic acid deficiency, niacin deficiency, hypercalcemia, neurosyphilis, human immunodeficiency virus infection), or substance-induced conditions.
- Cognitive deficits do not occur exclusively during the course of a delirium.
- Disturbance is not better accounted for by another Axis I disorder (e.g., major depressive disorder, schizophrenia).

Adapted from Diagnostic and statistical manual of mental disorders, 4th ed. Washington, DC: American Psychiatric Association, 1994.

blood count, chemistry panel, thyroid function tests, serologic testing for syphilis, vitamin B_{12} and folate levels, urinalysis, chest radiograph, electrocardiogram, computed tomography or magnetic resonance imaging of the head).

Treatment

The treatment of reversible causes of cognitive impairment is directed toward the underlying cause (e.g., thyroid hormone replacement, discontinuation of medication, evacuation of subdural hematoma). For Alzheimer's dementia, treatment consists of supportive care, treatment of behavioral symptoms, and treatment to preserve memory and cognitive function.

Supportive Care. The objective of supportive care for the patient with Alzheimer's disease is to maximize physical, mental, and social activity in a safe environment. Fundamental safety issues relate to whether the patient should live independently, with family, in an assisted living setting, or in a nursing home and whether safe driving is possible. In each of these settings, environmental interventions are often necessary to enhance safety, such as preventing accidental wandering outside the home and measures to prevent falls and burns (see Chapter 10). Proper personal hygiene, nutrition, and exercise should be ensured. Consistent daily routines and surroundings enhance the patient's sense of stability. Stimulation and orientation can be enhanced by arranging for attractive and colorful surroundings; large clocks, calendars, and familiar photographs; visits by family, friends, children, and pets; individual and group therapy; open space for free movement; daily walks; and structured social events. The patient may benefit from participation in activities in which failure is unlikely (e.g., reminiscing, listening to music, watching television). The use of traditional restraints or drug therapy should be minimized by using pillows, reclining chairs, wedge cushions, pads, and mittens.

Family members and other caregivers experience substantial stress in caring for patients with Alzheimer's disease. The clinician should therefore devote time to family education and counseling to help caregivers cope with emotional, logistical, or medical problems. The clinician should also refer patients to local self-help and support groups, lectures, and other community resources for families of patients with Alzheimer's disease (see "Resources" section later in this chapter). Some caregivers may require more intensive clinical interventions or psychotherapy. Stresses associated with medical decisions about terminal care can be reduced by arranging advance directives and durable power of attorney before the patient's cognition is severely impaired. Legal, economic, and social services are available in most communities to help families cope with special problems related to case management and with arranging specialized services such as home nursing or physical therapy. Clinicians should have access to information about local area agencies on aging, adult day care and respite care centers, and nursing homes with specialized units for patients with Alzheimer's disease.

Treatment of Behavioral Symptoms. Dementia is often accompanied by depression, and appropriate antidepressant medications should be prescribed in selected patients (see earlier discussion of depression). Agents should be selected to minimize anticholinergic effects on cognition and to decrease the risk of falls. Many patients suffering from dementia experience agitation, delusions, or hallucinations. Neuroleptic agents (e.g., haloperidol) can be helpful in some patients with severe agitation, hallucinations, or paranoia but, because of their effects on cognition and orthostatic hypotension, should be avoided or used in low doses to control mild behavioral symptoms, such as restlessness and uncooperativeness. Short courses of short-acting benzodiazepines (e.g., oxazepam, lorazepam, temazepam) and other agents listed earlier in this chapter (see "Anxiety") may be helpful in treating mild behavioral symptoms but may also affect cognition.

Treatment of Cognition. Vasodilators (e.g., ergoloid mesylates, nimodipine) have been used in an attempt to improve cognition, but studies of effectiveness have produced mixed results. Cholinesterase inhibitors, such as physostigmine, have proven effective in improving short-term memory. One recently approved agent, tacrine hydrochloride, was shown in some studies to improve cognitive test scores at doses of 40–160 mg/day for 6–8 weeks, but a significant improvement in functional status was not demonstrated (12, 13). Other similar agents (e.g., velnacrine maleate) are currently under study.

OFFICE AND CLINIC ORGANIZATION

The office or clinic interested in screening for impaired functional status, depression, or dementia should maintain a supply of appropriate screening instrument forms. Patient education materials on relevant mental health topics (see "Resources" section of this chapter) should be easily accessible so that the clinician can hand them to the patient, family member, or caregiver as part of counseling. The office should maintain a listing of community resources for patients with impaired functional status, including relevant social service agencies; physical, occupational, and speech-language therapists; and home health and respite care services. Referral arrangements for mental health professionals offering a variety of psychotherapeutic methods should be available.

RESOURCES—PATIENT EDUCATION MATERIALS

Anxiety

American Academy of Family Physicians
8880 Ward Parkway
Kansas City, MO 64114-2797
800-944-0000
   "Anxiety" (brochure 1559); "Stress" (brochure 1513).

Krames Communications
1100 Grundy Lane
San Bruno, CA 94066-3030
800-333-3032
   "A Guide to Managing Stress" (brochure 1108); "Couple Troubles" (1244); "Coping With Change" (1252).

National Institute of Mental Health
5600 Fishers Lane, Room 15C05
Rockville, MD 20857
301-443-4513
   "Mental Health/Mental Illness: A Consumer's Guide to Services" (brochure 92-0214).

Depression

Agency for Health Care Policy and Research
Publications Clearinghouse
P.O. Box 8547
Silver Spring, MD 20907
800-358-9295
   "Depression is a Treatable Illness: A Patient's Guide" (brochure 93-0553).

American Academy of Family Physicians
8880 Ward Parkway
Kansas City, MO 64114-2797
800-944-0000
   "Depression: You Don't Have To Feel This Way" (brochure 1547); "Grieving: Facing Illness, Death and Other Losses" (brochure 1535).

American Academy of Pediatrics
141 Northwest Point Blvd.
P.O. Box 927
Elk Grove Village, IL 60000-0927
800-443-9016
   "Surviving: Coping With Adolescent Depression and Suicide" (brochure HE0046).

Depression Awareness, Recognition, and Treatment (D/ART) Program
National Institute of Mental Health
5600 Fishers Lane, Room 10-85
Rockville, MD 20857
301-443-4140, 800-421-4211
   "Depression: Effective Treatments Are Available" (brochure, English/Spanish ADM 93-3590); "Depression: What You Need to Know" (brochure ADM 91-1543); "Depressive Illnesses: Treatments Bring New Hope" (booklet ADM 94-3612); "What to Do When a Friend Is Depressed: A Guide for Students" (pamphlet ADM 89-1628); "If You're Over

65 and Feeling Depressed" (booklet ADM 89-1653); "Plain Talk About Depression" (brochure ADM-89-1639); "A Consumer's Guide to Mental Health Services" (booklet ADM 87-0214). (These publications also available from Consumer Information Center, Pueblo, CO, 81009.)

National Alliance for the Mentally Ill
2101 Wilson Boulevard, Suite 302
Arlington, VA 22201
800-950-6264

National Foundation for Depressive Illness
20 Charles Street
New York, NY 10014
   Information about centers that specialize in treating depressive disorders.

National Institute of Mental Health
Public Inquiries and Publications
301-443-4513

National Mental Health Association
1021 Prince Street
Alexandria, VA 22314-2971
800-969-6642
   The national headquarters can put patients or clinicians in touch with local chapters that can recommend private practitioners.

Cognitive Impairment

Alzheimer's Association
70 E. Lake Street, Suite 600
Chicago, IL 60601-5997
312-853-3060, 800-621-0379

Alzheimer's Disease and Related Disorders Association
919 N. Michigan Ave., Suite 1000
Chicago, IL 60611
800-272-3900
   Information about support groups and literature.

Alzheimer's Disease Education and Referral Center
P.O. Box 8250
Silver Spring, MD 20907
800-438-4380

American Academy of Family Physicians
8880 Ward Parkway
Kansas City, MO 64114-2797
800-944-0000
   "Memory Loss With Aging: What's Normal, What's Not" (brochure 1519).

National Association for Home Care
519 C Street, NE
Washington, DC 20002
202-547-7424

National Council on the Aging
600 Maryland Avenue, SW
West Wing 100
Washington, DC 20024
800-424-9046

National Institute on Aging
Public Information Office
Federal Building, Room 6C12
Bethesda, MD 20892
301-496-1752
"Age Page—Forgetfulness in Old Age: It's Not What You Think."

SUGGESTED READINGS

Functional Status

American College of Physicians, Health and Public Policy Committee. Comprehensive functional assessment for elderly patients. Ann Intern Med 1988;109:70–72.
Stewart AL, Ware JE Jr, eds. Measuring functioning and well-being: the medical outcomes study approach. Durham, NC: Duke University Press, 1992.

Self-Esteem

Branden N. Honoring the self: the psychology of confidence and respect. Toronto: Bantam, 1983.
Jacoby M. Shame and the origins of self-esteem: a Jungian approach. London: Routledge, 1994.
Jung CG. The basic writings of C.G. Jung. Princeton, NJ: Princeton University Press, 1990.

Anxiety

Roy-Byrne P, Wingerson D, Cowley D, Dager S. Psychopharmacologic treatment of panic, generalized anxiety disorder, and social phobia. Psychiatr Clin North Am 1993;16:719–735.
Walley EJ, Beebe DK, Clark JL. Management of common anxiety disorders. Am Fam Phys 1994;50:1745–1753.

Depression

Depression in primary care: volume I. Detection and diagnosis (AHCPR Publication No. 93-0550), volume II. Treatment of major depression (AHCPR Publication No. 93-0551). Rockville, MD: Agency for Health Care Policy and Research, 1993. Order free copies at 800-358-9295.
National Institutes of Health. Diagnosis and treatment of depression in late life. JAMA 1992;268:1018–1024.

Cognitive Impairment

Gugel RN. Behavioral approaches for managing patients with Alzheimer's disease and related disorders. Med Clin N Amer 1994;78:861–867.
Kluger A, Ferris SH. Scales for the assessment of Alzheimer's disease. Psychiatr Clin N Amer 1991;14:309–326.
National Institute on Aging. Working with your older patients: a clinician's handbook. Bethesda, MD: National Institute on Aging, 1995. Order copies by calling 301-496-1752.

Roth ME. Advances in Alzheimer's disease: a review for the family physician. J Fam Pract 1993;37:593–607.

REFERENCES

1. World Health Organization constitution. In: Basic documents. Geneva: World Health Organization, 1948.
2. Patrick DL, Erickson P. Assessing health-related quality of life for clinical decision-making. In: Walker SR, Rosser RM, eds. Quality of life assessment: key issues in the 1990s. Dordrecht, the Netherlands: Kluwer Academic Publishers, 1993:11–63.
3. Health data on older Americans, United States, 1992. Series 3, No. 27. Hyattsville, MD: National Center for Health Statistics, 1992.
4. Chrousos GP, Gold PW. The concepts of stress and stress system disorders. JAMA 1992;267:1244–1252.
5. Diagnostic and statistical manual of mental disorders, 4th ed. Washington, DC: American Psychiatric Association, 1994.
6. Hamilton M. The assessment of anxiety states by rating. Br J Med Psychol 1959;32:50.
7. Ornish D, Brown SE, Scherwitz LW, Billings JH, et al. Can lifestyle changes reverse coronary heart disease? The Lifestyle Heart Trial. Lancet 1990;336:129–133.
8. Clum GA, Surls R. A meta-analysis of treatments for panic disorder. J Consult Clin Psychol 1993;61:317–326.
9. Zung WWK, Broadhead WE, Roth ME. Prevalence of depressive symptoms in primary care. J Fam Pract 1993;37:337–344.
10. Depression in primary care: volume I. Detection and diagnosis. AHCPR Publication No. 93-0550. Rockville, MD: Agency for Health Care Policy and Research, 1993.
11. National Institute on Aging. Progress report on Alzheimer's disease, 1993. NIH Publication No. 93-3409. Bethesda, MD: National Institutes of Health, 1993.
12. Gauthier S, Bouchard R, Lamontagne A, et al. Tetrahydroaminoacridine-lecithin combination treatment in patients with intermediate-stage Alzheimer's disease. N Engl J Med 1990;322:1272–1276.
13. Davis KL, Thal LJ, Gamzu ER, et al. A double-blind, placebo-controlled multicenter study of tacrine for Alzheimer's disease. N Engl J Med 1992;327:1253–1259.

17. What to Do with Abnormal Screening Test Results

STEVEN H. WOOLF

INTRODUCTION

This chapter examines what clinicians should do when they receive abnormal results from screening tests. The specific screening tests considered are the history, physical examination, and laboratory procedures discussed in Chapters 2–4. Collectively, these maneuvers screen for a broad range of conditions, including risk factors and preclinical states for coronary artery disease, cancer, endocrine and metabolic disorders, hematologic abnormalities, urologic and renal disorders, infectious diseases, impaired hearing and vision, mental illness, impaired functional status, and childhood developmental disorders.

A thorough discussion of how to evaluate and treat each of these problems is clearly beyond the scope of a single chapter, since these disorders constitute much of the practice of internal medicine, pediatrics, ophthalmology, otolaryngology, urology, psychiatry, social work, and other disciplines (e.g., audiology, speech pathology). Despite these limitations, this chapter on follow-up is included to emphasize its importance in the practice of health promotion and disease prevention. Screening without proper follow-up constitutes incomplete care. Too many persons undergo screening without receiving a clear explanation of the results or without arrangements for proper follow-up. In the most tragic example of this problem, patients develop advanced stage cancer, despite having undergone prior screening, because their physicians did not receive laboratory results or misinterpreted the findings, or because patients did not understand or act on the clinician's recommendations (e.g., failing to return for repeat screening or to visit a specialist). Preventive medicine does not end with the ordering of a test but with careful patient education to explain the results and with comprehensive medical evaluation of abnormalities. Difficulties in ensuring this follow-up represent the principal disadvantage of community screening at shopping centers, worksites, and schools, when conducted by persons who are not responsible for the patient's ongoing care.

Even the patient's physician may face difficulties in providing thorough follow-up. A common obstacle is lack of knowledge, since clinicians must remain informed of current literature and practice guidelines to keep abreast of the latest treatment options. As most physicians know, it is much easier to order a test than to maintain this knowledge base. Some failures in follow-up are due to simple forgetfulness. Clinicians may not remember when a patient is due for screening or that test results have not returned from the laboratory. Health maintenance schedules and flow sheets (Chapter 22) and reminder systems for clinicians and patients (Chapter 26) can help to minimize these oversights. Even when test results are available, another form of forgetfulness can lead to incomplete follow-up. Physicians often remember only parts of the algorithm for evaluating results. They may remember that a patient with a positive syphilis test requires antibiotic therapy but may forget that sexual partners and the public health department need to be notified. They may order a scrotal ultrasound examination for a man with a palpable testicular mass but forget to measure blood levels of alpha-fetoprotein or beta-human chorionic gonadotropin. They may refer a patient whom they have diagnosed with advanced prostate cancer to a urologist but forget to arrange for cancer education and support group services.

The purpose of this chapter is to remind the clinician of the types of follow-up interventions that may be necessary when patients have abnormal screening test results. Space limitations make it impossible to review the proper algorithm for selecting tests and treatments for each potential problem detected by screening. Instead, the tables that follow present the key options in a menu format to remind the clinician of the possible choices, *but not to suggest that each item is always necessary or how they should be selected*. The clinician should consider the natural history of the disease and consult the suggested readings for guidance in making these choices. The main purpose of each table is to remind the clinician of the options to consider.

Each section below provides seven types of information:

1. *Abnormal screening test result*: the abnormalities on screening that are usually first recognized by the clinician. Techniques for performing the screening tests are discussed in Chapters 2–4.

2. *Diagnostic studies that* may *be indicated*: the laboratory tests, imaging studies, or other diagnostic maneuvers that *might* be ordered to confirm the diagnosis, by ruling out false-positive results or other conditions in the differential diagnosis, or to test for common coexisting conditions. *It is rarely appropriate to order all tests listed in this section.* As in any diagnostic exercise, tests should be selected according to a rational plan that reflects an understanding of the pathophysiology of the disease rather than by resorting to a "shotgun" approach. Usually, only one or two tests are necessary initially to determine the general class of

the disorder (e.g., microcytic versus normocytic/macrocytic anemia, primary versus secondary hypothyroidism); additional tests can then be ordered selectively to help clarify the diagnosis. The accuracy of the test and its proven effectiveness in improving outcomes should be considered in selecting the best test. Although the history and physical examination are not specifically listed here, the need for many tests can be avoided by obtaining a more detailed history or by checking for relevant physical examination findings.

3. *Treatment options that* may *be indicated*: treatment modalities and educational interventions that *may* be indicated, depending on the results of testing. As with the previous section, *patients rarely require all treatment options*. The appropriate interventions depend on the diagnosis, available evidence regarding effectiveness, and the patient's preferences. Although not always listed in each section, patient education is essential (a) to ensure that patients or parents understand the diagnosis and the potential benefits and harms of treatment and (b) to consider this information and their personal preferences to make an informed decision about which treatment option to pursue. See "Shared Decision Making" in Chapter 19.

4. *Potential referrals and consultations*: specialists and community resources that may be helpful in selecting or performing diagnostic tests and treatments. This section first lists physician specialists with relevant expertise and then lists other health professionals and community resources that can provide assistance. (Public health departments are listed under "nonphysician" resources, although they often employ physicians with public health, preventive medicine, or other training.) Although primary care physicians with adequate proficiency in managing the problem often do not need to involve medical specialists in the patient's care, failure to include certain health professionals, social workers, or community resources can sometimes lead to incomplete care in cases requiring expertise or services outside the primary care provider's capabilities.

5. *Follow-up*: monitoring and surveillance after the patient has undergone initial testing and treatment. Clinicians caring for the patient, especially primary care providers, should ensure that arrangements for follow-up are made with the patient. Although not specifically listed in each section, follow-up almost always includes periodic history taking and physical examinations to check for signs and symptoms of new complications. Also listed in this section are blood tests, imaging studies, and other diagnostic maneuvers to confirm the adequacy of treatment or to detect early complications. *Once again, it is rarely necessary to perform all of the tests listed in this section.* In most cases, there is little scientific evidence regarding the optimal interval for follow-up examinations.

6. *Resources*: brochures and booklets that will provide patients with information about the disorder and relevant diagnostic studies. This section also includes telephone numbers to clearinghouses and resource centers that can provide patients with additional information and physicians with rapid answers to questions. By addressing specific diseases, the patient education materials listed here differ from those listed in other chapters of this book, which generally describe screening tests or health promotion advice for patients who have not re-

ceived an abnormal screening test result or developed disease. The resources in this chapter for persons with specific health problems include only a portion of the hundreds of high-quality patient education materials available to the public; they are cited to illustrate what is available and not necessarily to discourage the use of other publications.

7. *Suggested readings*: references that will provide the clinician with further background on how to select appropriate diagnostic tests and treatment options and additional sources for background reading.

This chapter addresses abnormal results for only certain screening tests. Some screening tests may reveal disorders that are discussed in other chapters of this book, such as overweight (Chapter 9), alcohol or other drug abuse (Chapter 13), dental disease (Chapter 15), depression (Chapter 16), and cognitive impairment (Chapter 16). Please refer to these chapters for information about recommended interventions and educational materials for patients with these problems. Other screening tests omitted here include tests that are not routinely performed on asymptomatic persons or that are specifically discouraged as screening tests (see Chapter 21).

SCREENING SUGGESTIVE OF CARDIOVASCULAR RISK FACTORS

Hypertension (Table 17.1)

Table 17.1

Abnormal Screening Test Results	Diagnostic Studies That *May* Be Indicated	Treatment Options That *May* Be Indicated	Potential Referrals/ Consultations	Follow-Up
Elevated blood pressure as defined in Table 3.2	Complete blood count Chemistry panel Urinalysis Electrocardiogram Echocardiogram Chest radiograph Renal imaging	*Nonpharmacologic therapy* Reduced dietary sodium Reduced caloric intake Reduced alcohol intake Exercise Weight management Surgery for structural causes (e.g., renal artery stenosis) *Pharmacologic therapy* Diuretics, beta-blockers, angiotensin-converting enzyme inhibitors, calcium antagonists, alpha-receptor blockers	*Physicians:* Cardiologist, ophthalmologist, nephrologist, endocrinologist *Non-Physicians:* Dietitian, substance abuse counselor	Blood pressure measurements, patient compliance, side effects to medications, other barriers to compliance, positive reinforcement for adherence

RESOURCES—PATIENT EDUCATION MATERIALS

American Academy of Family Physicians
8880 Ward Parkway
Kansas City, MO 64114-2797
800-944-0000
   "High Blood Pressure: Things You Can Do To Help Lower Yours" (brochure 1541).

American Heart Association
7320 Greenville Avenue
Dallas, TX 75231
214-373-6300
   "About High Blood Pressure" (brochure 50-052D: English, Spanish); "Ten Command-
   ments for the Patient With High Blood Pressure (wallet card 58-005C: English, Spanish); "Doctors Answer Your Questions About Blood Pressure" (reduced reading level
   brochure 64-1025); "Salt, Sodium, and Blood Pressure" (brochure 50-065B); "Cooking
   Without Your Salt Shaker" (book 53-002A); "About High Blood Pressure in Children"
   (brochure 50-045A); "About High Blood Pressure in Adolescents" (brochure 50-049A);
   "About High Blood Pressure in African Americans" (brochure 50-1105).

National Heart, Lung, and Blood Institute
High Blood Pressure Information Line
800-575-WELL

National High Blood Pressure Education Program
P.O. Box 30105
Bethesda, MD 20824-0105
301-251-1222
   "Eat Right to Help Lower Your High Blood Pressure" (brochure, NIH Pub No. 92-3289).

SUGGESTED READINGS

Joint National Committee on Detection, Evaluation, and Treatment of High Blood Pressure.
   The fifth report of the Joint National Committee on Detection, Evaluation, and Treat-
   ment of High Blood Pressure (JNC V). Arch Intern Med 1993;153:154–183.
The physician's guide: improving adherence among hypertensive patients. (NIH Pub. No.
   NN250). Bethesda, MD: National Heart, Lung, and Blood Institute.

Lipid Disorders (Table 17.2)

Table 17.2

Abnormal Screening Test Results	Diagnostic Studies That *May* Be Indicated	Treatment Options That *May* Be Indicated	Potential Referrals/ Consultations	Follow-Up
Elevated total or LDL-cholesterol, low HDL-cholesterol	Total cholesterol (repeat) Lipoprotein analysis	*Nonpharmacologic therapy* Step I low-fat diet Step II low-fat diet Weight reduction Exercise *Pharmacologic therapy* Bile acid sequestrants Nicotinic aicd HMG CoA reductase inhibitors Fibric acids Probucol	*Physician:* Endocrinologist, cardiologist *Non-Physicians:* Dietitian	Adherence to dietary plan, exercise and weight management, monitoring of side effects of cholesterol-lowering drugs, cholesterol and/or lipoprotein levels

Legend: LDL, low-density lipoprotein; *HDL,* high-density lipoprotein, *HMG CoA,* hydroxymethylglutaryl-coenzyme A.

RESOURCES—PATIENT EDUCATION MATERIALS

American Academy of Family Physicians
8880 Ward Parkway
Kansas City, MO 64114-2797
800-944-0000
"Cholesterol: What You Can Do To Lower Your Level" (brochure 1503).

American Heart Association
7320 Greenville Avenue
Dallas, TX 75231
214-373-6300
"Cholesterol and Your Heart" (brochure 50-1038); "Dietary Treatment of Hypercholesterolemia" (brochure 64-9545).

National Cholesterol Education Program
NHLBI Education Programs Information Center
P.O. Box 30105
Bethesda, MD 20824-0105
301-951-3260
"So You Have High Blood Cholesterol" (booklet 93-2922); "Step By Step: Eating to Lower Your High Blood Cholesterol" (booklet 94-2920).

SUGGESTED READINGS

Expert Panel on Detection, Evaluation, and Treatment of High Blood Cholesterol in Adults. Summary of the second report of the National Cholesterol Education Program (NCEP) Expert Panel on Detection, Evaluation, and Treatment of High Blood Cholesterol in Adults (Adult Treatment Panel II). JAMA 1993;269:3015–3023.

Levine GN, Keaney JF Jr, Vita JA. Cholesterol reduction in cardiovascular disease: clinical benefits and possible mechanisms. N Engl J Med 1995;332:512–521.

National Cholesterol Education Program. Report of the Expert Panel on Blood Cholesterol Levels in Children and Adolescents. Pediatrics 1992;89:525–584.

Asymptomatic Coronary Artery Disease (Table 17.3)

Table 17.3

Abnormal Screening Test Results	Diagnostic Studies That *May* Be Indicated	Treatment Options That *May* Be Indicated	Potential Referrals/ Consultations	Follow-Up
Electrocardiographic changes suggestive of silent ischemia	Ambulatory electrocardiographic monitoring Exercise stress testing Myocardial perfusion scintigraphy Stress echocardiography Coronary angiography	Antianginal medical therapy Coronary artery revascularization Percutaneous transluminal coronary angioplasty Atherectomy Behavior modification	*Physicians:* Cardiologist, nuclear medicine physician, cardiac surgeon *Non-Physicians:* Dietitian, trainer	Resting/stress electrocardiogram; stress myocardial perfusion scintigraphy

RESOURCES—PATIENT EDUCATION MATERIALS

Chek Med Systems, Inc.
1027 Mumma Road
Wormleysburg, PA 17043-9933
800-451-5797

"Cardiac Catheterization" (brochure English MC-03; Spanish MSC-03); "The Exercise and Thallium Stress Test" (brochure, English MC-08; Spanish MSC-08).

National Heart, Lung, and Blood Institute
Education Programs Information Center
P.O. Box 30105
Bethesda, MD 20824-0105
301-951-3260

"Facts About Coronary Heart Disease" (brochure 93-2265).

SUGGESTED READINGS

American College of Sports Medicine. Guidelines for exercise testing and prescription. Malvern, PA: Lea & Febiger, 1991.

Chou TM, Amidon TM. Evaluating coronary artery disease noninvasively—which test for whom? West J Med 1994;161:173–180.

Deedwania PC, Carbajal EV. Silent myocardial ischemia: a clinical perspective. Arch Intern Med 1991;151:2373–82.

Pepine CJ, Kern MJ, Boden WE. Advisory group reports on silent myocardial ischemia, acute intervention after myocardial infarction, and postinfarction management. Am J Cardiol 1992;69:41B–46B.

Zaret BL, Wackers FJ. Nuclear cardiology. N Engl J Med 1993;329:775–783.

SCREENING SUGGESTIVE OF NEOPLASIA

Breast Cancer (Table 17.4)

Table 17.4

Abnormal Screening Test Results	Diagnostic Studies That *May* Be Indicated	Treatment Options That *May* Be Indicated	Potential Referrals/ Consultations	Follow-Up
Abnormal breast examination/ mammogram	Comprehensive, magnification, or spot-compression mammography Fine-needle aspiration cytology Ultrasound Stereotactic biopsy Open biopsy with frozen-section examination Liver function tests Chest radiograph Computerized tomogram	Partial breast resection Axillary node dissection Modified radical mastectomy Chemotherapy Radiation therapy Hormonal therapy	*Physicians:* General surgeon, oncologist, radiologist, pathologist, radiation therapist *Non-Physicians:* Pain center, counseling and support groups, dietitian, home care services, social services	Breast examination/ mammography, pelvic examination, chest radiograph, liver function tests, tumor markers

RESOURCES—PATIENT EDUCATION MATERIALS

American Institute for Cancer Research
1759 R Street, NW
Washington, DC 20069
800-843-8114, 202-328-7744
"Questions and Answers About Breast Lumps and Breast Cancer" (booklet).

Krames Communications
1100 Grundy Lane
San Bruno, CA 94066-3030
800-333-3032
"Breast Lumps: A Guide to Understanding Breast Problems and Breast Surgery" (booklet English 1019; Spanish 1060); "Breast Biopsy" (booklet 1156); "Breast Surgery: From Biopsy to Reconstruction" (booklet 1291).

National Cancer Institute
Building 31, Room 10A24
Bethesda, MD 20892
800-4-CANCER

"What You Need To Know About Breast Cancer" (NIH Publication No. 93-1556); "Helping Yourself During Chemotherapy: 4 Steps for Patients" (NIH Publication No. 94-3701); "Radiation Therapy And You: A Guide to Self-Help During Treatment" (booklet 92-2227).

SUGGESTED READINGS

Donegan WL. Evaluation of a palpable breast mass. N Engl J Med 1992;327:937–941.

Harris JR, Lippman ME, Veronesi U, Willett W. Breast cancer. N Engl J Med 1992; 327:390–398.

Greenall MJ. Current controversies in the surgical management of breast cancer. Ann Oncol 1994;5 Suppl 4:39–43.

Olson LK. Interpreting the mammogram report. Am Fam Phys 1993;47:396–403.

Overmoyer BA. Chemotherapy in the management of breast cancer. Cleve Clin J Med 1995;62:36–50.

Shapiro CL, Henderson IC. Adjuvant therapy of breast cancer. Hematol-Oncol Clin N Amer 1994;8:213–231.

Colorectal Cancer (Table 17.5)

Table 17.5

Abnormal Screening Test Results	Diagnostic Studies That *May* Be Indicated	Treatment Options That *May* Be Indicated	Potential Referrals/ Consultations	Follow-Up
Palpable mass on digital rectal examination Positive fecal occult blood test Polyp/mass on screening sigmoidoscopy	Colonoscopy Air-contrast barium enema Biopsy Carcinoembryonic antigen Complete blood count Liver function tests Chest radiography Abdominal/pelvic computerized tomogram	Polyp resection/ fulguration En bloc surgical resection Adjuvant radiation therapy Adjuvant chemotherapy	*Physicians:* Gastroenterologist, oncologist, general surgeon, radiation therapist *Non-Physicians:* Pain center, counseling and support groups, dietitian, home care services, social services	Colonoscopy/ air-contrast barium enema, fecal occult blood test, carcino-embryonic antigen

RESOURCES—PATIENT EDUCATION MATERIALS

American Cancer Society
1599 Clifton Road, NE
Atlanta, GA 30329
800-227-2345, 404-320-3333
"Facts on Colorectal Cancer" (brochure English 2004; Spanish 2703).

Channing L. Bete Co., Inc.
200 State Road
South Deerfield, MA 01373-0200
800-628-7733
"Living With Colorectal Cancer (brochure T12823A).

Krames Communications
1100 Grundy Lane
San Bruno, CA 94066-3030
800-333-3032
"Colorectal Health" (brochure 1226); "Colonoscopy" (brochure 5007).

National Cancer Institute
Building 31, Room 10A24
Bethesda, MD 20892
800-4-CANCER
"Helping Yourself During Chemotherapy: 4 Steps for Patients" (NIH Publication No. 94-3701); "Radiation Therapy and You: A Guide to Self-Help During Treatment" (booklet 92-2227).

SUGGESTED READINGS

Bond JH, for American College of Gastroenterology. Polyp guideline: diagnosis, treatment, and surveillance for patients with nonfamilial colorectal polyps. Ann Intern Med 1993;119:836–843.
DeCosse JJ, Tsioulias GJ, Jacobson JS. Colorectal cancer: detection, treatment, and rehabilitation. CA 1994;44:27–42.
Moertel CG. Chemotherapy for colorectal cancer. N Engl J Med 1994;330:1136–1142.

Cervical Cancer (Table 17.6)

Table 17.6

Abnormal Screening Test Results	Diagnostic Studies That *May* Be Indicated	Treatment Options That *May* Be Indicated	Potential Referrals/ Consultations	Follow-Up
Squamous epithelial cell abnormalities (e.g., dysplasia, cervical intraepithelial neoplasia, carcinoma-in-situ), glandular cell abnormalities (e.g., adenocarcinoma), squamous cell carcinoma, or Papanicolaou class III–V	Colposcopy Endocervical curettage Cervical punch biopsy Diagnostic conization Endometrial sampling Loop electrosurgical excision	Local excision Cryotherapy Carbon dioxide laser vaporization Loop electrosurgical excision Hysterectomy/ radical lymphadenec-tomy Radiation therapy	*Physicians:* Cytopathologist, gynecologist, oncologist, radiotherapist *Non-Physicians:* Pain center, counseling and support groups, dietitian, home care services, social services	Papanicolaou smear, colposcopy

RESOURCES—PATIENT EDUCATION MATERIALS

American Academy of Family Physicians
8880 Ward Parkway
Kansas City, MO 64114-2797
800-944-0000
　　"Pap Smears: What They Are and What The Results Mean" (brochure 1539).

National Cancer Institute
Building 31, Room 10A24
Bethesda, MD 20892
800-4-CANCER
"What You Need To Know About Cervical Cancer" (brochure 91-2047); "Radiation Therapy
And You: A Guide to Self-Help During Treatment" (booklet 92-2227).

SUGGESTED READINGS

Cervical cytology: evaluation and management of abnormalities. ACOG Technical Bulletin
　　No. 183. Washington, DC: American College of Obstetricians and Gynecologists, 1993.
Kurman RJ, Hensen DE, Herbst AL, Noller KL, Schiffman MH, for the 1992 National Cancer
　　Institute Workshop. Interim guidelines for management of abnormal cervical cytology.
　　JAMA 1994;271:1866–1869.
National Cancer Institute Workshop. The revised Bethesda system for reporting
　　cervical/vaginal cytologic diagnoses: report of the 1991 Bethesda workshop. Acta Cytol
　　1992;36:273–275.
Seminars in Oncology 1994;21(Z): (Entire issue devoted to the treatment of cervical dysplasia
　　and cancer.)

Prostate Cancer (Table 17.7)

Table 17.7

Abnormal Screening Test Results	Diagnostic Studies That *May* Be Indicated	Treatment Options That *May* Be Indicated	Potential Referrals/ Consultations	Follow-Up
Abnormal digital rectal examination, prostate-specific antigen level, transrectal ultrasound	Prostate-specific antigen level Transrectal ultrasound Fine-needle biopsy Pelvic/ abdominal computed tomogram Radionuclide bone scan	Watchful waiting Radical prostatectomy External-beam radiation therapy Interstitital radiation therapy Hormonal therapy	*Physicians:* Urologist, oncologist, radiologist, nuclear medicine specialist, radiotherapist *Non-Physicians:* Pain center, counseling and support groups, dietitian, home care services, social services	Prostate-specific antigen level, other tumor markers, bone scan, chemistry panel, computerized tomogram

RESOURCES—PATIENT EDUCATION MATERIALS

American Cancer Society
1599 Clifton Road, NE
Atlanta, GA 30329
404-320-3333, 800-ACS-2345
    "Facts on Prostate Cancer" (brochure 2654).

Agency for Health Care Policy and Research
Publications Clearinghouse
P.O. Box 8547
Silver Spring, MD 20907
800-358-9295
    "Treating Your Enlarged Prostate" (brochure 94-0584).

Krames Communications
1100 Grundy Lane
San Bruno, CA 94066-3030
800-333-3032
    "Living With Prostate Cancer" (booklet 1375).

National Cancer Institute
Office of Cancer Communications
Building 31, Room 10A24
Bethesda, MD 20892
800-4-CANCER
    "What You Need to Know About Prostate Cancer" (NIH Pub No. 93-1576); "Radiation
    Therapy And You: A Guide to Self-Help During Treatment" (booklet 92-2227).

SUGGESTED READINGS

Catalona WJ. Management of cancer of the prostate. N Engl J Med 1994;331:996–1004.

Oral Cancer (Table 17.8)

Table 17.8

Abnormal Screening Test Results	Diagnostic Studies That *May* Be Indicated	Treatment Options That *May* Be Indicated	Potential Referrals/ Consultations	Follow-Up
Suspicious lesion on oral cavity examination	Oral exfoliative cytology Toluidine blue/ tolonium chloride mucosal staining Biopsy	Surgical resection Neck dissection Radiation therapy Chemotherapy	*Physicians:* Otolaryngologist, oral-maxillofacial surgeon, plastic surgeon, dermatologist, oncologist, radiation therapist, radiologist *Non-Physicians:* Dentist, pain center, counseling and support groups, dietitian, home care services, social services	Clinical monitoring

RESOURCES—PATIENT EDUCATION MATERIALS

American Cancer Society
1599 Clifton Road, NE
Atlanta, GA 30329
404-320-3333, 800-ACS-2345
　　"Facts on Oral Cancer" (brochure English 2630; Spanish 2706).

National Oral Health Information Clearinghouse
1 NOHIC Way
Bethesda, MD 20892-3500

National Cancer Institute
Office of Cancer Communications
Building 31, Room 10A24
Bethesda, MD 20892
800-4-CANCER
　　"What You Need To Know About Oral Cancer" (brochure 93-1574); "Helping Yourself During Chemotherapy: 4 Steps for Patients" (NIH Publication No. 94-3701); "Radiation Therapy And You: A Guide to Self-Help During Treatment" (booklet 92-2227).

SUGGESTED READINGS

Schantz SP, Harrison LB, Hong WK. Cancer of the head and neck. In: Devita VT Jr, Hellman S, Rosenberg SA, eds. Cancer: principles and practice of oncology, 4th ed. Philadelphia: JB Lippincott, 1993:574–630.
Seminars in Oncology 1994;21(3): (Entire issue devoted to head and neck cancer.)

Testicular Cancer (Table 17.9)

Table 17.9

Abnormal Screening Test Results	Diagnostic Studies That *May* Be Indicated	Treatment Options That *May* Be Indicated	Potential Referrals/ Consultations	Follow-Up
Palpable scrotal mass	Scrotal ultrasound Beta-human chorionic gonadotropin Alpha-fetoprotein Orchiectomy Chest radiograph Chest computerized tomogram	Radical/partial orchiectomy Retroperitoneal lymph node dissection Radiation therapy Chemotherapy	*Physicians:* Radiologist, urologist, oncologist, radiation therapist, general surgeon *Non-Physicians:* Pain center, counseling and support groups, home care services, social services	Beta-human chorionic gonadotropin Alpha-fetoprotein Chest/abdominal computerized tomogram

RESOURCES—PATIENT EDUCATION MATERIALS

American Cancer Society
1599 Clifton Road, NE
Atlanta, GA 30329
404-320-3333, 800-ACS-2345
    "Facts on Testicular Cancer" (brochure 2645).

National Cancer Institute
Office of Cancer Communications
Building 31, Room 10A24
Bethesda, MD 20892
800-4-CANCER
    "What You Need to Know About Testicular Cancer" (booklet 93-1565); "Helping Yourself During Chemotherapy: 4 Steps for Patients" (NIH Publication No. 94-3701); "Radiation Therapy And You: A Guide to Self-Help During Treatment" (booklet 92-2227).

SUGGESTED READINGS

Einhorn LH, Richie JP, Shipley WU. Cancer of the testis. In: Devita VT Jr, Hellman S, Rosenberg SA, eds. Cancer: principles and practice of oncology, 4th ed. Philadelphia: JB Lippincott, 1993:1126–1151.

Skin Cancer (Table 17.10)

Table 17.10

Abnormal Screening Test Results	Diagnostic Studies That *May Be* Indicated	Treatment Options That *May* Be Indicated	Potential Referrals/ Consultations	Follow-Up
Suspicious lesion on skin examination	Complete skin examination Biopsy (punch, incisional, excisional) Complete blood count Liver function tests Chest radiograph	*Nonmelanomatous skin cancer* Excision Mohs' micrographic surgery Cryotherapy Topical chemotherapy Curettage and electrodesiccation Laser vaporization Radiation therapy *Melanomatous skin cancer* Excision Prophylactic lymph node dissection Chemotherapy	*Physicians:* Dermatologist, plastic surgeon, oral-maxillofacial surgeon, oncologist, radiation therapist *Non-Physicians:* Pain center, counseling and support groups, dietitian, home care services, social services	Complete blood count, chemistry panel, chest radiograph, liver function tests, abdominal computerized tomogram

RESOURCES—PATIENT EDUCATION MATERIALS

American Cancer Society
1599 Clifton Road, NE
Atlanta, GA 30329
404-320-3333, 800-ACS-2345
    "Facts on Skin Cancer" (brochure 2049).

Channing L. Bete Co., Inc.
200 State Road
South Deerfield, MA 01373-0200
800-628-7733
    "Living With Skin Cancer" (brochure T37259A).

National Cancer Institute
Office of Cancer Communications
Building 31, Room 10A24
Bethesda, MD 20892
800-4-CANCER
    "What You Need To Know About Skin Cancer" (brochure 94-1563); "What You Need To Know About Melanoma" (brochure 93-1563); "What You Need To Know About Moles and Dysplastic Nevi" (brochure 93-3133); "Helping Yourself During Chemotherapy: 4 Steps for Patients" (NIH Publication No. 94-3701).

SUGGESTED READINGS

Kuflik AS, Schwartz RA. Actinic keratosis and squamous cell carcinoma. Am Fam Phys 1994;49:817–820.

National Institutes of Health Consensus Development Conference. Diagnosis and treatment of early melanoma 1992 Jan 27-29;10(1):1–26.

Pariser DM, Phillips PK. Basal cell carcinoma: when to treat it yourself, and when to refer. Geriatrics 1994;49:39–44.

Runkle GP, Zaloznik AJ. Malignant melanoma. Am Fam Phys 1994;49:91–98.

SCREENING SUGGESTIVE OF ENDOCRINE AND METABOLIC DISORDERS

Diabetes Mellitus (Table 17.11)

Table 17.11

Abnormal Screening Test Results	Diagnostic Studies That *May* Be Indicated	Treatment Options That *May* Be Indicated	Potential Referrals/ Consultations	Follow-Up
Elevation of plasma glucose ($\geq$200 mg/ dL), fasting plasma glucose $\geq$140 mg/ dL	Fasting plasma glucose Glucose tolerance test Glycosylated hemoglobin Lipid profile Serum creatinine Urinalysis Thyroid function tests Electrocardiogram	Diabetic diet Exercise *Medications* Oral hypogly- cemic agents Insulin Pneumococcal/ influenza vaccination	*Physicians:* Endocrinologist, ophthalmologist, neurologist, nephrologist, cardiologist *Non-Physicians:* Podiatrist, dietitian, home care services, social services	Physical findings, fasting plasma glucose, glycosylated hemoglobin, urinalysis, creatinine clearance, ability to self-monitor blood/urine glucose and ketones

RESOURCES—PATIENT EDUCATION MATERIALS

American Academy of Family Physicians
8880 Ward Parkway
Kansas City, MO 64114-2797
800-944-0000
   "Diabetes: Taking Charge of Your Diabetes" (brochure 1530); "Diabetes And Your Body: How To Take Care of Your Eyes and Feet" (brochure 1553).

Krames Communications
1100 Grundy Lane
San Bruno, CA 94066-3030
800-333-3032
   "Type I Diabetes" (booklet 1465); "Type II Diabetes" (brochure English 1472; Spanish 1480).

National Diabetes Information Clearinghouse
1 Information Way
Bethesda, MD 20892-3560
301-468-2162

"Insulin-Dependent Diabetes" (booklet NIH No. 94-2098); "Noninsulin-Dependent Diabetes" (booklet NIH No. 92-241).

SUGGESTED READINGS

National Diabetes Information Clearinghouse, P.O. Box NDIC, 9000 Rockville Pike, Bethesda, MD, 20892, 301-468-2162

American Diabetes Association. Office guide to diagnosis and classification of diabetes mellitus and other categories of glucose intolerance. Diabetes Care 1993;16(Suppl 2):4.

American Diabetes Association. Standards of medical care for patients with diabetes mellitus. Diabetes Care 1993;16(Suppl 2):10–13.

Kerr CP. Improving outcomes in diabetes: a review of the outpatient care of NIDDM patients. J Fam Pract 1995;40:63–75.

U.S. Centers for Disease Control and Prevention. The prevention and treatment of complications of diabetes: a guide for primary care practitioners. NIH Publication No. 93-3464. Atlanta: U.S. Public Health Service, 1991.

Thyroid disorders (Table 17.12)

Table 17.12

Abnormal Screening Test Results	Diagnostic Studies That *May* Be Indicated	Treatment Options That *May* Be Indicated	Potential Referrals/ Consultations	Follow-Up
Thyroid function test suggestive of hypothyroidism or hyper-thyroidism	Thyroxine (T$_4$) Free thyroxine index Triiodothyronine (T$_3$) Sensitive/ ultrasensitive thyroid stimulating hormone Thyroxine-binding globulin Antithyroglobulin antibodies Antimicrosomal antibodies Radionuclide thyroid scan Radiographic bone age (newborn) Chest radiograph (newborns)	*Thyroid replacement* Levothyroxine Liothyronine Liotrix Natural thyroid hormone preparations *Antithyroid medications* Propylthiouracil Methimazole Radioactive iodine therapy Subtotal thyroidectomy Adjunctive therapy Beta-adrenergic blockers Calcium channel blockers	Endocrinologist, nuclear medicine specialist, surgeon, ophthalmologist	Thyroid function tests, pediatric growth and development

SUGGESTED READINGS

American Academy of Pediatrics Section on Endocrinology and Committee on Genetics, American Thyroid Association Committee on Public Health. Newborn screening for congenital hypothyroidism: recommended guidelines. Pediatrics 1993;91:1203–1209.

Klein I, Becker DV, Levey GS. Treatment of hyperthyroid disease. Ann Intern Med 1994; 121:281–288.

Rogers DG. Thyroid disease in children. Am Fam Phys 1994;50:344–350.

Singer PA, Cooper DS, Levy EG, Ladenson PW, Braverman LE, Daniels G, et al. Treatment guidelines for patients with hyperthyroidism and hypothyroidism. JAMA 1995;273: 8008–812.

Surks MI, Chopra IJ, Mariash CN, Nicoloff JT, Solomon DH. American Thyroid Association guideline for use of laboratory tests in thyroid disorders. JAMA 1990;263:1529–1532.

Toft AD. Thyroxine therapy. N Engl J Med 1994;331:174–180.

Phenylketonuria (Table 17.13)

Table 17.13

Abnormal Screening Test Results	Diagnostic Studies That *May* Be Indicated	Treatment Options That *May* Be Indicated	Potential Referrals/ Consultations	Follow-Up
Elevated serum phenylalanine level	Serum phenylalanine Serum tyrosine Serum dihydropteridine reductase Urinary pteridines Urinary phenylalanine metabolites	Parental education and counseling Dietary phenylalanine restriction	*Physicians:* Geneticist, endocrinologist, developmental specialist *Non-Physicians:* Dietitian	Phenylalanine levels, physical and neuro-behavioral development

RESOURCES—PATIENT EDUCATION MATERIALS

March of Dimes Birth Defects Foundation
P.O. Box 1657
Wilkes-Barre, PA 18703
800-367-6630
    "PKU: Phenylketonuria" (information sheet).

National Center for Education in Maternal and Child Health
2000 15th Street North, Suite 701
Arlington, VA 22201-2617
    "New Parents Guide to PKU" (B335).

SUGGESTED READINGS

Goodman SI, Greene CL. Inborn errors of metabolism. In: Hathaway WE, Hay WW Jr, Groothuis JR, Paisley JW, eds. Current pediatric diagnosis and treatment, 11th ed. Norwalk, CT: Appleton and Lange, 1993:885–905.

Metalon R, Michalis K. Phenylketonuria: screening, treatment and maternal PKU. Clin Biochem 1991;24:337–342.

Lead Toxicity (Table 17.14)

Table 17.14

Abnormal Screening Test Results	Diagnostic Studies That *May* Be Indicated	Treatment Options That *May* Be Indicated	Potential Referrals/ Consultations	Follow-Up
Blood lead ≥15 mcg/ dL	Complete blood count Serum iron, iron binding capacity, ferritin Blood urea nitrogen/ creatinine Urinalysis Edetate disodium calcium provactive chelation test Abdomen/long bone radiographs	Parent education and counseling Notification of health department Screening of household members Patient/family relocation Environmental lead hazard control *Chelation therapy* Succimer Edetate disodium calcium Dimercaprol D-penicillamine	*Physicians:* Neurologist *Non-Physicians:* Public health department, environmental specialist, community outreach worker, psychologist, social worker, dietitian, housing and environmental agencies	Blood lead measurements

RESOURCES—PATIENT EDUCATION MATERIALS

Channing L. Bete Co., Inc.
200 State Road
South Deerfield, MA 01373-0200
800-628-7733
    "About Lead Poisoning" (brochure English T18028A; Spanish T43075A).

National Institute of Environmental Health Sciences
Office of Communications
P.O. Box 12233
Research Triangle Park, NC 27709
919-541-3345
    "Lead and Your Health" (booklet NIH Pub No. 92-3465).

U.S. Centers for Disease Control and Prevention
1600 Clifton Road, NE
Atlanta, GA 30333
    "Important Facts About Childhood Lead Poisoning Prevention" (brochure).

SUGGESTED READINGS

American Academy of Pediatrics Committee on Environmental Health. Lead poisoning: from screening to primary prevention. Pediatrics 1993;92:176–183.

Preventing lead poisoning in young children. Atlanta: U.S. Centers for Disease Control and Prevention, 1991.

SCREENING SUGGESTIVE OF HEMATOLOGIC DISORDERS

Anemia (Table 17.15)

Table 17.15

Abnormal Screening Test Results	Diagnostic Studies That *May* Be Indicated	Treatment Options That *May* Be Indicated	Potential Referrals/ Consultations	Follow-Up
Low hemoglobin or hematocrit concentration	Complete blood count with peripheral smear Reticulocyte count Red-cell distribution width Iron, iron binding capacity, ferritin, transferrin Hemoglobin electrophoresis Thyroid function tests Folate/B_{12} Schilling test Lead level Coombs test Fecal occult blood test Bone marrow aspiration	Treatment of underlying cause Ferrous sulfate (for iron-deficiency anemia), folate/B_{12} for persons with deficiency, etc.	*Physicians:* Hematologist, pathologist, geneticist, gastroenterologist *Non-Physicians:* Dietitian	Hemoglobin/ hematocrit, nutrient status

RESOURCES—PATIENT EDUCATION MATERIALS

American Academy of Family Physicians
8880 Ward Parkway
Kansas City, MO 64114-2797
800-944-0000
    "Anemia: When Low Blood Iron Is The Cause" (brochure 1562).

SUGGESTED READINGS

Brown RG. Determining the cause of anemia: general approach, with emphasis on microcytic hypochromic anemias. Postgrad Med 1991;89(6):161–170.

Wintrobe MM, Lukens JN, Lee GR. The approach to the patient with anemia. In: Lee GR, Bithell TC, Foerster J, Athens JW, Lukens JN, eds. Clinical hematology, 9th ed. Malvern, PA: Lea & Febiger, 1993:715–744.

Hemoglobinopathies (Table 17.16)

Table 17.16

Abnormal Screening Test Results	Diagnostic Studies That *May* Be Indicated	Treatment Options That *May* Be Indicated	Potential Referrals/ Consultations	Follow-Up
Abnormal hemoglobin electrophoresis, isoelectric focusing, or high-performance liquid chromatography	Hemoglobin analysis Complete blood count Iron studies	Genetic counseling Nutritional counseling Prophylactic penicillin therapy Pneumococcal vaccination Transfusion therapy Splenectomy Chelation therapy Folic acid supplementation Bone marrow transplantation Testing of family members	*Physicians:* Hematologist, pathologist, geneticist *Non-Physicians:* Social services	Periodic check-ups, routine childhood immunizations, need for social support services

RESOURCES—PATIENT EDUCATION MATERIALS

Agency for Health Care Policy and Research
Publications Clearinghouse
P.O. Box 8547
Silver Spring, MD 20907
800-358-9295
    "Sickle Cell Disease in Newborns and Infants" (93-0564).

March of Dimes Birth Defects Foundation
P.O. Box 1657
Wilkes-Barre, PA 18703
800-367-6630
    "Sickle Cell Disease" and "Thalassemia" (information sheets).

National Association for Sickle Cell Disease
800-421-8453

National Center for Education in Maternal and Child Health
2000 15th Street North, Suite 701
Arlington, VA 22201-2617
    "Parents Handbook for Sickle Cell Disease" (F060); "Thalassemia Among Asians" (English F043; Chinese F055; Korean F056; Laotian F057; Vietnamese F059).

SUGGESTED READINGS

Agency for Health Care Policy and Research. Clinical practice guideline for sickle cell disease: screening, diagnosis, management, and counseling in newborns and infants. AHCPR Pub. No. 93-0562. Rockville, MD: Agency for Health Care Policy and Research, 1993. (To order, call 800-358-9295.)

Giardina PJ, Hilgartner MW. Update on thalassemia. Pediatr Rev 1992;13:55–62.

Lukens JN. The thalassemias and related disorders: quantitative disorders of hemoglobin synthesis. In: Lee GR, Bithell TC, Foerster J, Athens JW, Lukens JN, eds. Clinical hematology, 9th ed. Malvern, PA: Lea & Febiger, 1993:1102–1145.

Management and therapy of sickle cell disease (booklet 92-2117). Bethesda, MD: National Heart, Lung, Blood Institute. (To order, call 301-951-3260.)

SCREENING SUGGESTIVE OF INFECTIOUS DISEASES

Syphilis (Table 17.17)

Table 17.17

Abnormal Screening Test Results	Diagnostic Studies That *May* Be Indicated	Treatment Options That *May* Be Indicated	Potential Referrals/ Consultations	Follow-Up
Positive Rapid Plasma Reagin (RPR) or Venereal Disease Research Laboratory (VDRL) test	Fluorescent treponemal antibody test-absorbed (FTA-ABS) Microhemagglutination assay for antibodies to *Treponema pallidum* (MHA-TP) Hemagglutination treponemal test for syphilis (HATTS) Darkfield examination/direct fluorescent antibody test of tissue or exudates Lumbar puncture HIV antibody Screening for other sexually transmitted diseases	Parenteral benzathine penicillin G Doxycycline Tetracycline Erythromycin Notification, evaluation and treatment of sexual partners (parents, if patient is child) Notification of health department	*Physicians:* Infectious disease specialist, neurologist, ophthalmologist *Non-Physicians:* Public health department, social worker, child protective services (if patient is child)	Serologic examinations

RESOURCES—PATIENT EDUCATION MATERIALS

American Social Health Association
P.O. Box 13827
Research Triangle Park, NC 27709-3827
919-361-8400
    "STD (VD): Questions and Answers" (English, Spanish).

Channing L. Bete Co., Inc.
200 State Road
South Deerfield, MA 01373-0200
800-628-7733
    "What Everyone Should Know About Syphilis and Gonorrhea" (brochure T38414A).

Krames Communications
1100 Grundy Lane
San Bruno, CA 94066-3030
800-333-3032
> "Sexually Transmitted Diseases" (booklet 1181); "Condoms and STDs" (booklet, English 1422; Spanish 1423); "Safer Sex" (booklet 1267).

National Institute of Allergy and Infectious Diseases
Office of Communications
National Institutes of Health
Bethesda, MD 20892
301-496-5717
> "Syphilis" (brochure 92-909I); "An Introduction to Sexually Transmitted Diseases" (brochure 92-909A).

National STD Hotline
800-227-8922

SUGGESTED READINGS

U.S. Centers for Disease Control and Prevention. 1993 sexually transmitted diseases treatment guidelines. MMWR 1993;42(RR-14).

Gonorrhea (Table 17.18)

Table 17.18

Abnormal Screening Test Results	Diagnostic Studies That *May* Be Indicated	Treatment Options That *May* Be Indicated	Potential Referrals/ Consultations	Follow-Up
Positive gonorrhea culture or indirect assay	Rapid Plasma Reagin (RPR)/ Venereal Disease Research Laboratory (VDRL) test HIV test Chlamydia screening	*Antibiotic therapy* Ceftriaxone Cefixime Ciprofloxacin Ofloxacin Sexual abstinence during treatment Notification, evaluation, and treatment of sexual partners (parents, if patient is child) Notification of health department	*Physicians:* Infectious disease specialist, gynecologist *Non-Physicians:* Public health department, social worker, child protective services (if patient is child)	Clinical monitoring

RESOURCES—PATIENT EDUCATION MATERIALS

American Social Health Association
P.O. Box 13827
Research Triangle Park, NC 27709
919-361-8400

"Stopping Gonorrhea, The Clap" (brochure): "STD (VD): Questions and Answers" (English, Spanish).

Channing L. Bete Co., Inc.
200 State Road
South Deerfield, MA 01373-0200
800-628-7733
"What Everyone Should Know About Syphilis and Gonorrhea" (brochure T38414A).

Krames Communications
1100 Grundy Lane
San Bruno, CA 94066-3030
800-333-3032
"Sexually Transmitted Diseases" (booklet 1181); "Condoms and STDs" (booklet, English 1422; Spanish 1423); "Safer Sex" (booklet 1267).

National Institute of Allergy and Infectious Diseases
Office of Communications
National Institutes of Health
Bethesda, MD 20892
301-496-5717
"Gonorrhea" (brochure 92-909D); "An Introduction to Sexually Transmitted Diseases" (brochure 92-909A).

National STD Hotline
800-227-8922

SUGGESTED READINGS

U.S. Centers for Disease Control and Prevention. 1993 sexually transmitted diseases treatment guidelines. MMWR 1993;42(RR-14).

Chlamydia (Table 17.19)

Table 17.19

Abnormal Screening Test Results	Diagnostic Studies That *May* Be Indicated	Treatment Options That *May* Be Indicated	Potential Referrals/ Consultations	Follow-Up
Positive chlamydial culture or indirect assay	Chlamydial cell culture Nonculture test (repeat) Screening for HIV/other sexually transmitted diseases	*Antibiotic therapy* Doxycycline Ofloxacin Erythromycin Azithromycin Sexual abstinence during treatment Notification, evaluation, and treatment of sexual partners (parents, if patient is child) Notification of health department	*Physicians:* Infectious disease specialist *Non-Physicians:* Public health department, social worker, child protective services (if patient is child)	Repeat chlamydial culture

RESOURCES—PATIENT EDUCATION MATERIALS

American Social Health Association
P.O. Box 13827
Research Triangle Park, NC 27709-3827
919-361-8400
   "Some Questions and Answers About Chlamydia" (brochure); "Some Questions and Answers About NGU" (brochure); "STD (VD): Questions and Answers" (English, Spanish).

Channing L. Bete Co., Inc.
200 State Road
South Deerfield, MA 01373-0200
800-628-7733
   "What Everyone Should Know About Chlamydia" (brochure T14738A).

Krames Communications
1100 Grundy Lane
San Bruno, CA 94066-3030
800-333-3032
   "Sexually Transmitted Diseases" (booklet 1181); "Condoms and STDs" (booklet, English 1422; Spanish 1423); "Safer Sex" (booklet 1267).

National Institute of Allergy and Infectious Diseases
Office of Communications
National Institutes of Health
Bethesda, MD 20892
301-496-5717
   "Chlamydia" (brochure 92-909B); "An Introduction to Sexually Transmitted Diseases" (brochure 92-909A).

National STD Hotline
800-227-8922

SUGGESTED READINGS

Majeroni BA. Chlamydial cervicitis: complications and new treatment options. Am Fam Phys 1994;49:1825–1829.
U.S. Centers for Disease Control and Prevention. 1993 sexually transmitted diseases treatment guidelines. MMWR 1993;42(RR-14).
U.S. Centers for Disease Control and Prevention. Recommendations for the prevention and management of Chlamydia trachomatis infections, 1993. MMWR 1993;42(RR-12).

Human Immunodeficiency Virus (HIV) Infection (Table 17.20)

Table 17.20

Abnormal Screening Test Results	Diagnostic Studies That *May* Be Indicated	Treatment Options That *May* Be Indicated	Potential Referrals/ Consultations	Follow-Up
Confirmed Western blot/ immuno- fluorescent antibody test	CD4 T-lymphocyte count Complete blood count Chemistry panel Hepatitis B serology Toxoplasmosis titer Rapid Plasma Reagin (RPR)/ Venereal Disease Research Laboratory (VDRL) test Purified protein derivative (PPD)/anergy panel Papanicolaou smear Psychosocial evaluation	Posttest counseling Mental health treatment/crisis management Case management services Influenza, pneumococcal, hepatitis B, tetanus, mumps, rubella, measles, *Haemophilus influenza* type b vaccination *Antiretroviral therapy* Zidovudine (AZT) Didanosine (ddI) Zalcitabine (ddC) Stavudine *Pneumocystis carinii pneumonia prophylaxis* Trimethoprim- sulfamethoxazole Dapsone Aerosolized pentamidine isethionate Pyrimethamine- sulfadoxine *Toxoplasma gondii prophylaxis* Trimethoprim- sulfamethoxazole	*Physicians:* Infectious disease specialist, ophthalmologist, dermatologist, gastro- enterologist, neurologist, psychiatrist *Non-Physicians:* Local HIV case managment program, public health department, psychologist, social services, home care, dietitian	CD4 cell counts, complete blood count, Papanicolaou smear, psychosocial assessment, behaviors to reduce risk of transmission

Table 17.20—*continued*

Abnormal Screening Test Results	Diagnostic Studies That *May* Be Indicated	Treatment Options That *May* Be Indicated	Potential Referrals/ Consultations	Follow-Up
		Dapsone- pyrimethamine *Mycobacterium avium intracellulare prophylaxis* Rifabutin Isoniazid chemoprophylaxis Notification of health department Referral of sexual/ needle partner, children, parents (if patient is young child)		

RESOURCES—PATIENT EDUCATION MATERIALS

CDC National AIDS Hotline
800-342-AIDS(English)
800-344-SIDA (Spanish)
800-AIDS-TTY (TDD/TTY)

Pediatric and Pregnancy AIDS Hotline
212-430-3333

National Pediatric HIV Resource Center
800-362-0071

AIDS Clinical Trials Information Service
800-TRIALS-A

Agency for Health Care Policy and Research
Publications Clearinghouse
P.O. Box 8547
Silver Spring, MD 20907
800-358-9295
    "Understanding HIV" (brochure 94-0574); "HIV and Your Child" (brochure 94-0576).

American Red Cross
General Supply Division
7401 Lockport Place
Lorton, VA 22079
800-969-8890
    "Living With HIV Infection" (brochure 329548).

Krames Communications
1100 Grundy Lane
San Bruno, CA 94066-3030
800-333-3032
    "Understanding HIV Infection and AIDS" (booklet English 1231; Spanish 1265).

National Institute of Allergy and Infectious Diseases
Office of Communications
Building 31, Room 7A50
9000 Rockville Pike
Bethesda, MD 20892
301-496-5717
   "Testing Positive for HIV: How To Help Yourself" (booklet, NIH Publication No. 93-3323); "HIV Infection and AIDS" (brochure 92-909F).

RESOURCES—PROFESSIONAL EDUCATION

American Academy of Family Physicians
HIV Telephone Consultation Service
800-933-3413
   Every state also has an AIDS hotline with information about HIV-specific resources, counseling, and testing services.

U.S. Centers for Disease Control and Prevention
National AIDS Clearinghouse
P.O. Box 6003
Rockville, MD 20849-6003
800-458-5231

SUGGESTED READINGS

Agency for Health Care Policy and Research. Managing early HIV infection: quick reference guide for clinicians. AHCPR Pub. No. 94-0573. Rockville, MD: Agency for Health Care Policy and Research, 1994. (Order free copies at 800-342-AIDS or 800-358-9295.)

Gallant JE, Moore RD, Chaisson RE. Prophylaxis for opportunistic infections in patients with HIV infection. Ann Intern Med 1994;120:932–944.

Infectious Disease Clinics of North America 1994;8(2): (Entire issue devoted to management of infection in HIV disease).

U.S. Centers for Disease Control and Prevention. Public Health Service guidelines for counseling and antibody testing to prevent HIV infection and AIDS. MMWR 1987;36:509–515.

U.S. Centers for Disease Control and Prevention. Guidelines for prophylaxis against pneumocystis carinii pneumonia for persons infected with human immunodeficiency virus. MMWR 1989;38:S-5.

U.S. Centers for Disease Control and Prevention. Guidelines for prevention of transmission of human immunodeficiency virus and hepatitis B virus to health-care and public-safety workers. MMWR 1989;38(Suppl 6):1–37. (Published erratum appears in MMWR 1989;38:746.).

U.S. Centers for Disease Control and Prevention. 1993 revised classification system for HIV infection and expanded surveillance case definition for AIDS among adolescents and adults. MMWR 1992;41(RR-17).

U.S. Centers for Disease Control and Prevention. Recommendations of the Advisory Committee on Immunization Practices (ACIP): use of vaccines and immune globulins in persons with altered immunocompetence. MMWR 1993;42(RR-4).

U.S. Centers for Disease Control and Prevention. 1993 sexually transmitted diseases treatment guidelines. MMWR 1993;42(RR-14).

U.S. Centers for Disease Control and Prevention. 1994 revised guidelines for the performance of CD4+ T-cell determinations in persons with human immunodeficiency virus (HIV) infections. MMWR 1994;43(RR-3).

Tuberculosis (Table 17.21)

Table 17.21

Abnormal Screening Test Results	Diagnostic Studies That *May* Be Indicated	Treatment Options That *May* Be Indicated	Potential Referrals/ Consultations	Follow-Up
Reactive tuberculin skin test	Mantoux test (for persons with positive multiple-puncture test) Isolation/culture of *M. tuberculosis* Drug-susceptibility testing Chest radiograph Sputum cytology HIV antibody	Isoniazid Rifampin Ethambutol Pyrazinamide Directly observed therapy Notification of health department	*Physicians:* Infectious disease specialist, pulmonologist *Non-Physicians:* Public health department, social services, community outreach workers	Clinical monitoring

RESOURCES—PATIENT EDUCATION MATERIALS

American Academy of Pediatrics
Publications Department
141 Northwest Point Blvd.
P.O. Box 927
Elk Grove Village, IL 60009-0927
800-433-9016
   "Patient Medication Instructions: Isoniazid" (PM1015).

American Lung Association
1740 Broadway
New York, NY 10019
212-315-8700, 800-586-4872
   "Facts About Tuberculosis" (brochure 1091).

Krames Communications
1100 Grundy Lane
San Bruno, CA 94066-3030
800-333-3032
   "Understanding Tuberculosis" (brochure, English 9863; Spanish 9864).

RESOURCES—PROFESSIONAL EDUCATION

American Thoracic Society
1740 Broadway
New York, NY 10019-4374

U.S. Centers for Disease Control and Prevention
National Center for Prevention Services
Division of Tuberculosis Elimination
Atlanta, GA 30333

SUGGESTED READINGS

Advisory Council for the Elimination of Tuberculosis. Initial therapy for tuberculosis in the era of multidrug resistance. MMWR 1993;42(RR-7).
American Thoracic Society. Treatment of tuberculosis and tuberculosis infection in adults and children. Am J Respir Crit Care Med 1994;149:1359–1374.
Ciesielski SD. BCG vaccination and the PPD test: what the clinician needs to know. J Fam Pract 1995;40:76–80.

SCREENING SUGGESTIVE OF HEARING AND VISION DISORDERS

Abnormal Hearing (Table 17.22)

Table 17.22

Abnormal Screening Test Results	Diagnostic Studies That *May* Be Indicated	Treatment Options That *May* Be Indicated	Potential Referrals/ Consultations	Follow-Up
Abnormal hearing examination/ audiometry/ newborn screening	Audiometry Speech recognition threshold Brainstem auditory evoked responses Tympanogram Rapid Plasma Reagin (RPR)/ Venereal Disease Research Laboratory (VDRL) test Rubella (newborns)	Antibiotics (children) Tympanostomy (children) Hearing aids (analog, hybrid, digital) *Assistive devices* Listening devices Alerting devices Signaling devices Telecommunications devices for the deaf (TDD) Information devices Cochlear implants Referral to community resources	*Physicians:* Otolaryngologist, neurologist *Non-Physicians:* Audiologist, speech-language pathologist, school system. Information about local speech-language pathologists and audiologists can be obtained by calling the American Speech-Language-Hearing Association HELPLINE, 800-638-8255 (voice or TDD), 301-897-8682 (Maryland, Alaska, Hawaii)	Hearing threshold, fit and function of hearing aid, speech and language development (children), school performance (children)

RESOURCES—PATIENT EDUCATION MATERIALS

American-Speech-Language-Hearing Association
10801 Rockville Pike
Rockville, MD 20852
800-638-8255, 301-897-5700

"Treatment for Hearing Problems," "Hearing Impairment and the Audiologist," "Can We Talk? A Guide to Your Child's Speech and Hearing," "How Does Your

Child Hear and Talk?," "How to Buy a Hearing Aid," "Noise In Your Workplace" (brochures).

Krames Communications
1100 Grundy Lane
San Bruno, CA 94066-3030
800-333-3032
"Hearing Aids: A Guide to their Wear and Care" (booklet 1045).

National Institute on Deafness and Other Communication Disorders Information Clearinghouse
1 Communications Avenue
Bethesda, MD 20892-3456
800-241-1044, 800-241-1055 (TTY)
"Hearing and Hearing Loss" (information packet DC-103); "Hearing and Older People" (fact sheet DC-24); "Deafness, Hearing, and Hearing Disorders Organizational Resources, 1994" (DC-84); information for physicians also available.

SUGGESTED READINGS

Joint Committee on Infant Hearing. Joint Committee on Infant Hearing 1994 position statement. Pediatrics 1995;95:152–156.
Zazove P, Kileny PR. Devices for the hearing impaired. Am Fam Phys 1992;46:851–858.

Impaired Visual Acuity (Table 17.23)

Table 17.23

Abnormal Screening Test Results	Diagnostic Studies That *May* Be Indicated	Treatment Options That *May* Be Indicated	Potential Referrals/ Consultations	Follow-Up
Abnormal visual acuity testing	Formal acuity testing Ophthalmoscopy Retinoscopy Visual evoked response testing Visual field/ perimetry	Corrective lenses Treatment of underlying cause of amblyopia Patching Strabismus surgery	*Physicians:* Ophthalmologist *Non-Physicians:* Optometrist, optician, school system, speech-language therapist	Visual acuity, ocular alignment (children)

RESOURCES—PATIENT EDUCATION MATERIALS

American Academy of Pediatrics
Publications Department
141 Northwest Point Blvd.
P.O. Box 927
Elk Grove Village, IL 60009-0927
800-433-9016
"Your Child's Eyes" (brochure HE0143).

American Optometric Association
243 North Lindbergh Boulevard
St. Louis, MO 63141
  "Answers to Questions About Common Vision Conditions" (brochure).

Krames Communications
1100 Grundy Lane
San Bruno, CA 94066-3030
800-333-3032
  "Total Eye Care" (booklet 1322); "A Guide to Understanding Strabismus and Amblyopia" (booklet 1010).

National Institute on Aging
NIA Information Center
P.O. Box 8057
Gaithersburg, MD 20898-8057
800-222-2225
  "Aging and Your Eyes."

SUGGESTED READINGS

Newell FW. Ophthalmology: principles and concepts, 7th ed. St. Louis: Mosby Year Book,
  1992:409–422.
Rubin SE, Nelson LB. Amblyopia: diagnosis and management. Ped Clin N Amer
  1993;40:727–735.

SCREENING SUGGESTIVE OF DEVELOPMENTAL DISORDERS

Abnormal growth and development (Table 17.24)

Table 17.24

Abnormal Screening Test Results	Diagnostic Studies That *May* Be Indicated	Treatment Options That *May* Be Indicated	Potential Referrals/ Consultations	Follow-Up
History or physical examination findings or developmental screening suggestive of developmental disorder	Complete blood count Chemistry panel Lead level Metabolic screening Thyroid function tests Chromosomal testing Urinalysis Stool analysis Upper/lower gastrointestinal imaging Electroencephalogram Cerebral imaging Psychometric testing Hearing/vision assessment Family assessment	Nutritional counseling Maternal/ family counseling Treatment of underlying cause of develop- mental delay or failure to thrive	*Physicians:* Orthopedic surgeon, physiatrist, geneticist, ophthalmologist, otolaryngologist, child neurologist, child psychiatrist *Non-Physicians:* Speech-language therapist, nurse, dietitian, social worker, physical therapist, occupational therapist, psychologist, special educator, school system	Anthropometric measurements, behavior, psychometric testing

RESOURCES—PATIENT EDUCATION MATERIALS

American Academy of Pediatrics
Publications Department
141 Northwest Point Blvd.
P.O. Box 927
Elk Grove Village, IL 60009-0927
800-433-9016
  "Learning Disabilities and Children: What Parents Need to Know" (brochure HE0063).

March of Dimes Birth Defects Foundation
P.O. Box 1657
Wilkes-Barre, Pennsylvania, 18703
800-367-6630

National Institute of Mental Health
5600 Fishers Lane, Room 15C05
Rockville, MD 20857
301-443-4513
  "Learning Disabilities" (NIH Publ No. 93-3611).

National Institute on Deafness and Other Communication Disorders Information
Clearinghouse
1 Communications Avenue
Bethesda, MD 20892-3456
800-241-1044, 800-241-1055 (TTY)
 "Update on Developmental Speech and Language Disorders" (DC-76).

SUGGESTED READINGS

First LR, Palfrey JS. The infant or young child with developmental delay. N Engl J Med 1994;330:478–483.
Levy SE, Hyman SL. Pediatric assessment of the child with developmental delay. Ped Clin N Amer 1993;40:465–477.

18. Immunizations

STEVEN H. WOOLF

INTRODUCTION

Immunizations are one of the most successful examples of the primary prevention of disease. Infectious diseases that were, at the turn of the century, the leading causes of childhood death and disability are now relatively rare in the United States. Vaccination programs have been responsible for the global eradication of smallpox and are close to eliminating others (e.g., poliomyelitis) in the near future. Unfortunately, the reduced incidence in the United States of such diseases as pertussis and measles, achieved through decades of organized efforts to vaccinate children, has led to complacency among many clinicians and public officials regarding the continued importance of vaccinations. In recent years, this attitude and certain social policies have led to unfortunate lapses in immunization coverage and to the inevitable and unnecessary resurgence of these dangerous diseases.

For many years, inadequate immunization coverage among preschool children has been a particular problem in the United States, which has had lower early childhood immunization rates than virtually any other industrialized nation (and a large number of developing countries) (1). A nine-city survey in 1991 found that only 10–38% of two-year-old children were properly immunized (2). Recent surveys have shown higher coverage, perhaps in response to a national initiative to increase preschool immunization; as of 1993, 67% of two-year-old children had been completely immunized (3). Inadequate immunization coverage is not limited to children. The current burden of suffering from vaccine-preventable diseases may even be higher in adults. An estimated 50,000–70,000 adults die each year in the United States from pneumococcal infection, influenza, and hepatitis B, whereas fewer than 100 children die annually from diseases targeted by childhood immunizations.

The causes of inadequate immunization are multifactorial, including limited access to immunization services, vaccine cost, and patient disinterest. One of the most disturbing barriers to adequate immunization, however, is the failure of health professionals to recognize when patients need to be immunized. In 1988, 60% of the infants who had not been adequately immunized had completed three well-child visits by eight months of age (4). This problem has many elements. First, many providers do not routinely check the immunization status of patients. Second, clinicians are often unclear about who and when to immunize, due in part to frequent changes in recommendations and vaccine products. The recommended childhood immunization schedule has undergone major revisions six times since 1989, due to changes in schedules, numbers of recommended doses, and the introduction of new vaccines.

A third cause of provider failures in vaccinating patients is misconceptions about contraindications. Vaccinations are often inappropriately postponed by physicians because children have mild illnesses, low-grade fever, or other innocuous symptoms. Misconceptions about contraindications appear to be common. A survey of primary care physicians found that 27% would incorrectly defer diphtheria-tetanus-pertussis (DTP) vaccination in a child with allergic rhinitis and that 45% would not offer the vaccine if the child had developed a fever of 103°F after the preceding immunization. About 40% believed incorrectly that a child whose mother is pregnant should not receive measles-mumps-rubella (MMR) vaccine and that simultaneous administration of multiple vaccines (DTP, oral trivalent live attenuated poliomyelitis [OPV] vaccine, MMR, *Haemophilus influenzae* type b [HiB]) was contraindicated (1). Another study of a measles outbreak revealed that 38% of the patients who acquired measles had been immunized previously with trivalent OPV and/or DTP at a time when MMR could have been given, suggesting that the providers were under the mistaken impression that MMR was contraindicated (5).

Finally, providers can contribute to poor immunization coverage by failing to emphasize its importance with patients. Studies suggest that the physician's attitude can play an important role in patient compliance. In one survey, 28% of parents cited the physician's recommendation as the reason they had their children immunized with DTP. Of those who decided against immunization, 16% indicated that they were waiting for their physician's approval and 4% reported that their physician had advised against the immunization (6).

This chapter reviews the indications and contraindications for routine childhood and adult vaccinations. It focuses on commonly used vaccines in the primary care setting and those that offer the greatest protective public health benefits among asymptomatic persons. Vaccines for selected population groups (e.g., rabies vaccine), for international travelers, and for postexposure prophylaxis are not emphasized. Patients with altered immune competence (e.g., patients with cancer, acquired immunodeficiency syndrome) require special immunization protocols (7) that are not discussed in this chapter. This chapter also does not discuss vaccination of persons with acute illnesses or of pregnant women, outside of standard contraindications.

The recommendations in this chapter are generally consistent with the guidelines issued by major authorities (Advisory Committee on Immunization Practices of the Centers for Disease Control and Prevention, American Academy of Pediatrics, American College of Physicians, American Academy of Family Physicians, U.S. Preventive Services Task Force) at the time of publication; important differences in official recommendations are noted below in discussions of specific vaccines. Because of the frequency with which vaccine products and recommendations undergo change, however, readers are encouraged to consult current guidelines for further details.

GENERAL PRINCIPLES

Vaccines are generally recommended for age groups at risk for the disease at the youngest age at which a person is known to develop an adequate postvaccination antibody response. Suggested ages for childhood immunizations (Table 18.1) are approximate and not mandatory (e.g., most immunizations recommended for infants at two months of age can be given at 6–10 weeks of age). Nonetheless, immunizations should generally be given at the earliest recommended age at which the child presents to the clinician. Partial doses or doses given too frequently may dampen the antibody response and should not be counted as part of a primary series. It is unnecessary to restart an interrupted series of a vaccine or toxoid or to add extra doses. Intramuscular injections are generally administered in the anterolateral aspect of the thigh in infants and in the deltoid muscle in older children and adults; they should not be administered in the gluteal muscles at any age. Further details about vaccine handling and injection technique are provided in the references at the end of this chapter.

Simultaneous administration of most vaccines does not impair antibody responses or increase rates of adverse reactions (8). In fact, simultaneous administration is an important public health strategy, potentially increasing immunization coverage by an estimated 9–17% (9). Immune globulin may interfere with viral replication and antibody response of certain live virus vaccines. Administration of MMR or its component vaccines should be delayed for 3–11 months after the administration of immune globulins, depending on the type of preparation and its dose; specific guidelines for spacing administration are provided elsewhere (10). If MMR vaccination precedes immune globulin administration, it need not be readministered if the interval between immunizations is longer than 14 days.

Appropriate contraindications to vaccination are listed in Table 18.2. It is important for the clinician to recognize that mild illnesses, low-grade fever, penicillin allergy, prematurity, family history of allergies, and current antibiotic therapy are generally *unfounded reasons for deferring vaccina-*

Table 18.1
Childhood Immunization Schedule

Vaccine	Dose (ml)	Birth	2 Months	4 Months	6 Months	12 Months	15 Months	4–6 Years	11–16 Years
DTP	0.5/i.m.		DTP-1	DTP-2	DTP-3		DTP-4[a]	DTP-5[a]	Td
OPV	0.5/p.o.		OPV-1	OPV-2	OPV-3[b]			OPV-4	
MMR	0.5/s.c.						MMR[c]		MMR[d]
HiB	0.5/i.m.								
HbOC			HiB-1	HiB-2	HiB-3		HiB-4		
PRP-T			HiB-1	HiB-2	HiB-3		HiB-4		
PRP-OMP			HiB-1	HiB-2			HiB-3		
		Birth (before hospital discharge)	1–2 Months	4 Months	6–18 Months				
HBV	See								
Option 1	Table	HBV-1	HBV-2			HBV-3			
Option 2	18.6		HBV-1	HBV-2		HBV-3			

Adapted from U.S. Centers for Disease Control and Prevention. General recommendations on immunization: recommendations of the Advisory Committee on Immunization Practices. MMWR 1994;43:RR-1.

Legend: DTP = *Diphtheria-tetanus-pertussis toxoid*; OPV = *Trivalent oral polio vaccine*; inactivated polio vaccine is indicated for some high-risk children (see text); MMR = *Measles-mumps-rubella vaccine*; HiB = *Haemophilus influenzae type b*; HbOC = HibTITER; Lederle-Praxis Biologicals; PRP-T = ActHIB, OmniHIB; Pasteur Merieux, SmithKline Beecham, Connaught; PRP-OMP = PedvaxHIB; Merck Sharp and Dohme; i.m. = *intramuscular*, s.c. = *subcutaneous*; p.o. = *oral*.

[a]This dose can be administered as early as 12 months of age, provided that the interval since the previous DTP dose is at least six months, and some experts recommend giving this dose at 18 months of age. Diphtheria, tetanus, and *acellular* pertussis (DTaP) vaccine is preferred over whole-cell vaccine for the 4th and 5th doses of the DTP series. DTaP is only licensed for use at 15 months of age or greater.

[b]This dose may be administered at 6–18 months of age.

[c]Measles vaccination may begin as young as six months in outbreak areas where cases are occurring among children less than one year of age. Children vaccinated before their first birthday, however, should be revaccinated at 12–15 months of age (with a spacing of at least one month after the first dose) and should receive the customary second dose before school entry. *Varicella vaccine*, which was licensed shortly before publication of this book, is recommended for children 12–18 months of age, preferably at the same time that MMR is administered.

[d]The second dose of MMR should be administered *either* at 4–6 years of age (generally before entry to primary school) or at 11–12 years of age (generally before entry to middle or junior high school). Physicians should check state statutes regarding specific school requirements.

tion. Anaphylactic reactions to certain vaccines (e.g., DTP, hepatitis B vaccine) or vaccine components have been reported on rare occasions. Hypersensitivity to vaccines can occur in reaction to vaccine antigen, animal proteins, antibiotics (e.g., neomycin), preservatives (e.g., thimerosal), or stabilizers contained in the vaccine. The most common animal protein allergen is egg protein, which is present in measles, mumps, influenza, and

Table 18.2
Contraindications, Precautions, and Misconceptions Regarding Childhood Immunizations

Vaccine	Contraindications	Precautions[a]	Incorrect Contraindications
All	Anaphylactic reaction to a vaccine or its constituent		Mild-moderate local reaction (soreness, redness, swelling) following a dose
	Moderate or severe illnesses, with or without a fever		Mild acute illness, with or without a low-grade fever
			Current antimicrobial therapy
			Convalescent phase of illnesses
			Prematurity
			Recent exposure to an infectious disease
			History of penicillin or other nonspecific allergies, or family history of such allergies
DTP/DTaP	Encephalopathy within 7 days of administration of previous dose	History of fever > 105°F, collapse or shock-like state (hypotonic-hyporesponsive episode), or inconsolable crying lasting ≥ 3 hrs during a 48-hour period after receiving DTP or DTaP	Fever < 105°F or high-pitched cry following previous dose
			Family history of seizures
		History of seizures withín 3 days of receiving DTP or DTaP[b]	Family history of adverse event following DTP administration
			Family history of sudden infant death syndrome
OPV	Known altered immunodeficiency (e.g., HIV infection) or household contact with immunodeficient person	Pregnancy	Breastfeeding
			Current antimicrobial therapy
			Diarrhea

Vaccine	True contraindications	Precautions	Not contraindications (may be vaccinated)
IPV	Anaphylactic reaction to neomycin or streptomycin	Pregnancy	Breastfeeding Current antimicrobial therapy Diarrhea
MMR	Anaphylactic reaction to egg ingestion or neomycin[c] Pregnancy Known altered immunodeficiency (except HIV infection)	Recent immune globulin administration[d] Thrombocytopenia	Tuberculosis, or positive tuberculin skin test Simultaneous tuberculin skin testing[e] Breastfeeding Pregnancy of recipient's mother Immunodeficient family member or household contact HIV infection Nonanaphylactic reactions to egg or neomycin
HiB	None identified	None identified	History of HiB disease
HBV	Anaphylactic reaction to common baker's yeast	None identified	Pregnancy

Adapted from Ad Hoc Working Group for the Development of Standards for Pediatric Immunization Practices. Standards for pediatric immunization practices. JAMA 1993;269:1817–22; U.S. Centers for Disease Control and Prevention. General recommendations on immunization: recommendations of the Advisory Committee on Immunization Practices. MMWR 1994;43:RR-1. Legend: DTP = Diphtheria-tetanus-pertussis (whole cell) toxoid; DTaP = Diphtheria-tetanus-pertussis (acellular) toxoid; OPV = Trivalent oral polio vaccine; IPV = Inactivated polio vaccine; MMR = Measles-mumps-rubella vaccine; HiB = Haemophilus influenzae type b vaccine; HBV = Hepatitis B vaccine.

[a]Although not a contraindication, the benefits and risks of administering the vaccine under these conditions should be carefully reviewed. Some of these precautions were once considered absolute contraindications.

[b]Whether and when to administer DTP to children with proven or suspected neurologic disorders should be decided on an individual basis.

[c]Persons with a history of anaphylactic reactions following egg ingestion should be vaccinated only with extreme caution. Protocols developed for such patients should be consulted (J Pediatr 1983;102:196–199; J Pediatr 1988;113:504–506).

[d]The number of months required depends on the type and dose of immune globulin; see MMWR 1994;43(RR-1):15–17.

[e]Measles vaccination may temporarily suppress tuberculin reactivity. If testing cannot be done on the day of MMR vaccination, the test should be postponed for 4–6 weeks.

other vaccines. Most patients who are able to eat eggs safely may receive these vaccines. They are, however, contraindicated in most persons with a history of anaphylactic reactions to egg products, including a history of hives, swelling of the mouth or throat, difficulty breathing, hypotension, or shock; protocols have been developed to vaccinate such persons (11). Neomycin-containing antibiotics are contraindicated in persons with a history of anaphylactic reactions to neomycin. The most common allergy to neomycin, delayed-type hypersensitivity manifested as contact dermatitis, is not a contraindication to receiving these vaccines.

PARENTAL EDUCATION AND COUNSELING

Many children do not receive vaccines because their parents or guardians do not appreciate the importance of immunizations, timely administration, or maintaining complete personal immunization records. It is therefore important for clinicians to explain the purpose of immunizations, the diseases that they prevent, and the rationale for the recommended immunization schedules. They should be counseled about the importance of obtaining immunizations at the recommended ages and should be urged to bring the child's immunization record to each visit. As with other forms of patient education, counseling about immunizations should be culturally sensitive. Children with inadequate immunization coverage often come from families of low socioeconomic status; their parents may have low educational levels or may not understand the clinician's language. Clinicians should take special measures under these circumstances (e.g., obtaining assistance from translators) to ensure that parents obtain accurate information.

Federal legislation (National Childhood Vaccine Injury Act) has required since 1992 the distribution of vaccine information pamphlets before administering measles, mumps, rubella, diphtheria, tetanus, pertussis, or polio vaccines. Specially prepared "Vaccine Information Statements" developed by the U.S. Centers for Disease Control of Prevention must be used (a provision that allowed private physicians to develop their own versions of the pamphlet was terminated in 1994). The mandated educational materials provide information about the disease, the benefits and harms of the vaccine, the recommended immunization schedule, indications for delaying or not administering the vaccine, potential postimmunization complications and ways to reduce them, and addresses and telephone numbers for reporting adverse effects (if the physician fails to do so) and for obtaining federal compensation under the National Vaccine Injury Compensation Program. Information statements for hepatitis B and HiB vaccines are available for optional use. The pamphlets are available in English, Spanish, French, and Vietnamese. Further information about these requirements can be obtained from the National Immunization Program at the U.S. Centers for Disease Control and Prevention in Atlanta, GA.

Diphtheria-Tetanus-Pertussis (DTP) Vaccine

Since the introduction of the DTP vaccine in the late 1940s, diphtheria and tetanus have become rare diseases in the United States (less than five and about 50–70 cases per year, respectively), with most cases occurring in adults who have not completed a primary immunization series. Both diphtheria and tetanus are associated with high case-fatality rates (5–10% and 25–30%, respectively). Booster doses every 10 years are recommended to maintain antibody levels, but there is little direct evidence that this practice reduces the incidence of clinical disease, since most tetanus cases occur in persons without a clear history of primary vaccination. Completion of the primary series in children and unimmunized adults is the important priority.

Pertussis is also considerably less common in the United States than in previous years, due largely to the efficacy of pertussis vaccine. Nonetheless, nearly 12,000 cases occurred in the United States during 1989–1991, and the highest annual total since 1967 (over 6,500 cases) occurred in 1993 (12). During this period, about two-thirds of cases among children under 4 years of age occurred in patients with inadequate immunization. Pertussis vaccination efforts have been curtailed in some communities because of public concerns about risks of neurologic complications from the vaccine. What is often less apparent to lay persons is that the disease itself poses a far greater risk to children than the vaccine. Nearly 70% of infants infected by pertussis require hospitalization (12). The importance of the vaccine has been underscored by the serious pertussis outbreaks that have occurred in communities and countries in which pertussis vaccination coverage has been reduced. Attack rates among children during these outbreaks have been directly related to the adequacy of vaccine coverage. During one outbreak, for example, the incidence of pertussis was 30%, 50%, and 82%, respectively, for children who had received three to five, one to two, or zero doses of pertussis vaccine (13). Long-term trends since 1976 suggest an overall increase in the incidence of pertussis.

Indications

DTP vaccination is indicated in all children, except those with the contraindications listed in Table 18.2, beginning at 6 weeks to 2 months of age. Because the vaccine may cause adverse reactions and because the incidence and severity of pertussis decreases with age, pertussis vaccination is not recommended after age 7. Tetanus-diphtheria (Td) toxoid boosters are indicated every 10 years in adolescents and adults who have completed a primary series.

Administration

The full DTP series consists of four doses, the first three doses given at four to eight-week intervals and the fourth dose given six to 12 months after the third dose (preferably at 15 months of age) to maintain adequate immunity during the preschool years. The recommended immunization schedule is presented in Table 18.1. Children who are behind on immunizations should be vaccinated according to the schedule in Table 18.3 if they are under age 7

Table 18.3
Recommended Schedule for Infants and Children under Age 7 Not Immunized at the Recommended Time in Early Infancy

Timing	Vaccine(s)	Comments
First visit: 2–11 months of age ≥ 12 months of age	DTP-1, OPV-1, HiB-1,[a] HBV-1 DTP-1, OPV-1, MMR-1, HiB-1,[a] HBV-1	DTP, OPV, MRR, and possibly HiB (see text) should be administered simultaneously if appropriate for age
Second visit: 1 month after first visit	DTP-2, HiB-2,[a] HBV-2	
Third visit: 1 month after second visit	DTP-3, HiB-3,[a] OPV-2	
Fourth visit: 6 weeks after third visit	OPV-3	
Fifth visit: ≥ 6 months after third visit	DTP-4,[b] HiB-4,[a] HBV-3	
Preschool (4–6 years)[c]	DTP-5,[b] OPV-4, MMR-2[d]	Preferably at or before school entry
14–16 years	Td	Repeat every 10 years throughout life

Adapted from U.S. Centers for Disease Control and Prevention. General recommendations on immunization: recommendations of the Advisory Committee on Immunization Practices. MMWR 1994;43:RR-1. *Legend*: DTP = *Diphtheria-tetanus-pertussis (whole cell) toxoid*; OPV = *Trivalent oral polio vaccine*; MMR = *Measles-mumps-rubella vaccine*; HiB = Haemophilus influenzae *type b vaccine*; HBV = *Hepatitis B vaccine*, Td = *Tetanus-diphtheria toxoid.*

[a]The number of required HiB doses in the initial series depends on the age of the child. Children 2–6 months of age require three doses, if HbOC or PRP-T is used, or two doses of PRP-OMP (see Table 18.1 for description of HiB vaccine product names). Children 7–11 months of age require two doses, and children 12–14 months of age require one dose. Children in all of these age groups (2–14 months of age) require a booster dose at 12–15 months of age (12–18 months for children who first present at 7–11 months of age), provided the booster is given at least two months after the prior dose. If the child is 15–59 months of age, only a single dose is required. HiB vaccine is generally not administered after the fifth birthday.

[b]Diphtheria, tetanus and *acellular* pertussis vaccine (DTaP) is preferred for the 4th and 5th doses.

[c]The preschool dose is not necessary if the fourth dose of DTP and third dose of OPV are administered after the fourth birthday.

[d]The second MMR dose may be given at entry to middle or junior high school (check state requirements for school entry).

or the schedule in Table 18.4 if they are age 7 or older. Adults should be immunized according to the schedule in Table 18.5.

Once the primary DTP series is started, interruptions in the recommended schedule or delays in administering subsequent doses do not require restarting the series. Thus, persons who received a partial series in the past need only complete the schedule. The booster (fifth) dose, which is normally given at age 4–6, is unnecessary if the fourth dose in the primary series is given after age 4.

Acellular pertussis vaccine (DTaP), which causes fewer side effects than whole-cell DTP, was licensed in 1991 as the preferred agent for the fourth and fifth doses in children previously vaccinated with whole-cell DTP. (Whole-cell vaccine can also be used for the fourth and fifth doses.) DTaP is not licensed for use in children less than 15 months or over 7 years of age. In 1993, the U.S. Food and Drug Administration licensed the use of combined diphtheria-tetanus (DT) toxoids, whole-cell pertussis, and HiB (TETRAMUNE, Lederle-Praxis; or PRP-T [ActHIB, OmniHIB; Pasteur Merieux, SmithKline Beecham, Connaught] reconstituted with DTP vaccine produced by Connaught) when indications for these vaccines coincide. Premature infants should be vaccinated at their chronological age from birth.

For reasons mentioned earlier, persons over age 7 should undergo primary immunization with the Td toxoid used for adults rather than with DTP. The first two doses can be given 4–8 weeks apart, and the third dose can be given 6–12 months after the second dose.

Table 18.4
Recommended Immunization Schedule for Children Beginning Immunizations at Age 7 or Older

Timing	Vaccine(s)
First visit	Td-1,[a] OPV-1,[b] MMR-1
Second visit: 6–8 weeks after first visit	Td-2, OPV-2,[b] MMR-2[c]
Third visit: 6 months after second visit	Td-3, OPV-3[b]
10 years after Td-3 and every 10 years thereafter	Td

Adapted from U.S. Centers for Disease Control and Prevention. General recommendations on immunization: recommendations of the Advisory Committee on Immunization Practices. MMWR 1994;43:RR-1. *Legend*: Td = *Tetanus-diphtheria-toxoid*; OPV = *Trivalent oral polio vaccine*; MMR = *Measles-mumps-rubella vaccine*.

[a]DTP doses given to children under age 7 who remain incompletely immunized at age 7 or older should be counted as prior Td exposures (e.g., a child who previously received two doses of DTP needs one dose of Td to complete a primary series).

[b]When polio vaccine is given to individuals age 18 or older, inactivated polio virus is preferred. OPV-3 may be given as soon as 6 weeks after OPV-2.

[c]The second dose is indicated for children with no documentation of live measles vaccination after the first birthday and should be given at least one month after the first dose.

Table 18.5
Immunization Schedule for Adults[a]

Vaccine	Indications	Dose (ml)/Route	Schedule	Contraindications
Td	*Primary series*: adults who have not received a primary series *Booster*: all adults	0.5/i.m.	*Primary series*: 2 doses, 1–2 mos apart, 3rd dose 6–12 mos later *Booster*: every 10 years[b]	History of neurologic reaction or severe hypersensitivity after prior dose
HiB	May be considered in splenic dysfunction or HIV infection	0.5/i.m.[c]	One dose	History of anaphylactic reaction to vaccine or its constituents; moderate or severe illnesses
Influenza	Adults age 65 and older, other persons at increased risk of complications from influenza (see text)	0.5/i.m.	Annual dose in fall (see text)	Anaphylactic allergy to eggs[d]; acute febrile illness
Pneumococcal polysaccharide	Adults age 65 and older, other persons at increased risk of pneumococcal disease and its complications (see text)	0.5/s.c. or i.m.	One dose[e]	Known hypersensitivity to vaccine components; less than six years since prior pneumococcal vaccination
Measles	Adults without evidence of immunity (see text); persons given killed measles vaccine, 1963–1967	0.5/s.c.	One dose[f]	Anaphylactic reaction to egg ingestion or neomycin[d]; pregnancy; known immunodeficiency (except HIV infection)
Mumps	Adults without evidence of immunity (see text)	0.5/s.c.	One dose	Anaphylactic reaction to egg ingestion or neomycin[d]; pregnancy; known immunodeficiency (except some persons with HIV infection)

Rubella	Adults, especially women of childbearing age, without documented immunity (see text)	0.5/s.c.	One dose	Pregnancy; anaphylactic reaction to neomycin; immune deficiency (except HIV infection); acute febrile illness
Inactivated Polio	Unimmunized or partially immunized adults	0.5/s.c. (inactivated vaccine)	*Primary series:* 2 doses 4–8 wks apart, 3rd dose 6–12 mos after 2nd	Anaphylactic reaction to neomycin or streptomycin
Hepatitis B	Health care workers and others at high risk (see text)	See Table 18.6	Three doses at 0, 1, and 6 months	History of anaphylactic reaction to vaccine or its constituents

Adapted from Task Force on Adult Immunization. Guide for adult immunization, 3rd ed. Philadelphia: American College of Physicians, 1994. *Legend:* Td = *Tetanus-diphtheria toxoid;* HiB = Haemophilus influenza *type b;* i.m. = *Intramuscular;* s.c. = *Subcutaneous.*

[a]Does not include adult immunizations for travelers (see text).

[b]The American College of Physicians recommends that a single Td booster at age 50, for those who have completed the full five-dose pediatric series, is equally acceptable as decennial dosing.

[c]Optimal dose in adults had not been determined.

[d]Persons with a history of anaphylactic reactions following egg ingestion should be vaccinated only with extreme caution. Protocols developed for such patients should be consulted (J Pediatr 1983;102:196–199; J Pediatr 1988;113:504–506).

[e]Revaccination is indicated in selected patients (see text).

[f]Adults requiring two doses include those entering college or other educational settings, those beginning employment in health care settings who will have direct contact with patients, and travelers to areas with endemic measles.

Adverse Effects

Local reactions (e.g., erythema, induration) and mild systemic reactions (e.g., fever, drowsiness, irritability, anorexia) are common after the administration of DTP or its component antigens but are less common after administration of DTaP. DTP may also cause febrile convulsions (a benign complication in normal children). Infrequently, children experience moderate or severe systemic reactions (e.g., high fever, persistent crying, hypotonic-hyporesponsive episodes, brief seizures), but these appear to be without sequelae. Severe neurologic events, such as prolonged seizures or encephalopathy, occur at a rate of 0–10 cases per million doses of vaccine and may lead to permanent brain damage. A recent Institute of Medicine review concluded that the balance of evidence supported a causal association between DTP vaccine and chronic brain damage in children who developed encephalopathy within seven days of vaccination, but the evidence was inadequate to infer causality in other cases of chronic nervous system dysfunction (14). Anaphylactic reactions to DTP vaccine are also rare. Arthus-type reactions to tetanus toxoid can occur, especially in adults who have received frequent tetanus toxoid boosters. Thus, Td boosters should be avoided in patients who have completed a primary series or have received a booster dose within the previous five years. They should also be avoided in patients who have experienced Arthus reactions and received a dose within the past 10 years.

Precautions and Contraindications

Precautions and contraindications to DTP vaccine are listed in Table 18.2. In general, pertussis vaccine should not be given to patients with unstable neurologic conditions, such as uncontrolled seizure disorders or progressive encephalopathy. Stable neurologic conditions, such as cerebral palsy and well-controlled seizures, are not contraindications. A history of a single seizure that was not temporally related to DTP does not contraindicate vaccination, especially if the seizure can be explained by other factors. Parents of infants and children with personal or family histories of seizures should be informed that the vaccine increases the risk of simple febrile seizures but that the latter have not been shown to produce long-term health effects. Acetaminophen (15 mg/kg at the time of vaccination and every 4 hours for 24 hours) should be given to children with such histories to reduce the likelihood of postvaccination fever.

    When an infant or child returns for the next DTP dose, the physician should question the parent or guardian about adverse events that may have occurred after the previous dose. DTP should not be given if the parent describes an anaphylactic reaction that occurred immediately after the dose, or an unexplained encephalopathy that developed within seven days of the dose. The precautions listed in Table 18.2 identify situations in which DTP should *probably* not be given. These events, although generally not associated with permanent sequelae, were once considered absolute contraindications to pertussis vaccination. Vaccination is now considered appropriate in these patients, however, if the risks of pertussis in the community are especially high. If pertussis vaccine is contraindicated, DTP should be replaced with DT in children under age 7, or with Td (which contains a smaller amount of diphtheria toxoid) in persons age 7 or older.

The only contraindications to Td are a history of a severe neurologic or hypersensitivity reaction following a previous dose, and moderate to severe illness.

Measles-Mumps-Rubella (MMR) Vaccine

Measles can be a severe disease, often complicated by middle ear infection or bronchopneumonia. About 20% of cases and nearly 30% of measles-related deaths occur in adults. The incidence of measles has fallen dramatically since 1963, when the vaccine was first licensed and routine childhood vaccination instituted. A resurgence of measles occurred in the United States between 1989 and 1991, however, when measles accounted for 55,622 cases, 11,251 hospitalizations, and 132 deaths (4). Although this epidemic occurred primarily among unvaccinated preschool children, a substantial number of school-aged children (most of whom were vaccinated) and adults were affected. Other data suggested that measles could spread among highly vaccinated school populations, largely because 2–5% of vaccine recipients remained susceptible after a single dose. In 1989, this information prompted a national effort to expand childhood immunization coverage and the addition of a second dose of measles vaccine to the childhood immunization schedule, given either at preschool or on entry to middle or junior high school (see Table 18.1).

Mumps vaccine was introduced in 1967, and since then the incidence of the disease has decreased substantially. Nonetheless, about 4000–5000 cases of mumps occur each year in the United States. Mumps is primarily a disease of school-aged children, although the relative incidence among persons over age 15 has increased in recent years. The risks are of particular concern to postpubertal males who have not had mumps, since orchitis occurs in 40% of cases.

About 200–1000 cases of rubella infection are reported annually in the United States. Although about half of cases are subclinical, rubella infection may be associated with significant morbidity in adults; the greatest risk is when infection occurs in pregnant women, in whom vertical transmission to the fetus can produce congenital rubella syndrome. Rubella vaccination of children was introduced in 1969, after which the incidence of new cases fell from 30:100,000 to 0.1:100,000 by 1988. Several large outbreaks of rubella occurred between 1990 and 1991, however, and the incidence of congenital rubella syndrome increased 15-fold. Despite current vaccination efforts, 6–11% of women of childbearing age still lack immunity to the disease. Thus, in addition to universal rubella vaccination of children, pregnant women are routinely screened for rubella susceptibility, and vaccination is offered postpartum to those who are susceptible.

Indications

All children (at least 12 months of age) and nonpregnant adults, with the exception of those with the contraindications listed in Table 18.2 and 18.5, should receive MMR vaccine if they are susceptible to measles, mumps, or rubella infection. Persons are considered susceptible to measles (or mumps) if they lack documentation of a physician-diagnosed illness, laboratory evidence of immunity, or receipt of two doses of live measles vaccine (or one dose of mumps vaccine). Recipients of killed measles vaccine (a product used in 1963–1967) should be revaccinated to avoid the severe atypical form of disease that can occur in such persons after exposure to natural measles. Most persons born before 1957 are likely to have already been infected with measles and mumps and are generally not considered susceptible. Measles vaccine may be given to older persons, however, if there is reason to believe that they are susceptible. Persons are considered susceptible to rubella if they lack documentation of vaccination on or after the first birthday or laboratory evidence of immunity; physician diagnosis is not considered evidence of immunity because the clinical presentation of rubella often resembles other illnesses. The Advisory Committee on Immunization Practices recommends that, unless it can be assured that susceptible women will return for vaccination, persons who may be immune to rubella but lack adequate documentation of immunity should be vaccinated, rather than first performing serologic testing for rubella antibodies (15). Such testing should generally be performed, however, at the first clinical encounter with women of childbearing age.

Administration

The recommended immunization schedule for MMR is presented in Table 18.1. Children who are behind on immunizations should be vaccinated according to the schedule in Table 18.3 if they are under age 7 or the schedule in Table 18.4 if they are age 7 or older. Adults should be immunized according to the schedule in Table 18.5. As noted earlier, MMR should be administered at least 14 days before, or deferred for 3–11 months after, administration of immune globulin because passively acquired antibodies may interfere with the response to the vaccine; guidelines for spacing the immunizations based on the type and dose of immune globulin are provided elsewhere (10). Many persons will receive two doses of mumps and rubella vaccine because of the two-dose schedule for MMR administration. There is no evidence that repeat administration of these vaccines is harmful nor affects immunity. MMR is therefore the preferred vaccine for individuals who are susceptible to measles, mumps, or rubella and who lack contraindications.

Adverse Effects

Primary vaccination with measles vaccine may be associated with mild fever and a transient rash, beginning 7–12 days after vaccination and usually lasting several days. About 5–15% of patients develop a fever greater than 103°F. Neurologic complications, including encephalitis and encephalopathy, reportedly occur in less than one case per million doses administered (an incidence rate lower than the rate for encephalitis of unknown etiology). Mild, self-limited thrombocytopenia may occur in 1 out of 30,000 doses of MMR vaccine. Recipients of killed vaccine may be more likely to experience local and systemic reactions after revaccination with live measles vaccine.

On rare occasions, mumps vaccination can produce parotitis and lymphadenopathy. Allergic reactions such as rash and pruritus, which are usually brief, are reported occasionally. Very rarely, manifestations of central nervous system involvement (e.g., febrile seizures, aseptic meningitis, unilateral nerve deafness, encephalitis) occur; almost all of these cases resolve uneventfully, and none have been linked conclusively to vaccines used in the United States. Recipients of rubella vaccine can develop low-grade fever, a rash lasting 1–2 days, and lymphadenopathy that may persist 1–2 months after vaccination. About 25% of adult recipients report arthralgias, usually occurring 1–3 weeks after immunization and lasting up to 3 days, and about 10% of adult recipients develop arthritis. These rheumatologic complications appear to be more common in women than in children. Rubella vaccination of adult women may also be associated with an increased risk of chronic arthritis (16). Rarely, transient peripheral neuritis is reported following rubella vaccination.

Precautions and Contraindications

Precautions and contraindications to MMR are listed in Table 18.2. Measles, mumps, and rubella vaccines should not be given to females known to be pregnant or who might become pregnant within 3 months after vaccination. No cases of congenital rubella syndrome have been documented among infants born to women who inadvertently received rubella vaccine during pregnancy. Thus, although rubella vaccination should be avoided during pregnancy, there is insufficient evidence of risk to justify termination of pregnancy if a pregnant woman inadvertently receives the vaccine. Children of pregnant women can safely receive MMR vaccine without risk to the mother or fetus. Although MMR vaccination of persons with moderate or severe illness should be postponed, minor illnesses such as upper respiratory infection, with or without a low-grade fever, do not preclude vaccination.

Hypersensitivity reactions to MMR vaccine are rare and generally consist of wheal-and-flare or urticarial reactions at the injection site. Although measles and mumps vaccines (but not rubella vaccine) contain egg protein, persons are not at increased risk of complications unless they have a history of anaphylactic egg allergies. A history of allergies to chicken or feathers also does not increase risk. Measles, mumps, and rubella vaccines contain about 25 µg of neomycin, and therefore true neomycin hypersensitivity is a contraindication.

Polio Vaccine

Poliomyelitis, a disease that once crippled or killed millions of persons, has become a rare disease in industrialized nations because of routine polio vaccination. In the United States, the number of annual cases has fallen from about 20,000 in 1954 (the year before the vaccine was introduced) to four in 1992. All current cases in the United States are due to vaccine-associated poliomyelitis; the last episode of spread of wild poliovirus in this country occurred in 1979. No new cases of wild-type virus have been reported in the Western Hemisphere since 1991, and global eradication of the disease may be possible by the turn of the century.

Indications

Polio vaccine should be administered to all children and susceptible adults, except those with the contraindications listed in Table 18.2 and 18.5.

Administration

Available vaccines include OPV and enhanced-potency inactivated poliovirus (IPV) vaccines. The recommended childhood immunization schedule for OPV is presented in Table 18.1 and contraindications are listed in Table 18.2. Children who are behind on immunizations should be vaccinated according to the schedule in Table 18.3 if they are under age 7 or the schedule in Table 18.4 if they are age 7 or older. Adults should be immunized according to the schedule in Table 18.5. Trivalent OPV is the vaccine of choice for all infants, children, and adolescents (less than 18 years of age), if there are no contraindications to OPV. A 6-week interval is required between doses of trivalent OPV. IPV should be used for persons over 18 years of age and for immunocompromised children or those who have close (e.g., household) contact with immunocompromised persons.

Adverse Effects

Rare cases of paralysis have been reported in recipients of OPV and their contacts (the estimated overall risk is 1:1–2.5 million); unimmunized adults should be advised of the small risk of acquiring the disease from children or other close contacts receiving OPV. The rare occurrence of Guillain-Barré syndrome has been associated with OPV in some studies, but subsequent investigations have not confirmed this association. No serious side effects of IPV have been documented. IPV may contain trace amounts of streptomycin and neomycin, and it therefore poses a potential risk to persons with a history of anaphylactic reactions to these antibiotics.

Precautions and Contraindications

Precautions and contraindications to polio vaccine are listed in Table 18.2.

Haemophilus Influenzae Type B Vaccine

Haemophilus influenzae type b can cause serious bacterial diseases among children, such as meningitis, pneumonia, septic arthritis, epiglottitis, and sepsis. These illnesses occur primarily among children less than five years of age. Although severe disease is most common in children 6–12 months of age, about 20–35% of cases of severe disease occur in children 18 months of age or older. The introduction of conjugated HiB vaccine in the late 1980s was followed by a decline in the incidence of invasive disease. Among children less than age 5, the incidence fell from 41:100,000 in 1987 to 2:100,000 in 1993 (17). Compliance with HiB immunization guidelines has been difficult in recent years because of the rapid introduction of new vaccine products, frequently changing recommendations, and schedules that vary with the age at which immunization is initiated. Nonetheless, surveys suggest that HiB coverage in two-year-old children increased from 28% in 1992 to 71% by the first quarter of 1994 (18). The introduction of combined DTP-HiB vaccines should help improve coverage.

Indications

A complete HiB vaccination series is indicated in all infants and children below age 15 months and in certain high-risk adults. A single dose is indicated in children 15 months to 5 years of age. Children who have had HiB disease when they were less than 24 months of age should still receive HiB vaccine, since most fail to mount an immune response to clinical disease. Children 24 months of age or older who have had reliably diagnosed invasive disease do not need vaccination. The vaccine is not given after age 5 except in special circumstances, such as human immunodeficiency virus (HIV) infection, asplenia, sickle cell disease, and chemotherapy for Hodgkin's lymphoma. Household and day care center contacts of patients with HiB disease should receive rifampin postexposure prophylaxis (if one of the contacts is a child less than one year of age or an older child who has not been fully vaccinated).

Administration

Four different vaccines are currently licensed in the United States. Diphtheria CRM_{197} Protein Conjugate (HbOC), Meningococcal Protein Conjugate (PRP-OMP), Polyribosylribitol Phosphate-Tetanus Toxoid Conjugate (PRP-T), and Diphtheria Toxoid Conjugate (PRP-D). (PRP-D, the original vaccine, is not licensed for primary immunization of children less than 15 months of age but can be used as a booster, beginning at 12 months of age.) Current evidence suggests that these products can be used interchangeably. In 1993, the Food and Drug Administration also licensed the use of combined DT toxoids, whole-cell pertussis vaccine, and HiB (TETRAMUNE, Lederle-Praxis; or PRP-T [ActHIB, OmniHIB; Pasteur Merieux, SmithKline Beecham, Connaught] reconstituted with DTP vaccine produced by Connaught) when indications for both vaccines coincide.

The recommended immunization schedule for HiB vaccination is presented in Table 18.1. Children who are behind on HiB immunizations (and are under age 5) should be vaccinated according to the schedule in Table 18.3. Adults should be immunized according to the indications and schedule in Table 18.5. Intervals between HiB doses should be at least 1 month.

The dosage for rifampin prophylaxis is 20 mg/kg (maximum of 600 mg) orally once daily for 4 days; the dose for infants less than 1 month of age should probably be 10 mg/kg/day in divided doses.

Adverse Effects

Serious complications from HiB vaccine are unusual. Redness or swelling occurs in less than 2% of recipients, and a fever of 101.3°F or greater occurs in about 1% of recipients. Severe hypersensitivity reactions are rare.

Hepatitis B Vaccine

Hepatitis B is a serious public health problem in the United States. About 200,000–300,000 cases of acute infection occur annually and about

18,000–30,000 of these patients develop chronic disease. About 4000–5000 persons die each year from hepatitis B, due largely to cirrhosis or hepato-cellular carcinoma (19). About one million Americans are thought to be infectious carriers. The incidence of the disease did not decline after the introduction of hepatitis B vaccine in 1982 and the institution of a program to vaccinate persons with specific risk factors for hepatitis B infection and the offspring of infected mothers. In 1990, because of the failure of vaccination recommendations to have modified disease incidence and because about 30% of cases of hepatitis B were occurring in persons without identifiable risk factors, the U.S. Public Health Service modified its high-risk strategy and recommended universal infant vaccination and more intensive screening of adults (including universal screening of pregnant women). The recommendation for universal infant vaccination has since been endorsed by other groups, including the American Academy of Pediatrics and the American Academy of Family Physicians, and infant vaccination is required by law in some states. The public health impact and cost-effectiveness of the policy, and its relative benefits compared to universal vaccination of adolescents, remain uncertain, however, and continue to be widely debated among researchers and practitioners (20).

Indications

The Advisory Committee on Immunization Practices recommends vaccinating all infants, as well as high-risk adolescents and adults. (It recommends universal vaccination of adolescents in communities with a high incidence of intravenous drug use, sexually transmitted diseases, or teenage pregnancy; universal screening of pregnant women is also recommended.) In general, persons at markedly increased risk of acquiring hepatitis B include intravenous drug users; homosexual and heterosexual persons with multiple partners; health care workers and others with potential exposure to blood products; hemodialysis and hemophilia patients; recipients of certain blood products; household contacts or sexual partners of hepatitis B carriers; inmates of long-term correctional institutions; immigrants from certain countries (e.g., China, Southeast Asian countries, African countries, the Philippines, Haiti, Eastern European countries); other population groups (e.g., Alaskan Natives, Pacific Islanders) in which hepatitis B is common; and international travelers to these regions for whom sexual contact, exposure to blood, or residence longer than 6 months is likely.

Administration

The recommended infant immunization schedule for hepatitis B vaccine is presented in Table 18.1, and the recommended dosages are listed in Table 18.6. Two options for integrating infant immunizations with other vaccinations include starting the series at birth or at 1–2 months of age

Table 18.6
Recommended Doses of Currently Licensed Hepatitis B Vaccines

Group	Recombivax HB		Engerix-B	
	Intramuscular (μg)	(ml)	Intramuscular Dose (μg)	(ml)
Infants of HBsAg-negative mothers and children < age 11	2.5	0.5[a]	10	0.5
Infants of HBsAg-positive mothers; prevention of perinatal infection	5	0.5	10	0.5
Children and adolescents age 11–19	5	0.5	10	0.5
Adults ≥ age 20	10	1.0	20	1.0
Dialysis patients and other immuno-compromised persons	40	1.0	40	2.0

Adapted from U.S. Centers for Disease Control and Prevention. Hepatitis B virus: a comprehensive strategy for eliminating transmission in the United States through universal childhood vaccination. Recommendations of the Immunization Practices Advisory Committee (ACIP). MMWR 1991;40(RR-13). *Legend*: HBsAG = *Hepatitis B surface antigen*.

[a]0.5 ml are administered if the pediatric formulation of Recombivax HB (2.5 μg/0.5 ml) is used. 0.25 cc are administered if the standard formulation (10 μg/cc) is used. For further details, see MMWR 1993; 42:686–688.

(Table 18.1). Primary vaccination generally consists of three intramuscular doses. In older children and adults, the second dose is given 1 month after the first dose and the third dose 6 months after the first dose. The two currently licensed vaccines, Recombivax HB and Engerix-B, can be used interchangeably (at appropriate doses) throughout the series. (Plasma-derived vaccine is no longer distributed in the United States.) Engerix-B is also licensed for a four-dose series administered at 0 (at birth, before hospital discharge), 1, 2, and 12 months. The interval between the first and second dose should be at least 1 month, and the interval between the second and third doses should be at least 2 months. The second dose should be administered between 1 and 4 months of age, provided at least 1 month has elapsed since the first dose, and the third dose should be given by 6–18 months of age. Higher antibody titers are achieved when the last two doses are administered at least 4 months apart. Once they exceed 2000 g in weight, preterm infants can be immunized against hepatitis B according to their chronological age.

Persons who require postexposure prophylaxis against hepatitis B should be immunized according to the schedules in Tables 18.7 and 18.8. Infants born to hepatitis B surface antigen-positive mothers should receive their first dose of hepatitis B vaccine (and 0.5 ml of hepatitis B immune globulin [HBIG] intramuscularly at a different site) within 12 hours of

Table 18.7
Hepatitis B Virus Postexposure Recommendations

	Hepatitis B Immune Globulin (HBIG)		Hepatitis B Vaccine	
Exposure	Dose	Timing	Number of Doses	Timing
Perinatal	0.5 ml i.m.	As soon as possible (within 12 hours)	3	Within 7 days (preferably within 12 hours); repeat at 1 and 6 months of age
Sexual	0.06 ml/kg i.m. (maximum of 5 ml)	Within 14 days of contact	3	First dose at time of HBIG; repeat in 1 and 6 months
Acute hepatitis B in household contact		As soon as		
< 12 mos of age	0.5 ml i.m.	possible	3	At time of exposure,
≥ 12 mos of age[a]	—	—	3	then 1 and 6 mos later
Percutaneous or permucosal—See Table 18.8				

Adapted from U.S. Center for Disease Control and Prevention. Hepatitis B virus: a comprehensive strategy for eliminating transmission in the United States through universal childhood vaccination. Recommendations of the Immunization Practices Advisory Committee (ACIP). MMWR 1991;40(RR-13). *Legend:* i.m. = *Intramuscular,* HBIG = *Hepatitis B immune globulin.*

[a]Patients ≥ 12 months of age need not be vaccinated unless the index case becomes a carrier or the household is in a high-risk category.

birth, and the second and third vaccine doses should be given at 1 and 6 months of age, respectively. (If the four-dose, Engerix-B schedule is used, the third and fourth doses are administered at 2 and 12–18 months of age, respectively.) If the mother's hepatitis B surface antigen status is unknown, the same schedule is used, except that HBIG is not administered; if the mother is found to be positive for hepatitis B surface antigen, HBIG is given to the infant as soon as possible but not later than 1 week after birth.

The anterolateral thigh is the preferred site for intramuscular injection of hepatitis B vaccine in infants and young children. The deltoid muscle is the preferred site in adults. Intramuscular injections in the buttocks result in lower seroconversion rates. Hepatitis B vaccine can be given simultaneously with DTP (or DTaP), OPV, MMR, and HiB at the same visit. Although half of adult recipients have low or undetectable hepatitis B antibody levels seven to ten years after vaccination, there is currently insufficient evidence to recommend booster doses in persons who have received a complete hepatitis B vaccination series.

Adverse Effects

The most common side effects are pain at the injection site (3–29%) and mild fever (1–6%). More serious complications are reported in less than

Table 18.8
Recommended Hepatitis B Prophylaxis After Percutaneous or Permucosal Exposure

Exposed Person	HBs-Ag-Positive Source	HBs-Ag-Negative Source	Source Not Tested or Unknown
Unvaccinated	1 dose of HBIG[a]; initiate hepatitis B vaccine series (see Table 18.5)	Initiate hepatitis B vaccine series (see Table 18.5)	Initiate hepatitis B vaccine series (see Table 18.5)
Previously vaccinated			
• Known responder	Test exposed person for anti HBs-Ag level: 1. If adequate,[b] no treatment 2. If inadequate, hepatitis B vaccine booster dose	No treatment	No treatment
• Known nonresponder	2 doses of HBIG, or 1 dose of HBIG plus 1 dose of hepatitis B vaccine	No treatment	If known high-risk source, may treat as if source were HBsAg-positive
• Response unknown	Test exposed person for anti HBs-AG: 1. If adequate,[b] no treatment 2. If inadequate, 1 dose of HBIG plus hepatitis B vaccine booster dose	No treatment	Test exposed person for anti HBs-Ag level: 1. If adequate,[b] no treatment 2. If inadequate, hepatitis B vaccine booster dose

Adapted from U.S. Centers for Disease Control and Prevention. Hepatitis B virus: a comprehensive strategy for eliminating transmission in the United States through universal childhood vaccination. Recommendations of the Immunization Practices Advisory Committee (ACIP). MMWR 1991;40(RR-13). *Legend:* HBIG = *Hepatitis B immune globulin*; HBsAg = *Hepatitis B surface antigen*; Anti-HBs-Ag = *Anti-hepatitis B surface antigen antibody.*

[a]HBIG dose = 0.06 ml/kg i.m.

[b]Adequate anti-HBsAg level = ≥ 10mIU.

1% of recipients. The principal side effects of HBIG are pain and swelling at the injection site. Urticaria, angioedema, and anaphylaxis have rarely been reported.

Influenza Vaccine

Since 1957, there have been at least 19 influenza epidemics in the United States in which more than 10,000 persons died. Influenza vaccine is prepared each year in an attempt to anticipate antigenic variation among influenza viruses. Two strains of influenza A and one strain of influenza B are selected based on circulating strains. These vaccines provide moderate antibody protection against influenza viruses with the same antigenic characteristics. Protective efficacy is estimated to be 65–80% in young adults but only 30–40% in preventing illness in older adults, who account for 80–90% of influenza deaths. The vaccine is estimated to have higher efficacy (50–60%) in preventing hospitalization and pneumonia in older adults. The vaccines do not protect against infection with antigenically dissimilar influenza strains.

Indications

Influenza vaccination is generally recommended for persons age 65 or older and those with medical conditions that increase the risk of complications from influenza. The latter include residents of nursing homes and other chronic care facilities housing persons with chronic medical conditions; patients with chronic pulmonary or cardiovascular conditions, including children with asthma; patients who have required regular medical follow-up or hospitalization during the previous year because of chronic metabolic diseases (e.g., diabetes mellitus), renal dysfunction, hemoglobinopathy, or immunosuppression; and children and adolescents receiving long-term aspirin therapy who may therefore be at risk of developing post-influenza Reye's syndrome. Vaccination is also indicated for persons who can transmit influenza to high-risk patients, such as health care personnel, employees of nursing homes and other chronic care facilities who have contact with patients, home care providers for high-risk patients, and household contacts of high-risk persons. Influenza vaccination should be administered to persons who request the vaccine but is not routinely indicated for healthy young adults and children.

Administration

Influenza vaccine is administered annually, preferably before the beginning of the influenza season (mid-October to mid-November). Physicians should begin vaccinating high-risk patients in September, if the vaccine is available. Whole-virus and split-virus vaccines can be administered to all patients over age 12; only split-virus preparations should be used for patients age 12 or younger. The pediatric dose is 0.25 ml in children 6 to 35 months of age, and 0.5 ml intramuscularly in patients 3 years of age or older. Children less than 9 years of age who require influenza vaccine and have not received it previously should receive two doses, at least 1 month apart, before the influenza season. Influenza and pneumococcal vaccination can be performed at the same visit.

Amantadine and/or rimantadine should be given prophylactically to residents of institutions housing high-risk patients in which an influenza A outbreak occurs; older adults, and others at high risk, in whom immunization is contraindicated; older adults, and others at high risk, who have been exposed recently to influenza A but are unimmunized or only recently immunized; and immunocompromised patients and others expected to have a suboptimal response to immunization. The dose of amantadine is 100 mg orally daily for persons age 65 or older, 100 mg orally twice daily for persons ages 9 to 64, and 4.4–8.8 mg/kg/day orally (not to exceed 150 mg daily) in children; the dose should be reduced for patients with renal dysfunction or those who experience side effects. The dose of rimantadine is 100 mg orally twice daily in adults (50 mg orally twice daily for persons with adverse effects such as hepatic or renal dysfunction) and 5 mg/kg orally once daily (not to exceed 150 mg daily) in children under age 10. Prophylactic amantadine or rimantadine is given daily for the duration of the influenza season. When used as an adjunct in controlling community outbreaks, these agents are given daily for only 2 weeks (or until approximately 1 week after the outbreak has ended).

Adverse Effects

Adverse reactions to influenza vaccine are generally mild, consisting of discomfort at the injection site for up to two days. Immediate allergic reactions (e.g., urticaria, angioedema) are rare and are usually related to allergies to egg proteins. Fever, malaise, and myalgia, usually lasting 6 to 48 hours, have been infrequently reported. Although Guillain-Barré syndrome was associated with the use of the "swine flu" vaccine in 1976, annual surveillance in subsequent years has not demonstrated a clear association between influenza vaccination and neurologic complications.

Precautions and Contraindications

Contraindications to influenza vaccine are listed in Table 18.5.

Pneumococcal Vaccine

More than 200,000 cases of pneumococcal pneumonia occur annually in the United States, and about 40,000 persons die each year from pneumococcal disease and its complications. Mortality is expected to increase in the future due to the advancing age of the population, the effects of pneumococcal infection on patients with acquired immunodeficiency syndrome, and the emergence of antibiotic-resistant strains. The 14-valent polysaccharide vaccine was first licensed in 1977, and the current 23-valent vaccine was introduced in 1983. Most evidence suggests a protective efficacy of about 60% against invasive pneumococcal disease. Uncertainties about efficacy may account for low rates of immunization coverage (less than 15–20% of persons for whom pneumococcal vaccine is recommended) (21).

Indications

Pneumococcal vaccination is generally recommended once for persons age 65 or older and adults with medical conditions that increase their risk of acquiring pneumonia or experiencing complications. The latter include patients with chronic illnesses (e.g., cardiopulmonary disease, diabetes mellitus, alcoholism, cirrhosis), immunocompromised persons (e.g., patients with splenic dysfunction, sickle cell anemia, lymphoma, multiple myeloma, chronic renal failure, organ transplantation), persons infected with HIV, and residents of areas with an increased risk of pneumococcal disease (e.g., certain Native American populations). Children two or more years of age with chronic illnesses specifically associated with increased risk of pneumococcal disease or its complications (e.g., anatomic or functional asplenia, nephrotic syndrome, cerebrospinal fluid leaks, immunosuppression, HIV infection) should also receive pneumococcal vaccine. As of this writing, some groups are considering the need for routine pneumococcal vaccination beginning at age 55 because of evidence that this age group is more likely to mount an immune response than persons over age 65.

Administration

The recommended immunization schedule for pneumococcal vaccine is presented in Table 18.5. To improve vaccination coverage, physicians have been encouraged to use hospitalizations (e.g., at discharge), nursing home visits, and similar opportunities to administer the vaccine. Pneumococcal vaccine can also be given at the same time as influenza vaccination. Revaccination may be indicated for high-risk adult patients (e.g., asplenic persons) who received the 14-valent vaccine or received the 23-valent vaccine 6 or more years earlier. Revaccination is also indicated for adult patients thought to have rapid declines in antibody levels (e.g., patients with nephrotic syndrome or renal failure, and transplant recipients). Children with nephrotic syndrome, asplenia, or sickle cell disease should be revaccinated 3–5 years after the first dose if they are age 10 or younger at revaccination.

Adverse Effects

About half of vaccine recipients experience mild side effects (e.g., erythema, pain) at the injection site. Less than 1% report fever, myalgias, or severe local reactions. The estimated risk of anaphylactic reactions is 1:250,000 doses.

Precautions and Contraindications

Contraindications to pneumococcal vaccine are listed in Table 18.5.

Immunizations for Travelers

Patients traveling to other countries may require special immunizations against endemic diseases and/or chemoprophylaxis against malaria and other diseases. Some countries require an International Certificate of Vaccination against yellow fever. Immunoglobulin prophylaxis against hepatitis A and vaccination against hepatitis A, meningococcal disease, Japanese encephalitis, polio, plague, rabies, or typhoid fever may be indicated for travelers to certain countries. Depending on their destination, patients may also require counseling about measures to protect themselves against exposure to mosquitoes and arthropod vectors, risks from water and food, swimming and animal-related hazards, traveler's diarrhea, and motion sickness.

Clinicians who are unfamiliar with current recommendations for travel to specific countries can consult the latest edition of *Health Information for International Travel* (22), which is published yearly by the U.S. Centers for Disease Control and Prevention. Health professionals and patients can also obtain information by calling the U.S. Centers for Disease Control and Prevention automated travelers hotline (404-332-4559), which is accessible 24 hours a day from a touch tone telephone, or by fax; (404-332-4565). To write for information, see address in the "Resources" section later in this chapter. Other important local resources include local health departments, many of which operate travel medicine clinics (see Chapter 24), other health care facilities in the community offering immunization services for international travelers, and local infectious disease specialists with expertise in travel medicine.

Other Immunizations

Rabies vaccination is indicated as preexposure prophylaxis for persons whose occupations, travel, or recreational activities expose them to potentially rabid animals, and (along with human rabies immune globulin) as postexposure prophylaxis following certain bite wounds. *Tetanus prophylaxis* with tetanus immune globulin and/or toxoid is also indicated in certain patients with wounds that are potentially contaminated with tetanus spores. *Bacille Calmette-Guérin vaccine* is recommended in the United States only for certain children at high risk of acquiring tuberculosis. Its use among children and adults has been reconsidered because of the resurgence of tuberculosis and multidrug-resistant mycobacterial strains, but advisory groups recently recommended against expanded vaccination. Vaccines that were licensed only shortly before publication of this book include live attenuated *varicella vaccine* and killed-virus *hepatitis A vaccine*. Readers should consult current recommendations (see "Suggested Readings" for this chapter) regarding the proper use of these agents. As of this writing, the new varicella vaccine is recommended for children between 12 and 18 months of age (and for children between 18 months and 12 years of age who were not immunized previously and have not already had chicken pox). Persons age 13 or older without a history of varicella should receive two doses 4–8 weeks apart.

ORGANIZATION OF OFFICE OR CLINIC

Special procedures are often necessary in the office or clinic to provide comprehensive immunization services (23). The absence of such procedures may account for a large proportion of missed opportunities in vaccinating eligible patients. In response to this problem, standards for pediatric immunization practices (SPIP) (9) and objectives for adult

Table 18.9
Standards for Pediatric Immunization Practices

1. Immunization services are readily available.
2. There are no barriers or unnecessary prerequisites to the receipt of vaccines.
3. Immunization services are free or available for a minimal fee.
4. Providers use all clinical encounters to screen and, when indicated, immunize children.
5. Providers educate children and guardians about immunization in general terms.
6. Providers question children or guardians about contraindications and, before immunizing a child, inform them in specific terms about the risks and benefits of the immunizations their child is to receive.
7. Providers follow only true contraindications.
8. Providers administer simultaneously all vaccine doses for which a child is eligible at the time of each visit.
9. Providers use accurate and complete recording procedures.
10. Providers co-schedule immunization appointments in conjunction with appointments for other child health services.
11. Providers report adverse events following immunization promptly, accurately, and completely.
12. Providers operate a tracking system.
13. Providers adhere to proper procedures for vaccine management.
14. Providers conduct semiannual audits to assess immunization coverage levels and to review immunization records in the patient populations they serve.
15. Providers maintain up-to-date, easily retrievable medical protocols at all locations where vaccines are administered.
16. Providers operate with patient-oriented and community-based approaches.
17. Vaccines are administered by properly trained individuals.
18. Providers receive ongoing education and training on current immunizations recommendations.

From Ad Hoc Working Group for the Development of Standards for Pediatric Immunization Practices. Standards for pediatric immunization practices. JAMA 1993;269:1817–1822.

immunization (24) have been issued by the National Vaccine Advisory Committee. These standards suggest organizational practices to help providers ensure timely and comprehensive immunization of all appropriate patients (Table 18.9). The SPIP have been endorsed by the U.S. Public Health Service and the American Academy of Pediatrics. They were developed in collaboration with a 35-member working group that represented 22 public and private agencies and that had input from state and local health departments, physician and nursing organizations, and public and private providers. Although these recommendations were originally developed to improve the delivery of childhood immunizations, the same office procedures can also enhance the delivery of adult immunizations. Many SPIP recommendations are cited in the following discussion:

- *Vaccine product management:* Office or clinic procedures for handling and storage of vaccines should be designed to comply with the recommendations in the manufacturer's package inserts. The SPIP recommended daily monitoring of the temperature at which vaccines are stored and the expiration date of each vaccine.

- *Minimization of waiting time:* Office procedures to minimize waiting time can reduce the role of lengthy delays as a barrier to receiving immunizations. The SPIP recommend reducing waiting time to less than 30 minutes and making immunizations available on a walk-in basis, for both new and established patients. They advise against the practice of requiring children to undergo well-child examinations, physical examinations, or vital sign measurement before being vaccinated. According to the SPIP, observing the child's general state of health, asking the parent or guardian if the child is well, and questioning them about potential contraindications are all that is necessary to determine the appropriateness of immunizations.

- *Use of appropriate contraindications:* Systems should be in place to ensure that parents are asked routinely about adverse events following prior immunizations and that proper precautions or contraindications (Table 18.2) are considered before administering any vaccine. The SPIP recommend posting up-to-date immunization protocols at all locations where vaccines are administered. Vaccines should only be administered by individuals with proper training and/or supervision.

- *Opportunistic screening and vaccination:* Clinicians can use most clinical encounters (including emergency department visits and hospitalizations) to consult the immunization record and ask patients whether immunizations are up-to-date. In general, all needed vaccines should be administered simultaneously. MMR vaccine should always be used in combined form for routine childhood immunizations. The SPIP also recommend checking the immunization status of children who accompany patients during office or clinic visits.

- *Reminder systems:* Reminder systems can be helpful in ensuring that children return on time for their next immunization. Manual or automated systems can be used to trigger postcard, letter, or telephone reminders for patients to schedule their next vaccination appointment (see Chapters 22, 23, and 26 for further details about the use of reminder systems).

- *Minimization of costs:* Charges for vaccinations have been identified as a major barrier to immunizations, especially among poor patients. The SPIP recommend that immunization services in the public sector should be free of charge and in the private sector should be limited to the cost of the vaccine and a "reasonable administrative fee."

Other important measures to expand immunization coverage include efforts to target high-risk groups, such as children at risk of delayed or missed immunization and those whose parents are of lower socioeconomic status, less educated, or young.

MEDICAL RECORD DOCUMENTATION

Physicians are required by statute to record the following information about childhood immunizations: name of vaccine, date of administration, manufacturer, lot number, signature and title of person administering the vaccine, and address where the vaccine was given. In addition, a flow sheet or other chart inserts are often helpful in quickly reviewing the immunization history to determine whether the patient's immunizations are up-to-date. Adverse reactions to immunizations should be described in detail in the medical record. Health care providers are required by law to report selected adverse events occurring after vaccination with DTP, DT, Td, MMR, MR, measles, OPV, and IPV. Reportable events, which are specified elsewhere (25), are generally those requiring the patient to seek medical attention. The information should be reported to the Vaccine Adverse Event Reporting System, which is operated by the U.S. Centers for Disease Control and Prevention and the Food and Drug Administration. Report forms and assistance can be obtained by calling 800-822-7967 or writing Vaccine Adverse Event Reporting System, P.O. Box 1100, Rockville, MD 20849.

Communication with other health care providers: Clinicians administering immunizations who are not the patient's primary care provider (e.g., public health department, emergency department, or subspecialty physicians) should adopt procedures to notify the patient's primary care provider. Often, this is accomplished by recording the immunization on the child's personal immunization record card (an official immunization card has been adopted by every state), specifying the vaccine given, date of administration, and name of provider. The SPIP also recommend informing the child's regular health care provider directly and, if a parent fails to bring the child's immunization card, issuing a new card that describes all current and previous immunizations. Participation in local immunization registries provides another important means of sharing vaccination records. State-based computerized immunization information systems are currently being developed in many states.

The SPIP include other recommendations that may help improve immunization practices but that may be difficult for some providers to implement. These include confirming the accuracy of immunization records by checking the patient's personal records or contacting previous providers, maintaining separate medical records of preschool children to facilitate assessment of coverage, periodic sorting of these records to remove inactive files, maintaining records of other primary care services received with immunizations to facilitate "coscheduling," and conducting semiannual audits to assess immunization coverage.

RESOURCES—PATIENT EDUCATION MATERIALS
General

American Academy of Family Physicians
8880 Ward Parkway
Kansas City, MO 64114-2797
800-944-0000
> "Childhood Vaccines: What They Are And Why Your Child Needs Them" (brochure 1532); "Immunizations" (brochure 735).

American Academy of Pediatrics
Publications Department
141 Northwest Point Blvd.
P.O. Box 927
Elk Grove Village, IL 60009-0927
800-433-9016
> "Immunization Protects Children" (brochure English IS5081; Spanish IS5082).

U.S. Centers for Disease Control and Prevention
Division of Immunization
Atlanta, GA 30333
404-639-3747
> "Immunization of Adults: A Call To Action."

National Institute on Aging
NIA Information Center
P.O. Box 8057
Gaithersburg, MD 20898-8057
800-222-2225
> " 'Shots' for Safety."

State and local health departments
> "Parent's Guide to Childhood Immunizations."

Diphtheria-Tetanus-Pertussis Vaccine

Academy of Family Physicians
8880 Ward Parkway
Kansas City, MO 64114-2797
800-944-0000
> "Diphtheria, Tetanus, and Pertussis Vaccine (DTP): What You Need to Know Before Your Child Gets the Vaccine" (fact sheet 926). Originally produced by the U.S. Centers for Disease Control and Prevention.

American Academy of Pediatrics
Publications Department
141 Northwest Point Blvd.

P.O. Box 927
Elk Grove Village, IL 60009-0927
800-433-9016

"Diphtheria, Tetanus, and Pertussis Vaccine (DTP): What You Need To Know Before Your Child Gets the Vaccine" (fact sheet, English HE0113; Spanish HE0121); "Tetanus and Diphtheria Vaccine (Td): What You Need To Know Before You or Your Child Gets The Vaccine" (fact sheet HE0144). Both publications were produced originally by the U.S. Centers for Disease Control and Prevention.

National Institute on Aging
Building 31, Room 5C27
Bethesda, MD 20892
301-496-1752

"Age Page—'Shots' for Safety."

Measles–Mumps–Rubella Vaccine

American Academy of Family Physicians
8880 Ward Parkway
Kansas City, MO 64114-2797
800-944-0000

"Measles, Mumps, and Rubella Vaccine (MMR): What You Need To Know Before You or Your Child Gets The Vaccine" (fact sheet, product 928). Originally produced by the U.S. Centers for Disease Control and Prevention.

American Academy of Pediatrics
Publications Department
141 Northwest Point Blvd.
P.O. Box 927
Elk Grove Village, IL 60009-0927
800-433-9016

"Measles, Mumps, and Rubella Vaccine (MMR): What You Need To Know Before You or Your Child Gets The Vaccine" (fact sheet, English HE0114;Spanish HE0122). Originally produced by the U.S. Centers for Disease Control and Prevention.

Polio Vaccine

American Academy of Family Physicians
8880 Ward Parkway
Kansas City, MO 64114-2797
800-944-0000

"Polio Vaccine: What You Need To Know Before You or Your Child Gets The Vaccine" (fact sheet, product 927). Originally produced by the U.S. Centers for Disease Control and Prevention.

American Academy of Pediatrics
Publications Department
141 Northwest Point Blvd.
P.O. Box 927
Elk Grove Village, IL 60009-0927
800-433-9016

"Polio Vaccine: What You Need To Know Before You or Your Child Gets The Vaccine" (fact sheet, English HE0115; Spanish HE0123). Originally produced by the U.S. Centers for Disease Control and Prevention..

Haemophilus Influenzae Type B Vaccine

American Academy of Pediatrics
Publications Department
141 Northwest Point Blvd.
P.O. Box 927
Elk Grove Village, IL 60009-0927
800-433-9016

> "Haemophilus Influenzae Type b: What Parents Need to Know" (brochure, English HE0119; Spanish HE0151); "Haemophilus Influenzae Type b Fact Sheet" (English HE0117; Spanish HE0152).

Hepatitus B Vaccine

American Academy of Pediatrics
Publications Department
141 Northwest Point Blvd.
P.O. Box 927
Elk Grove Village, IL 60009-0927
800-433-9016

> "Hepatitis B: What Parents Need to Know" (brochure, English HE0120; Spanish HE0142); "Hepatitis B Fact Sheet" (English HE0118; Spanish 0140).

American Liver Foundation
1425 Pompton Avenue
Cedar Grove, NJ 07009
800-223-0179

> "Hepatitis A, B & C: Liver Diseases You Should Know About."

American Social Health Association
P.O. Box 13827
Research Triangle Park, NC 27709-3827
919-361-8400

> "Hepatitis B: The Sexually Transmitted Disease With No Cure."

National Center for Education in Maternal and Child Health
2000 15th Street North, Suite 701
Arlington, VA 22201-2617

> "Hepatitis B" (English F040; Chinese F041; Korean F042; Laotian F043; Vietnamese F046).

National Center for Prevention Services
Information Services Office (E-06)
Centers for Disease Control
Atlanta, GA 30333

> "Why Does My Baby Need Hepatitis B Vaccine?" Also available from state and local health departments.

National Institute of Allergy and Infectious Diseases
Office of Communications
National Institutes of Health
Bethesda, MD 20892

> "Hepatitis" (booklet 92-909E).

Influenza Vaccine

American Lung Association
1740 Broadway

New York, NY 10019
212-315-8700, 800-586-4872
    "Be A Fighter: Knock Out the Flu Before the Flu Knocks You." (brochure 1262.)

Food and Drug Administration
Information and Outreach Staff
HFE-88, Room 16-63
5600 Fishers Lane
Rockville, MD 29857
301-443-3170
    "Flu Shots: Do You Need One?" (FDA90-3175).

National Institute of Allergy and Infectious Diseases
9000 Rockville Pike
Bethesda, MD 20892
301-496-5717
    "Flu."

National Institute on Aging
Building 31, Room 5C27
Bethesda, MD 20892
301-496-1752
    "Age Page—What To Do About Flu."

Pneumococcal Vaccine

American Lung Association
1740 Broadway
New York, NY 10019
212-315-8700, 800-586-4872
    "Pneumonia? Not Me." (brochure 1326).

National Institute on Aging
Building 31, Room 5C27
9000 Rockville Pike
Bethesda, MD 20892
301-496-1752
    "Age Page—'Shots' for Safety," "Facts For Patients About Pneumococcal Disease" (pa-
    tient tear-off pads), "The Pneumonia Vaccine: It's Worth a Shot."

National Institute on Aging Information Center
P.O. Box 8057
Gaithersburg, MD 20898-8057
800-222-2225
    Brochures listed above also available from this resource.

Immunizations for Travelers

U.S. Centers for Disease Control and Prevention
National Center for Prevention Services
Division of Quarantine
Travelers' Health Section
Atlanta, GA 30333

U.S. Centers for Disease Control and Prevention
Automated Travelers' Hotline
404-332-4559 (accessible 24 hours a day from a touch-tone telephone)
404-332-4565 (FAX)

Rabies Vaccine

National Institute of Allergy and Infectious Diseases
Office of Communications
Building 31, Room 7A50
9000 Rockville Pike
Bethesda, MD 20892
301-496-5717
"Rabies" (pamphlet).

RESOURCES—PROFESSIONAL EDUCATION MATERIALS

American Academy of Family Physicians
8880 Ward Parkway
Kansas City, MO 64114-2797
800-944-0000
"Recommendations for Hepatitis B Preexposure Vaccination and Postexposure Prophylaxis" (product 966).

Connaught Laboratories
Swiftwater, PA 18370
800-822-2463
Information for physicians on reconstitution of HiB vaccine (PRP) and DTP (Connaught, Inc.).

SUGGESTED READINGS

General

Advisory Committee on Immunization Practices. Recommended childhood immunization schedule—United States, January, 1995.

Advisory Committee on Immunization Practices. General recommendations on immunization. MMWR 1994;43:RR-1.

Age charts for periodic health examination (reprint no. 510). Kansas City, MO: American Academy of Family Physicians, 1994.

American Academy of Pediatrics, Committee on Infectious Diseases. Recommended schedule for immunization of healthy infants and children. Pediatrics 1994;94:131.

Gardner P, Schaffner W. Immunization of adults. N Engl J Med 1993;328:1252–1258.

Immunization Practices Advisory Committee. Update on adult immunization: recommendations of the Immunization Practices Advisory Committee. MMWR 1991;40(RR-12).

Report of the Committee on Infectious Diseases, 23rd ed. Elk Grove Village, IL: American Academy of Pediatrics, 1994.

Task Force on Adult Immunization. Guide for adult immunization, 3rd ed. Philadelphia: American College of Physicians, 1994.

U.S. Preventive Services Task Force. Guide to clinical preventive services, 2nd ed. Baltimore: Williams & Wilkins, in press.

Diphtheria–Tetanus–Pertussis Vaccine

U.S. Centers for Disease Control and Prevention. Diphtheria, tetanus, and pertussis: recommendations for vaccine use and other preventive measures. Recommendations of the Immunization Practices Advisory Committee (ACIP). MMWR 1991;40:RR-10.

U.S. Centers for Disease Control and Prevention. Pertussis vaccination: acellular pertussis vaccine for reinforcing and booster use—supplementary ACIP statement. Recommendations of the Immunization Practices Advisory Committee (ACIP). MMWR 1992;41:RR-1.

U.S. Centers for Disease Control and Prevention. Pertussis vaccination: acellular pertussis vaccine for the fourth and fifth doses of the DTP series. Update to supplementary ACIP statement. Recommendations of the Immunization Practices Advisory Committee. MMWR 1992;41:RR-15.

U.S. Centers for Disease Control and Prevention. FDA approval of use of a new Haemophilus b conjugate vaccine and a combined diphtheria-tetanus-pertussis and Haemophilus b conjugate vaccine for infants and children. MMWR 1993;42:296–298.

Measles–Mumps–Rubella Vaccine

U.S. Centers for Disease Control and Prevention. Measles prevention: recommendations of the Immunization Practices Advisory Committee (ACIP). MMWR 1989;38:S-9.

U.S. Centers for Disease Control and Prevention. Mumps prevention: recommendations of the Immunization Practices Advisory Committee (ACIP). MMWR 1989;38:22.

U.S. Centers for Disease Control and Prevention. Rubella prevention: recommendations of the Immunization Practices Advisory Committee (ACIP). MMWR 1990;39:RR-15.

Polio Vaccine

American Academy of Pediatrics, Committee on Infectious Diseases. Administration of the third dose of oral poliomyelitis vaccine at 6 to 18 months of age. Pediatrics 1994;94:774–775.

U.S. Centers for Disease Control and Prevention. Poliomyelitis prevention. MMWR 1982;31:22–26,31–34.

U.S. Centers for Disease Control and Prevention. Poliomyelitis prevention: enhanced-potency inactivated poliomyelitis vaccine—supplementary statement. MMWR 1987;36:795–798.

Haemophilus Influenze Type B Vaccine

U.S. Centers for Disease Control and Prevention. Haemophilus b conjugate vaccines for prevention of Haemophilus influenza type b disease among infants and children two months of age and older: recommendations of the Immunization Practices Advisory Committee (ACIP). MMWR 1991;40:RR-1.

U.S. Centers for Disease Control and Prevention. FDA approval of use of a new Haemophilus b conjugate vaccine and a combined diphtheria-tetanus-pertussis and Haemophilus b conjugate vaccine for infants and children. MMWR 1993;42:296–298.

Hepatitis B Vaccine

U.S. Centers for Disease Control and Prevention. Hepatitis B virus: a comprehensive strategy for eliminating transmission in the United States through universal childhood vaccination. Recommendations of the Immunization Practices Advisory Committee (ACIP). MMWR 1991;40(RR-13). [Copies of this report can be obtained from Hepatitis Branch, Centers for Disease Control and Prevention, Mailstop A33, 1600 Clifton Road, Atlanta, GA 30333, 404-639-2339.]

American Academy of Pediatrics, Committee on Infectious Diseases. Universal hepatitis B immunization. Pediatrics 1992;89(4 Pt 2):795–800.

Influenza Vaccine

Advisory Committee on Immunization Practices. Prevention and control of influenza, part I, vaccines: recommendations of the Advisory Committee on Immunization Practices (ACIP). MMWR 1994;43:RR-9.

Pneumococcal Vaccine

U.S. Centers for Disease Control and Prevention. Pneumococcal polysaccharide vaccine: recommendations of the Immunization Practices Advisory Committee. MMWR 1989; 38:64–68,73–76.

Other Vaccines

Centers for Disease Control and Prevention. Licensure of varicella virus vaccine, live. MMWR 1995;44:264.

Immunization Practices Advisory Committee. Rabies prevention—United States, 1991. MMWR 1991;40(RR-3).

Lieu TA, Cochi SL, Black SB, Halloran E, Shinefield HR, Holmes SJ, Wharton M, Washington AE. Cost-effectiveness of a routine varicella vaccination program for U.S. children. JAMA 1994;271:375–381.

National Association of State Public Health Veterinarians. Compendium of animal rabies control, 1994. MMWR 1994;43 (RR-10):1–9.

REFERENCES

1. Zimmerman RK, Giebink GS. Childhood immunizations: a practical approach for clinicians. Am Fam Phys 1992;45:1759–1772.
2. U.S. Centers for Disease Control and Prevention. Retrospective assessment of vaccination coverage among school-aged children: selected U.S. cities, 1991. MMWR 1992; 41:103–107.
3. U.S. Centers for Disease Control and Prevention. Vaccination coverage of 2-year-old children—United States, 1993. MMWR 1994;43:705–709.
4. Mustin HD, Holt VL, Connell FA. Adequacy of well-child care and immunizations in U.S. infants born in 1988. JAMA 1994;272:1111–1115.
5. Hutchins SS, Escola J, Markowitz LE, et al. Measles outbreak among unvaccinated preschool-aged children. Pediatrics 1989;83:369–374.
6. 1979 Immunization Survey. Vol. 1. Atlanta: Centers for Disease Control, 1979:120-1, 180-1.

7. U.S. Centers for Disease Control and Prevention. Recommendations of the Immunization Practices Advisory Committee (ACIP): Use of vaccines and immune globulins in persons with altered immunocompetence. MMWR 1993;42:RR-4.

8. King GE, Hadler SC. Simultaneous administration of childhood vaccines: an important public health policy that is safe and efficacious. Pediatr Infect Dis J 1994;13:394–407.

9. Ad Hoc Working Group for the Development of Standards for Pediatric Immunization Practices. Standards for pediatric immunization practices. JAMA 1993;269:1817–1822.

10. U.S. Centers for Disease Control and Prevention. General recommendations on immunization: recommendations of the Advisory Committee on Immunization Practices (ACIP). MMWR 1994;43(RR-1):15–17.

11. Greenberg MA, Birx DL. Safe administration of mumps-measles-rubella vaccine in egg-allergic children. J Pediatr 1988;113:504–506.

12. U.S. Centers for Disease Control and Prevention. Resurgence of pertussis—United States, 1993. MMWR 1993;42:952–953,959–960.

13. Broome CV, Preblud SR, Bruner B, et al. Epidemiology of pertussis, Atlanta, 1977. J Pediatr 1981;98:362–367.

14. Institute of Medicine. DTP vaccine and chronic nervous system dysfunction: a new analysis. Washington, DC: National Academy Press, 1994.

15. U.S. Centers for Disease Control and Prevention. Rubella prevention. MMWR 1990;39:R-15.

16. Institute of Medicine. Adverse effects of pertussis and rubella vaccines. Washington, DC: National Academy Press, 1991.

17. U.S. Centers for Disease Control and Prevention. Progress toward the elimination of Haemophilus influenzae type b disease among infants and children—United States, 1987–1993. MMWR 1994;43:144–148.

18. U.S. Centers for Disease Control and Prevention. Vaccination coverage of 2-year-old children—United States, January–March, 1994. MMWR 1994;44:142–143, 149–150.

19. Mahoney FJ, Burkholder BT, Matson CC. Prevention of hepatitis B virus infection. Am Fam Phys 1993;47:865–872.

20. Loewenson PR, White KE, Osterholm MT, MacDonald KL. Physician attitudes and practices regarding universal infant vaccination against hepatitis B infection in Minnesota: implications for public health policy. Pediatr Infect Dis J 1994;13:373–378.

21. Fedson DS, Harward MP, Reid RA, Kaiser DL. Hospital-based pneumococcal immunization: epidemiologic rationale from the Shenandoah study. JAMA 1990;264:1117–1122.

22. Health information for international travel, 1994. HHS Publication No. (CDC) 94-8280. Atlanta: U.S. Centers for Disease Control and Prevention, 1994.

23. Zimmerman RK. The role of family physicians in immunization. Arch Fam Med 1994;3:225–227.

24. Fedson DS. Adult immunization: summary of the National Vaccine Advisory Committee Report. JAMA 1994;272:1133–1137.

25. U.S. Centers for Disease Control and Prevention. National Childhood Vaccine Injury Act: requirements for permanent vaccination records and for reporting of selected events after vaccination. MMWR 1988;37:197–200.

19. Chemoprophylaxis

STEVEN H. WOOLF

INTRODUCTION

Chemoprophylaxis in preventive medicine is the use of drugs, nutritional and mineral supplements, or other natural substances by asymptomatic persons to prevent future disease. It does not include using such agents to treat symptomatic illnesses or in persons with a prior history of the disorder. This chapter examines the use of medications for preventive chemoprophylaxis. (Examples of other agents used for preventive chemoprophylaxis are the use of iron supplements in menstruating or pregnant women or in young children to decrease the risk of iron-deficiency anemia, fluoride supplements to decrease the risk of dental caries, folic acid supplements to decrease women's risk of giving birth to children with neural tube defects, and beta carotene and antioxidants to reduce the risk of cancer and heart disease. Only some of these practices are fully supported by current evidence.)

This chapter examines the most commonly recommended drugs for preventive chemoprophylaxis: postmenopausal estrogen to prevent osteoporosis and heart disease, and aspirin to prevent heart disease, stroke, and possibly cancer. The chapter examines the role of these drugs in primary prevention (i.e., for asymptomatic persons). The use of aspirin in patients with known cardiovascular disease and the use of estrogen to control postmenopausal symptoms are not discussed.

SHARED DECISION MAKING

Shared decision making plays an important role in counseling patients about chemoprophylaxis, as well as about other medical interventions with complex benefits and harms. *Shared decision making* refers to the process of providing patients with information about potential outcomes in a manner that empowers them to make individual choices based on their personal preferences. This approach differs from the older, more paternalistic practice in which physicians told patients "what to do." It is especially relevant to the interventions discussed in this chapter, because they involve drugs with important side effects and complications.

The inappropriateness of the paternalistic approach is understood by realizing that medical decisions involve both objective and subjective elements. The objective elements are the facts about the potential benefits and harms of various options. They are based largely on scientific and clinical information and are often best assessed by health professionals. However, the next step in decision making is to determine which option is best for the particular patient, which depends on a subjective assessment of the relative importance of benefits and harms in one's life. The latter, at least in part, is a matter of personal preference and is best determined by the patient. The paternalistic clinician who simply tells patients "what to do" intrudes on the subjective part of decision making. Clinicians who feel justified in doing so assume, often incorrectly, that patients lack knowledge and would share the same opinions that they assign to potential benefits and harms if they had the same knowledge. Studies have confirmed that physician estimations of patient preferences and knowledge are often inaccurate.

The primary professional responsibility of the clinician who practices shared decision making is to frame the objective elements of the decision: provide the patient with the latest evidence about the potential benefits and harms of available options, the probability of those outcomes, and the quality of the evidence on which the information is based. Summarizing this information in a balanced presentation that does not introduce personal biases is often difficult. The tone and body language used by the clinician and the emphasis given to certain facts can expose the clinician's biases and distort the patient's understanding of the topic. Current research is exploring the use of various tools, such as carefully designed "objective" fact sheets (see Fig. 21.1), videotapes, and interactive videodiscs, which clinicians can use to provide patients with a balanced discussion of the topic.

The next step in shared decision making is the subjective component, in which the patient arrives at a decision by considering the relative importance of the potential benefits and harms. The proper role of the clinician in helping the patient to make a decision is variable, depending on the patient's wishes and personality. Some independent, well-empowered patients reach conclusions immediately after the "information presentation" without further assistance from the clinician. Many patients make better decisions if the clinician helps to structure the decision making process. For example, the clinician can say, *"So, in summary, this treatment will lower your risk of cancer by about 50%, but there is also a 10% chance that it will cause blurred vision. To make this decision, you will have to balance the benefits of lowering your risk of cancer against the risk of poor vision."* This assistance in framing the issues will help many patients to reach a conclusion. Others will still have difficulty in weighing the options and will ask clinicians for their advice or will request that they make the decision for them.

Clinicians who engage in shared decision making are often surprised by their patients' choices, reflecting the differences between patient preferences and professional values in the face of the same facts. It is important for clinicians to respect the choices made by patients and not try to "talk them out of it." Disapproving comments (e.g., *Are you sure about this?*) and nonverbal communication (e.g., raised eyebrows, frowning) are inappropriate. Clinicians who think that the patient has made the wrong decision should ask themselves whether objective or subjective "errors" led to the decision. If there is a problem with the objective element, meaning that the clinician believes that the patient was influenced by incomplete or inaccurate facts about the benefits and harms, the clinician should remedy this problem by providing more accurate information. But if the problem is with the subjective element, meaning that the patient understands the facts but has demonstrated a value judgment that differs from that of the clinician, it is inappropriate for the clinician to suggest that such conclusions are "wrong" and impose his or her personal preferences on the patient. The choices made by well-informed patients are, by definition, the best choices, and interference by health professionals is disrespectful, inappropriate, and often counterproductive.

ESTROGEN REPLACEMENT THERAPY

Loss of ovarian estrogens following menopause is associated with decreased bone density, elevated blood cholesterol, increased risk of coronary artery disease, and postmenopausal symptoms (e.g., hot flashes, atrophic vaginitis). In addition to the unpleasantness of these symptoms, the biologic effects of estrogen deficiency contribute to substantial morbidity and mortality from osteoporotic fractures and heart disease. Estrogen replacement can reduce the risk of osteoporotic fractures by enhancing bone mineral content and can reduce the risk of ischemic heart disease, in part by improving serum lipid profiles and fibrinogen levels. Unopposed oral estrogens (estrogens without a combined progestin) generally raise the serum level of high-density lipoproteins and decrease the level of low-density lipoproteins; estrogens in combination with progestin have the same effect but raise high-density lipoproteins less dramatically; and transdermal estrogen does not appear to substantially change lipid profiles. (Although not addressed directly in this chapter, estrogen replacement also reduces vasomotor symptoms, atrophic vaginitis, and, possibly, some adverse psychological features associated with menopause.)

Estrogen replacement therapy is not without risks. The use of unopposed estrogen increases the risk of developing endometrial hyperplasia and cancer. This risk can be reduced by adding a combined progestin for at least twelve days of the cycle, but it is unclear whether progestins limit the beneficial effects of estrogen on heart disease. Although progestins have no significant effect on lowering low-density lipoproteins, increases in high-density lipoproteins may be blunted by some progestin formulations, and the overall effect on risk of myocardial infarction and other heart disease outcomes awaits the results of ongoing clinical trials (1). Estrogen may also increase the risk of breast cancer, but current evidence is inconclusive regarding the magnitude of this risk. The body of evidence to date suggests that, if a risk exists, it affects primarily women who have taken estrogens for 10 or more years. The effects of progestins on breast cancer risk are uncertain.

Compliance with estrogen replacement therapy can be difficult because of the long-term nature of therapy and the attendant costs. Common barriers to compliance include dislike of taking tablets, fear of cancer, and continued menstruation or spotting. The average wholesale costs of estrogen replacement therapy are about $100–$200 per year.

Official Recommendations

Most groups (including the U.S. Preventive Services Task Force, Canadian Task Force on the Periodic Health Examination, American College of Obstetricians and Gynecologists, American College of Physicians, and American Academy of Family Physicians) advise physicians to discuss the benefits and harms of estrogen replacement therapy with perimenopausal and postmenopausal women. Reviews of the data by the U.S. Preventive Services Task Force, Canadian Task Force on the Periodic Health Examination, and American College of Physicians have concluded, however, that there is insufficient evidence to make a blanket recommendation for or against routine hormone replacement in postmenopausal women.

Essentials of Counseling

Physicians should provide perimenopausal and postmenopausal women with information about the potential benefits and harms of estrogen replacement therapy. In general, women should not be told that they should or should not start taking estrogen. Instead, the principles of shared decision making should be used to arrive at a decision. The information provided in Table 19.1 may be helpful in framing the objective elements of the decision. Written brochures (see "Resources—Patient Education Materials" section later in this chapter) may also be helpful in providing background reading as the woman considers her options. Women at increased risk of coronary artery disease should understand that they are more likely than other women to benefit from estrogen replacement therapy. The distinctions between relative and absolute risk (see Chapter 1) should also be clarified. For example, the average 65–74-year-old woman faces a 0.6% risk

Table 19.1
Estimated Benefits and Harms of Estrogen Replacement Therapy

Potential Outcomes	Estimated Magnitude	
	Unopposed Estrogen	Estrogen/Progestin
	Benefits	
Decreased risk of coronary artery disease	About 35% risk reduction	Magnitude of benefit uncertain
Decreased risk of osteoporotic fractures	About 25% reduction in risk of hip fractures and about 50% reduction in risk of vertebral fractures	Magnitude of benefit uncertain
	Harms	
Endometrial cancer	Eightfold increase in risk after 10–20 years of use; little effect on mortality because endometrial cancer is generally curable; 20% lifetime probability of hysterectomy	No increase in risk
Breast cancer	Available evidence is inconsistent, but suggests that risk may be increased by about 25% after 10–20 years of treatment	Available evidence is inconsistent but suggests that increased risk is comparable to unopposed estrogen and could be larger
Other side effects	5–10% risk of bloating, headache, and breast tenderness; 35–40% risk of uterine bleeding	Dose-related increase in bloating, weight gain, irritability, and depression due to progestin; 30–50% risk of uterine bleeding in first 8–12 months

Adapted from American College of Physicians. Guidelines for counseling postmenopausal women about preventive hormone therapy. Ann Intern Med 1992;117:1038–1041.

of dying from a hip fracture. Thus, although estrogen replacement therapy might decrease the risk of hip fractures by 60%, the absolute risk of dying from a hip fracture would be reduced by only 0.36%. Some women may benefit from knowing their bone mineral content and risk of osteoporosis as an aid in decision making about estrogen replacement. See Chapter 21 regarding the limitations of bone densitometry and other imaging studies as screening tests for osteoporosis.

Women who choose to take estrogen replacement should be prescribed an estrogen-progestin regimen, unless they have undergone a hysterectomy. The most common estrogen-progestin regimens are *continuous combined therapy* (estrogen and progestin daily) or *continuous sequential therapy* (estrogen on days 1–25 of the menstrual cycle and progestin starting on days 10–13 and continuing through day 25). Estrogen is usually given once a day as 0.625 mg of conjugated equine estrogen (Premarin) or its equivalent (0.02 mg of ethinyl estradiol [Estinyl], 0.625 mg of estropipate [Ogen], 1 mg of micronized estradiol [Estrace]). Progestin is usually given daily as medroxyprogesterone acetate (2.5 mg for continuous combined therapy or 5–10 mg for continuous sequential therapy) or its equivalent (2.5–5.0 mg of norethindrone). Women should be advised that continuous sequential therapy is often accompanied by continued menstruation. Continuous combined therapy is more likely to achieve amenorrhea, but there is a 30–50% chance of breakthrough bleeding in the first eight to twelve months of therapy. The dose of medroxyprogesterone is typically increased to 5.0 or 10.0 mg per day if women experience spotting or irregular bleeding. Women who have undergone a hysterectomy can take unopposed estrogens, with the possible exception of women with a history of endometrioid ovarian tumors or endometriosis.

Estrogen can also be administered as transdermal patches, which deliver 0.5 mg or 1 mg of estradiol per day and are applied twice a week. The patch is applied to the skin of the lower abdomen or buttocks. Transdermal estrogen is delivered directly into the systemic circulation, thereby avoiding first-pass metabolism in the liver, but the physiological effects of this decrease in hepatic metabolism are currently uncertain. The transdermal route of administration is generally preferred for women who are intolerant to oral preparations and women with a history of hypertension, venous thromboembolism, or stable liver disease, but evidence to support these preferences is limited. Transdermal patches may also be especially advantageous in women who smoke. It is currently unclear whether transdermal estrogen improves lipid levels, and thus oral preparations may be preferred in women with hypercholesterolemia.

Some physicians recommend that women undergo a pelvic examination before starting treatment and, if no progestin is prescribed, an endometrial biopsy. On any regimen, an endometrial biopsy is probably necessary if the patient has repeated episodes of suspicious vaginal bleeding (for women on continuous combined therapy: heavy, prolonged, or frequent bleeding, or bleeding that occurs after the first 10 months during which breakthrough bleeding is expected; for women on continuous sequential therapy: bleeding on days of the cycle other than those during which withdrawal bleeding is expected). Vaginal bleeding is more suspicious if it occurs after amenorrhea has been established. See Chapter 21 regarding the role of endometrial biopsy.

Contraindications

Women should not be prescribed estrogen if they have a prior or current history of breast cancer, although there has been recent speculation that such a history might not preclude therapy in the future. Other absolute contraindications include known or suspected pregnancy and a prior history of thrombophlebitis while taking hormone replacements. Relative contraindications include endometrial cancer, undiagnosed abnormal vaginal bleeding, and active thrombophlebitis. There is no evidence that estrogen replacement therapy increases the risk of venous thrombosis in postmenopausal women, but such a history is often identified as a relative contraindication. Because of current uncertainty regarding the effects of progestins on the risk of ischemic heart disease, combination therapy may be less advisable than unopposed estrogen therapy in women with multiple cardiac risk factors.

ASPIRIN PROPHYLAXIS

Studies suggest that asymptomatic men who take aspirin daily can reduce their risk of developing coronary artery disease in the future. (Its role in the treatment of men and women with known cardiovascular disease, such as prior myocardial infarctions, transient ischemic attacks, or strokes, and its role in the prevention of preeclampsia, for which it may also be effective, is beyond the scope of this book.) The principal evidence regarding aspirin use in asymptomatic persons comes from a British and American clinical trial, both of which studied healthy male physicians (2, 3). The American study reported a 44% reduction in the incidence of myocardial infarction (from about 0.4% to 0.2%) in men who took 325 mg of aspirin every other day. There was no improvement in cardiovascular mortality, but there were insufficient deaths in the study to demonstrate a statistically significant difference. The British study reported no difference in myocardial infarctions or mortality at a dose of 500 mg daily. The generalizability of these findings to women is uncertain. A large clinical trial involving over 40,000 female health professionals, which is currently in progress, is expected to provide direct evidence regarding the benefits of aspirin in women.

The value of aspirin in the primary prevention of cerebrovascular disease and cancer is currently under study. The principal benefit appears to lie in the prevention of embolic strokes and seems most appropriate in persons with risk factors for cerebrovascular disease. Evidence from some observational studies suggests that aspirin may reduce the risk of colorectal cancer, but this hypothesis needs to be confirmed in prospective controlled trials.

The adverse effects of routine aspirin use are not insignificant, because its antiplatelet activity may increase the risk of gastrointestinal and intracranial bleeding. The relationship between aspirin use and gastrointestinal bleeding appears to be dose-related. At doses as low as 75 mg daily, a small but statistically significant increase in bleeding has been observed;

this risk is doubled at 300 mg daily and increased by about 500% at doses of 1800–2400 mg daily (4). The previously mentioned American trial reported a statistically significant increase in the incidence of gastrointestinal hemorrhage requiring transfusion among the men who took aspirin. The above studies also reported a trend toward an increased incidence of hemorrhagic stroke in the group taking aspirin, but the increase was not statistically significant and the absolute risk of hemorrhagic stroke was low (less than 0.3%).

Official Recommendations

The U.S. Preventive Services Task Force and the Canadian Task Force on the Periodic Health Examination found insufficient evidence to recommend for or against counseling patients to take aspirin prophylaxis. The American Heart Association has stated that aspirin prophylaxis is prudent in middle-aged and older men whose risks of a first myocardial infarction are sufficiently high to warrant the potential adverse effects of long-term aspirin use. Each of these groups and the American Academy of Family Physicians emphasize the need for individualized decision making in which the patient considers the potential benefits and harms of aspirin.

Essentials of Counseling

Physicians should discuss the potential benefits and harms of routine aspirin use with men over age 40. (Women who are interested in routine aspirin use should understand that there is no direct evidence that it benefits women or that the benefits outweigh the risks.) The principles of shared decision making should be followed to arrive at a decision. Written brochures (see "Resources—Patient Education Materials" later in this chapter) may also be helpful in summarizing the benefits and harms. Patients should understand that the benefits of aspirin are more likely to outweigh the risks of bleeding if they are at increased risk of coronary artery disease or embolic strokes.

Patients who choose to begin aspirin prophylaxis should take 325 mg daily or every other day. Although a dose as low as 75 mg daily may be adequate to achieve the desired antiplatelet activity, further research is necessary to determine the optimal dose. Use of aspirin preparations that are diluted, enteric-coated, or buffered; cimetidine or other H_2 blockers; and antacids may decrease the risk of gastrointestinal discomfort and bleeding.

Contraindications

Routine aspirin use should be reconsidered in patients with a history of peptic ulcer disease or gastrointestinal bleeding, cerebral hemorrhage, history of uncontrolled hypertension, a bleeding diathesis, allergy to aspirin, liver or kidney disease, or diabetic retinopathy.

ORGANIZATION OF OFFICE OR CLINIC

Offices or clinics that provide counseling about chemoprophylaxis should offer relevant patient education materials (see "Resources—Patient Education Materials" later) in the waiting area and in the examining room, so that the physician can hand the brochures directly to the patient after counseling.

MEDICAL RECORD DOCUMENTATION

Physicians should document in the medical record that the patient was counseled about chemoprophylaxis. If the patient chooses to forego treatment, the physician should document this decision and should note in the record that the patient received adequate information about potential benefits and harms. See Chapters 3 and 4 regarding reminder systems to ensure that women receive breast cancer screening on schedule, which is especially important for women taking estrogen.

RESOURCES—PATIENT EDUCATION MATERIALS

Estrogen Replacement Therapy

American Academy of Family Physicians
8880 Ward Parkway
Kansas City, MO 64114-2797
800-944-0000
> "Osteoporosis in Women" (brochure 1510); "Every Woman's Guide to Osteoporosis" (brochure 1179); "Osteoporosis in Women: Keeping Your Bones Healthy and Strong" (brochure 1510).

Arthritis Foundation
P.O. Box 19000, Drawer AI
Atlanta, GA 30326
800-283-7800
> "Osteoporosis" (brochure 4191).

Krames Communications
Order Department
1100 Grundy Lane
San Bruno, CA 94066-9821
800-333-3032
> "Hormone Replacement Therapy" (brochure 1364).

National Arthritis and Musculoskeletal and Skin Diseases Information Clearinghouse
P.O. Box AMS
9000 Rockville Pike
Bethesda, MD 20892
301-495-4484

National Institute on Aging
NIA Information Center
P.O. Box 8057
Gaithersburg, MD 20898-8057
800-222-2225
    "Should You Take Estrogen?"

National Osteoporosis Foundation
1150 17th Street, NW, Suite 500
Washington, DC 20036-4603
202-223-2226
    "Stand Up To Osteoporosis."

Aspirin

American Heart Association
Office of Scientific Affairs
7272 Greenville Avenue
Dallas, TX 75231-4596
800-242-8721
    "Aspirin and Cardiovascular Diseases." (publication 64-9609).

RESOURCES—PROFESSIONAL EDUCATION MATERIALS

American College of Physicians
Department of Scientific Policy
Independence Mall West
Sixth Street at Race
Philadelphia, PA 19106-1572
    "Guidelines for Counseling Postmenopausal Women About Preventive Hormone Therapy." See also Ann Intern Med 1992;117:1038–1041.

American Heart Association
Office of Scientific Affairs
7272 Greenville Avenue
Dallas, TX 75231-4596
800-242-8721
    "Aspirin as a Therapeutic Agent in Cardiovascular Disease."

SUGGESTED READINGS

Belchetz PE. Hormone treatment of postmenopausal women. N Engl J Med 1994;330:1062–1071.
Canadian Task Force on the Periodic Health Examination. Periodic health examination, 1991 update: 6. Acetylsalicylic acid and the primary prevention of cardiovascular disease. Can Med Assoc J 1991;145:1091–1095.
Grady D, Rubin SM, Pettiti DB, Fox CS, Black D, Ettinger B, et al. Hormone therapy to prevent disease and prolong life in postmenopausal women. Ann Intern Med 1992;117:1016–1037.
Lufkin EG, Ory SJ. Relative value of transdermal and oral estrogen therapy in various clinical situations. Mayo Clin Proc 1994;69:131–135.

REFERENCES

1. The Writing Group for the PEPI Trial. Effects of estrogen or estrogen/progestin regimens on heart disease risk factors in postmenopausal women: the Postmenopausal Estrogen/Progestin Interventions (PEPI) trial. JAMA 1995;273:199–208.
2. Steering Committee of the Physicians' Health Study Research Group. Final report on the aspirin components of the ongoing Physicians' Health Study. N Engl J Med 1989;321:129–135.
3. Peto R, Gray R, Collins R, Wheatley K, Hennekens C, Jamrozik K, Warlow C, Hafner B, Thompson E, Norton S, et al. Randomized trial of prophylactic daily aspirin in British male doctors. Br Med J 1988;296:313–316.
4. Prichard PJ, Kitchingman GK, Hawkey CJ. Gastric mucosal bleeding: what dose of aspirin is safe? Gut 1987;28:A1401.

20. Self-Examination of the Breasts, Skin, and Testes

STEVEN H. WOOLF

INTRODUCTION

Cancer of the breast, skin (malignant melanoma), and testes have relatively good prognoses when diagnosed at an early stage. In addition to obtaining periodic cancer screening by physicians, the public has been advised for many years to perform monthly self-examinations at home to help detect malignant or premalignant conditions at a curable stage. Health professionals have been encouraged to devote time during clinical encounters to train and remind patients how to correctly perform self-examination.

The appropriateness of these recommendations is not universally accepted, however. As is discussed in more detail below, performing and teaching self-examination have not been shown in prospective studies to reduce morbidity or mortality and may have unintended adverse effects. Abnormalities detected by patients on self-examination, most of which are false-positives, often generate physician office visits, biopsies, and other procedures. While awaiting their follow-up appointments and biopsy results, patients may experience anxiety over the possibility of having cancer.

The controversy over self-examination is reflected in the discrepant recommendations of various groups. The American Cancer Society recommends that all women over age 20 and all postpubertal males perform monthly breast or testicular self-examination, respectively. According to the American Cancer Society, American Academy of Family Physicians, and American College of Obstetricians and Gynecologists, physicians should routinely teach their female patients breast self-examination technique. The American Academy of Dermatology, American Cancer Society, and the National Institutes of Health Consensus Development Conference on Malignant Melanoma recommend that physicians also teach patients how to perform skin self-examination. Other groups, however, have different recommendations. The U.S. Preventive Services Task Force and Canadian Task Force on the Periodic Health Examination, for example, found insufficient evidence to recommend for or against breast, skin, or testicular self-examination.

This chapter examines both sides of the controversy. For those clinicians interested in teaching self-examination to their patients, the chapter also discusses current methods for teaching self-examination and how to enhance compliance. The inclusion of these sections, however, does not imply an endorsement of self-examination by the editors. The chapter focuses on the examination of three organs—breasts, skin, and testes—for which self-examination is most commonly recommended. Self-examination of the oral cavity, eyes, and other parts of the body is recommended less frequently, supported by fewer scientific data, and therefore not discussed in this chapter. Screening for cancer through clinical examinations and laboratory screening tests (e.g., mammography) are discussed in Chapters 3 and 4.

THE CONTROVERSY OVER SELF-EXAMINATION

The primary debate over self-examination relates to whether it reduces morbidity or mortality. There is currently no direct evidence from controlled prospective studies that persons who practice self-examination have longer survival from cancer than those who do not. There is some indirect evidence, however, primarily related to self-detection of breast cancer. Most breast cancers are first discovered by patients and not their physicians [1]. As discussed in recent reviews [2, 3], observational studies suggest that breast cancers detected through self-examination are likely to be smaller and less advanced, to have less axillary node involvement, and to be associated with higher survival rates than cancers detected by other means [4–7]. Similarly, a thin malignant melanoma (less than 0.76 mm thickness) carries little risk of metastatic spread to other sites, but 10-year survival drops off to 66% if it is only slightly thicker (1.7–3.6 mm) at diagnosis; a grave prognosis is associated with more advanced lesions [8, 9].

Skeptics cite several problems with this evidence. First, some observational studies [2, 10–12] found no benefit from self-examination (although many of these studies suffered from design limitations themselves) [1]. Second, even in studies that reported a benefit, the higher survival rates associated with self-examination may reflect statistical artifacts (e.g., lead-time, length, or selection biases) rather than an actual reduction in mortality. In *lead-time bias*, survival appears to be longer simply because the cancer was diagnosed at an earlier age and not because death was postponed. In *length bias*, self-examination preferentially detects slowly growing tumors rather than aggressive malignancies, producing an artificially higher estimate of survival rates. *Selection bias* reflects the tendency of persons who practice self-examination to come from a more health-conscious population than the general public, making it unclear whether health practices other than self-examination (e.g., low dietary fat or alcohol intake) are more directly responsible for the observed benefits.

A third limitation relating to breast self-examination data is that many, if not most, women engaging in this practice also undergo screening by physicians and routine mammography, making it difficult to isolate the benefits attributable to self-examination. Fourth, in the case of testicular cancer, survival is good even without screening. About 60–80% of testicular seminomas are diagnosed at stage I without screening (13). Current survival rates approach 100% for early-stage disease and are over 80% for most other stages of testicular cancer (14). Given these potential biases, the only study design that can convincingly demonstrate the effectiveness of self-examination is a controlled, prospective study that compares morbidity and mortality rates in persons who do and do not perform self-examination. Such studies are currently underway in the United Kingdom and Russia for the evaluation of breast self-examination.

Proponents of self-examination cite other benefits of the practice. Introducing self-examination at an early age may make patients more familiar with the appearance and texture of their breasts, skin, and testes, thereby enabling more accurate and prompt detection of malignant changes later in life. Self-examination is inexpensive and empowers patients to take a more active role in the care of their body. In rural areas or other regions of the country with limited access to physicians or imaging centers (e.g., facilities for mammography or scrotal ultrasound), self-examination may provide the only available means of early detection. These potential benefits have not been proven.

The seeming harmlessness and low cost of self-examination are also debated. The examination skills of patients are often less sensitive and specific than those of clinicians trained in physical examination techniques and familiar with the physical characteristics of suspicious lesions. For example, although breast examination by physicians has a reported sensitivity of 45–63% (see Chapter 3), the reported sensitivity of breast self-examination is only 12–26%; higher rates (about 40%) are reported for younger women (under age 40) (15). The sensitivity of skin self-examination in detecting cancer is unknown. One study reported that its sensitivity in detecting large nevi was only 68% (16), suggesting an even lower sensitivity in detecting more subtle, malignant lesions.

Self-examination is thought to have a low positive predictive value: a large proportion of abnormalities found by the patient are likely to be benign conditions or normal tissue. For statistical reasons outlined in Chapter 4, the chances of false-positive results are even greater when the target condition is rare. In the case of testicular self-examination, the incidence of testicular cancer is extremely low (less than 3:100,000) (8), making it far more likely that abnormal findings on testicular self-examination will be benign conditions (e.g., epididymitis, spermatocele, hydrocele) than cancer. The low positive predictive value of self-examination has led some to worry that it may lead to an overdetection of harmless findings and to the unnecessary anxiety, discomfort, and cost of follow-up office visits and biopsies for benign lesions (17).

Other potential harms of self-examination have also been discussed. Persons who perform self-examination may mistakenly conclude that, if they do not find an abnormality, routine examinations by physicians are unnecessary. A particular concern for women is that this misunderstanding about breast self-examination might lead to poorer compliance with routine physician examination and mammography screening. Another concern is that a negative workup for an abnormality detected through self-examination might be misjudged by the patient as a reason to discontinue further screening. There is no evidence to support these concerns nor to suggest that they could not be remedied by proper patient education. In fact, some studies suggest that women who perform breast self-examination are more health-conscious and therefore more likely than other women to comply with physician screening examinations (1).

Another focus of controversy is whether standardized self-examination is more sensitive or specific than incidental detection. Many lesions detected by patients are discovered during bathing, dressing, and other routine activities. It is unclear whether the detection rate that occurs with these normal activities differs appreciably from that of self-examination performed according to a schedule (e.g., monthly) or to the step-by-step techniques recommended by experts.

Recommendations that clinicians incorporate self-examination instructions into routine visits have also drawn criticism. Many practitioners lack enthusiasm for teaching self-examination. In one survey, for example, 82% of physicians were unfamiliar with how to teach testicular self-examination or had not thought about it (18). There are several key objections to teaching self-examination. First, a thorough demonstration of self-examination technique is time-consuming; busy clinicians often lack the time for such counseling or do so at the expense of other forms of health education. A second concern is the lack of evidence that teaching is effective. Although some studies suggest that teaching self-examination improves patient knowledge levels and self-reported performance of self-examination, other studies have shown no effect (19). Self-reports of performance may not correlate with actual performance or improved detection; knowing how to perform the examination does not necessarily correlate with practice. In a national survey, 88% of women age 18 or older reported that they knew how to perform breast self-examination, but only 43% of the same sample reported performing the procedure at least 12 times each year (20). A third concern, as discussed below, is recidivism: patients who begin practicing self-examination on the advice of their physician often do not continue the practice over time, or do so incorrectly.

These concerns aside, self-examination clearly has the *potential* to reduce morbidity and mortality through early detection. No study has convincingly demonstrated that self-examination is ineffective or results in more harm than good, and there is suggestive evidence of potential benefits. In the case of breast cancer, for example, between 50% and 90% of tumors are first detected by patients and not clinicians. Studies of women undergoing regular breast cancer screening with clinical breast examinations and mammography report that 13–17% of cancers are detected by patients between screenings. Although theoretical harms from self-examination have been raised, the risks and costs of this simple practice are certainly far less than those of expensive or invasive clinical procedures that are routinely used in patient care despite similarly inadequate supporting evidence.

PROPER TECHNIQUE

Clinicians should consider these issues in deciding whether to devote time to teaching patients how to perform self-examination. For those interested in doing so, Tables 20.1–20.3 summarize the key instructions that patients are generally given. The absence of meaningful scientific data makes it difficult to know whether each of these steps is necessary. Few self-examination protocols have been validated in studies that measured clinical outcomes. Studies using intermediate outcomes have often produced conflicting results regarding the importance of specific self-examination procedures. For example, it is unclear whether women performing breast

Table 20.1
Instructions for Breast Self-Examination

• Don't check your breasts during your period. The best time is 3–7 days after your period ends.

• Lie on your back, place a towel or pillow under your right shoulder, and place your right hand behind your head. Examine your right breast and armpit with your left hand. Repeat with the left breast. You can use a "concentric" approach to make sure you examine the entire breast: Press the pads of your three middle fingers flat against the breast, moving gently in a circular motion, starting at the outermost top edge of the breast and spiraling in toward the nipple. Think of your breast as an imaginary clock face. Begin at the outermost rim at 12 o'clock, then move to 1 o'clock, and so on around the circle back to 12. Examine every part of the breast, from the armpit area to the breast bone, up to the collar bone, and back to the armpit. Feel for knots, lumps, thickenings, indentations, or swellings.

• Stand in front of a mirror. With arms at your sides and then raised above your head, look for changes in the size, shape, and contour of each breast. Look for swelling, bulges, puckering, dimpling, skin irritation or sores, changes in nipples, nipple discharge, or changes in skin texture.

If there are lumps, knots, nipple discharge, or other suspicious changes, contact your doctor.

Table 20.2
Instructions for Skin Self-Examination

Visual exam

- Undress completely and look at your body in a well-lighted room. Have a spouse or partner help you check the parts of your body that are difficult to see, or use a large hand mirror.
- The first time you do the self-examination, locate all moles, birthmarks, scars, spots, bumps, and lumps. It may be helpful for future reference to measure the width of unusual pigmented lesions (moles) and to mark their location on a body diagram.
- At future examinations, look for any changes in the size, shape, or color of these spots. Then look for new moles or sores.
- Lift your scalp hair and look at the skin underneath. A hand-held mirror or the assistance of a spouse or friend is often helpful to see the entire scalp. A hand-held blow dryer, turned to a cool setting, can be used to lift the hair and expose the scalp.
- Look closely at your face, neck, and ears. Men with facial hair should also look at the skin underneath.
- Look at your arms and hands, including the palms, front and back sides, spaces between the fingers, and fingernails. In front of a mirror, hold up your arms, bent at the elbows, with the palms facing you, to examine the back of your forearms and elbows.
- Look at your chest and abdomen. Looking in the mirror, lift your arms over your head with the palms facing each other. Look at each side of your body, including the hands and arms, underarms, and the sides of your trunk, thighs, and lower legs.
- Using a full-length mirror to help get a complete view, look at pubic areas, legs, and feet. With your back to the mirror, check the back of your neck and arms, the back itself, your buttocks, backs of your thighs, and lower legs.
- Sit down and prop up one leg on a chair or stool in front of you. Use a hand-held mirror to examine the inside of the propped-up leg, beginning at the groin area and moving the mirror down the leg to your foot. Also check the bottom of the feet and the spaces between the toes. Repeat the procedure with the other leg.

Touch exam

- Run your fingers over your whole body (including your scalp), feeling for lumps, bumps, or rough spots.
- Feel the back of your arms and shoulders.

Contact your doctor if you notice a change in a mole or other skin marking or if you have a new unexplained mole, skin lump, ulcer, or unhealed sore that has appeared since your last examination.

Adapted from Griffith HW. Instructions for Patients, 5th ed. Philadelphia: WB Saunders, 1994:571, and Friedman RJ, Rigel DS, Silverman MK, Kopf AW, Vossaert KA. Malignant melanoma in the 1990s: the continued importance of early detection and the role of physician examination and self-examination of the skin. CA 1991;41:201–226.

self-examination achieve a higher lump detection rate using the "vertical-strip" or "concentric-circle" method to completely palpate the breasts (21), although some studies suggest the vertical-strip method provides greater coverage.

The lack of evidence of an optimal self-examination protocol should be kept in mind in interpreting the recommendations of some experts that patients perform a series of specific self-examination procedures in special positions, using certain equipment, and sometimes with the assis-

Table 20.3
Instructions for Testicular Self-Examination

- Perform the examination after a warm bath or shower, while your hands are still warm.
- Examine each testicle gently with both hands. The index and middle fingers should be placed underneath the testicle, while the thumbs are placed on top. Roll the testicle gently between the thumbs and fingers.
- Your testicles should feel smooth, rubbery, and slightly tender. Surfaces should be smooth and without lumps. It is common for one testicle to be larger than the other.
- Feel for any abnormal hard lumps, nodules, or swelling on the front or side of the testicle.
- The epididymis is a cord-like structure on the top and back of the testicle. Do not confuse the epididymis with an abnormal lump.

If you find a lump, nodule, swelling, or dull ache, or if you notice another change, contact your doctor.

Adapted from National Cancer Institute. Testicular self-examination NIH Publication No. 94-2636. Bethesda, MD; National Cancer Institute, 1994.

tance of spouses or friends. Some instructions for skin self-examination specify six examination positions and the need for a full-length and hand-held mirror, blow dryer, two chairs, and an examination partner (5). Although common sense suggests that following these instructions would help patients examine themselves more carefully, there is no evidence that they achieve higher detection rates than more limited self-examinations. Quite the contrary, complex instructions may discourage patients from performing self-examination. Finally, there is no evidence to support the common advice to perform self-examination every month; no studies have determined whether monthly self-checks achieve higher detection rates than less frequent examinations.

COMPLIANCE

Most persons who are advised to perform monthly self-examinations do not do so. Reported compliance rates are about 20–35% for breast self-examination (2), 20% for skin self-examination (22), and 5–8% for testicular self-examination (15, 23). Moreover, a large proportion of persons who receive counseling or training to perform self-examination do not maintain the habit over time. Persons are more likely to perform self-examination if they fear cancer and believe that they are susceptible, believe that self-examination is an effective screening tool, understand how to perform the procedure, and have confidence in their examination skills (self-efficacy). The principal barriers include the absence of these beliefs, as well as fears of finding an abnormality, embarrassment, lack of time, and forgetting to do so. Poor compliance is sometimes due to misconceptions, such as believing that cancer can be detected early by simply paying attention to symptoms or that a healthy lifestyle is fully protective against cancer. Some barriers are related to age. Breast self-examination and the recognition of suspicious lesions by older women can be impaired by poor visual acuity, tactile sensation, and range of motion. Testicular and breast self-examination by adolescent boys and girls, respectively, can be influenced by embarrassment and uncomfortable feelings about body image.

Teaching patients how to perform self-examination, by itself, is unlikely to be effective if the clinician does not also address these concerns. Thus, along with teaching technique, clinicians should assess the patient's understanding of the rationale for self-examination, attitudes and beliefs about cancer and early detection, perceived self-efficacy, and relevant fears and anxieties about detecting cancer. Practical constraints, such as lack of time, privacy, or reminders to perform self-examination, should be addressed. The physical and cognitive limitations of older adults should receive special attention. Once this information has been gathered, the clinician's counseling about self-examination should be tailored to the patient's concerns. This may include correcting misconceptions about cancer, reassuring the patient that his or her self-examination technique is correct, suggesting reminder systems, and altering instructions for patients with physical limitations.

Many physicians lack the time, skills, or interest to properly teach self-examination. Trained nurses, physician assistants, and other counselors in the office or clinic are often better prepared and more capable than physicians of ensuring that patients fully understand examination technique and of reevaluating self-examination skills at future visits.

Patient education materials are often useful to help patients remember when to perform self-examination and to remind them of the proper technique. Although pamphlets (see "Resources—Patient Education Materials" later in this chapter) are often used to supplement counseling, videotapes and films are sometimes more effective in demonstrating examination technique. Self-examination can be taught in group settings, but current evidence is equivocal regarding the relative superiority of individual versus group counseling. Finally, patients need reminders and reinforcements to continue performing self-examination. Studies have shown that reassessment and retraining in breast self-examination may achieve higher breast lump detection rates (23). Thus, after teaching patients how to perform self-examination, clinicians may find it useful to reassess their performance and proficiency at a later date.

OFFICE AND CLINIC ORGANIZATION

Offices and clinics in which self-examination is taught should have private examination rooms in which the technique can be demonstrated. Some practices use models, diagrams, and illustrations as teaching aids. Patient education materials that reinforce and explain further the technique of self-examination and that define abnormal results should be easily accessible to hand to the patient; a list of such materials is provided below. Photographs of malignant and premalignant skin lesions, included either in office teaching aids or patient education literature, may help the patient identify important skin findings.

MEDICAL RECORD DOCUMENTATION

Clinicians who teach self-examination to patients should note the activity in the medical record, preferably on a flow sheet.

RESOURCES—PATIENT EDUCATION MATERIALS

Breast Self-Examination

American Cancer Society
1599 Clifton Road, NE
Atlanta, GA 30329
800-227-2345, 404-320-3333
"How to Do Breast Self Examination" (brochure, English 2088; Spanish 2674); "Triple Touch: How To Examine Your Breasts" (F-362); "For Women Only" (shower card, 2028).

Skin Self-Examination

National Cancer Institute
Office of Cancer Communications
Building 31, Rm 10A24
Bethesda, MD 20892
800-4-CANCER
"What You Need to Know About Skin Cancer" (brochure 94-1563).

Testicular Self-Examination

American Cancer Society
1599 Clifton Road, NE
Atlanta, GA 30329
800-227-2345, 404-320-3333
"For Men Only: Testicular Cancer and How To Do TSE" (brochure 2093); "For Men Only" (testicular self-examination shower card, 2028).

Krames Communications
1100 Grundy Lane
San Bruno, CA 94066-3030
800-333-3032
"Testicular Self-Examination" (brochure 1225).

National Cancer Institute
Office of Cancer Communications
Building 31, Rm 10A24
Bethesda, MD 20892
800-4-CANCER
"Testicular Self-Examination" (brochure 94-2636).

Oral Cavity Self-Examination

American Association of Oral and Maxillofacial Surgeons
9700 West Bryn Mawr Avenue
Rosemont, IL 60018
800-467-5268

REFERENCES

1. Foster RS Jr, Worden JK, Costanza MC, Solomon LJ. Clinical breast examination and breast self-examination. Cancer 1992;69:1992–1998.
2. Champion V. The role of breast self-examination in breast cancer screening. Cancer 1992;69:1985–1991.
3. Baines CJ. Breast self-examination. Cancer 1992;69(7 Suppl.):1942–1946.
4. Hill D, White V, Jolley D, Mapperson K. Self examination of the breast: is it beneficial? Meta-analysis of studies investigating breast self examination and extent of disease in patients with breast cancer. Br Med J 1988;297:271–275.
5. Foster RS, Constanza MC. Breast self-examination practices and breast cancer survival. Cancer 1984;53:999–1005.
6. Huguley CM, Brown RL, Greenberg RS, Clark WS. Breast self-examination and survival from breast cancer. Cancer 1988;62:1389–1396.
7. Kuroishi T, Tominaga S, Ota J, Horino T, Taguchi T, Ishida T, et al. The effect of breast self-examination on early detection and survival. Jpn J Cancer Res 1992;83:344–350.
8. Friedman RJ, Rigel DS, Silverman MK, Kopf AW, Vossaert KA. Malignant melanoma in the 1990s: the continued importance of early detection and the role of physician examination and self-examination of the skin. CA 1991;41:201–226.
9. National Institutes of Health Consensus Development Panel on Early Melanoma. Diagnosis and treatment of early melanoma. JAMA 1992;268:1314–1319.
10. O'Malley MS, Fletcher SW. Screening for breast cancer with breast self-examination. JAMA 1987;257:2197–2203.
11. Le Geyte M, Mant D, Vessey MP, Jones L, Yudkin P. Breast self examination and survival from breast cancer. Br J Cancer 1992;66:917–918.
12. Locker AP, Casildine J, Mitchell AK, Blamey RW, Roebuck EJ, Elston CW. Results from a seven-year programme of breast self-examination of 89,010 women. Br J Cancer 1989;60:401–405.
13. Westlake SJ, Frank JW. Testicular self-examination: an argument against routine teaching. Fam Pract 1987;4:143–148.
14. Richie JR. Detection and treatment of testicular cancer. CA 1993;43:151–175.
15. O'Malley MS, Fletcher SW. Screening for breast cancer with breast self-examination. JAMA 1987;257:2197–2203.
16. Gruber SB, Roush GC, Barnhill RL. Sensitivity and specificity of self-examination for cutaneous malignant melanoma risk factors. Am J Prev Med 1993;9:50–54.
17. Goldbloom RB. Self-examination by adolescents. Pediatrics 1985;76:126–128.
18. Sayger SA, Fortenberry JD, Beckman RJ. Practice patterns of teaching testicular self-examination to adolescent patients. J Adolesc Health Care 1988;9:441–442.
19. Dachs RJ, Garb JL, White C, Berman J. Male college students' compliance with testicular self-examination. J Adolesc Health Care 1989;10:295–299.
20. Piani A, Schoenborn C. Health promotion and disease prevention: United States, 1990. National Center for Health Statistics. Vital Health Stat 1993;10(185):59.
21. Murali ME, Crabtree K. Comparison of two breast self-examination techniques. Cancer Nurs 1992;15:276–282.

22. Friedman LC, Bruce S, Webb JA, Weinberg AD, Cooper HP. Skin self-examination in a population at increased risk for skin cancer. Am J Prev Med 1993;9:359–364.
23. Neef N, Scutchfield FD, Elder J, Bender SJ. Testicular self-examination by young men: an analysis of characteristics associated with practice. J Am Coll Health 1991;39:187–190.
24. Pinto BM. Training and maintenance of breast self-examination skills. Am J Prev Med 1993;9:353–358.

21. What Not to Do and Why

STEVEN H. WOOLF

INTRODUCTION

Not every potential preventive intervention is a good idea, although virtually every screening test has advocates who believe it should be performed on all patients, even in the absence of supporting evidence. There is a tendency in medicine to adopt unproven clinical practices because of their *potential* benefit to the patient. Studies to obtain persuasive proof of benefit often require over a decade to complete, during which time large numbers of patients may suffer enormous morbidity or mortality. Advocates of investigational cancer screening tests, for example, often argue that it is unethical to withhold tests that can detect early-stage cancer and to watch thousands of unscreened persons die from metastatic disease while awaiting the results of clinical trials. Aside from economic arguments, they argue, what is the harm in offering these potentially lifesaving tests while awaiting the completion of definitive studies?

These questions reflect the common tendency in medicine to overlook the potential adverse effects of health promotion or disease prevention efforts (1). It is sometimes counterintuitive to believe that such well-intentioned activities could result in more harm than good, and yet the potential harms can be significant. In the case of screening, as discussed in the introduction to Chapter 4, the potential harms include immediate complications from the test procedure (e.g., perforation during sigmoidoscopy) and the "cascade effect" produced by positive test results. That is, positive test results often require follow-up diagnostic procedures that are potentially uncomfortable or harmful to the patient (e.g., colonoscopy, breast biopsy). Falsely positive screening results can generate unnecessary anxiety, creating psychological morbidity that persists until the error is corrected. Screening can sometimes disclose clinically insignificant disease, exposing the patient unnecessarily to the risks and costs of treatment. Falsely negative results can give the patient an unfounded sense of security and may lead to the mistaken conclusion that further preventive measures (e.g., returning for repeat screening, modifying unhealthy behaviors) are unnecessary.

Other preventive services can also have harmful effects. Although immunizations generally produce only minor side effects (e.g., fever, local

448

discomfort at injection site), some vaccines can produce serious allergic reactions and other rare complications (e.g., paralytic poliomyelitis, Guillain-Barré syndrome) (see Chapter 18). Certain chemoprophylactic regimens (e.g., estrogen replacement therapy, aspirin prophylaxis) can cause major health problems, such as cancer, gastrointestinal hemorrhage, and stroke (see Chapter 19). Even patient education and counseling can be harmful if the patient is given incorrect information. Health behavior counseling can produce unnecessary psychological morbidity if the patient's risk of disease or need to modify behaviors is exaggerated.

As discussed in more detail in Chapter 27, important ethical concerns are raised by exposing patients to these risks. Patients receiving preventive services are generally asymptomatic, and therefore their care raises different ethical issues than does the care of symptomatic patients. Symptomatic patients visit clinicians seeking relief from discomfort or other health complaints that they have identified as problems. Exposing them to interventions with potential risks, if preceded by informed consent, is appropriate in light of the greater harm caused by their illness and the patients' desire for relief of symptoms. In the case of preventive services, however, the health problem and the need for intervention are usually raised by the clinician and not the patient. In this instance, the possibility of exposing an otherwise healthy individual to complications gives clinicians an extra responsibility to ensure that the benefits outweigh the risks.

The potential harms of preventive interventions are also important to society. Although an individual patient may be willing to undergo screening even though the potential harms outweigh the potential benefits, it is inappropriate for health policy officials or national medical organizations to encourage population-wide screening with such tests. Those concerned with public policy are responsible for ensuring that preventive interventions result in more good than harm for society at large. In an era of limited health care resources, it is difficult to justify expenditures for preventive services of unproven effectiveness, which may come at the expense of other services of proven benefit. The cost of financing routine ultrasound screening in low-risk pregnancies, for example, might mean that screening mammography, prenatal care, childhood immunizations, or other important services would be curtailed.

These concerns help explain why certain preventive services, despite having the potential to help patients, may nonetheless be discouraged by national health agencies and organizations. The decision to advise against certain preventive measures is often difficult and requires careful analysis of scientific evidence to determine the probability of potential benefits and harms. The detailed scientific arguments for recommending against specific maneuvers and the citations to relevant studies are beyond the scope of this chapter. The reader is referred to the reports of the U.S. Preventive Services Task Force (2) and the Canadian Task Force on the Periodic Health Examination (3) for the detailed rationale and relevant citations. Suggested readings at the end of the chapter provide further background on specific preventive measures.

This chapter examines screening tests that, according to the best evidence currently available, physicians should avoid performing on a routine basis. The list is not exclusive—a complete catalogue of inappropriate preventive services would number in the hundreds—this chapter therefore limits its discussion to the most commonly considered screening tests. Recommendations against performing these procedures are based on current evidence, which often is lacking because properly designed effectiveness studies have not been performed. Future research may demonstrate the effectiveness of the screening tests discussed in this chapter. Recommendations against performing these maneuvers on a routine basis are not meant to exclude their appropriate use in the diagnostic evaluation of patients with presenting complaints or in the screening of high-risk individuals.

ROUTINE BATTERIES

Commonly used screening test batteries include blood chemistry panels and complete blood counts that are performed routinely on asymptomatic persons. As discussed in more detail in Chapter 4, the probability of false-positive results is large when multiple tests are ordered at once. When ordered without indication, blood chemistry panels and other test batteries performed on asymptomatic persons are therefore more likely to erroneously produce abnormal findings, thus generating unnecessary diagnostic workups. Studies have shown that such testing practices also have little influence on clinical decision making. Further, even when the tests detect a true abnormality, there is little evidence that early detection results in improved outcome for the patient. The routine use of test batteries, because of the frequency with which they are ordered, accounts for billions of dollars in unnecessary health care expenditures in the United States.

ROUTINE SCREENING URINALYSES

Over 85 million urinalyses are ordered or performed in doctors' offices each year in the United States. Chemical (dipstick) and microscopic examination of the urine can detect a large number of urinary and other disorders by first detecting pyuria, hematuria, proteinuria, glycosuria, ketonuria, urinary crystals, casts, and other abnormalities. Of these, the conditions for which routine urinalysis of asymptomatic persons may be most beneficial is occult bacteriuria and diabetes mellitus. The early detection of asymptomatic bacteriuria may be important in young children, for whom permanent urologic abnormalities may be prevented through early treatment, but urine screening tests with adequate predictive value and supporting evidence of effectiveness are lacking. No prospective studies have shown that routine urinalyses improve health outcomes in asymptomatic persons, nor is there evidence that screening urinalyses are effective in reducing mortality from renal, bladder, or other urologic cancers. Because the prevalence of urinary disorders in healthy persons is low, routine urinalyses have a high probability of producing falsely positive results. Follow-up of abnormal results may generate a cascade of additional tests, including further urine studies, blood tests, imaging studies of the kidneys and bladder, and invasive procedures (e.g., cystoscopy).

PROSTATE-SPECIFIC ANTIGEN

Prostate-specific antigen (PSA) is often elevated in men with prostate cancer, and the American Cancer Society has recommended annual PSA testing of all men over age 50 (over age 40 for African American men and men with a positive family history). An important limitation of the test, however, is its poor specificity for clinically significant disease; abnormal results are often due to benign conditions (e.g., hypertrophy, prostatitis). Even when the findings are due to cancer, many carcinomas detected by PSA testing are unlikely to progress or manifest clinical symptoms in the patient's lifetime. Autopsy studies indicate that 30% of men over age 50 have histologic evidence of prostate cancer, far more than would be expected based on the prevalence of clinically apparent disease. Due to the frequently indolent behavior and slow growth of most prostate tumors, men with cancers detected through screening are often more likely to die of other causes (e.g., coronary artery disease) than of prostate cancer. Recent evidence suggests that prostate cancers detected by PSA screening often have features associated with progression (e.g., increased tumor volume, extracapsular penetration, poorly differentiated cells), but these findings lack sufficient predictive value to determine with certainty which cancers will remain latent and which will progress.

The most important problem with PSA screening is the lack of evidence that early detection and treatment of prostate cancer lower morbidity or mortality or that the benefits of treatment outweigh its potential harms. Randomized controlled trials comparing treatment with watchful waiting are currently in progress. Radical prostatectomy and radiation therapy can produce serious complications, such as incontinence, impotence, and death. While these risks may be justified in the treatment of potentially lethal prostate cancers, their appropriateness in treating cancers that are unlikely to progress is doubtful. Studies of watchful waiting suggest that men with localized prostate cancer may have a ten-year survival rate of 85–90% without treatment. Population-wide PSA testing of the 28 million American men over age 50 would subject large numbers of patients to these procedures, with uncertain benefit, and the effort would cost society billions of dollars each year. Given the slow growth of most tumors, the risk of iatrogenic complications from treatment, and current evidence that treatment results in more harm than good when life expectancy is less than 10 years, screening is especially difficult to justify in men over age 70. In the face of such uncertainties, PSA testing should not be ordered routinely on all men. Instead, physicians should first provide eligible patients (men age 50–70) with information about the potential benefits and harms of PSA testing and treatment before determining whether they want the test. See Chapter 19 for a discussion of "shared decision making," and see the conclusion of this chapter for a discussion of how to help patients decide about PSA testing.

OTHER SERUM TUMOR MARKERS

Other serum tumor markers can be elevated in persons with cancer of the pancreas, ovary, liver, and testes. Although these markers are used primarily to diagnose or monitor cancer treatment in patients with known or suspected disease, they are occasionally suggested as screening tests for asymptomatic persons. CA-125, for example, is often elevated in women with ovarian cancer and has been suggested as a screening test. It lacks sensitivity in asymptomatic women (about 50–85%), however, and its effect on clinical outcomes is unproven. CA 19-9 is often elevated in persons with pancreatic cancer (sensitivity of 70–80%), but its sensitivity for detecting early-stage disease in asymptomatic persons may be much lower. The low specificity of the test and the low prevalence of pancreatic cancer limit the positive predictive value of tumor marker screening, producing a high likelihood of false-positive results. Positive test results cannot be reliably confirmed through ultrasound imaging of the pancreas because of its limitations in detecting small lesions (see "Abdominal Ultrasound" later in this chapter). Combining tumor marker measurement with ultrasound screening may improve its sensitivity and specificity, but the clinical benefit and cost-effectiveness of this approach on a population-wide basis have not been fully evaluated.

ILLICIT DRUG SCREENING

About 15 million working Americans have their urine tested for illegal drugs each year. Although serum and urine assays for certain drugs play an important role when evaluating patients with evidence of intoxication, substance abuse, or unexplained neurologic or psychiatric symptoms, its use for routine screening of asymptomatic persons is more controversial, for several reasons. First, the accuracy of commonly used screening assays is limited, resulting in a high likelihood of false-positive results (about 30–60% for many urine drug assays). A positive result also provides little information on the individual's pattern of drug use. Second, positive screening test results can have serious personal, occupational, social, and legal consequences for the patient. Screening for illicit drugs without consent raises important ethical issues by violating the individual's privacy and confidentiality. Third, although it is clear that drug abuse and misuse account for enormous harms to the individual and society, there is little scientific evidence that early detection of drug abuse improves outcomes for the patient or enhances public safety. (Some employers have reported that urine drug testing improves productivity and reduces the frequency of worksite accidents.) Urine drug screening is mandatory for many government and transportation workers and for many private employees.

CHEST RADIOGRAPHY

Over 16 million chest radiographs are ordered or performed in doctors' offices each year in the United States. Screening chest radiography can detect early-stage lung cancer and therefore was once widely performed as a routine screening test. Multicenter clinical trials in the 1970s and 1980s, however, demonstrated that early detection of lung cancer through screening chest radiography and sputum cytology does not lower lung cancer mortality. Critics of these studies argue that the trials were not designed to evaluate the efficacy of chest radiography alone, that current radiographic technology is more sensitive, and that patients who smoke are more likely to benefit. Nonetheless, virtually no medical organization or health agency recommends routine chest radiography screening for lung cancer. Its use to screen for tuberculosis is sometimes suggested for persons who are unlikely to follow up on tuberculin skin test results (e.g., inmates of correctional institutions), but the clinical benefit of this practice has not been evaluated.

ABDOMINAL ULTRASOUND

Modern refinements in ultrasound technology have enhanced its sensitivity and specificity in detecting intra-abdominal pathology. It has therefore been suggested as a potential screening test for pancreatic cancer, ovarian cancer, and abdominal aortic aneurysms. Its sensitivity and specificity is probably poorest in detecting pancreatic cancer, for which there is also little evidence that early detection improves clinical outcome. Its positive predictive value in detecting ovarian cancer in asymptomatic women is also low, perhaps as low as 3%, but accuracy may be improved by obtaining transvaginal and color-Doppler views and by combining the results with serum tumor marker measurement (see discussion earlier in chapter). For ovarian cancer as well, however, there is little evidence that early detection improves outcome. Abdominal ultrasound has good sensitivity and specificity (80–100% and almost 100%, respectively) in detecting abdominal aortic aneurysms, a condition for which there is reasonable evidence that early detection improves outcome. Arguments against screening rest primarily on concerns about cost-effectiveness.

PERIPHERAL ARTERY EXAMINATION

Digital palpation of pedal pulses is a poor screening test for vascular disease, and Doppler ultrasound examination has been suggested by some proponents as a more accurate means of screening for peripheral arterial disease. The sensitivity and specificity of the test in asymptomatic persons are uncertain, however. There is also little evidence that early detection of peripheral arterial disease results in improved outcome, and the cost-effectiveness of such an approach has not been properly evaluated.

BONE DENSITY MEASUREMENT

Technological advances in bone densitometry have made it possible to accurately measure the mineral content of bones and thereby estimate the future risk of osteoporotic fractures. Although bone densitometry may have an important role when evaluating symptomatic patients, its potential effectiveness as a screening test is limited. Its ability to discriminate reliably between women who will or will not develop fractures is uncertain. The interventions that are generally recommended for women with decreased bone mineral content—estrogen replacement therapy, calcium supplementation, physical activity—are generally recommended irrespective of whether they have undergone bone density measurement. The principal purpose of screening for osteoporosis is to provide women with stronger arguments for following this advice (and for justifying the risks and side effects of hormone therapy). Although some women may be persuaded to take estrogen after being told that their bone density is low, most official groups have concluded that this provides insufficient grounds to recommend the potentially costly practice of routine bone density screening of all perimenopausal or postmenopausal women.

PULMONARY FUNCTION TESTING

Screening spirometry is sometimes included in comprehensive preventive examinations, especially those offered to business executives and in worksite screening programs. There is good evidence that thorough pulmonary function testing is accurate in detecting obstructive and restrictive pulmonary disease—it is, in fact, the reference standard that defines these conditions—but there is little evidence that early detection of chronic obstructive pulmonary disease or other lung disorders results in improved clinical outcomes. Smoking cessation requires urgent attention regardless of lung function test results. In certain occupational settings, early detection of pulmonary disease may identify harmful worksite exposures and inhalation risks. In the typical primary care setting, however, the cost-effectiveness of routinely performing this test, especially in nonsmokers, is doubtful. Simple pulmonary function tests, such as the measurement of peak-flow rates, are more cost-effective but less accurate in detecting pulmonary disease.

COLPOSCOPY

Colposcopy, the examination of the cervix under magnification to facilitate inspection, acetoacetate washing, and biopsy, is often performed as a follow-up test when patients have abnormal Papanicolaou cytology results. Some proponents have suggested using colposcopy as the initial screening test for cervical cancer to improve the sensitivity of screening. Few studies have examined colposcopy screening under these conditions, however; currently reported sensitivities and specificities are poor (about 30–45% and 70%, respectively). Moreover, the technique requires expensive equipment, specialized training, and may be more uncomfortable than the routine Papanicolaou examination. Its cost-effectiveness as a routine screening test has also not been evaluated.

ENDOMETRIAL BIOPSY

Endometrial biopsy is commonly performed on women with symptoms (e.g., abnormal vaginal bleeding) or laboratory results associated with uterine cancer (e.g., endometrial dysplasia or cancer on cervical cytology). Some proponents have suggested performing routine endometrial biopsy on all postmenopausal women or on selected high-risk groups (e.g., women taking estrogen replacement therapy). The technique has become more feasible in recent years with the introduction of soft plastic catheters that make aspiration curettage more comfortable. Nonetheless, there is little evidence regarding the sensitivity and specificity of endometrial biopsy in asymptomatic women. There are also few data to suggest that screening for endometrial cancer improves clinical outcome, which is generally good even without screening. In most cases, endometrial cancer is highly responsive to treatment, and early detection is common because most patients develop bleeding or spotting early in the course of disease.

TONOMETRY

An estimated 2.5 million persons in the United States suffer from glaucoma, the second leading cause of irreversible blindness. The principal screening tests for glaucoma are measurement of intraocular pressure (IOP), visual field testing, and evaluation of the optic disc. These measures are intended to detect elevated IOP and lower it with medications, but no studies have proven that these interventions reduce visual field loss or the incidence of blindness. IOP is common in the general population and is not specific to glaucoma; an estimated 70–97% of persons with elevated IOP will never develop the disease. Moreover, IOP measurement, visual field testing, and optic disc evaluation often have lower sensitivity and specificity when performed by primary care clinicians than by ophthalmologists and other eye specialists. Applanation and air puff noncontact tonometers are more accurate than Schiötz tonometers in measuring IOP, but they are generally unavailable in primary care offices and clinics. Similarly, although visual field testing, ophthalmoscopy, and evaluation of the optic disc can be performed by primary care physicians, the tests are generally more accurate when performed by eye specialists. Comprehensive eye examinations by eye specialists typically include additional tests, such as automated perimetry, direct ophthalmoscopy, nerve fiber layer analysis, and other evaluations of the optic nerve. For these reasons, primary care clinicians should refer patients who need glaucoma screening to an appropriate eye care specialist.

CONCLUSION

Many of the tests discussed in this chapter are specifically requested by patients based on information that they have received from relatives or friends, articles, television programs, or other lay media. A challenge faced by the clinician who feels that the screening test is inappropriate is providing the patient with a convincing explanation of why it should not be performed. Many patients are unsatisfied with arguments about inadequate evidence of benefit, since the value of detecting a disease seems intuitively obvious. Concerns about false-positive results may also seem irrelevant to the patient. The clinician's responsibility in this setting is to provide the patient with accurate and balanced information about the benefits and harms of testing and the rationale for discouraging the test. If, after receiving this information, the patient still wants the test, the physician faces a challenging conflict in responsibilities. As the patient's agent, some would argue that the physician's responsibility is to respect the patient's wishes and provide the test. Others would argue that the physician's responsibility to do no harm and to act as a "gatekeeper" over society's limited health care resources requires the physician to deny the patient's request. Physicians should decide on the basis of their own practice values which approach is best suited for them.

An important resource in helping patients with these decisions is patient education materials designed to review the advantages and disadvantages of a test. For example, as noted earlier, it is generally recommended that men who are eligible for the PSA test receive information about the benefits and harms of screening and treatment before undergoing testing. It is often difficult for the physician to present the facts objectively without revealing his or her biases (e.g., emphasizing the importance of early detection, minimizing the weaknesses in the evidence, dismissing the potential harms of treatment, or vice versa). Patient education materials that present information in a balanced fashion have been developed for this purpose. Figure 21.1 is an example of such a handout; although the data in the example are no longer current (4), its format illustrates how information about benefits and harms can be summarized for patients. See Chapter 23 for information about the role of a similar tool in modifying PSA test-ordering practices at a large health maintenance organization. Researchers at Dartmouth University (Foundation for Informed Medical Decision Making, Hanover, New Hampshire) have developed a videotape and interactive videodisc program for educating patients about PSA testing and other topics requiring shared decision making.

Patient education about the screening tests in this chapter should include a discussion of primary prevention rather than focusing only on testing. Patients who request screening tests are obviously concerned about the target condition and may not recognize that personal health behaviors are more likely to prevent diseases than testing. For example, the woman who requests bone densitometry to "prevent osteoporosis" may not realize that exercise, calcium supplementation, and estrogen replacement therapy are far more likely to prevent the disease. The patient who wants a carotid artery ultrasound examination should instead be encouraged to stop smoking and control blood pressure and cholesterol values. The patient's interest in screening is sometimes an indication that they are not truly asymptomatic. A request for a blood count or chemistry profile, for example, may arise from symptoms of depression, fatigue, poor appetite, or other somatic complaints that warrant a more detailed history and diagnostic workup; the physician who simply orders the requested screening test without exploring the reasons for the request may overlook an important problem. Finally, the request for a screening test provides an opportunity to educate the patient about signs and symptoms of early disease that should warrant a call to the physician. For example, the patient who is told that endometrial biopsy screening is unnecessary

---

Patient Information
PSA (prostate-specific antigen) Screening for Prostate Cancer

Before having the PSA (prostate-specific antigen) blood test, you should know the answers to the following questions:

1. QUESTION: How big a problem is prostate cancer for me? (How likely am I to die of prostate cancer, compared to dying of something else?)

ANSWER: Prostate cancer is common in older men, and can cause death. Current estimates indicate that a 50-year-old American man has an approximately 40% (4 in 10) chance of developing cells that look like prostate cancer under the microscope, a 10% (1 in 10) chance of having symptoms and being diagnosed with prostate cancer, and a 2% to 3% (2 to 3 in 100) chance of dying from prostate cancer.

Compared with the 2% to 3% (2 to 3 in 100) chance of dying from prostate cancer, a 50-year-old American man has a greater than 20% (2 in 10) chance of dying from other cancers and a greater than 50% (1 in 2) chance of dying from cardiovascular (heart and blood vessel) disease.

2. QUESTION: Am I better off having the test, or not having it? (Since I have no symptoms of prostate cancer, is there any evidence that having the screening test will increase my life expectancy, or improve my quality of life, compared to not having the test?)

ANSWER: No one knows for certain the answer to this question. At present, there is no scientific evidence that screening for prostate cancer by PSA testing, or by any other test, will increase your life expectancy, or improve your quality of life if you have no symptoms.

The PSA test can help to detect prostate cancer. However, approximately 95% (95 in 100) of the prostate cancer detected by PSA testing will not cause death, and approximately 75% (75 in 100) of the prostate cancer detected by PSA testing will never cause symptoms.

Some physicians believe that PSA screening will be beneficial because some fatal prostate cancer might theoretically be detected and treated successfully in an early stage.

Other physicians believe that PSA screening will be harmful because the majority of patients with prostate cancer found by PSA testing will be treated unnecessarily, and because there is no evidence that any treatment now available for early prostate cancer can prolong life.

All physicians agree that well-designed, scientific studies of prostate cancer treatment and PSA screening will be required to resolve this disagreement.

3. QUESTION: If I do have the test, what are the immediate consequences to me if I have an abnormal test?

ANSWER: If you have the PSA test, there is an 8% to 14% (8 to 14 in 100) chance that the result will be *outside the normal range*. If your PSA test result is *outside the normal range*, most urologists will recommend a test called "transrectal ultrasound" (a sound-wave test by means of a probe inserted into the rectum). Depending on the results of transrectal ultrasound, a second test called a "needle biopsy of the prostate gland" may be recommended.

If you have a test result that is *outside the normal range*, there is an approximately 11% to 33% (11 to 33 in 100) chance that you will subsequently receive a recommendation to receive a treatment for prostate cancer (either a "radical prostatectomy" or "radiation therapy"). Radical prostatectomy is a surgical procedure to completely remove the prostate gland. Radiation therapy involves the use of radiation to kill prostate cancer cells. The risks to you of radical prostatectomy and radiation therapy are shown in the Table.

Figure 21.1. Patient information on PSA screening. Although some of the data in the text are no longer current (4), the handout illustrates how information about benefits and harms can be summarized for the patient. From Hahn DL, Roberts RG. PSA screening for asymptomatic prostate cancer: truth in advertising. J Fam Pract 1993;37:432–436.

should also be educated about contacting the doctor if she notices abnormal vaginal bleeding.

The busy clinical encounter often does not provide enough time to address all of these issues in sufficient detail. Listed below are patient education materials on the target conditions discussed in this chapter. Patients who are advised against receiving screening tests can take these materials

4. QUESTION: If I have a normal PSA test result, will I have less chance of dying from prostate cancer, compared with someone who has an abnormal test result, or is not tested?

ANSWER: No one knows for certain the answer to this question. If you have a normal PSA test result, it is unknown whether your risk of dying from prostate cancer is different from someone who has an abnormal result, or from someone who has never had a PSA test.

Normal PSA values may be found in 25% (1 in 4 chance) to 45% (45 in 100 chance) of men with localized prostate cancer, so having a normal PSA test result does not guarantee the absence of prostate cancer. Also, a man with an enlarged prostate, but no prostate cancer, has a 33% (1 in 3) chance of having an abnormal PSA test result.

5. QUESTION: What do the experts recommend? What does my own doctor think?

ANSWER: The PSA test is recommended by some doctors and some experts, and is not recommended by other doctors and other expert groups. The American Cancer Society recommends PSA testing yearly for all men over 50 years old. This recommendation is based on the opinions of a group of experts. The United States Preventive Services Task Force, the International Union Against Cancer, and consensus conferences in Sweden, France, and Canada do not recommend PSA testing, or any other form of screening for prostate cancer. These recommendations are based on an evaluation of the available scientific evidence by other groups of experts.

Risks Associated with Radical Prostatectomy and Radiation Therapy

Risk	Likelihood	
	Radical Prostatectomy	Radiation Therapy
Death	2 in 100	0 in 100
Nonfatal thromboembolism (blood clot to the lungs)	10 in 100	0 in 100
Impotence (inability to have an erection)	20 in 100	40 in 100
Incontinence (dribbling, or uncontrollable loss of urine)	5 in 100	8 in 100
Rectal injury (radical prostatectomy) or intestinal injury (radiation therapy)	3 in 100	12 in 100
Urethral stricture (scar tissue narrowing the urine tube in the penis)	1 in 10	6 in 100
Lymphedema (swelling due to radiation damage to lymph nodes)	—	1 in 10
No complications	1 in 2	1 in 4

Overall, *by consenting to a PSA test* (even before the results are known), you should recognize that you are accepting a 0.2% (1 in 500) to 2.6% (2 to 3 in 100) chance that a urologist will recommend that you have a radical prostatectomy or radiation therapy.

Conclusion

Your decision whether to have PSA testing should be based on (1) your personal situation and (2) your understanding of the risks and benefits of PSA testing. Providing this information to you before you decide about PSA testing is part of a process called "informed consent." Despite disagreement about PSA recommendations, all experts and physicians agree that you should be fully informed about the possible benefits and known risks before you decide about PSA testing. Consider discussing PSA testing with your physician.

Figure 21.1. *Continued.*

home to learn more about primary prevention and how to detect the early signs of disease.

RESOURCES—PATIENT EDUCATION MATERIALS

Prostate Cancer

American Institute for Cancer Research
1759 R Street, NW
Washington, DC 20069
800-843-8114, 202-328-7744
    "Reducing Your Risk of Prostate Cancer" (brochure E42-BHP).

National Cancer Institute
Office of Cancer Communications
Building 31, Room 10A16
9000 Rockville Pike
Bethesda, MD 20892
800-4-CANCER
    "What You Need To Know About Prostate Cancer" (brochure 1576).

Ovarian Cancer

American Cancer Society
1599 Clifton Road, NE
Atlanta, GA 30329
404-320-3333, 800-227-2345
    "Facts On Ovarian Cancer" (brochure 88-100M).

National Cancer Institute
Office of Cancer Communications
Building 31, Room 10A16
9000 Rockville Pike
Bethesda, MD 20892
800-4-CANCER
    "What You Need To Know About Ovarian Cancer" (brochure 91-1561).

Pancreatic Cancer

National Cancer Institute
Office of Cancer Communications
Building 31, Room 10A16
9000 Rockville Pike
Bethesda, MD 20892
800-4-CANCER
    "What You Need To Know About Cancer of the Pancreas" (brochure 92-1560).

Lung Cancer

National Cancer Institute
Office of Cancer Communications
Building 31, Room 10A16
9000 Rockville Pike
Bethesda MD 20892
800-4-CANCER
    "What You Need To Know About Lung Cancer" (brochure 93-1553).

Peripheral Vascular Disease

Chek Med Systems, Inc.
1027 Mumma Road
Wormleysburg, PA 17043-9933
800-451-5797
    "Peripheral Vascular Disease" (brochure English MC-16; Spanish MSC-16).

Osteoporosis

American Academy of Family Physicians
8880 Ward Parkway
Kansas City, MO 64114-2797
800-944-0000
"Osteoporosis in Women: Keeping Your Bones Healthy and Strong" (brochure 1510).

Krames Communications
Order Department
1100 Grundy Lane
San Bruno, CA 94066-9821
800-333-3032
"Every Woman's Guide to Osteoporosis" (brochure 1179).

National Institute on Aging
NIA Information Center
P.O. Box 8057
Gaithersburg, MD 20898-8057
800-222-2225
"Osteoporosis: The Bone Thinner."

National Osteoporosis Foundation
1150 17th Street, NW, Suite 500
Washington, DC 20036-4603
202-223-2226
"Stand Up To Osteoporosis."

Endometrial Cancer

American Cancer Society
1599 Clifton Road, NE
Atlanta, GA 30329
404-320-3333, 800-227-2345
"Facts on Uterine Cancer" (brochure 2708).

National Cancer Institute
Office of Cancer Communications
Building 31, Room 10A16
9000 Rockville Pike
Bethesda, MD 20892
800-4-CANCER
"What You Need To Know About Cancer of the Uterus" (brochure 91-1562).

Glaucoma

American Optometric Association
243 North Lindbergh Boulevard
St. Louis, MO 63141
"Answers to Questions About Common Vision Conditions" (brochure) and "Glaucoma" (fact sheet).

National Eye Institute
Scientific Reporting Branch
Building 31, Room 6A32
Bethesda, MD 20892
301-496-5248
  "Don't Lose Sight of Glaucoma: Information for People at Risk" (NIH Pub No. 91-3251)
  and "Glaucoma."

SUGGESTED READINGS

Preferred practice pattern: the comprehensive eye examination in an otherwise asymptomatic adult. San Francisco: American Academy of Ophthalmology, 1988.

Routine cancer screening. Committee Opinion No. 128. Washington, DC: American College of Obstetricians and Gynecologists, 1993.

American College of Physicians. Screening for ovarian cancer: recommendations and rationale. Ann Intern Med 1994;121:141–142.

American Medical Association, Council on Scientific Affairs. Scientific issues in drug testing. JAMA 1987;257:3110–3114.

Carlson KJ, Skates SJ, Singer DE. Screening for ovarian cancer. Ann Intern Med 1994;121:124–131.

Crapo RO. Pulmonary-function testing. N Engl J Med 1994;331:25–29.

DeCew JW. Drug testing: balancing privacy and public safety. Hastings Center Report 1994;24:17–23.

Eddy DM. Screening for lung cancer. Ann Intern Med 1989;111:232–237.

Floren AE. Urine drug screening and the family physician. Am Fam Phys 1994;49:1441–1447.

Frame PS, Fryback DG, Patterson C. Screening for abdominal aortic aneurysm in men ages sixty to eighty years: a cost-effectiveness analysis. Ann Intern Med 1993;119:411–416.

Hockstad RL. A comparison of simultaneous cervical cytology, HPV testing, and colposcopy. Fam Pract Res J 1992;12:53–60.

Kozak BE. Diagnostic imaging in peripheral vascular disease. Ann Vasc Surg 1992;6:393–401.

Kramer BS, Brown ML, Prorok PC, Potosky AL, Gohagan JK. Prostate cancer screening: what we know and what we need to know. Ann Intern Med 1993;119:914–923.

Mettlin C, Jones G, Averette H, Gusberg SB, Murphy GP. Defining and updating the American Cancer Society guidelines for the cancer-related checkup: prostate and endometrial cancers. CA 1993;43:42–46.

National Cancer Institute Cooperative Early Lung Cancer Detection Program: summary and conclusions. Am Rev Respir Dis 1984;130:565–567.

Ostlere SJ, Gold RH. Osteoporosis and bone density measurement methods. Clin Orthoped Rel Res 1991;271:149–163.

Shapiro MF, Greenfield S. The complete blood count and leukocyte differential count: an approach to their rational application. Ann Intern Med 1987;106:65–74.

Steinberg W. The clinical utility of the CA 19-9 tumor-associated antigen. Am J Gastroenterol 1990;85:350–355.

Thoeni RF, Blankenberg F. Pancreatic imaging: computed tomography and magnetic resonance imaging. Radiol Clin N Amer 1993;31:1085–1113.

U.S. Preventive Services Task Force. Guide to clinical preventive services. Baltimore: Williams & Wilkins, 1996.

REFERENCES

1. Woolf SH, Kamerow DB. Testing for uncommon conditions: the heroic search for positive test results. Arch Intern Med 1990;150:2451–2458.
2. U.S. Preventive Services Task Force. Guide to clinical preventive services. Baltimore: Williams & Wilkins, 1996.
3. Canadian Task Force on the Periodic Health Examination. The Canadian guide to clinical preventive health care. Ottawa: Canada Communication Group, 1994.
4. Hahn DL, Roberts R. PSA screening (letter). J Fam Pract 1994;39:12.

Putting Prevention

Recommendations into

Practice

22. Developing a Health Maintenance Schedule

PAUL S. FRAME

INTRODUCTION

A health maintenance schedule is a series of interventions offered to patients at defined intervals, depending on their age, gender, and risk factors, for the primary or secondary prevention of disease. The interventions can include procedures (e.g., screening tests, immunizations), history taking, and counseling. The health maintenance schedule is a general guide for providers which can be modified, depending on the circumstances of individual patients. Designing and using a health maintenance schedule are essential tasks in primary care medicine. Preventive care does not happen by itself. The primary care clinician or group is unlikely to provide appropriate preventive care to most patients without a schedule that indicates which services are indicated and when.

Taking the time to carefully construct a health maintenance schedule is an important and sometimes intimidating task for the primary care clinician (1). It is important because caring for patients when they are well, in addition to when they are sick, and preventing illness whenever possible are the essence of what distinguishes primary care from specialty medicine. Designing the health maintenance schedule is intimidating because of the conflicting demands, expectations, constraints, and costs that the practitioner or group must face in designing the schedule.

This chapter presents a strategy for developing a health maintenance schedule and implementing it in practice. The discussion begins with an examination of the barriers to implementing prevention in practice, because the design of the health maintenance schedule must be sensitive to these barriers to be acceptable to the provider and applicable to patient care.

BARRIERS TO PREVENTION

The barriers to implementing preventive services that affect the development of a health maintenance schedule include: (a) lack of time, (b) uncertainty about the value of screening tests, and (c) conflict of expert recommendations.

Lack of time is a paramount concern in primary care. A busy clinician sees 25–35 patients per day, and at each patient visit the question must be asked, "Is health maintenance up-to-date?" Time does not permit clinicians to offer all preventive services to all patients. The health maintenance schedule must be sensitive to these time constraints by including only worthwhile interventions that are feasible in the practice setting and by allowing the provider to determine quickly which preventive services are indicated.

Uncertainty about the value of preventive services is another barrier. If the clinician does not believe a test or intervention is worthwhile, he or she is unlikely to do it consistently in practice. The primary care clinician should adopt criteria for preventive interventions that must be met before a particular intervention will be considered worthwhile for the practice (2). An example of such criteria is provided in Table 22.1. The health maintenance schedule should be consistent with this policy by including only those preventive services that meet the practice's criteria of effectiveness.

Conflict between expert groups provides a further obstacle to preventive medicine. Although there is a core of agreement within the recommendations of expert groups, there are also many disagreements (3). Specialists often recommend intensive preventive efforts in their particular specialty that do not meet screening criteria that are applicable to the general population. Their perspective is understandable, in that they frequently see the complications of late-stage disease and naturally would like to see them prevented. Primary care clinicians, on the other hand, who are often responsible for doing the screening, encounter a different, healthier population and should not be afraid to require evidence of benefit before blindly accepting "expert" recommendations. Evidence-based recommendations generally offer the best advice. The U.S. Preventive Services Task Force's (USPSTF) *Guide to Clinical Preventive Services* (4) is the most complete source of evidence-based preventive recommendations, but other excellent evidence-based guidelines are also available (5, 6).

Table 22.1
Screening Criteria

1. The condition must have a significant effect on the quality or quantity of life.
2. Acceptable methods of treatment must be available.
3. The condition must have an asymptomatic period in which detection and treatment significantly reduces morbidity and/or mortality.
4. Treatment in the asymptomatic phase must yield a superior result to that obtained by delaying treatment until symptoms appear.
5. Tests that are acceptable to patients must be available at reasonable cost to detect the condition in the asymptomatic period.
6. The incidence of the condition must be sufficient to justify the cost of screening.

Table 22.2
Pearls for Developing a Health Maintenance Schedule

1. Get maximum provider input in the developmental process.
2. Develop a minimum, not a maximum, schedule.
3. Allow individual provider variation above the minimum.
4. Make the schedule relevant to the local patient population and feasible to implement in the practice.
5. Remember that the development of the schedule is an ongoing dynamic process.
6. Remember that screening frequency is determined by the rate of progression of the disease and the sensitivity of the screening test.
7. Remember that a person's risk status influences the cost-effectiveness of screening for a given disease, not screening frequency.

In the end, the providers must agree with the implicit recommendations in their practice's health maintenance schedule. After all, they are the ones who must do the work and will experience the rewards and frustrations that come with the effort. It is therefore important for each clinician in the group to participate in the three steps in developing a health maintenance schedule: (a) establishing a group process, (b) determining which interventions to include in the schedule, and (c) deciding on the recommended frequency for each of the interventions. Table 22.2 lists the most important principles for each step.

ESTABLISHING THE GROUP PROCESS

Most clinicians practice in groups. Even physicians in solo practice work closely with nurses and other health professionals. Thus, a process is needed for the group to reach consensus on the content of the health maintenance schedule. In larger groups, there may be several providers with a particular interest in prevention. One of them is a logical choice to be the leader and to take charge of developing the schedule. Although there is no one method for forging consensus that will be right for all groups, several common principles apply:

1. *Have as many providers as possible involved in the process.* Ideally, all members of the group should participate, unless the group is very large. Remember, providers are not likely to perform procedures on the health maintenance schedule that they do not believe are worthwhile. Being involved in the developmental process is the best way to help people understand the rationale for each intervention. Depending on the size and dynamics of the group, it also may be desirable to have nurses and nonmedical personnel involved in addition to physicians.

2. *The goal is to develop a minimum acceptable protocol, not to develop consensus.* The schedule cannot list every preventive service recommended by an expert

group. One group alone, the USPSTF, has issued about 20 recommendations for low-risk adults and a similar number for children. In addition, there are numerous recommendations for patients with risk factors. It would be impossible for the providers in a practice to reach consensus on an identical schedule, nor is it necessary that they be in complete agreement. What is necessary is that a *minimum* standard be accepted for the group. Providers who wish to add other procedures or use more frequent intervals should be allowed to do so. In reality, however, screening is hard work, and most providers will be challenged to comply with even the minimum schedule for all patients.

3. *Don't be afraid to try an intervention for a specified time and reevaluate its value at a later date.* Developing a health maintenance schedule is a dynamic process that should result in changes to the document over time. If a major controversy over the schedule develops within the practice, make a temporary decision about what to include but also make a commitment to reevaluate the issue at a later date. The experience of either doing or not doing the intervention over time will help inform peoples' opinions about whether the schedule needs to be revised.

CHOOSING SPECIFIC INTERVENTIONS

Most practices will use a set of published guidelines (e.g., USPSTF recommendations) as the starting point for deciding which interventions to include in their schedule. It may be useful, however, to compare the recommendations of several groups before deciding on controversial interventions (3). Figure 22.1 is a "preventive care timeline," developed by the U.S. Public Heath Service, which summarizes the core preventive services recommended by most of these groups. From an organizational standpoint, it is useful to consider interventions for different age groups separately. Developing separate schedules for children (e.g., under age 16), young adults (e.g., ages 16–39), middle-aged adults (e.g., ages 40–64), and older adults (e.g., age 65 and older) may be helpful.

The rationale for each potential recommendation should be understood. Providers should not hesitate to question or be critical of any recommendation, regardless of its acceptance in the medical community. Medicine has many examples of accepted screening interventions, such as pelvic examinations for the detection of ovarian cancer, that are not supported by scientific evidence. In addition to the scientific validity of the recommendation, the providers should consider the relevance of the recommendation to their local patient population and the feasibility of implementing the recommendation under current practice conditions.

The definition of preventive services on the schedule may need special clarification. Whereas the meaning of some maneuvers (e.g., blood pres-

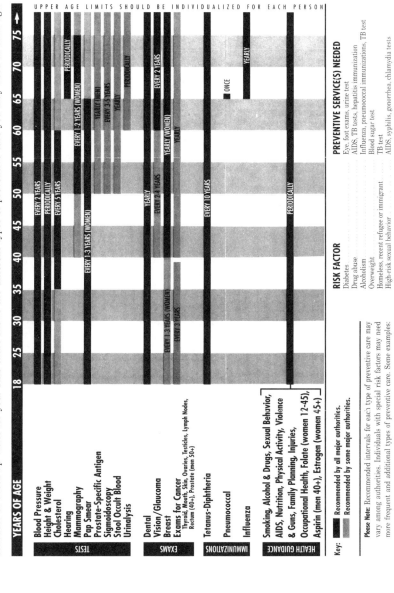

Figure 22.1. "Preventive Care Timeline," from "Put Prevention Into Practice" Education and Action Kit. Washington, DC: U.S. Public Health Service, 1994.

sure measurement) is obvious, the exact, operational meaning of other recommendations (e.g., counseling regarding nutrition and healthy eating habits) could have multiple interpretations. Is this a brief reminder to the patient to "eat well" or a lengthy dietary assessment? If the providers cannot decide exactly what they mean by a recommendation or how they will implement it, they probably should not include it in the schedule.

Keep the schedule simple. There is a strong tendency when developing health maintenance schedules to become idealistic and include a variety of noble interventions with marginal evidence of benefit. As a general rule, if an adult or pediatric schedule cannot be clearly outlined (in a flow sheet or table) on a single page, it is too complex. It will not be used in practice on a regular basis. An excessively complicated schedule frustrates practitioners, and they are likely to ignore it altogether, omitting worthwhile as well as marginal interventions.

The basic schedule should focus on interventions applicable to the general, low-risk population. A few interventions relevant to large, high-risk groups (e.g., influenza vaccination) might be included, but attempts to include most high-risk recommendations should be avoided. Such fine-tuning of the schedule is unnecessary in practice; clinicians individualize health maintenance to the particular patient, regardless of the standard protocol. This is partly because each patient has a unique set of risk factors and concurrent diagnoses, but it also reflects such factors as patient preferences. It is virtually impossible to include all these factors in a preset schedule. Rather, the schedule should be seen as a basic guide to be modified, augmented, or pruned to reflect the needs of the individual patient. A complete list of recommended high-risk interventions (such as those found in the *Guide to Clinical Preventive Services*) is a valuable reference to have available in the practice, but it should not be included in the basic health maintenance schedule.

FREQUENCY OF INTERVENTIONS

Most health maintenance schedules specify the frequency for carrying out procedures, not just a list of recommended procedures. For some recommendations, such as certain immunizations, the proper timing of the intervention is well-established. For some preventive services, such as smoking cessation counseling, there is no logical or scientific basis for specifying a frequency. For most preventive interventions, however, the evidence supports an acceptable range of frequencies (e.g., every 1–3 years for Papanicolaou smears).

The two most appropriate determinants of screening frequency are the sensitivity of the screening test and the rate of progression of the disease, not the incidence of (risk of acquiring) the disease. For example, consider a cancer with a slow rate of progression of 10 years from dysplasia to an incurable stage. If a screening test with a sensitivity of 80% is performed every 3 years, the first screening will detect 80% of cases, the second will detect 80% of the remainder (96% of cases), and the third will detect 80% of the remainder (99% of cases). The same proportion of cases will be detected, regardless of the patient's risk of acquiring the disease, unless the rate of progression of the disease or the sensitivity of the test changes. Thus, the health maintenance schedule should not recommend a shorter interval between screening tests for persons at high risk of disease simply because they are at higher risk. High-risk patients should receive more intensive outreach efforts to ensure their involvement in the practice's health maintenance program, but they need not be screened more frequently. A person's risk status does influence the cost-effectiveness of screening, however. Screening for tuberculosis, for example, will have a very low yield in an affluent suburban population but is very important in a prison population. Thus, risk status influences the decision of whether or not to screen more than it affects the decision of how often to screen.

For many preventive interventions, a frequency cannot be specified based on scientific evidence and must be determined by the providers. An excessively frequent interval will increase costs and take time away from other important tasks. In addition, more frequent testing increases the probability of generating false-positive results and unnecessary workups. Too long a screening interval will increase the risk of missing important disease. Since the group will have to make an arbitrary decision about the recommended frequency that will appear in the schedule, the concept of a minimum schedule with tolerance of individual variation is again useful.

The proper frequency of health maintenance *visits*, an issue separate from the frequency of doing specific procedures, is a subject of much controversy. The appropriateness of the "annual physical" has been debated since the 1940s, and the proper schedule for well-child examinations has received greater attention in recent years. There is little scientific evidence to determine an optimal visit schedule, and the timing of such visits cannot always be inferred from the recommended frequency of tests and immunizations for a given age group. Obviously, a clinician-patient visit is more than the sum of the procedures performed. The provider has the opportunity to determine how the patient is feeling in general, and it is possible that the history will disclose occult symptoms that would otherwise have been overlooked. Infrequent visits can disrupt the continuity of care. Moreover, many patients who are told to schedule another checkup in 1 year do not return for 2 or more years.

In practical terms, the question is whether adults need to be seen annually or whether health maintenance visits every 2 or possibly 3 years would be equally effective for some, especially younger, patients. There are no scientific data to answer this question. In the author's 20 years of experience in family practice, healthy patients under age 50 do not appear to have suffered from only being seen every 2 years instead of annually. Noncompliant patients fail to keep appointments, regardless of whether they are told to return in 1 or 2 years. Of course, all patients need a reminder mechanism for appointment intervals longer than about 3 months. (Reminder systems are discussed in more detail in the next chapter and in Chapter 26.)

IMPLEMENTING A HEALTH MAINTENANCE SCHEDULE

The best health maintenance schedule is useless unless it is implemented consistently on a regular basis. In order to offer health maintenance to all patients, the group must use tools to remind providers what to do for each patient and must have a quality assurance mechanism to monitor compliance with the schedule. The most commonly used health maintenance tracking system is the flow sheet in the patient's medical record (7), examples of which appear in Figures 22.2–22.4. Figures 22.2 and 22.3 are blank and sample versions of a flow sheet developed by the U.S. Public Health Service for its nationally disseminated "Put Prevention Into Practice" Education and Action Kit. Computerized tracking and reminder systems have also been developed to provide an automated health maintenance flow sheet (see Chapter 26).

Establishing a flow sheet-based tracking system for health maintenance requires a large initial investment of time and energy by the practice. Flow sheets must be placed in the charts and filled out for all patients. Physicians, nurses, and other staff must become familiar with the use and format of the flow sheet, and patients must become accustomed to the new questions. The process becomes easier over time, as patients and providers become familiar with the system and data entry is limited to only recently received preventive services. Gratification from the effort also comes over time, as providers begin to see enhanced compliance with preventive care recommendations, risk factors reduced, behaviors changed, and early, curable cancers detected.

Figure 22.4 shows the health maintenance flow sheet used by the author until 1993, when a computerized tracking system was installed. The dots to the right of each intervention indicate the health maintenance schedule. When a preventive service is performed, the provider writes the appropriate month and year at the top of the column that corresponds to the patient's age. Multiple entry codes, defined at the bottom of the figure, keep the provider appraised of the status of each health maintenance procedure (a simple "yes/no" coding is inadequate to describe the range of possible situations). The provider can individualize the flow sheet to the

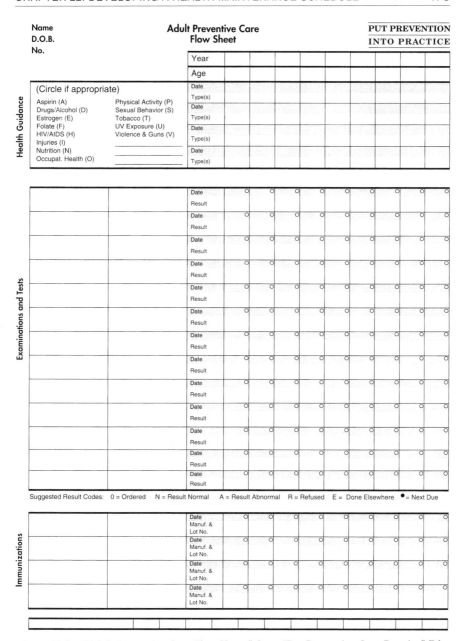

Figure 22.2. "Adult Preventive Care Flow Sheet," from "Put Prevention Into Practice" Education and Action Kit. Washington, DC: U.S. Public Health Service, 1994. Blank form.

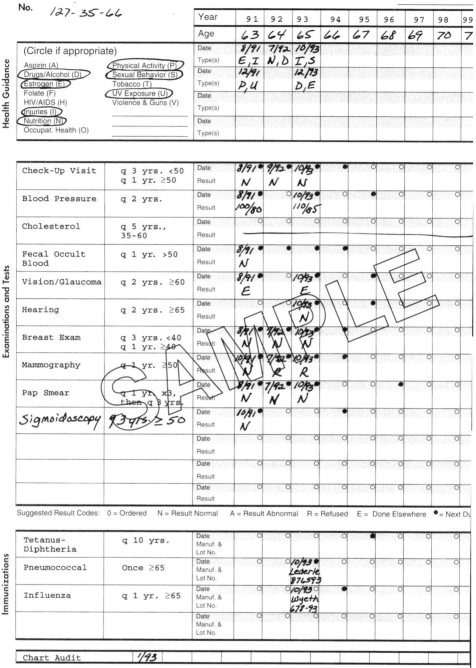

No. 127-35-66

	Year	91	92	93	94	95	96	97	98	99
	Age	63	64	65	66	67	68	69	70	7

Health Guidance

(Circle if appropriate)

Aspirin (A)   (Physical Activity (P))
(Drugs/Alcohol (D))   (Sexual Behavior (S))
(Estrogen (E))   Tobacco (T)
Folate (F)   (UV Exposure (U))
HIV/AIDS (H)   Violence & Guns (V)
(Injuries (I))
(Nutrition (N))
Occupat. Health (O)

	91	92	93	94	95	96	97	98	99
Date	8/91	7/92	10/93						
Type(s)	E, I	N, D	I, S						
Date	12/91		12/93						
Type(s)	P, U		D, E						
Date									
Type(s)									
Date									
Type(s)									

Examinations and Tests

			91	92	93	94	95	96	97	98	99
Check-Up Visit	q 3 yrs. <50	Date	8/91●	9/92●	10/93●	●	○	○	○	○	○
	q 1 yr. ≥50	Result	N	N	N						
Blood Pressure	q 2 yrs.	Date	8/91●	○	10/93●	○	●	○	○	○	
		Result	100/80		110/85						
Cholesterol	q 5 yrs., 35-60	Date	○	○	○	○	○	○	○	○	
		Result									
Fecal Occult Blood	q 1 yr. >50	Date	8/91●	●	●	●	○	○	○	○	
		Result	N								
Vision/Glaucoma	q 2 yrs. ≥60	Date	8/91●	○	10/93●	○	○	○	○	○	
		Result	E		E						
Hearing	q 2 yrs. ≥65	Date	○	○	10/93●	○	●	○	○	○	
		Result			N						
Breast Exam	q 3 yrs. <40	Date	8/91●	7/92●	10/93●	●	○	○	○	○	
	q 1 yr. ≥40	Result	N	N	N						
Mammography	q 1 yr. ≥50	Date	10/91●	7/92●	10/93●	●	○	○	○	○	
		Result	N	R	R						
Pap Smear	q 1 yr. x3, then q 3 yrs.	Date	8/91●	7/92●	10/93●	○	○	●	○	○	
		Result	N	N	N						
Sigmoidoscopy	q 3 yrs. ≥ 50	Date	10/91●	○	○	○	●	○	○	○	
		Result	N								
		Date	○	○	○	○	○	○	○	○	
		Result									
		Date	○	○	○	○	○	○	○	○	
		Result									

Suggested Result Codes: 0 = Ordered   N = Result Normal   A = Result Abnormal   R = Refused   E = Done Elsewhere   ● = Next Du

Immunizations

			91	92	93	94	95	96	97	98	99
Tetanus-Diphtheria	q 10 yrs.	Date / Manuf. & Lot No.	○	○	○	○	●	○	○	○	
Pneumococcal	Once ≥65	Date / Manuf. & Lot No.	○	○	10/93● Lederle 876593	○	○	○	○	○	
Influenza	q 1 yr. ≥65	Date / Manuf. & Lot No.	○	○	10/93○ Wyeth 678-93	●	○	○	○	○	
		Date / Manuf. & Lot No.	○	○	○	○	○	○	○	○	

Chart Audit	1/93								

Figure 22.3. "Adult Preventive Care Flow Sheet," from "Put Prevention Into Practice" Education and Action Kit. Washington, DC: U.S. Public Health Service, 1994. Completed form illustrating the use of the flow sheet for a hypothetical patient. A similar flow sheet is available for children.

476

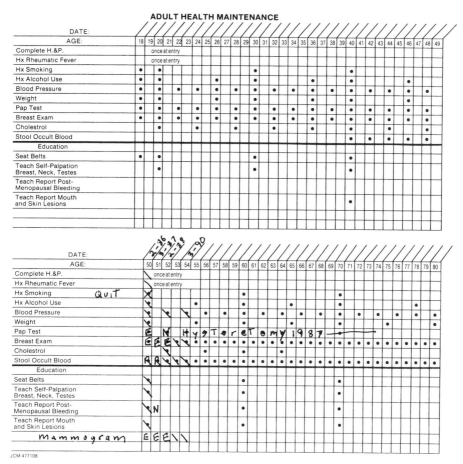

Figure 22.4.   Manual health maintenance flow sheet. Use of flow sheet and recording codes are illustrated. *Legend*: \, Test done, result normal; *R*, Patient refused test; *N*, Test not indicated; *X*, Test done, result abnormal; *E*, Test done elsewhere. Extra lines at the bottom allow addition of new tests or individualization of the flow sheet. Reproduced in a modified version with permission from Frame PS. A critical review of adult health maintenance; Parts 1–4. J Fam Pract 1986;22:29–39, 417–422, 511–520;23:29–39.

particular patient by adding or deleting procedures or by writing notes about the patient. The completed flow sheet allows the provider to determine at a glance, at each patient visit, whether health maintenance is up-to-date or what specific procedures are indicated.

When creating a new health maintenance flow sheet, always leave several extra blank lines at the bottom. This allows the addition of new procedures in the future and individualization of the protocol for specific patients.

HEALTH IS YOUR RESPONSIBILITY

Your lifestyle and habits determine to a large degree whether you will be healthy or will be at high risk for serious illness and accidents. Only you can decide if you will lead a healthy or destructive lifestyle.

SOME IMPORTANT ACTIONS YOU CAN TAKE INCLUDE:

1. Do not smoke tobacco.

2. Wear seatbelts whenever you ride in an automobile.

3. Drink alcohol in moderation, if at all, and never drive when you have been drinking.

4. Exercise regularly.

5. Be aware of the stresses and tensions in your life. Reduce non-essential stress.

Tri-County Family Medicine has a health maintenance program we want everyone involved in. You should have a complete physical examination when you first come to Tri-County and also, of course, if you are not feeling well or have a medical problem.

The focus of our health maintenance program, however, is on periodic checkups for a few specific diseases by tests of proven value. For most people this will mean a checkup every two years if you are under age 50 and every year for those over age 50. The complete program is shown on the back of this page.

CERTAIN PROBLEMS REQUIRE YOUR COOPERATION AT HOME

1. If you are overweight, now is the best time to start a diet.

2. Check regularly for new lumps, especially in the mouth, neck and groin. Report these to your doctor if they persist more than one month.

3. WOMEN: A. Check your breasts for lumps every month.
              B. Report vaginal bleeding after menopause.

4. MEN: Check for lumps in the testicles.

| TRI-COUNTY FAMILY MEDICINE PROGRAM |

Red Jacket Street	Park Avenue	61 State Street	North Church Street	East Naples Street
Dansville, N.Y. 14437	Cohocton, N.Y. 14826	Nunda, N.Y. 14517	Canaseraga, N.Y. 14822	Wayland, N.Y. 14572
(716) 335-6041	(716) 384-5310	(716) 468-2528	(607) 545-8333	(716) 728-5131

Figure 22.5.   Example of a patient health maintenance handout.

Patient education materials can enhance compliance with the health maintenance schedule. We have used the health maintenance handout shown in Figure 22.5 for this purpose. The handout is purposefully brief. The front of the handout emphasizes patient responsibilities and lifestyles that only the patient can change; the back provides a copy of the flow sheet for those patients who are interested. Health maintenance diaries

Personal Prevention Record

This Personal Prevention Record will help you keep track of the preventive care that you have received or will need in the future. With the help of your clinician, fill in how often you need each type of preventive care. For some types of preventive care, you may want to fill in a goal. Write in the date each time you receive preventive care. You may use the remaining space in each box to record other information (such as results of tests and the clinician's or clinic's name).

Type of Preventive Care	Enter Dates, Results and Other Information Below						
Weight Date							
Every ___ **months / years** **Goal** ___ **lbs.**							
Blood Pressure Date							
Every ___ **months / years** **Goal** ___ / ___							
Cholesterol Date							
Every ___ **months / years** **Goal** ___ **mg / dL**							
Tetanus (td) Shot Date							
Every 10 years							
Pneumococcal Shot Date							
Once at age 65							
Influenza Shot Date							
Every year starting at 65							
Dental Visits Date							
Every ___ **months / years**							

Figure 22.6.   Excerpt from "Personal Health Guide," "Put Prevention Into Practice" Education and Action Kit. Washington, DC: U.S. Public Health Service, 1994.

Continued on next page

Preventive Care For Women

Type of Preventive Care	Enter Dates, Results and Other Information Below					
Breast Exam　　Date						
By Clinician Every ____ Year(s)						
Mammogram　　Date						
Every ____ Year(s)						
Pap Smear　　Date						
Every ____ Year(s)						

Additional Preventive Care

Type of Preventive Care	Enter Dates, Results and Other Information Below					
Date						
Every ____ months / years						
Date						
Every ____ months / years						
Date						
Every ____ months / years						
Date						
Every ____ months / years						

Figure 22.6. *(continued)*

that are kept by the patient have been developed to allow patients to monitor their own compliance with the health maintenance schedule and to empower them to modify behavioral risk factors (8). "Personal Health Guides" for children and adults (an excerpt of which is shown in Figure 22.6) have been developed for this purpose by the U.S. Public Health Service, as part of its national "Put Prevention into Practice " campaign, and are being disseminated by the American Academy of Pediatrics, American Academy of Family Physicians, and other groups. These personal health guides are discussed in more detail in the next chapter.

Another patient intervention to enhance compliance with the health maintenance schedule is reminder systems, which are discussed in more detail in Chapters 23 and 26. In its simplest form, a postcard reminder system can be used to prompt patients who do not already have appointments for acute problems to return for health maintenance. For example, a "tickler" file extending at least 2 years into the future can be maintained. When the provider sees a patient and wants to schedule a follow-up health maintenance visit, a notation such as "RV 1 year, send card" can be written on the top of the encounter form, prompting the receptionist to place a reminder postcard in the file for mailing in the desired month. Other types of reminder systems, including computerized systems, are discussed in Chapter 26.

CONCLUSION

Developing and implementing a health maintenance schedule requires start-up and ongoing group commitment and cooperation. The schedule should include only preventive procedures of proven effectiveness. It should provide a minimum base for the group, with the understanding that it will be individualized, depending on the particular patient and provider. A structured approach should be developed to ensure that the health maintenance schedule is followed with all patients. This usually includes a flow sheet or computerized tracking system, patient involvement and recall, and a mechanism for monitoring and quality assurance. Once established and used, a health maintenance schedule is a source of pride and satisfaction. It is the linchpin of a true, comprehensive primary care practice.

RESOURCES

Put Prevention Into Practice
National Health Information Center
P.O. Box 1133
Washington, DC 20013-1133
    Information about the "Put Prevention Into Practice" campaign.

U.S. Government Printing Office
Superintendent of Documents
Mail Stop: SSOP
Washington, DC 20402-9328

>"Put Prevention Into Practice" action kit. Includes a clinician's handbook, flow sheets (Fig. 22.2), chart alert stickers, prescription pads, post-it note pads, reminder post cards, office posters, and "Personal Health Guides" for patients (Fig. 22.6).

American Academy of Family Physicians
8880 Ward Parkway
Kansas City, MO 64114-2797
800-944-0000

>The "Put Prevention Into Practice" kit or its enclosures (described above) can be ordered with American Academy of Family Physicians logos: Action Kit (No. 1999); "Clinicians Handbook" (No. 1980); "Personal Health Guide for Adults" (No. 1958); "Child Health Guide" (No. 1972).

American Academy of Pediatrics
Publications Department
P.O. Box 927
Elk Grove Village, Il 60009-0927
800-433-9016

>The "Put Prevention Into Practice" kit or its enclosures (described above) can be ordered with American Academy of Pediatrics logos: "Clinicians Handbook" (MA0070); "Child Health Guide" (HE0004).

REFERENCES

1. Frame PS. Health maintenance in clinical practice: strategies and barriers. Am Fam Physician 1992;45:1192–1200.
2. Frame PS. A critical review of adult health maintenance; Parts 1–4. J Fam Pract 1986;22:29–39, 417–422, 511–520;23:29–39.
3. Hayward RA, Steinberg EP, Ford DE, et al. Preventive care guidelines: 1991. Ann Intern Med 1991;114:758–783.
4. U.S. Preventive Services Task Force. Guide to clinical preventive services, 2nd ed. Baltimore: William & Wilkins, 1996.
5. Canadian Task Force on the Periodic Health Examination. The Canadian guide to clinical preventive health care. Ottawa, Canada: Canada Communications Group, 1995.
6. Eddy DM, ed. Common screening tests. Philadelphia: American College of Physicians, 1991.
7. Prislin MD, Vandenbark MS, Clarkson QD. The impact of a health screening flowsheet on the performance and documentation of health screening procedures. Fam Med 1986;18:290–292.
8. Dickey LL, Petitti D. Assessment of a patient-held minirecord for adult health maintenance. J Fam Pract 1990;31:431–438.

23. How to Organize a Practice for the Development and Delivery of Preventive Services

ROBERT S. THOMPSON, STEVEN H. WOOLF, STEPHEN H. TAPLIN,
BRUCE V. DAVIS, THOMAS H. PAYNE, MICHAEL E. STUART, and
EDWARD H. WAGNER

INTRODUCTION

Although the process of developing practice recommendations for primary and secondary prevention is an arduous task, it is small compared to the task of "making it happen" in day-to-day office practice. As summarized by Pommerenke and Dietrich, "The status quo is difficult to change, and medical practice is no exception." (1) Often, the magnitude of the problem is underestimated. Lewis (2) examined 32 studies of what primary care physicians said they did in clinical prevention practice. For immunizations, cancer screening, and lifestyle counseling, physicians consistently overestimated what they did (by two to sixfold) when compared to audits or patient reports, and the overall level of performance was generally low.

Improving the delivery of preventive services requires hard work. Simply informing clinicians about recommended practices is generally ineffective in changing behavior unless accompanied by a comprehensive, behaviorally oriented implementation strategy. In 1984, a review of the continuing education literature concluded that programs imparting knowledge alone were ineffective in changing physician behavior. In 1992, this same group reported that interventions using multifactorial practice-enabling strategies (facilitating desired changes at the practice site) and reinforcing strategies (with reminders or feedback) consistently improved physician performance and, in some instances, patient health care outcomes (3). This chapter describes how such approaches can be used by individual practitioners or larger groups to implement clinical preventive services.

The recommendations are based on the behavioral models of Green and colleagues (4) and on the authors' empirical experience at trying to "make it happen" over the last 20 years at Group Health Cooperative of

483

Puget Sound (GHC) in Seattle, Washington (5). GHC is currently the nation's largest consumer-governed health maintenance organization:
388,000 enrollees and 800 physicians in the Puget Sound area and 486,000
enrollees in Washington and Idaho. In the past 20 years, a comprehensive
implementation program at GHC has substantially improved the delivery
of preventive services. In 1972, there were no organizational guidelines for
physical examinations, disease screening, or risk factor identification and
counseling. By 1988–1989, after instituting a comprehensive program,
women age 50 and older enrolled at GHC had a 32% lower incidence of
late-stage breast cancer when compared to the preprogram period
(1983–1984). Immunizations for six-month-old GHC children are now at
least 80% complete. Bicycle safety helmet use by children increased 10-
fold during the period of 1987–1992, accompanied by a 67% decrease in
head injuries (5). Similar successes have been reported by other practices
around the country that have adopted systems for putting prevention into
practice (6), including a comprehensive implementation system for preventive services that is being promoted at over 200 primary care practices
in New England (7).

CONCEPTUAL FRAMEWORK FOR PREVENTIVE CARE IMPLEMENTATION

The successful implementation of a prevention program in the office or
clinic requires an organized approach that addresses the specific barriers
in the practice that interfere with delivery. A number of strategies have
been proposed in the literature (7). Figure 23.1 depicts a unifying intervention model based on the work of Green and others (4, 9, 10) and derived from the principles of social learning theory, academic detailing,
self-efficacy, and total quality management. This model has provided a
convenient format for organizing the thinking at GHC about how to deliver clinical preventive services. The model recognizes enabling, predisposing, and reinforcing factors that influence provider behavior. *Enabling
factors* include the skills and resources that are needed to perform the task
and/or the presence of organizational and practice-level infrastructure to
facilitate performance. *Predisposing factors* make the provider amenable to
behavior change. These factors include the practitioner's values, beliefs,
attitudes, confidence, and own health practices. Confidence influences
the provider's sense of self-efficacy that the task can be performed properly (e.g., offering persuasive smoking cessation advice) and will be accepted by the patient (e.g., overcoming the anxiety that routinely asking
about domestic violence is an unwarranted intrusion). *Reinforcing factors*
encourage behavior change over time. Examples of reinforcement include
peer support, observing evidence of results, and other feedback from patients and colleagues.

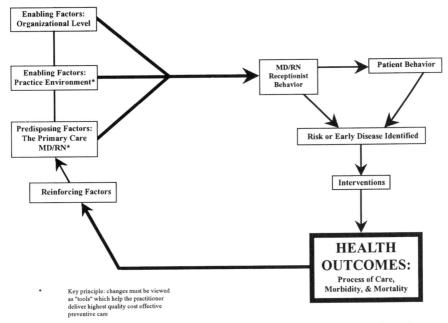

Figure 23.1. Program/Guideline Implementation Model. *Enabling factors* include the possession of skills to perform the tasks entailed in providing clinical preventive services and the presence of practice-level and organizational-level infrastructure to support service delivery. *Predisposing factors* include providers' values, beliefs, attitudes, perceptions, and personal health practices. *Reinforcing factors* include peer support, evidence of results, and feedback from patients and colleagues.

The combination of enabling and predisposing factors facilitates practitioner behavior change (Fig. 23.1), which can then lead to improved identification of risk factors and early-stage disease. An improvement in health outcomes is the ultimate objective. The feedback of these results from patients and colleagues reinforces the process and amplifies the cycle when intervention is successful. The flow depicted by the arrows in Figure 23.1 is a dynamic equilibrium; enabling factors and predisposing factors are capable of acting in concert with or in opposition to one another. For example, the predisposition of the practitioner to counsel about smoking cessation will have to be very high to succeed if there is no reimbursement for providing the service, the clinic is "swamped" with patients, no routine questions are asked to assess patient smoking status, and the practice's chief executive officer is a smoker. Conversely, the prospects for success are higher if the practice enforces a no-smoking policy and if practitioners are well-acquainted with the stages of smoking cessation, have role-played effective counseling techniques, and feel confident in their ability to assist patients in quitting.

Practice activities directed at increasing enabling, predisposing, and reinforcing factors must be viewed by practitioners as helpful to improving the quality of patient care or the interventions will not be accepted and the process will fail. The following discussion presents examples of enabling, predisposing, and reinforcing factors that can be modified in the office or clinic to improve the practice's delivery of preventive services.

Enabling Factors

Organizational Environment and Commitment

The firm commitment of the medical director, chief executive officer, and other practice managers to the cause of prevention is of major importance to successful implementation of preventive services. Making the case for an organized preventive medicine policy can be difficult. Although a straightforward presentation of the facts and figures will usually suffice in convincing the medical director or practice manager, it may occasionally be necessary to argue that programs will prove cost-effective, improve marketing, or that health assessments will attract new patients to the practice.

Leadership commitment takes many forms but generally includes a change in policy (e.g., emphasizing the importance of preventive care in organizational goals, routinely addressing preventive care issues at practice meetings, emphasizing prevention in written materials for patients) and the commitment of organizational resources (e.g., funds, staff) to implement those policies. A vision of the ideal is critical in defining the goals of the program. The GHC goals are listed in Table 23.1, which outlines a vi-

Table 23.1
The Vision: Group Health Cooperative of Puget Sound Goals for Prevention

A. The preventive care system is epidemiologically determined, population-based, and directed to the major causes of morbidity and mortality for which there is evidence that intervention will improve health outcomes.
B. The system of care functions at multiple levels.
　(1) **Primary care.** Physicians and other personnel in primary care have a high sense of confidence that they bring to the tasks of assisting patients in identifying choices and making behavior changes and of attending to patients' disease screening and immunization needs.
　(2) **Infrastructure level in primary care.** Quality information critical to success is available (a) at initiation; (b) during; and (c) at the conclusion of a visit; as well as (d) later for tracking and patient/clinician reminder functions.
　(3) **Organizational level.**
　(4) **External community.**
C. Necessary information is automated and used prospectively to the maximum extent feasible.
D. **Patient (consumer) involvement.** The benefits and risks of specific behavior changes, immunizations, and screening tests are examined interactively through discussion, written materials, videotapes, etc.

sion of what the ideal preventive care delivery system should look like by the year 2000. A series of steps, usually taken a few at a time, are generally necessary before such goals can be achieved.

Other organizational changes are frequently necessary. For example, designating an individual or small committee to provide leadership in analysis, discussion, and selection of preventive services is critical to success. A "prevention coordinator" can be assigned to take responsibility for implementing preventive care in the practice. This individual need not be a physician; nurses, medical assistants, office managers, or receptionists are often more successful at coordinating activities and talking informally with staff to identify problems. The management should encourage activities that involve all office staff in the prevention program. The setting can be as informal as once monthly "preventive care rounds." Staff involvement in preventive care demonstration or research projects can be a powerful factor in building organizational commitment. Offering health risk appraisals or lifestyle counseling to staff can help reinforce a health promotion "culture" within the office.

It is important for management to allow staff sufficient time and resources to conduct outcomes research and to evaluate the extent to which preventive services are being provided to patients in the practice. Without this information, the practice will lack essential benchmarks for identifying inadequacies in care and for measuring progress toward quality improvement. The analysis can focus on a specific question, such as "How are we doing on performing Papanicolaou smears on all women from ages 18 to 70?" The information is typically obtained by examining a systematically sampled or consecutive series of patient charts. Information that may be poorly documented in charts (e.g., whether patients were advised by their physician to stop smoking) can be obtained by distributing a brief patient survey or by asking a sample of patients about their receipt of services when they check in for office visits. A timetable for implementing changes, including a specific start date for initiating the program, can help ensure that the practice achieves steady progress toward its goals.

Another management responsibility is to ensure effective and efficient use of appointment time. Patient education and other preventive services cannot be provided if office visits are too short or poorly organized. Broadly speaking, two different approaches to this problem may be taken. One approach suggests that a single visit is insufficient for a complete periodic health examination or preventive checkup. Geiger and colleagues (6) suggested a model in which preventive health examinations are divided into two 30–45 minute visits. The first visit is devoted to a history and physical examination to identify needed preventive services. The second appointment, about two weeks after the first, is devoted to reporting test results and offering appropriate counseling. Prior to the second visit, patient education materials are selected, based on the patient's needs, and inserted in the chart before the appointment. Patients who call the office to schedule a "complete physical" or Papanicolaou smear are encouraged to schedule the two-visit appointment.

Others may find this approach inapplicable to their practice setting and patient population. A second approach focuses on gathering the requisite information from patients and offering patient education outside the encounter period: before the visit, at the end of the visit, in follow-up, or as part of a reminder function. In this approach, a complete health evaluation visit can be accomplished in a 30-minute appointment. Coordination of this system relies on computer-based or paper-based (e.g., hand tickler file) scheduling.

Rules or procedures can be introduced by management to improve the provision of medical services. Examples include rules that require justification for ordering certain laboratory tests, imaging procedures, or antibiotics. Alternatively, administrative changes may dictate the type of information collected at patient encounters or the types of services covered by the health plan. Since physicians are unlikely to provide preventive services for which there is inadequate reimbursement, it may become necessary for management to negotiate with managed care plans and other payers to ensure adequate coverage for preventive care.

Practice-Level Environment

Dietrich and colleagues (7) identified three characteristics of practices that influence the delivery of preventive services. First, primary care practices consist of teams of professionals, including receptionists, physicians, nurses, and other allied health professionals. Services are delivered most effectively when the skills and opportunities of each team member are utilized to achieve the practice's goals rather than relying on one individual (e.g., the physician) to complete all tasks. Second, office teams depend on routines for conducting much of their work. Preventive services that are incorporated into office routines are more likely to be delivered in a consistent manner. Third, no two practices are alike in terms of their needs, strengths, and limitations. Implementation strategies therefore need to be tailored to the particular conditions facing each practice.

These observations led Dietrich and his colleagues to propose a tailored approach to enhancing the delivery of preventive services in individual practices. In the four-step Preventive GAPS (Goals-Assessment-Planning-Starting) Approach, the practice (a) establishes explicit preventive care *goals* that identify which preventive services patients should receive; (b) *assesses* the extent to which these goals are currently being met, primarily by reviewing charts and examining current office procedures to determine how tasks are currently performed (e.g., which team members perform them, when they are performed); (c) *plans* improvements, often by designing new tools for performing tasks, identifying a more suitable time in the visit to perform the tasks, or selecting a more appropriate staff member to carry them out; and (d) *starting* and maintaining the new system, including an evaluation component to determine subsequently whether the practice goals are being met.

This model stresses the importance of a team approach, with organized roles and responsibilities for staff. Various members of the practice staff can contribute to the prevention program by incorporating selected tasks into their daily routines. Receptionists, for example, can ask female patients about their Papanicolaou smear or mammography status when they arrive for an office visit. Nurses or medical assistants can ask about smoking when vital signs are obtained. In the end, if these efforts by multiple individuals are properly coordinated, preventive services can be delivered more thoroughly and systematically than if one individual (e.g., the physician) assumes complete responsibility. The involvement of the entire team in problem-solving also helps to identify innovative methods for getting the job done that might not be considered by physicians or nurses working alone on the problem. For example, rather than relying on the physician to flip through the chart in the examination room to verify that screening and immunizations are up-to-date, the nurse or medical assistant can fill out a medical record flow sheet before the visit and place a self-adhesive note on the front of the chart to alert the physician about needed services.

When such approaches are used, the following additional enabling factors often emerge as critical:

Identity. Since clinical preventive care services are numerous and encompass primary and secondary prevention, it is useful to give these services a name. This provides an organizational shorthand for speaking about them, increases their visibility within the practice setting, and lends coherence to the efforts. The "Lifetime Health Monitoring Program" is the name GHC applies to a schedule of recommended physical examination visits and the primary and secondary preventive services delivered at these visits.

Guidelines. The next enabling step is to inform and remind providers about recommended preventive services. This lends clarity and consistency to program efforts and provides guidance for new and temporary staff members. The guidelines may be developed and compiled by one or more individuals in the practice and periodically updated. Alternatively, they may be adopted from one or more professional societies (American Academy of Family Physicians (11), American College of Obstetricians and Gynecologists), scientific review groups (U.S. Preventive Services Task Force

(12), American College of Physicians (13), Canadian Task Force on the Periodic Health Examination (14)), or advocacy groups (American Cancer Society (15)). (The authors of this chapter prefer the use of scientifically based guidelines on preventive care to those from other sources.) As part of its "Put Prevention into Practice Education and Action Kit" (see "Resources" at the end of the chapter), the U.S. Public Health Service has published a handbook (16) and wall chart for clinicians that summarizes the recommendations of all major authorities.

A philosophy for selecting clinical preventive services is important to success; it helps to separate the "wheat from the chaff." Chapter 22 discusses this selection process in detail. The GHC philosophy is that guideline and program development should be epidemiologically based and incorporate both the "needs" (diseases and risks) and "wants" (desires) of the enrollees to the maximum extent possible. In general, preventive services (especially secondary prevention) must be held to a higher standard of proof than is applied to treatment of sick patients with symptoms, because in the former case the clinician seeks out the patient. The implicit message of the clinician offering a screening test is, "I have something 'good' for you." Given the potential psychic and physical harms triggered by the investigation of positive test results, which may be ultimately shown to be false-positives, the clinician must remember the maxim, *primum non nocere*, and require a high degree of proof of efficacy and effectiveness before launching screening efforts.

See Chapter 22 for details on how to reach consensus within the practice on appropriate guidelines and how to convert guidelines into a health maintenance schedule for patients and flow sheets for patient charts. Flow sheets for children and adults have been developed by the U.S. Public Health Service for its "Put Prevention Into Practice Education and Action Kit" (see "Resources" at end of chapter, and Fig. 22.2) and have been endorsed by numerous medical organizations. At GHC, the preventive care guidelines are brief and flexible to allow the clinician to tailor them to the individual patient. Management theory supports the importance of involving the intended users in the planning of change. GHC guidelines are routinely developed by volunteer doctors, nurses, and other providers and are subsequently sent to and discussed with all relevant medical providers (17).

The practice should make copies of its health maintenance schedule readily available in the office or clinic to communicate clear goals for all office staff. Doing so also promotes teamwork and helps coordinate care. Copies of the protocol can be posted in examination rooms and other parts of the office. At GHC, multiple presentations to staff are made to demonstrate the rationale for the guidelines and their application in practice. The health maintenance schedule can also be shared with patients; the recommendations, captured in lay terminology and appropriate languages, can be summarized in fliers, posters, displays on the waiting room bulletin board, or letters, thereby helping patients to anticipate and request needed preventive services.

Continuing Education. As mentioned above, multifactorial continuing education approaches, which emphasize enabling and reinforcing factors along with providing information, show promise for improving practitioner implementation of clinical preventive services (3). As is detailed below, a comprehensive continuing education program can be woven into a variety of practice activities, including computer-generated reminders, feedback, role playing, modeling exercises, printed materials, and didactic presentations. Examples of topics covered at GHC continuing education courses include effective strategies for patient behavior change, cancer screening controversies (e.g., colon and prostate cancer), practice-based injury prevention maneuvers, prevention and the menopause, domestic violence, how to help patients stop smoking, the role of a low-fat diet and antioxidants in health, and computer applications for individual patient and population-based care.

The focus of educational course offerings at GHC and other practices is shifting from the pure conveyance of information to more sophisticated and effective strategies for patient and practitioner behavior change. For example, numerous studies have demonstrated that academic detailing is an effective means of modifying physician behavior (10, 18, 19). The method consists of a series of brief, face-to-face encounters where specific educational messages are transmitted. Typically, the academic detailer (often an "educational influential," a local expert frequently consulted by colleagues) schedules a 10–15 minute visit with the physician. A detailer for cholesterol screening might ask, "Do you know what the major cut points are for increased risk?" He or she would then briefly review them and leave the recipient with a fact sheet that summarizes the information. At GHC, combining these approaches with individualized feedback has helped implement guidelines on cholesterol screening and drug therapy (20) and on prostate-specific antigen screening for prostate cancer (21). In both approaches, clinical leaders at 28 GHC outpatient facilities were trained in the methods of academic detailing. Workshops used case presentations with role playing to teach techniques for academic detailing and for providing practitioners with feedback through newsletters and individual contacts.

Physical Layout and Patient Flow Characteristics. The layout of the practice and the direction of patient flow influence the delivery of preventive services. These considerations have been detailed by Pommerenke and Dietrich (1, 22), who suggested tracing the patient's path through the office or clinic to identify opportunities for providing and reinforcing preventive care. They grouped these opportunities into factors to consider before, during, and after the encounter.

Factors that are relevant *before* the encounter include smoke-free waiting rooms, posters and other educational messages, contact with the receptionist, and the length of waiting time. As already noted, registration at the receptionist's desk provides an opportunity to systematically check the status of specific preventive services. During the fall, for example, the receptionist can ask all older adult patients whether they have received an influenza vaccination and make an appropriate notation in the chart. The display of examination room or waiting area posters in the implementation of preventive services has great potential but little formal assessment. Posters can emphasize the importance of the issue and convince patients that "we are interested and committed; the subject is one that you can discuss with us." The display of bicycle safety helmet posters in physicians' offices was an important component of a successful Seattle-area campaign to boost helmet use (23). The American Medical Association's Coalition of Physicians Against Domestic Violence distributes certificates of membership and powerful posters on the subject. Other waiting room interventions are also possible. Bulletin boards and display racks with patient education materials can be updated each month to emphasize specific prevention themes.

The before-visit period provides an important opportunity to collect relevant health and historical information. Questionnaires can be completed by patients at home or in the waiting room to provide practitioners with information about risk factors and prior screening tests. A health risk appraisal (see Chapter 1) can also be completed, providing both the patient and clinician with a convenient summary of risks and disease screening needs. The computed results can be mailed to the patient and placed in their charts. At GHC, a series of four questionnaires are used at health maintenance visits for children, adolescents, adults, and seniors. Scientifically validated questions are incorporated whenever possible. Figure 23.2 presents one page from the senior health questionnaire.

Procedures *during* the encounter can aid routine questioning and counseling about important health issues (e.g., smoking status, domestic violence) and the status of screening and immunizations. The first opportunity for such inquiries occurs when the nurse or medical assistant obtains vital signs before placing the patient in an examination room. Asking about one or two specific preventive services can be incorporated into the nurses' routine, thereby ensuring more systematic inquiry than relying on the physician to ask. Establishing a routine to ensure that physicians assess risks and disease screening needs is also essential to ensure consistency. Properly maintained flow sheets (Chapter 22) and problem lists, displayed prominently in the medical record, are an essential prerequisite for this

How much in the **last month** were you distressed or bothered by...
(Check the correct box for each statement below)

	Not at all	A little bit	Moderately	Quite a bit	Extremely
feeling low in energy or slowed down					
blaming yourself for things					
feeling lonely or blue					
sleep that was restless or disturbed					
feeling hopeless about the future					
feeling everything was an effort					
	0	1	2	3	4

DEPRESSION SCREENING SECTION

HEALTH HABITS AND RISKS

Y N Physician Comments

1. Do you exercise regularly?
   If yes, what exercises ? _____
   How many times per week? _____
   For how long? _____
2. Do you smoke cigarettes now?
   If you quit, please indicate month and year. Mo____ Yr____
   If you smoke now, how many cigarettes per day?_____
   How long have you smoked? _____
3. Are you overweight?
4. Do you drink alcoholic beverages?
   If yes, how many per week?
   (1 drink=1 glass of beer, wine, or hard liquor drink)
   ___ 7 or less ___ 8-14 ___ 15 or more
   If yes, have you ever:
   Felt the need to cut down on your drinking?
   Felt annoyed by criticism of your drinking?
   Had guilty feelings about your drinking?
   Taken a morning eye opener?
5. When was your last complete eye exam? _____
6. Do you use seatbelts?
7. Is the hot water from your tap too hot to hold your hand under comfortably?
8. Does your house have: a smoke detector?
                            a fire extinguisher?

FUNCTIONAL ASSESSMENT/PLANNING FOR THE FUTURE

1. Do you have difficulty with:
   Y N
   | | | |
   dressing
   bathing
   getting in and out of bed
   using the bathroom
   eating
   doing household chores
   shopping

Y N

2. ☐ ☐ Do you drive? If no, how do you get where you want to go?
3. ☐ ☐ If you need help or someone to talk with, is there someone you can call?
4. ☐ ☐ Do you manage your own finances?
5. ☐ ☐ Do you have a will?
6. ☐ ☐ Have you signed a living will or power of attorney?
   ☐ ☐ If no, do you know where to get assistance in acquiring one?

CHECKLIST OF FEELINGS: Developed from Johns Hopkins symptom check list applied to GHC enrollees. If score of 10+ follow-up with the Geriatric Depression Scale and/or specific questions to ascertain if the patient has current major depression. All patients with score of 10+ will benefit from counseling about increasing activity levels. For patients with current major depression also consider the use of medications.

Figure 23.2. One page from the Lifetime Health Monitoring Program Health Questionnaire for Age 65 and Over, Group Health Cooperative of Puget Sound.

task, and physicians or other office staff should ensure that they are kept current.

Since many clinicians are too preoccupied and busy to carefully examine flow sheets during the examination, it is useful for office staff to place manually or computer-generated notices, preprinted self-stick removable notes, or prominent chart stickers on the outside cover of the chart to call attention to specific risk factors and tests that need attention. Such reminder systems have proven effective in increasing the use of preventive services in office practice (24, 25, 26). Preprinted self-stick notes and colorful chart stickers for 16 health problems are available in the "Put Prevention Into Practice Education and Action Kit" distributed by the U.S. Public Health Service. As suggested by Dietrich and colleagues (7), such notes can be used to call attention to special barriers identified by office staff in their discussions with patients (e.g., "afraid mammogram hurts"). Posted signs (e.g., "Ask all patients about smoking") and wall charts that summarize guidelines and algorithms may also help remind the examiner about anticipatory guidance, health behaviors, and screening tests to discuss with patients. At GHC, we have developed a series of anticipatory guidance, risk factor, and immunization reminder sheets to be used at well-child visits from 14 days to 12 years of age.

As discussed in Chapter 26, a variety of computerized tracking and reminder systems are being developed and implemented to help remind providers about needed preventive services (27). At GHC, an automated clinical information system (Fig. 23.3) with advice modules and a reminder function has been developed to link existing data systems and is

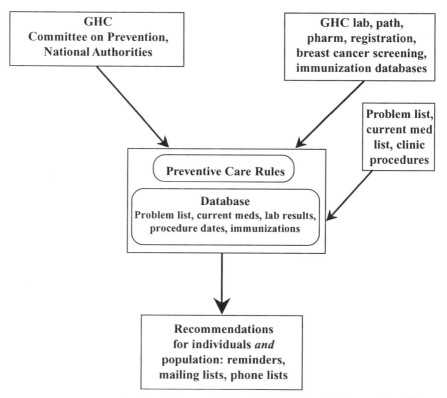

Figure 23.3.   Automated clinical information system, Group Health Cooperative of Puget Sound.

being piloted at a local medical center. The prototype produces problem lists, including risk factors and diagnoses, current medication lists, immunizations, and results of laboratory and screening tests. It allows preventive care guidelines to be applied both to individual enrollees and to the entire population of patients cared for by the practitioner's team. Enrollees not satisfying preventive care guidelines can be mailed reminders or telephoned. Practitioners are spared the effort of sorting through hundreds of charts to determine which patients in their practice need preventive care maneuvers. See Chapter 26 for more details about computerized reminder systems for preventive care.

Procedures to consider *after* the encounter include the provision of written materials and resource lists on the subject at hand, explicit directions for tests or procedures, follow-up telephone calls and reminder systems, formal contracts for behavior change (e.g., starting a fitness program), attention to insurance coverage and billing codes (see Chapter 25), and payment schedules. "Prescription" forms for preventive care are available in the "Put Prevention Into Practice Education and Action Kit" to help clinicians establish contracts with patients and provide written instructions for making lifestyle changes. The prescriptions are printed on pressure-sensitive paper so that a copy can be placed in the patient's chart. As discussed in earlier chapters, ready access to relevant patient education materials increases the likelihood that they will be distributed to patients. Other health professionals (nurses, nurse practitioners, physician assistants, dietitians) in the office or community can also play an important role in patient education. Practices can establish a system in which nurses instruct patients on breast self-examination or follow-up with patients on their efforts to stop smoking. Finally, on-site laboratory or imaging facilities can facilitate compliance with certain screening tests (e.g., mammography).

An important after-visit intervention is reminding the patient to return for follow-up visits and repeat screening. A useful first step is to have the patient leave the office with an appointment card for the next visit. Subsequent patient reminders can be provided in postcards or letters (generated by computer or manually), or can also be communicated in telephone follow-up calls that incorporate counseling and reinforcement along with the reminder. Simple postcard reminders prove surprisingly effective in boosting compliance for prevention activities. One study found that mailing a postcard reminder 10 days after a fecal occult blood test increased compliance by 25% (24). A postcard "tickler file" can be established by addressing a card at the time of the patient's visit and filing it under the month of the next desired visit. The reminder postcards are then mailed at the beginning of the month, or at the end of the month if the patient does not schedule an appointment.

Patient-held minirecords or diaries, pocket-sized booklets in which patients or parents keep track of preventive services, are an important empowerment tool that has proven successful in boosting immunization and cancer screening rates (28, 29). At GHC, wallet-sized schedules, minirecords of well-child visits, are given to parents to help them keep track of heights, weights, screening test results, and immunizations for each child. Pocket-sized minirecords for adults and children (*Personal Health Guide* and *Child Health Guide*) have been endorsed by the American Academy of Family Physicians and American Academy of Pediatrics and are distributed as part of the "Put Prevention Into Practice Education and Action Kit" (see "Resources" below). Recommendations in these minirecords about when to return for repeat screening include blank spaces to allow the physician to customize the instructions. To be used effectively, patients should be encouraged to keep their minirecords in a safe place and bring them back at each visit for reference and updating. The minirecords should be presented when patients check in for appointments. During the visit, the clinician or office staff should cross-check the information in the minirecord against the patient's chart, offer positive reinforcement for keeping entries up-to-date, and discuss selected topics from specific pages.

At GHC, computerized prospective reminders are a routine feature of the breast cancer screening program (30). Immunizations have been entered on a computerized tracking system since 1991, and the development of a reminder function is underway. For several years, computerized printouts of patients belonging to a particular physician's practice panel are combined with pharmacy information to identify high-risk candidates in need of influenza vaccinations each fall. Direct mail and telephone reminding, much of it performed by patient volunteers, has gradually increased the proportion of seniors vaccinated against influenza from 34% in 1984 to 70% in the winter of 1993–1994.

Predisposing Factors

The attitudes and perceived self-efficacy of primary care physicians and nurses are an important and frequently overlooked determinant of the quality of preventive care within a practice. Most family physicians, general internists, pediatricians, and primary care nurses tend to see case-finding, screening, anticipatory guidance, and counseling as an integral part of their practitioner role. For them, the issue is not whether primary and secondary preventive maneuvers are worth doing, but deciding which maneuvers are effective and how to incorporate them into the practice routine. For other, more skeptical providers, the feeling that prevention is a frustrating part of their practice or beyond their clinical responsibilities represents an important attitudinal barrier to compliance (9).

It is important to clarify the specific attitudinal barriers that affect the providers in the practice. Information about their knowledge and beliefs is essential to developing and implementing effective clinical preventive services. Physicians and nurses who are expected to implement guidelines must understand them, believe that they can be implemented, and value the results. Tailoring systems to these perceived barriers increases the prospects for success. For example, a GHC review of spousal abuse identification and management revealed that primary care providers lacked confidence in intervention skills, were fearful of causing offense, and were concerned about "lack of time." The data from this assessment of barriers provided a basis for improving the practice's detection and treatment efforts (31).

Clinician self-confidence (i.e., sense of self-efficacy) is a key to action on preventive services (32). A recent review of hundreds of continuing education studies observed that "the dissemination of clinical policies or practice guidelines alone showed a negative effect" but that physician performance was changed by specific protocols, workshops, "practice rehearsal" strategies, and feedback (3). The common theme in these interventions was the enhancement of practitioner self-confidence (self-efficacy) for incorporating new procedural and counseling skills into practice (22).

Confidence in procedural skills, such as performing sigmoidoscopy, can be increased through supervised training and practice. Confidence in counseling can be boosted through role playing. The National Cancer Institute has developed a high-quality training program that details a specific step-by-step approach to implementing smoking cessation in office practice. The training module includes role playing (33). At GHC, role playing was used in a 1991 course to improve the early detection of depression. A staff psychologist played the patient while a family practitioner demonstrated how the questioning could be integrated smoothly and efficiently into the office practice routine. Course attendees subsequently practiced applying the intervention.

To be adequately motivated, the practitioner must possess the belief that the proposed interventions will prove helpful in practice and not hinder necessary tasks. The primary care practitioner is on a rather rapid treadmill in day-to-day office practice. To the maximum extent possible, anything "new" should be substitutive. If a new responsibility is added, an older one should be removed, or the addition should increase the effectiveness or efficiency of services already being provided. For example, if the developers of new guidelines provide brief scripts to the clinician for dealing with increased patient demand, the intervention has a better chance of succeeding (22). Brief scripts (Fig. 23.4) are used at GHC to facilitate a balanced discussion of the benefits and risks of prostate-specific antigen and cholesterol screening.

PSA Screening Test (8)

I. THE DILEMMA OF PROSTATE CANCER SCREENING
- Autopsy studies show that approximately 30% of males greater than age 50 have foci of prostate cancer that is not clinically evident. Up to 70% of men over age 70 and 100% of men over age 90 have such a cancer;
- Less than one in forty of these cancers will act in a malignant fashion and will cause death;
- Screening measures currently cannot differentiate aggressive malignant lesions for "innocent" cancers, i.e., cancers that will not act in a malignant fashion;
- Increased case finding from aggressive screening is more likely to find cancers that are not going to cause death since they are much more prevalent.

II. PSA AS A SCREENING TEST
- Will increase case finding but cannot discriminate between clinically relevant and incidental cancers;
- PSA as a screening test has very poor specificity (59% in the Catalona study). Screening would result in numerous false positive tests and negative biopsies;
- There is no evidence that PSA screening would result in decreased mortality from prostate cancer;
- Estimates of the positive predictive value of PSA as a screening test range from an optimistic 40% to a perhaps more realistic 10%.

III. CONSEQUENCES OF THE DECISION TO SCREEN FOR PSA
A. There will be a significant cascade of intervention for those with PSAs greater than four (13% of men in Catalona's study) to proceed to sextant biopsies of the prostate.

B. Although most biopsies will be negative, a significant number will be positive. Those with positive biopsies will be asked to choose between radical prostatectomy and radiation therapy, both of which have significant risks:

Risk of Radical Prostatectomy	Risk of Radiation Therapy
• 1–2% surgical mortality	• 25–41% risk of impotence
• 25–84% risk of impotence	• 4.5–8% risk of urinary stricture
• 12–18% risk of urinary stricture	• 3–6% risk of incontinence
• 6–40% risk of incontinence	• 1–11% risk of rectal injury
• 3% risk of rectal injury	• 0.2–0.5% mortality (sepsis)

IV. IF YOUR PATIENT DECIDES TO HAVE PSA SCREENING, HE SHOULD KNOW:
1. There are no data to show that PSA screening leads to decreased mortality from prostate cancer;
2. If his test is positive (a value greater than four), the chances are about 70% that he will undergo the anxiety, expense, discomfort, and potential complications of prostate biopsies for no benefit;
3. If he were to have cancer found by PSA testing, it is likely that the cancer would never have progressed to become a "killer cancer," and that he would have undergone the risks of treatment without benefiting;
4. The operative mortality for radical prostatectomy is 1–2%;
5. The US Preventive Services Task Force and the Group Health Committee on Prevention do not advocate PSA screening.

Figure 23.4. Script used at Group Health Cooperative of Puget Sound to guide clinician counseling about PSA screening. (From Stuart ME, Handley MA, Thompson RS, Conger M, Timlin D. Clinical practice and new technology, Prostate-specific antigen (PSA). HMO Practice 1992;6(4):5–11.)

Reinforcing Factors

Even if predisposing and enabling factors make it possible for providers to introduce preventive services into practice routines, continued adherence to recommendations is likely to wane without further reinforcement. Peer support and feedback can provide the clinician with incentives to maintain and improve the quality of preventive care.

Peer Support

Peer support for the development and implementation of clinical preventive care programs can be provided by designating and repeatedly recognizing leadership, through newsletters emphasizing prevention issues, salary bonuses for performance, and other awards for excellence. At GHC, a plaque and small honorarium are awarded to the "Preventive Care Scholar" of the year. The individual is selected by his or her peers, and thus the award is an important symbol of their support.

Feedback

Practitioner behavior can also be changed by providing performance information. Physicians often change their behavior when they learn that their test ordering practices differ from those of their colleagues or the community standard of care (9). Reports on performance can be provided by colleagues or in computer printouts that compare individual performance with that of the whole practice (10). The medical education department at GHC distributes clinic-specific information about prostate-specific antigen testing every three months to the academic detailers at 28 GHC facilities. The 1992 ratios for testing male patients age 50 and older ranged from 1:28 to 1:2. This information is discussed at each clinic by the detailer. Feedback about patient outcomes is another important reinforcer of prevention programs and guidelines. In 1984 at GHC, influenza vaccinations were obtained by only 34% of patients age 65 and older. After instituting a program that publicized the results on an annual basis, the percentage increased to 70% by 1993–1994. Similar outcome feedback is now being used for childhood immunizations and breast cancer screening.

PROGRAM EVALUATION

How can a practice determine whether its efforts to develop and implement clinical preventive services are paying off? The answer to this question is largely a function of the initial objective of implementing the services in the first place, the length of time since implementation, and the availability of relevant data. Some of the main considerations are outlined in Figure 23.5, which groups potential evaluation measures into attitudes/knowledge, process of care, and health outcomes.

If the program is early in its implementation, informal surveys of practitioners and/or patients to measure their satisfaction with and concerns about the program may be sufficient. If practitioner attitudes (e.g., "asking about domestic violence is none of my business") were a major concern when starting the program, it is appropriate to monitor whether they change over time. If the program is targeted to screening procedures or identification and counseling for risks, a series of process of care measures may be helpful. Does mammography really increase? Is questioning about cigarette smoking routinely recorded as a vital sign? This information is usually obtained by medical record audits and chart reviews. Computerized systems can quickly produce data on compliance with recommended preventive services and can stratify the information for individual providers, clinics, or patient subgroups. If the program has been in place for a longer time, issues such as its effect on subsequent health outcomes, medical care utilization, and cost-effectiveness (34) may be available.

For clinicians, morbidity and mortality (health outcomes) are of particular interest in evaluating the success of clinical prevention programs. When evaluating screening programs, a series of commonly anticipated steps or markers may suggest that the program is effective. For example, it is customary to see increased case-finding early in cancer screening programs; the yearly incidence rate of breast cancer in women age 40 and older may triple. Next, the staging of the cases may show a "left shift" to earlier stages, followed by a decreased incidence of late-stage disease, and finally decreased mortality (35, 36). Decreased mortality is the "gold stan-

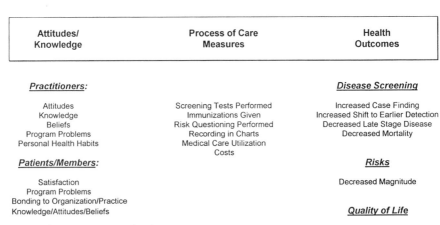

Figure 23.5. Program evaluation.

dard" for evaluating cancer screening programs, since it is free of the problems of lead time and length bias inherent in measures of case-finding and stage shifts. For example, studies of chest radiography screening for lung cancer in the 1960s and 1970s confirmed a marked left shift in staging but observed no effect on mortality (37).

If the prevention program is directed at reducing modifiable risk factors, a decrease in the prevalence of the risk factor may provide a satisfactory outcome measure for evaluation. For example, at GHC, the prevalence of cigarette smoking in adults was 25% in 1985; by 1994 it was 17%, with a rate in the surrounding community of 24% (5). Since studies of mortality take many years to complete, and most of the chronic diseases of interest cause considerable morbidity in the intervening years, evaluations should also focus on the quality of life and measures of health and functional status to fully evaluate effectiveness (see "Functional Status" in Chapter 16) (38).

Examples of program evaluation outcome measures used at GHC include: (a) attitudes of members and staff toward the breast cancer screening program (89% of enrollees rated the program as excellent to very good, 86% of physicians were satisfied with the program); (b) attitudes and beliefs of 38 GHC primary care physicians toward identification and management of domestic violence (61% felt that they lacked training, 72% believed they did not have enough time, and 55% were fearful that such questions would be offensive); (c) completed immunizations in children six months of age (80% coverage in the second quarter of 1994, ranging from 57% to 90% at the 28 GHC clinics); (d) smoke detector ownership among seniors (87%); and (e) fire extinguisher ownership among seniors (increased from 59% to 72% between 1984 and 1991).

CONCLUSION

The comprehensive approach outlined in this chapter may not be attainable in all practices. The adoption of individual components of the implementation plan may be the only practical option in such settings. Ultimately, however, a comprehensive approach is necessary for "making it happen" in clinical practice and for providing the highest quality of preventive care for all patients.

ACKNOWLEDGMENTS

The authors wish to thank James Toomey for his skill and patience during repeated manuscript drafts and his graphics preparation. The authors also wish to thank Nancy Snell, Kathleen Hall, and Eve Adams for their help with manuscript preparation.

RESOURCES

Superintendent of Documents
P.O. Box 371954
Pittsburgh, PA 15250-7954
202-512-2250

> The "Put Prevention Into Practice Education and Action Kit" includes a copy of the Clinician's Handbook of Preventive Services and multiple copies of the *Personal Health Guide, Child Health Guide,* patient reminder postcards, patient chart flow sheets, colored chart stickers, preprinted self-adhesive removable reminder notes, prevention prescription pads, a poster, and wall charts outlining recommended preventive services.

American Academy of Family Physicians
8880 Ward Parkway
Kansas City, MO 64114-2797
800-944-0000

> Custom versions of the "Put Prevention Into Practice Education and Action Kit" are also available from this specialty society: "Put Prevention into Family Practice" Action Kit (No. 1999); "Clinicians Handbook" (No. 1980); "Personal Health Guide for Adults" (No. 1958); "Child Health Guide" (No. 1972).

American Academy of Pediatrics
P.O. Box 927
Elk Grove Village, IL 60009-0927
800-433-9016

> Custom versions of the "Put Prevention Into Practice Education and Action Kit" are also available from this specialty society: "Clinicians Handbook" (MA0070); "Child Health Guide" (HE0004).

National Cancer Institute
Building 31, Room 10A24
Bethesda, MD 20892
800-4-CANCER

> "How to help your patients stop smoking. A National Cancer Institute Manual for Physicians" (NIH Pub. No. 92-3064).

SUGGESTED READINGS

Dietrich AJ, Woodruff CB, Carney PA. Changing office routines to enhance preventive care: the Preventive GAPS Approach. Arch Fam Med 1994;3:176–183.

McPhee SJ, Detmer WM. Office-based interventions to improve delivery of cancer prevention services by primary care physicians. Cancer 1993;72:1100–1112.

Taplin SH, Mandelson MT. Principles of cancer screening for clinicians. Primary Care 1992;19:513–533.

Thompson RS, Taplin SH, McAfee TA, Mandelson MT, Smith AE. Primary and secondary prevention services in clinical practice: twenty years' experience in development, implementation, and evaluation. JAMA 1995;273:1130–1135.

REFERENCES

1. Pommerenke FA, Dietrich A. Improving and maintaining preventive services, Part 1: Identifying barriers and opportunities by applying the Patient Path Model. J Fam Pract 1992;34:86–91.

2. Lewis CE. Disease prevention and health promotion practices of primary care physicians in the United States. Am J Prev Med 1988;4:9–16.
3. Davis DA, Thompson MA, Oxman AD, Haynes BR. Evidence for the effectiveness of CME: a review of 50 randomized controlled trials. JAMA 1992;268:1111–1117.
4. Green LW, Eriksen MP, Schor E. Preventive practices by physicians: behavioral determinants and potential interventions. Am J Prev Med 1988;4:101–107.
5. Thompson RS, Taplin SH, McAfee TA, Mandelson MT, Smith AE. Primary and secondary prevention services in clinical practice: twenty years' experience in development, implementation, and evaluation. JAMA 1995;273:1130–1135.
6. Geiger WJ, Neuberger MJ, Bell GC. Implementing the U.S. preventive services guidelines in a family practice residency. Fam Med 1993;25:447–451.
7. Dietrich AJ, Woodruff CB, Carney PA. Changing office routines to enhance preventive care: the Preventive GAPS Approach. Arch Fam Med 1994;3:176–183.
8. Jaen CR, Stange KC, Nutting PA. Competing demands of primary care: a model for the delivery of clinical preventive services. J Fam Pract 1994;38:166–171.
9. Lawrence RS. Diffusion of the US Preventive Services Task Force Recommendations into practice. J Gen Intern Med 1990;5(suppl.):S99–S103.
10. Walsh JME, McPhee SJ. A systems model of clinical preventive care: an analysis of factors influencing patient and physician. Health Educ Q 1992;19:157–175.
11. American Academy of Family Physicians, Commission on Public Health and Scientific Affairs. Age charts for periodic health examination (product No. 972). Kansas City, MO: American Academy of Family Physicians, 1994.
12. U.S. Preventive Services Task Force. Guide to clinical preventive services, 2nd ed. Baltimore: Williams & Wilkins, 1996.
13. Common screening tests. Philadelphia: American College of Physicians, 1991.
14. Canadian Task Force on the Periodic Health Examination. The Canadian guide to clinical preventive health care. Ottawa: Canada Communication Group, 1994.
15. American Cancer Society. Summary of American Cancer Society recommendations for the early detection of cancer in asymptomatic people. CA 1993;43:42–46.
16. Clinician's handbook of preventive services. Washington, DC: U.S. Public Health Service, 1994.
17. Thompson RS, Carter AP, Taplin SH. Health promotion in an HMO: Ad astra per aspera. HMO Practice 1989;3:82–88.
18. Avorn J, Soumerai SB. Improving drug-therapy decisions through educational outreach: A randomized controlled trial of academically based "detailing." N Engl J Med 1983;308:1457–1463.
19. Soumerai SB, Avorn J. Principles of educational outreach ("academic detailing") to improve clinical decision making. JAMA 1990;263:549–556.
20. Stuart ME, Handley MA, Chamberlain MA, Wallach RW, Penna PM, Stergachis A. Successful implementation of a guideline program for the rational use of lipid-lowering drugs. HMO Practice 1991;5:198–204.
21. Stuart ME, Handley MA, Thompson RS, Conger M, Timlin D. Clinical practice and new technology: prostate-specific antigen (PSA). HMO Practice 1992;6:5–11.
22. Pommerenke FA, Dietrich A. Improving and maintaining preventive services, Part 2: Practical principles for primary care. J Fam Pract 1992;34:92–97.
23. Bergman AB, Rivara FP, Richards DD, Rogers LW. The Seattle Children's Bicycle Helmet Campaign. Am J Dis Child 1990;144:727–731.
24. Thompson RS, Michnich ME, Gray J, Friedlander L, Bilson B. Maximizing compliance with Hemoccult screening for colon cancer in clinical practice. Med Care 1986;24:904–914.

25. McDowell J, Newell C, Rosser W. A randomized trial of computerized reminders for blood pressure screening in primary care. Med Care 1989;27:297–305.
26. Office of Disease Prevention and Health Promotion, U.S. Department of Health and Human Services. Office systems for promoting preventive care. An unpublished background paper for the U.S. Preventive Services' Coordinating Committee, May, 1992.
27. McDonald CH, Hui SL, Smith DM, Tierney WM, Cohen SJ, Weinberger M, et al. Reminders to physicians from an introspective computer medical record: a two-year randomized trial. Ann Intern Med 1984;100:130–138.
28. Dickey LL, Petitti D. A patient-held minirecord to promote adult preventive care. J Fam Pract 1992;34:457–463.
29. Dickey LL. Promoting preventive care with patient-held minirecords: a review. Patient Educ Coun 1993;20:37–47.
30. Thompson RS, Taplin SH, Carter AP, Schnitzer F. Cost effectiveness in program delivery. Cancer 1989;64:2682–2689.
31. Sugg N, Invi T. Opening Pandora's box: primary care physician's response to domestic violence. JAMA 1992;267:3157–3160.
32. Maiman LA, Becker MH, Liptak GS, Nazarian LF, Rounds KA. Improving pediatricians' compliance-enhancing practices: a randomized trial. Am J Dis Child 1988;142:773–779.
33. Glynn TJ, Manley MW. How to help your patients stop smoking. A National Cancer Institute manual for physicians (NIH Pub. No. 92-3064). Bethesda, MD: National Cancer Institute, 1991.
34. Doubilet P, Weinstein MC, McNeill BJ. Use and misuse of the term "Cost Effective" in medicine. N Engl J Med 1986;314:253–255.
35. Morrison AS. Screening in chronic disease. In: Kelsey J, Marmot M, Stolley P, Vessey M, eds. Monographs in epidemiology and biostatistics. Oxford University Press, New York, 1992;19:13–18.
36. Taplin SH, Mandelson MT. Principles of cancer screening for clinicians. Primary Care 1992;19:513–533.
37. Fontana RS. Screening for lung cancer; recent experience in the United States. In: Hansen HH, ed. Lung cancer. Boston: Martinus Nijhioff, 1986:91–111.
38. Jett AM, Davies AR, Cleary PD, et al. The functional status questionnaire: reliability and validity when used in primary care. J Gen Intern Med 1986;1(3):143–149.

24. Providing Preventive Care in the Public Health Department, Worksite, and Emergency Department

MARK B. JOHNSON, TEE L. GUIDOTTI, JULIAN ORENSTEIN,
THOM A. MAYER, and STEVEN H. WOOLF

Although much of the clinical practice of preventive medicine occurs in traditional primary care settings, such as the offices and clinics of pediatricians, family physicians, and internists, a significant proportion of preventive services are delivered in other practice environments. The inpatient setting is the most obvious example; as noted elsewhere in the book, if physicians remember to perform them, hospitalized patients can receive needed screening tests (e.g., Papanicolaou smears, mammography), counseling, and immunizations during their hospital stay.

The doctor's office and the hospital are not the only context in which health promotion and disease prevention are practiced, however. Preventive services are also delivered at public health departments, the worksite, and emergency departments. Primary care physicians and other health professionals often forget the important role played by health professionals at these delivery sites in providing clinical and patient education services. They also overlook the extent to which they can use these programs in routine medical care to complement and coordinate the delivery of clinical preventive services. Some patients can receive preventive care only at these sites, either because of limited access to care or the primary care practitioner's inability to provide preventive services. But even when patients receive their preventive care in the private practice environment, the scope and quality of care can often be expanded by collaborating with professionals in other settings.

This chapter reviews the types of preventive services offered at public health departments, the worksite, and emergency departments. Other important collaborations with community allied health resources, such as mental health professionals, social service agencies, substance abuse counselors, and dietitians, are discussed elsewhere in this book. The primary objectives of this chapter are to suggest ways in which practitioners can familiarize themselves with the preventive services that patients receive elsewhere, such as immunizations received at the public health or emergency department, and how they can use the resources and services offered at these sites to implement and reinforce preventive interventions. By understanding the types of preventive services that are offered and the organizational environment in which they are received, primary care clinicians can provide their patients with more meaningful advice about how to use these resources effectively and safely. Open communication between the primary care provider and public health, occupational medicine, and emergency medicine colleagues can avoid duplication and oversights in care and can ensure that programs are consistent with the medical needs and limitations of patients.

This chapter is also written for practitioners who occasionally practice in these settings. For example, the section on the emergency department is intended, in part, to remind physicians that they can provide preventive care when they see patients in the emergency department. Clinicians who sometimes work at employee health or public health department clinics may also find this chapter useful. The chapter is not intended, however, for practitioners who specialize in these fields, such as public health officials, emergency medicine specialists, and occupational health physicians. A complete discussion of how to provide preventive services in these settings is beyond the scope of a single chapter and is addressed in more detail elsewhere (e.g., references at end of chapter).

Providing Preventive Care in the Public Health Department

MARK B. JOHNSON

Public health departments have traditionally promoted health through the control of communicable diseases, health education, environmental sanitation, consumer protection, and the provision of medical and nursing services for the diagnosis, treatment, and prevention of diseases in hard-to-reach populations (1). Although clinical medicine and public health departments work in concert in dealing with the health of the public, it is often an uneasy relationship characterized by poor coordination. This may stem from the fact that, although they share a common goal, their focus is on different stages of the process. Unlike patient care, which seeks to provide the best possible outcome for the individual, public health seeks to optimize the health of the community. Surveillance and monitoring activities are used to identify and track the behavioral, communicable, and environmental factors that contribute to morbidity and mortality in the community. Clinicians play an important role in this process. Accurate surveillance data, for example, require the reliable and timely reporting of communicable diseases by providers in the community. Accurate birth and death certificates, completed by physicians, provide information that is vital to the formation of public policy and the allocation of health resources.

Public health activities are coordinated through a network of municipal, county, state, and federal agencies (2). Public health units are very diverse; no description adequately captures a "typical" health department. To understand fully the functions of one's local health department, both to assess how it can help provide preventive services and to determine how these programs interface with other services in the community, one must know its program structure and staffing pattern. It also helps to understand the legal, medical, and budgetary constraints within which the department operates. The clinician need not fully understand the complexities of the health department to work with it effectively, however. Knowing what services are available, where and when they are offered, and how much they cost is a good place to start.

To obtain this information, clinicians should contact the health department in their community and request a list of services available to the practitioner. Ideally, a direct line of communication should be established between the practitioner and specific individuals in the health department. The clinician should determine what resources are available at both the local and state levels. Examples of appropriate questions include:

- Does the health department provide supplemental food and nutrition programs for pregnant women, infants, and children (WIC Program)?

- Does the health department have clinics for family planning and prenatal care?

- Are there clinics and services for patients with sexually transmitted diseases, human immunodeficiency virus (HIV) infection, and acquired immunodeficiency syndrome (AIDS)?

- Does the health department provide foreign travel immunizations?

- What community classes are taught? Do they include such topics as smoking cessation, cholesterol reduction, weight management, blood pressure control, and injury prevention?

- Are there eligibility requirements for participants?

In addition to clinics and classes, clinicians should become acquainted with other services that may be available at their community health department. Case management services may be available for high-risk or adolescent pregnant women, or for patients with such diseases as tuberculosis. Does the health department assist in arranging social or other services for these patients? Does its staff oversee directly observed therapy (direct observation to verify that patients take antibiotics for tuberculosis or other forms of chemoprophylaxis)? What patient education materials, such as brochures, posters, videos, or models, are available? Does the health department have staff who can help identify, trace, and contact persons who may have been exposed to an environmental or communicable disease through household contacts, worksites, day care facilities, restaurants, sexual practices, or other lifestyle choices?

Health departments may also be able to provide technical information and expertise to private clinicians. In this sense, the health department can be used as a consultant. Due to their ongoing surveillance activities, most health departments are able to provide useful epidemiologic information of direct relevance to clinical practice, such as the prevalence of lead in the local environment, the risk of rabies in the local animal population, and the level of fluoride in the water supply. Most state and large local health departments publish periodic epidemiology bulletins with information on current disease trends in the community as well as national and state recommendations for preventing disease. These bulletins are usually free for local clinicians who wish to be on the mailing list. As part of the national network of public health agencies, local health departments can often provide resources from outside their immediate jurisdiction and from national health agencies (e.g., U.S. Centers for Disease Control and Prevention). They can serve as a local link between clinicians and state and national public health experts and reference laboratories.

Public health departments are also a common provider of clinical services. Most public health officials and policymakers work to assure that all residents within their jurisdiction have access to needed health care services, including preventive services. A 1992 National Association of County Health Officials study showed that the majority of responding health departments provide some clinical health services to the public (3). While few health departments provide comprehensive primary care services or are the only source of care for the medically indigent within their jurisdiction, most local health departments play some role as health care providers. Extrapolating the results of the survey to the general population suggests that approximately 40 million Americans receive one or more clinical services through their health department.

Surveys indicate that clinical preventive services are offered by over half of all health departments (Table 24.1) (3, 4). Some health departments provide comprehensive primary care coverage, but most limit their programs to preventive services, frequently provided in a preventive "pack-

Table 24.1
Services Provided at Local Health Departments

Reported Services	Health Departments with Active Programs
Prenatal care	59%
Home health care	50%
Assisting handicapped children	47%
Human immunodeficiency virus testing and counseling	57%
Laboratory services	43%
Family planning	60%
Prevention of chronic diseases	69%
Women, Infants, and Children (WIC) program services	69%
Sexually transmitted disease control	73%
Direct treatment	60%
Tuberculosis control	83%
Direct treatment	65%
Child health care services	84%
Immunization programs	92%

From Primary care assessment: local health departments' role in service delivery. Washington, DC: National Association of County Health Officials, 1992. National profile of local health departments. Washington, DC: National Association of County Health Officials, 1990.

age." Approximately 47% of responding health departments provide a package that includes immunizations, health education, tuberculosis screening and treatment, well-child visits, nutrition services for women and children, sexually transmitted disease screening, partner identification and treatment, and HIV testing and counseling.

The majority (68%) of local health departments offer personal health services to all persons living in their jurisdiction, contrary to the common misconception that public health departments offer services only to the medically indigent. The remaining departments may have eligibility limitations based on age, income, or both. In some states and for most federally funded programs, public health departments are mandated to provide services to all citizens regardless of their ability to pay. Health departments depend on a number of reimbursement mechanisms to pay for their services. The majority accept Medicaid. Most have a sliding-fee scale based on income eligibility criteria. A significant minority accept other third party payments, obtain Medicare reimbursement, charge fee-for-service, or charge no fees at all.

Although a health department may be actively involved in assuring that certain personal health services are available in their community, those services may not necessarily be provided on-site at the department or by the departmental staff. Increasingly, health departments contract clinical services to private providers or other public entities such as community health centers, a trend that will undoubtedly continue in light of current

economic and political realities. The public health work force often includes "physician extenders," such as registered nurses, nurse practitioners, physician assistants, nutritionists or dietitians, health educators, and
other allied health professionals. Although the overall number of public
health professionals is lower at suburban and rural health departments,
staffing patterns are similar.

Because of their emphasis on physician extenders, most health department clinics depend heavily on medical protocols and practice guidelines
in decision making and treatment. In addition, since much of the clinical
practice at health departments depends on federal funding, federal guidelines and protocols mandate how these programs should provide services
and treatments. This reliance on protocols increases the potential opportunities for preventive care. Rather than relying on individual practitioner
habits or practice patterns, in which preventive interventions can be overlooked, prevention is built into the mandated protocols. Audits are done
periodically to ensure adherence to the guidelines. Emphasizing prevention in practice guidelines and protocols and tying them to payment motivate clinical staff at public health departments to improve their prevention
efforts.

Private practitioners can benefit from a partnership with the public
health system by augmenting their preventive practices with the services of
allied health professionals, who can often provide care in a less costly, non-
competitive manner. Solo practitioners and small group practices may lack
the resources or practice size to justify providing these services in the office or clinic. This is particularly true in rural areas, where few allied
health professionals may practice. The clinician's local health department,
however, may have health educators, social workers, psychologists, nutritionists or dietitians, and others on staff or on contract who can provide
such services. As greater pressure is exerted on the health care system to
control costs, the private clinician may find the health department to be a
more cost-effective site for the delivery of preventive care than the office.
Patients may also be more receptive. Many clinicians find patients unprepared or unwilling to accept preventive services when they seek illness
care. Since many health department clients are not ill but are already seeking prevention services, they may be more receptive to health education
and other preventive interventions in this setting than in the doctor's office.

The practitioner must, however, appreciate the limitations under
which the local health department may be operating. Budgetary constraints, for example, may limit the number of staff available or may restrict clinic hours, so that follow-up of patients cannot be ensured. Practitioners should also coordinate their services with those provided by the

local health department to avoid redundancy in services provided and to assure that no patients "fall through the cracks."

Discussion

The role of the local health department will probably change with the dramatic restructuring of health care delivery systems that is sweeping the country. The need will continue, however, for communicable disease control, environmental health assessment and regulation, health policy development, community health assessment, and the assurance that the health needs of all are being met in a quality manner. Health departments' continued involvement in the provision of clinical health services will vary from state to state and from community to community. As the landscape changes, practitioners will need to remain familiar with the services and programs being provided by the health department in their community to manage effectively the health promotion and disease prevention needs of their patients.

Providing Preventive Care at the Worksite

TEE L. GUIDOTTI

Preventable chronic diseases are responsible for hugely escalating health care costs for employers. Corporations pay an estimated 30–40% of national health expenditures (5). The diseases that account for these costs share the same risk factors (especially smoking, substance abuse, and inactivity) as contemporary short-term diseases that contribute to sickness-related work absence (6). This observation has motivated a number of employers to introduce health promotion programs and to support employee fitness programs. Early programs in the 1970s proved very popular with employees and coincided with a general societal movement toward increased interest in fitness and taking responsibility for one's own health. In the 1980s, these programs became an accepted management practice and are today present in some form in almost all large employers and many medium-sized organizations (7). Health promotion programs are often perceived as an employee benefit that increases morale and attracts and holds good workers, at relatively little cost. They remain largely beyond the means of small employers, however, for reasons of cost, access, practicality, and diseconomies of small scale.

The anticipated benefits of worksite health promotion programs to employers are obvious: enhanced morale, cost-effective benefits to employees, and at least the hope of a reduction in both overall health care costs and sickness absence, if not a rise in productivity. An improvement in health outcomes has been demonstrated in some studies of worksite health promotion (8). The anticipated benefits to the worker are equally clear: a sound program of personal health enhancement that is subsidized. The potential gain for society is also great: to the extent that workers participate in programs that they could not easily access in other ways, these programs may increase vitality, productivity, and well-being while reducing the health risk (and, potentially, the costs) for the most economically productive segment of the population.

These anticipated benefits have focused attention on the potential for health promotion to help contain health care costs (8). A leadership group known as the Health Project Consortium (9) has proposed that health care costs could be brought under control by worksite health promotion interventions targeted to prevent disability and the loss of productive years of life, rather than the more traditional goals of extending life and preventing disease. The ability of such programs to achieve cost savings is uncertain, however. In its review, the Consortium could point to only eight out of 200 studies that showed convincing documentation of savings, despite reductions in sickness absence, outpatient costs, and hospitalization in some other studies. Obviously, the argument for worksite health promotion cannot rest entirely on economic grounds (10).

Content of Worksite Health Promotion Programs

The worksite is a particularly attractive venue for prevention-oriented activities. There may be little else in common among North Americans, but most adults are employed. More than 110 million persons are employed in the United States, and they care for an additional 100 million dependents (11). The employer therefore provides a means of reaching a large proportion of the population and an organizational framework for supporting health promotion activities. Since the social support system at work is one of the most important factors in most people's lives, it offers an incentive to participate in activities with fellow workers. For all these reasons, worksite health promotion programs have grown in popularity.

Current data on worksite health promotion activities are difficult to obtain (12). The most accurate data in recent years are from a series of studies (13–15), published in 1989 and 1993, reflecting the prevalence of worksite health promotion activities before 1992. As of 1992, an estimated 81% of private workplaces had one or more health promotion activities. The most frequently mentioned activities were, in descending order, injury prevention, physical fitness, smoking cessation, and stress management (15). Surveys in the 1980s indicated that screening programs in the form of health risk appraisals were offered by 24% of all worksites, compared to the older approach of clinical periodic health evaluations, which were offered by 77% of worksites (14). Screening activities were primarily directed at hypertension, cancer detection, fitness, and diabetes mellitus. There were more programs and greater employee participation overall in larger firms (more that 750 employees). The evidence from the 1980s and early 1990s suggested that worksite health promotion programs were rapidly increasing in number, with considerable room for growth (7, 12–14).

The recession and recovery of the early 1990s, with its emphasis on short-term cost savings and downsizing the work force, had exceptionally severe implications for employment and employee benefits. It is possible that the number and extent of health promotion programs actually shrank during the early 1990s. Because worksite health promotion has now assumed the status of a "tried and true" management technique, however, it is very likely that growth will resume with improvement in the economy.

Models for Worksite Programs

There are several specific models of worksite health promotion. Some of the more generally applicable models are discussed below.

Multiphasic health screening is a form of periodic health surveillance in which subjects undergo a battery of standard clinical tests for disease detection and risk factor characterization. These tests are often carried out in a routine manner, whenever possible are automated, and are usually provided by mobile units on-site in the workplace. The use of multiphasic health screening has fallen off considerably since the 1970s. Evaluation of such programs strongly suggested that they were not cost-effective, largely because there was little follow-up on the findings by employees or their physicians and because the proportion of false-positive results in a healthy work force is usually large (see discussion of positive predictive value in Chapter 4). Another reason is that such programs usually provided little individualized health education or any preventive intervention beyond communicating results to the worker's personal physician. The technology and systems that were developed for multiphasic screening, however, remain useful elements in more comprehensive programs.

Health risk appraisal is one such element, described in more detail in Chapters 1 and 2. The earliest health risk appraisal instruments were rapidly scored questionnaires that provided limited feedback to subjects, had little educational content, and were part of a multiphasic system that emphasized reporting to the worker's personal physician rather than changing individual behavior. They are much more sophisticated in design today and are oriented toward the individual worker as a person empowered to change his or her health risk through changing personal behavior. Health risk appraisal is now a common element in worksite health promotion programs, either to provide an initial or periodic assessment of overall health risk or in abbreviated form to target a specific outcome such as cardiovascular disease. It is sometimes coupled with additional outreach efforts, such as mail contact or nurse education telephone counseling, self-care books, and "electronic house calls" involving telecommunication technologies (e.g., electronic mail, Internet bulletin boards, cable television).

Health fairs are special events, often held in conjunction with company celebrations or community activities, in which basic screening services are offered free (usually blood pressure determination and blood cholesterol levels) and employees may visit booths, exhibits, or audiovisual presentations providing education on a variety of health-related topics. The overall atmosphere is celebratory and casual, making these events popular but usually best suited to introducing rather than sustaining health promotion programs.

Health education classes are a relatively primitive method but are often the first thought of managers who wish to initiate a program without committing themselves to an expensive undertaking. Classes are usually held during a lunch hour or on the employee's own time and often feature an outside educator discussing a topic of general interest. Often the topics are selected on the basis of recent incidents or concerns expressed by employees. Popular topics include heart health, cancer prevention, preventing substance abuse, smoking cessation, weight control, nutrition, stress reduction, travel, child care, and immunization. The most effective use of classes is to target a single topic in which there is local concern and to use it to provide a group of workers with the knowledge they need to solve their own health problems. Classes tend to work poorly when they are structured like school classes, with an emphasis on didactic lectures and instructing employees broadly in general health sciences. Classes seem to work better in communities or employee groups that are isolated but homogenous, when they are combined with other program elements, and when they have a casual social atmosphere.

Fitness programs are by far the most popular program elements and are seen by a substantial fraction of employees—usually younger and already fit—as a major employment benefit. Access to fitness facilities on-site or nearby in the workers' own home community is highly attractive to workers who are already persuaded of the benefits of fitness. It is also common for employees to organize their own informal fitness programs, such as lunch time aerobics, with management cooperation. In the past two decades most large companies have enthusiastically joined this trend, often installing well-equipped fitness facilities at their headquarters and major locations and hiring trainers and coordinators to staff them. These facilities are very expensive and are cost-effective only when large numbers of employees are concentrated in one place. An alternative is for the employer to pay for memberships in local fitness clubs or gyms, although the "team" identification with the employer tends to be less strong in this case. A key to the success of fitness programs beyond lunch time aerobics is to make available a variety of levels of involvement so that workers can individualize their regimens according to need, preference, and personal schedules. Regimented programs, as in the Japanese stereotype, invariably leave out many workers with different needs and are distasteful to American sensibilities of individualism.

"Corporate culture" programs are highly sophisticated campaigns that link the employers' image and identification with health and vitality. The emphasis is on energy, optimism, productivity, and teamwork. These campaigns weave health promotion elements throughout, including fitness programs, fundraising for health-related appeals, heart healthy cafeteria menus, and positive thinking.

Whatever model of health promotion program is undertaken, there are certain implicit principles that must be followed. Effective programs are easily accessible to employees, both geographically and culturally. They are adaptable to individual needs and emphasize personal responsibility and empowerment. They may contribute to a positive corporate culture and image, but they are not extensions of human resources departments or ways of monitoring employee behavior outside of work hours. It is never acceptable to break confidentiality with personal health information (see also Chapter 27). Employees who choose not to participate in designated activities such as fitness programs should not be coerced or made to feel that they are letting down "the team."

Worksite health promotion programs target those health-related behaviors that are most appropriate to employed persons, who are generally between ages 20 and 65 and are in good health. They tend to attract more youthful, physically fit, and middle-class workers who are already aware of health risk factors. Blue-collar workers, linguistically or ethnically isolated workers, and workers in rural areas or whose worksite is remote from headquarters (e.g., drivers, sales personnel, workers engaged in telecommuting) tend not to participate, although there is evidence that they stand to benefit as much or more than white-collar, urban workers. Access is also limited for those employed by small businesses, transiently employed persons, and employee dependents. Executives tend to prefer their own programs, but for ensuring motivation and credibility among employees it is important that the executives be seen to participate in worksite programs, at least nominally.

Targeted Behaviors

Specific health promotion activities are discussed in Section 2. The following discussion deals only with elements of risk factor modification that are common and important in worksite programs, with an emphasis on how they fit into the larger picture.

Nutrition and weight control is a very popular program element that taps into the nearly universal concern of North Americans about their weight and eating habits. Because weight reduction is best achieved through group reinforcement of diet and exercise behavior, it makes sense that such programs would be effective (16), although this remains unproven. Further, because objective nutritional education is hard to obtain in daily life in a society devoted to product marketing, the nutritional counseling component of such programs is very popular. Weight control programs dovetail well with other health promotion activities, particularly fitness and cardiovascular risk factor modification, and lend themselves well to campaigns and institutional changes (particularly "light" cafeteria menus). They are good ways to start or to introduce a more comprehensive health promotion program in the workplace. Predictably, they attract more women than men, although men may be more motivated by cardiovascular risk factor modification.

Fitness programs, as noted, are enormously popular but involve the heaviest investment in facilities. They can be started on a shoestring as lunch time aerobics and stepped up from there. Men, particularly, often see the facilities as an opportunity to regain or maintain athletic levels of fitness, but it is important that fitness programs encourage participation at all levels and discourage attitudes that promote a "gym mentality" of personal competition or cliquishness. Properly supervised, fitness-activity-related injuries are much less common than unsupervised sports-related injuries and on balance appear to reduce the risk of workplace injuries among participating workers, although this has been difficult to document.

Smoking cessation programs are common, popular, and often effective, especially when combined with a change in corporate smoking policies that reduces opportunities to smoke (17). They are an ethical necessity when smoking is abruptly prohibited in a facility or workplace. Because approximately one-third of smokers are thought to be sufficiently addicted to be unable or unwilling to quit on their own, corporate smoking cessation programs can provide a real community service.

Cardiovascular risk factor modification programs include all of the elements previously mentioned as well as regular cholesterol and blood pressure determinations. Managing individuals with clinical hypertension or major elevations in atherogenic blood cholesterol fractions is primarily a medical responsibility. Cardiovascular risk factor modification in worksite health promotion programs plays a supporting role in modifying the health risk of the great majority of persons with normal blood lipid phenotypes who can control their level of risk by simple dietary adjustments and exercise.

Substance abuse prevention is an important health education topic in worksite health promotion programs. Substance abuse *detection and control* should be left to corporate drug screening policies and employee assistance programs and kept strictly out of health promotion programs. Mixing the two is likely to risk cynicism and suspicion on the part of many workers. Combining the two, administratively or programmatically, will destroy the effectiveness of the health promotion program for little or no gain in substance abuse control.

Stress management is a popular theme in health promotion programs and is sometimes introduced during critical transitions in the company, especially during times of layoffs. The economic recession in the early 1990s placed greater pressures on workers as corporations engaged in downsizing, "re-engineering," and shifting from full-time to part-time workers. Behavioral techniques of stress reduction are valuable in all aspects of life, however. They are supportive when workers are making other changes in their lives or are involved in other health promotion programs that require difficult commitment, such as smoking cessation and weight reduction.

Worksite Health Promotion and the Primary Care Clinician

Worksite health promotion programs may play an extremely important and constructive role in an individual worker's health care (5). It is a solid adjunct to personal prevention at home and a healthy lifestyle. It is therefore useful for the worker's personal physician to know about the worker's participation in the worksite program and to take advantage of the opportunity the worksite program offers to target individual risk factors. Clinicians should ask their patients to describe the health promotion services available at their worksite. For example, a worksite health promotion program may be the most appropriate setting for prescribed exercise programs, for nutritional counseling, or for support in lifestyle changes such as smoking cessation or weight reduction.

Likewise, the worker's personal physician can play a helpful and supportive role in the worksite health promotion program. For older workers or those with risk factors, an evaluation prior to participating can reduce the risk of sudden exercise-induced problems in the unfit subject and of sports injuries. The clinician may also be able to target specific health risks that are best addressed through participation in the worksite program. In addition to traditional medical risk factors, such as overweight or elevated lipids, which might benefit from relevant worksite programs, the clinician may also become aware of emotional stresses at work or at home that could be addressed in worksite counseling and substance abuse programs.

Most worksite health promotion programs are not supervised directly by a physician on-site, although many have physicians as consultants or advisors. When there is a special need or opportunity, the worker's physician should not hesitate to contact the physician associated with the program in order to maximize the benefit and to minimize the risk of that worker participating in the program.

Providing Preventive Services in the Emergency Department

JULIAN ORENSTEIN, THOM A. MAYER and STEVEN H. WOOLF

Over 120 million patients visit emergency departments (EDs) each year in the United States. These clinical encounters offer important opportunities for the delivery of preventive services. Although treatments directed at the presenting injury or illness account for most of the care provided in EDs, patients can also receive a variety of preventive services. These include screening tests, patient education and counseling, the delivery of primary care services, and the updating of immunizations.

Screening

Screening tests are often performed in the ED as part of the evaluation of a patient's presenting complaints. Blood pressure measurements, for example, are performed in about 75% of ED visits (18), and recent legislation (19) mandates vital sign measurement in all patients. Testing for HIV infection and other sexually transmitted diseases (e.g., gonorrhea, chlamydial infection) accounts for a large proportion of diagnostic procedures performed in the ED. Follow-up interventions can be performed or arranged in the ED if the results are obtainable in the ED or from the laboratory during the patient's visit.

Counseling

ED staff have the opportunity to educate and counsel patients about personal health behaviors and other measures for preventing disease. Problems commonly seen in the ED provide important opportunities for counseling about tobacco use (e.g., bronchitis, angina), sexual practices (e.g., urethritis, pelvic inflammatory disease), and other health behaviors. Of these, injuries, which account for 35% of all ED visits (18), provide the best opportunity for preventive intervention. Recognizing this, the American College of Surgeons and the American College of Emergency Physicians have required the inclusion of an injury prevention component in all trauma center programs (20). Injury prevention is also required in the curriculum of emergency medicine residencies and pediatric emergency medicine fellowships.

Comprehensive ED injury prevention counseling addresses pre-event, event, and post-event factors that contribute to injury. Injured patients, and the parents of injured children, are especially receptive to such messages because they are able to appreciate the connection between pre-event risk factors and the injury event itself. Patients being seen for motor vehicle injuries, for example, can be counseled about the importance of driving safely, wearing seat belts, avoiding drinking and driving, and the potential legal consequences of violating motor safety laws. Parents of children with head injuries from falls can be informed about the need and legal requirements for such items as bicycle safety helmets and protective equipment for rollerblading. Other aspects of injury prevention counseling are discussed in Chapter 10.

Basic Primary Care

The growing population without access to primary care has shifted greater responsibility on EDs to provide basic health care services, forcing EDs to expand beyond their traditional mission. Nonurgent problems currently account for 55% of ED visits (18). The patient population that receives services from EDs typically includes disadvantaged persons with multiple risk factors, who have the greatest need for preventive care. The uninsured, homeless, and working poor, many of whom may lack the money or time to visit private physicians during working hours, often turn to the ED for basic health care services. ED staff often take advantage of these clinical encounters to provide preventive services that patients would otherwise not receive. Studies have demonstrated, for example, that the use of the ED in this manner can expand immunization coverage for children (21) and older adults (22); screening for hypertension (23), hypercholesterolemia (24), cervical cancer (25), and syphilis (26); and other forms of early detection.

Advantages of the Emergency Department in Providing Preventive Services

The ED offers several advantages as a setting for providing preventive care. First, patients who are acutely ill or injured are often more receptive to advice about measures for preventing future recurrences or complications. This time of crisis is often described as the "teachable moment." The vast majority of ED visits are initiated by the patient or family, which often further enhances patient compliance with follow-up recommendations. Second, in terms of injury prevention, the population served by EDs (i.e., injury victims) is a self-selected group whose members have demonstrated their need for injury prevention interventions. Third, the high-risk population with the greatest need for preventive services is more likely to interact with physicians in EDs than with those in private offices or other settings. The incidental ED visit may, in fact, provide the only opportunity for reaching these patients.

Disadvantages of the Emergency Department in Providing Preventive Services

There are important disadvantages, however, to providing preventive care in EDs (27). EDs are not designed to provide primary care services; they do so largely to compensate for deficiencies in the health care system. EDs are often overcrowded, and waiting times for stable patients can be lengthy (several hours in busy EDs). Test results obtained in the ED may be inaccurate; elevations in blood pressure may be secondary to pain or anxiety from the presenting problem (e.g. headache, extremity pain, abdominal pain) rather than to hypertension. EDs generally lack access to outpatient medical records and are unable to follow patients over time. They are often unable to act on abnormal laboratory results, locate and contact patients requiring follow-up, or reinforce previous health messages. One ED that performed cervical cancer screening reported that 177 telephone calls were necessary to reach 54 women with abnormal Papanicolaou smears (25).

ED screening efforts are generally ineffective unless follow-up can be carried out immediately. Thus, for example, screening for gonorrhea or chlamydial infection in the ED is often more successful than performing Papanicolaou smears or testing for HIV infection. Antibiotic treatment for the former can be offered readily during the same visit, whereas cervical cancer screening requires follow-up of cytology results and potential recall of the patient for repeat screening or referrals. Pretest and posttest HIV counseling requires considerable time and is often not feasible in busy EDs. Brief advice on safe sexual practices is possible, but effective counseling typically requires a lengthier discussion about the consequences of sexual activity, risk-taking behavior, and contraception. Further, such advice is more effective when given by a clinician with whom the patient has an established relationship than when delivered by a stranger, as is usually the case in the ED. Many states require that facilities offering HIV testing must provide timely counseling for patients with positive results (28), which is extraordinarily difficult in the ED setting. Finally, patients who receive care from several different EDs may receive conflicting and confusing instructions, rather than the consistent health education message that they would receive from a primary care provider. They rarely have an opportunity to develop a therapeutic alliance with a single clinician, thus rendering counseling and health promotion more difficult.

Theoretically, the ED can provide an appropriate setting for improving immunization coverage, since the need for vaccination can be identified and resolved in the same visit. Logistical problems, however, can interfere with this effort. In the absence of a tracking system or central vaccine registry, EDs lack a mechanism for determining which immunizations have already been received. In the ED, patients, parents, and other family members generally cannot remember the dates of previous immunizations and rarely bring personal immunization records with them when they visit the ED (29). Access to outpatient medical records is often difficult. Even if the vaccine is administered, poor communications between the ED and the patient's other physicians may leave the vaccination undocumented in the patient's long-term records.

Other characteristics of the ED interfere with the delivery of preventive care. ED physicians care for large numbers of patients, many of whom are critically ill, and often cannot spend time with stable patients to discuss personal health behaviors. The use of the ED for nonurgent problems draws personnel away from the primary mission of providing acute care and places greater demands on other ED staff. Financial, professional, and other resources are taxed further when the ED is used as a *de facto* public health clinic. In many cities, EDs have been forced to close because they were unable to cope with these stresses. Economic pressures have become especially great in inner cities, where the financial viability of EDs is tenuous because of high rates of unreimbursed care.

Discussion

Although some of these problems will not be solved without broad-based health care reform, individual EDs can often improve preventive care through special measures. To accomplish this end, adequate time, personnel, and resources need to be set aside by the hospital and ED administration to promote research, surveillance, and advocacy on health promotion issues. A "point" person should be assigned responsibility for prevention programs. That person would teach accurate recording of pre-event, event, and post-event factors related to injury counseling; maintain a high level of awareness of specific, local prevention initiatives; accumulate data on specific injuries, with links to regional Emergency Medical System data sets (or on a state or national level using E-codes) or agreed upon standards for research; conduct research directed at the epidemiology of injury and other preventable problems seen in the ED; participate with community efforts to promote local and state legislation to reduce injury and disease risks; and monitor the effectiveness of ED programs. The ED can promote greater attention to preventive issues by individual clinicians by adding preventive care items to checklists or chart inserts, adopting a manual or automated tracking system to identify outstanding laboratory results without follow-up, and improving communication with local practitioners to enhance the exchange of information about preventive care received by patients.

Aside from providing preventive care for individuals, EDs can also play a role in promoting community-based prevention. Our ED has recently implemented an *index case* program for school-based pediatric injury prevention, based on the assumption that classmates and playmates of seriously injured children are likely to be more receptive to injury prevention messages than other children. After obtaining consent from the parents of the injured child (index case), the ED injury prevention team that has cared for the child makes a presentation at the child's school. The speakers include the paramedics involved in the child's care, the emergency department resuscitation team, and the trauma team responsible for treatment and rehabilitation. In over 75% of cases, the family and the patient also participate. Assessments before and after the presentation suggest high receptivity to the injury prevention information program and substantial retention over the six-month period following the presentation.

By monitoring pre-event, event, and post-event modifiers, EDs can identify local conditions affecting safety and alert appropriate health, safety, and rescue agencies. School playgrounds and neighborhood parks, for example, are well-monitored, high-use areas where ED recommendations to remove a potential source of injuries are likely to be heeded. Similar advice about passive countermeasures, such as engineering or safety designs, may also be useful. Finally, EDs can be active in promoting legislation to prevent injuries and health risks. See Chapter 28 for further details about clinician involvement in community-based prevention activities.

REFERENCES

1. U.S. Department of Health and Human Services, Public Health Service. For a healthy nation: returns on investment in public health. Washington, DC: Government Printing Office, 1994.
2. U.S. Centers for Disease Control and Prevention and the National Association of County Health Officials. Blueprint for a health community: a guide for local health departments. Washington, DC: National Association of County Health Officials, 1994.
3. Primary care assessment: local health departments' role in service delivery. Washington, DC: National Association of County Health Officials, 1992.

4. National profile of local health departments. Washington, DC: National Association of County Health Officials, 1990.

5. Stokols D, Pelletier KR, Fielding JE. Integration of medical care and worksite health promotion. JAMA 1995;273:1136–1142.

6. Bertera RL. The effects of workplace health promotion on absenteeism and employment costs in a large industrial population. Am J Public Health 1990;80:1101–1105.

7. Office of Disease Prevention and Health Promotion. National survey of worksite health promotion activities. Washington, DC: U.S. Department of Health and Human Services, 1987.

8. Pelletier KR. A review and analysis of the health and cost-effective outcome studies of comprehensive health promotion and disease prevention programs at the worksite: 1991–1993 update. Am J Health Promotion 1993;8:350–362.

9. Fries JF, Koop CE, Beadle CE, Cooper PR, England MJ, Graves RF, Sokolov JJ, Wright D, Health Project Consortium. Reducing health care costs by reducing the need and demand for medical services. N Engl J Med 1993;329;321–325.

10. Russell LB. The role of prevention in health reform. N Engl J Med 1993;329:352–354.

11. Green LW, Cargo MD. The changing context of health promotion in the workplace. In: O'Donnell MP, Harris JS, eds. Health promotion in the workplace, 2nd ed. Albany, NY: Delmar Publishers, 1994:497–524.

12. Fielding J. Effectiveness of employee health improvement programs. J Occ Med 1982;24:907–916.

13. Fielding J. Frequency of health risk assessment activities at US workplaces. Am J Prev Med 1989;5:75–81.

14. Fielding J. Frequency of worksite health promotion activities. Am J Public Health 1989;79:16–20.

15. U.S. Department of Health and Human Services. 1992 national survey of worksite health promotion activities: summary. Am J Health Promotion 1993;7:452–464.

16. Jeffrey RW, Forster JL, French SA, Kelder SH, Lando HA, McGovern PG, Jacobs DR Jr, Baster JE. The healthy worker project: a work-site intervention for weight control and smoking cessation. Am J Public Health 1993;83:395–401.

17. Fielding J. Smoking control at the workplace. Ann Rev Public Health 1991;12:209–239.

18. McCaig LF. National Hospital Ambulatory Medical Care Survey: 1992 emergency department summary. Advance data from vital and health statistics; no. 245. Hyattsville, MD: National Center for Health Statistics, 1994.

19. Frew SA. Patient transfers: how to comply with the law. Dallas: American College of Emergency Physicians, 1991.

20. American College of Emergency Physicians. Guidelines for trauma care systems. Ann Emerg Med 1993;22:1079–1100.

21. Bell LM, Lopez NL, Pinto-Martin J, et al. Potential impact of linking an ED and hospital-affiliated clinics to immunize preschool age children. Pediatrics 1994;93:99–103.

22. Rodriguez RM, Baraff LJ. Emergency department immunization of the elderly with pneumococcal and influenza vaccines. Ann Emerg Med 1993;22:1729–1732.

23. Chernow SM, Iserson KV. Use of the emergency department for hypertension screening: a prospective study. Ann Emerg Med 1987;16:180–182.

24. Burns RB, Stoy DB, Feied CF, Nash E, Smith M. Cholesterol screening in the emergency department. J Gen Intern Med 1991;6:210–215.

25. Hogness CG, Engelstad LP, Linck LM, Schorr KA. Cervical cancer screening in an urban emergency department. Ann Emerg Med 1992;21:933–939.

26. Hibbs JR, Ceglowski WS, Goldberg M, Kauffman F. Emergency department-based surveillance for syphilis during an outbreak in Philadelphia. Ann Emerg Med 1993;22:1286–1290.

27. Avner JR. The difficulties in providing primary care in the emergency department. Pediatr Emerg Care 1992;8:101–102.

28. Siegel DM. Confidentiality. In: Henry GL, ed. Emergency medicine risk management. Dallas: American College of Emergency Physicians, 1991.

29. Goldstein KP, Kviz FJ, Daum RS. Accuracy of immunization histories provided by adults accompanying preschool children to a pediatric emergency department. JAMA 1993;270:2190–2194.

25. Reimbursement for Preventive Services

MICHAEL D. PARKINSON and PERRIANNE LURIE

INTRODUCTION

Inadequate payment for clinical preventive services represents a formidable barrier to both patients who seek appropriate care and to clinicians who strive to deliver it. Improved insurance coverage is a necessary, but not sufficient, factor in more widespread delivery and receipt of preventive screening, counseling, and immunization services. *Healthy People 2000*, the national health promotion and disease prevention objectives for the year 2000, articulates the following goal:

> Improve the financing and delivery of clinical preventive services so that virtually no American has a financial barrier to receiving, at a minimum, the screening, counseling and immunization services recommended by the U.S. Preventive Services Task Force. (1)

CURRENT STATUS OF REIMBURSEMENT FOR PREVENTIVE SERVICES

Health insurance in the United States is provided by a wide assortment of private and public organizations (2). The majority of the approximately 85% of Americans who have health insurance obtain it from their employer, which either purchases a group plan from an insurance company or insures its own employees.

Insurance coverage for preventive services has been determined to be the greatest single predictor of their delivery (3). The exact degree of payment for clinical preventive services is difficult to ascertain either for a population of individuals in a given health care plan, or even for an individual patient. For example, a preventive service may be paid for because it is delivered at the time of care for another medical condition or because the patient's condition is coded as if there were a medical diagnosis. Specific coverage for selected preventive services under various types of insurance plans in 1992 is summarized in Table 25.1 (4).

In general, screening procedures and laboratory tests are most likely to be reimbursed, physical examinations less reliably, and counseling interventions least of all. Counseling for behavioral risk factors, such as

Table 25.1
Percentage of Employees with Health Insurance in the Private Sector Who Are Covered for Selected Services, by Plan Type, 1992

	Type of Plan (%)			
Preventive Service	Conventional	HMO	PPO	POS
Adult Physical Examination	35	*	50	91
Mammography	73	97	83	94
Papanicolaou Smear	62	*	77	92
Child Immunizations	54	*	66	99
Well-Baby Care	50	*	69	99
Well-Child Care (age 1–4)	43	*	60	97

From Employer-sponsored health insurance in private sector firms in 1992. Washington, DC: Health Insurance Association of America, 1993. *Legend: *, HMOs are assumed to cover these services; *HMO*, health maintenance organizations; *PPO*, preferred provider organizations; *POS*, point-of-service health plans ("open-ended HMOs").

smoking cessation therapy, is rarely covered under traditional indemnity plans. Approximately 40% of health maintenance organization plans (covering approximately two-thirds of all health maintenance organization enrollees) include smoking cessation classes among their benefits (5).

In response to the rapid escalation in health care costs, employers are increasingly self-insuring; raising employee coinsurance, copayments, and deductible levels; and utilizing managed care plans. The federal Employee Retirement Income Security Act (ERISA) of 1974 exempts employers providing health insurance from state-legislated mandates for specific coverage, including preventive services.

Public insurance plans provide coverage for a few selected preventive services, usually as a result of specific federal or state mandates. As of 1994, Medicare, the federal health insurance plan for elderly and disabled Americans, covered pneumococcal vaccination, cervical cancer screening, mammography, and hepatitis B vaccination for at-risk individuals. Medicaid, the joint federal-state health insurance plan for the poor, varies widely in both coverage policy and income levels which qualify beneficiaries for enrollment. Preventive health services are mandated to be covered for all Medicaid-eligible children under age 21 through the Early and Periodic Screening, Diagnostic, and Treatment (EPSDT) program. Adult preventive services are an optional Medicaid benefit that only 19 states have chosen to cover. As is the case for other diagnostic and therapeutic interventions, Medicare, and particularly Medicaid, usually pay considerably less than private insurance plans for the same service.

BARRIERS TO FINANCING OF CLINICAL PREVENTIVE SERVICES

Despite significant progress in demonstrating the clinical effectiveness of preventive services in preventing or decreasing morbidity and mortality, the barriers to financing of clinical preventive services remain formidable. Historical, philosophical, scientific, and economic factors have contributed to the current lack of coverage for preventive services.

The philosophical foundation for indemnity health insurance in the United States was based upon the need to pay for hospitalization for destitute patients during the Great Depression. The primary objective of "health insurance" has been to pay for catastrophic, unpredictable hospitalization and outpatient illness care costs. In both private and public insurance plans, inexpensive and "predictable" preventive interventions have most often been specifically excluded from coverage.

Insurers, payers, and legislators have often required that preventive services, in addition to significantly reducing morbidity and mortality, also prove themselves to be "cost-effective." This greater degree of scrutiny is in part explained by the late entry of clinical preventive services into the medical market at a time of increased emphasis on health care cost containment. Proponents of expanded coverage for preventive services have criticized this "double standard," which has not traditionally been applied to curative services. Economic analyses can include a wide variety of costs, benefits, and relative measures of effectiveness, which complicate uniform policy making with respect to coverage. With the exception of selected immunizations, the majority of preventive services that have been studied have not been shown to save direct medical costs (6). Increasing patient and provider demand for reimbursement of preventive services, the application of more rigorous standards of clinical and cost-effectiveness to other diagnostic and therapeutic services, and the development of more uniform cost-effectiveness study criteria may alter the approach to coverage decisions for preventive services in the future.

The lack of clear consensus concerning which interventions are appropriate for asymptomatic, healthy patients has also deterred payers and insurers from covering preventive services. The U.S. Preventive Services Task Force's recommendations for clinically effective screening, counseling, and immunization interventions represent a major advance in the United States in this regard.

Physicians and other health care providers, through their daily interactions with patients and their professional relationships with policy makers and the medical community, can help promote improved reimbursement for preventive services. Understanding the cost estimates for appropriate preventive services is important in effectively arguing for their coverage in an era of cost containment. Likewise, with an increasing emphasis on outcomes research for all facets of medical care, the accurate coding and billing of these services are essential to evaluate their utilization and health- and cost-effectiveness. Both of these important barriers to improved reimbursement, namely costs and coding taxonomies, have recently been addressed.

COSTS OF PREVENTIVE SERVICES

The costs of a core set of preventive services for a well population, "packaged" into age and gender-specific periodic health examinations and based upon the 1989 recommendations of the U.S. Preventive Services Task Force, have been calculated (7). The services include periodic examinations by physicians, immunizations, laboratory tests, and other screen-

Table 25.2
Preventive Services Packages

Age (yrs)	Preventive Services		
	Immunizations[a]	Tests	Clinician Visits
0–5	5 DTP, 4 OPV, 2-3 HiB, 3 HBV, 2 MMR	1 Hematocrit, 2 Lead,[b] 1 Urinalysis	9
6–19	1 Td	Pap/pelvic[c] every 3 years[d,e]	5
20–39	1 Td every 10 years	Cholesterol every 5 years Pap/pelvic[c] every 3 years[d,e]	Every 3 years
40–49	1 Td every 10 years	Cholesterol every 5 years Pap/pelvic[c] every 3 years[d,e]	Every 2 years
50–64	1 Td every 10 years	Cholesterol every 5 years Pap/pelvic and mammogram every 2 years	Every 2 years
65+	1 Td every 10 years	Cholesterol every 5 years Mammogram every 2 years	Annually

From Preventive Services in the clinical setting: What works and what it costs. Special report to National Coordinating Committee on Clinical Preventive Services. Washington, DC: U.S. Public Health Service, Office of Disease Prevention and Health Promotion, 1993.

[a]DTP, diphtheria, tetanus, pertussis vaccine; OPV, oral polio vaccine; Hib, *Haemophilus influenzae* type b vaccine; HBV, hepatitis B vaccine; MMR, measles, mumps, rubella vaccine; Td, tetanus-diphtheria toxoid.

[b]Children at high risk of lead exposure.

[c]Females once sexually active.

[d]Once three annual negative smears obtained.

[e]Females of childbearing age with more than one sexual partner should have an annual Pap smear and screening for chlamydia and gonorrhea.

ing tests. All periodic health examinations include a history, blood pressure measurement, and risk assessment/health guidance. The content and periodicity of these visits for asymptomatic individuals without special risk factors is described in Table 25.2.

The estimated lifetime annual costs for providing these services was $78 per year for females and $55 per year for males in 1992 dollars. The 1992 premiums for adding these preventive services to private health insurance programs, assuming average participation rates of 50–90% based upon review of population and special studies, ranged from $11.66 to $15.98 per month for family coverage and $3.48 to $4.77 per month for single coverage. Because copayments and deductibles have been shown to have an adverse effect on the receipt of preventive services (3), these estimates were made using those utilization rates that occurred when no specific patient contribution was required. The additional premium costs for coverage of preventive services are relatively low, representing less than 3% of the 1990 average monthly premiums of $319 per month for family coverage and $148 for single coverage under the typical employer's insurance plan.

CURRENT STATUS OF CODING OF PREVENTIVE SERVICES

Physicians are reimbursed for preventive services in the same way that they are paid for all other medical services. The amount of reimbursement is determined by the patient's diagnoses and the number and type of procedures performed. In order to reimburse providers for care given to a particular patient and to set adequate rates for future reimbursement, payers need to have accurate information about these diagnoses and procedures. This information is provided to the payers through codes assigned to the diagnoses and procedures listed in the patient record. In some instances, these codes are assigned by the physician himself or herself; at other times a member of the office or hospital staff is responsible for code assignment. The physician is required to attest to the accuracy of the assigned codes, even if he or she was not responsible for the initial code assignment.

Physicians have inaccurately listed codes for diagnoses (e.g. "breast lump") in order to justify the use of a screening test (e.g. mammography), which was not otherwise reimbursable. Changes in reimbursement policies have made this practice unnecessary in many instances. Such practices should be discouraged for several reasons. In addition to being fraudulent, such misrepresentation reflects an inaccurate picture of the volume and nature of preventive services delivered. Regulators, payers, policy makers, and evaluators of health care plans may be dissuaded from improving reimbursement if the clinical significance and volume of preventive services are systematically underestimated.

Table 25.3
CPT Evaluation and Management [E/M] Codes for Preventive Medicine Services

NEW PATIENT

99381   Initial evaluation and management of a healthy individual requiring a comprehensive history, a comprehensive examination, the identification of risk factors, and the ordering of appropriate laboratory/diagnostic procedures, new patient; infant (age under 1 year)
99382   early childhood (age 1 through 4 years)
99383   late childhood (age 5 through 11 years)
99384   adolescent (age 12 through 17 years)
99385   age 18–39 years
99386   age 40–64 years
99387   age 65 years and older

ESTABLISHED PATIENT

99391   Periodic reevaluation and management of a healthy individual requiring a comprehensive history, comprehensive examination, the identification of risk factors and the ordering of appropriate laboratory/diagnostic procedures, established patient; infant (age under 1 year)
99392   early childhood (age 1 through 4 years)
99393   late childhood (age 5 through 11 years)
99394   adolescent (age 12 through 17 years)
99395   age 19–39 years
99396   age 40–64 years
99397   age 65 years and older

PREVENTIVE MEDICINE, INDIVIDUAL COUNSELING

These codes are used to report services provided to healthy individuals for the purpose of promoting health and preventing illness or injury.

Counseling and risk factor reduction interventions provided in conjunction with an initial or periodic preventive medicine visit will vary with age and should address such issues as family problems, diet and exercise, substance abuse, sexual practices, injury prevention, and dental health.

These codes are not to be used to report counseling and risk factor reduction visits provided to patients with symptoms or established illness. For counseling individual patients with symptoms or established illness, use the appropriate office, hospital or consultation, or other evaluation and management codes. For counseling of groups of patients with symptoms or established illness, use 99078.

99401   Counseling and/or risk factor reduction intervention(s) provided to a healthy individual; approximately 15 minutes
99402   approximately 30 minutes
99403   approximately 45 minutes
99404   approximately 60 minutes

PREVENTIVE MEDICINE, GROUP COUNSELING

99411   Counseling and/or risk factor reduction intervention(s) provided to healthy individuals in a group setting; approximately 30 minutes
99412   approximately 60 minutes

OTHER PREVENTIVE MEDICINE SERVICES

99420   Administration and interpretation of health risk assessment instrument (e.g., health hazard appraisal)
99429   Unlisted preventive medicine service

Physicians' Current Procedural Terminology, Fourth Edition (CPT-4)

The *Physicians' Current Procedural Terminology* (CPT), published by the American Medical Association, is a classification of procedures and services provided by physicians (8). It is used for the reporting of outpatient procedures and services to third-party payers and for physician billing of inpatient procedures and services. The Health Care Financing Administration (HCFA) Common Procedure Coding System (HCPCS) Level 1 is identical to CPT-4; HCPCS is used to determine not only HCFA reimbursement rates using the Resource-Based Relative Value Scale (RBRVS) but also private insurance rates using a "usual, customary, reasonable" fee schedule.

> Physicians' Current Procedural Terminology is a systematic listing of coding of procedures and services performed by physicians. Each procedure or service is identified with a five digit code. The use of CPT codes simplifies the reporting of services. With this coding and recording system, the procedure or service rendered by the physician is accurately identified. (8)

The first chapter of the 1994 edition of CPT-4 is devoted to evaluation and management (E/M) services and contains a section on preventive medicine services. These codes are to be used to report " . . . routine evaluation and management of adults and children when these services are performed in the absence of patient complaints . . . (These codes) do not include counseling, risk factor reduction interventions, or immunizations [which are classified elsewhere.] If risk management services are provided at the same session as a preventive medicine visit, both codes should be reported." (8, p. 65) The codes for preventive services are divided into general E/M codes and codes for counseling and/or risk factor reduction interventions (Table 25.3). The CPT "Medicine" chapter contains codes for "Immunization Injections" (90700–90749). These codes are listed in Table 25.4. Codes for "ancillary studies involving laboratory, radiology, or other procedures" are in the appropriate chapters (i.e., Radiology, Pathology, and Laboratory). Table 25.5 lists codes of particular relevance in these areas.

CPT is maintained by an editorial panel and an advisory committee that includes representatives from the various specialty societies and third-party payers. It is updated annually. Requests for modifications to CPT should be directed to the American Medical Association.

International Classification of Diseases, Ninth Revision, Clinical Modification (ICD-9-CM)

The *International Classification of Diseases, Ninth Revision, Clinical Modification* (ICD-9-CM) (9) is a statistical classification of diseases, injuries, and health-related conditions based on an expansion of the ninth revision of

Table 25.4
ICD-9-CM and CPT Codes for Prophylactic Vaccinations and Inoculations

Vaccination or Inoculation	ICD-9-CM Diagnosis Codes	CPT Procedure Codes[a]
Cholera alone	V03.0	90725
Typhoid-paratyphoid	V03.1	90714
Tuberculosis [BCG]	V03.2	90728
Plague	V03.3	90727
Tularemia	V03.4	90749*
Diphtheria alone	V03.5	90719
Pertussis alone	V03.6	90749*
Tetanus toxoid alone	V03.7	90703
Poliomyelitis	V04.0	90712 (live, oral)
		90713 (other)
Measles alone	V04.2	90705
Rubella alone	V04.3	90706
Yellow fever	V04.4	90717
Rabies	V04.5	90726
Mumps alone	V04.6	90704
Influenza	V04.8	90724
Viral hepatitis	V05.8	90731 (hepatitis B)
Diphtheria-tetanus-pertussis [DTP]	V06.1	90701
Diphtheria-tetanus-acellular pertussis	V06.8*	90700
Diphtheria-tetanus-pertussis (DTP) Haemophilus influenza type B (HiB)	V06.8*	90720
Measles-mumps-rubella [MMR]	V06.4	90707
Measles-mumps-rubella-varicella	V06.8*	90710
Diphtheria and tetanus [Td or DT]	V06.5	90702 (DT)
		90718 (Td)
Encephalitis vaccine	V05.0	90735
Pneumococcus	V03.82	90732
Meningococcus	V03.89	90733
Haemophilus influenza, type B [HiB]	V03.81	90737
Hepatitis A	V05.9*	90730
Prophylactic immunotherapy	V07.2	90741 (immune serum globulin)
		90742 (hyperimmune serum globulin)

[a]Physicians' current procedural terminology, fourth edition. Chicago: American Medical Association, 1994. CPT codes, descriptions, and two digit numeric modifiers only are copyright 1994 American Medical Association. All rights reserved.

*Nonspecific code

Table 25.5
ICD-9-CM and CPT Codes for Other Preventive Services

Procedure	ICD-9-CM Code	Title	CPT Code^a	Title
Examination and Testing:		Encounter for:		
Hemoglobin	V72.6*	Laboratory exam	85018	Hb, colorimetric
Hematocrit	V72.6*	Laboratory exam	85014	Hematocrit
Hearing	V72.1	Examination of ears and hearing	92551-92560	Audiology
Erythrocyte protoporphyrin	V72.6*	Laboratory exam	84202	RBC protoporphyrin, quantitative
			84203	RBC protoporphyrin, screen
Hemoglobin electrophoresis	V72.6*	Laboratory exam	83020	Hb electrophoresis
Thyroxine [T4]	V72.6*	Laboratory exam	84436	Thyroxine
Thyroid stimulating hormone [TSH]	V72.6*	Laboratory exam	84443	TSH
Phenylalanine	V72.6*	Laboratory exam	84030	Phenylalanine [PKU], blood
Blood pressure	V72.8*	Other specified exam	**	
Eye examination—amblyopia	V72.0*	Examination of eyes and vision	**	
Urinalysis—bacteriuria	V72.6*	Laboratory exam	81007	Bacteriuria screen
PPD	V72.6*	Laboratory exam	86580, 86585	Skin test, tuberculosis
Skin examination	V72.8*	Other specified exam	**	
Testicular examination	V72.8*	Other specified exam	**	
Rubella antibodies	V72.6*	Laboratory exam	**	
Serologic tests for syphilis	V72.6*	Laboratory exam	86781	FTA-Abs
Chlamydia testing	V72.6*	Laboratory exam	87110	Culture, chlamydia
Gonorrhea culture	V72.6*	Laboratory exam	**	
HIV testing	V72.6*	Laboratory exam	86311	HIV antigen test
			86701	HIV antibody detection
			86689	Confirmatory test
Papanicolaou smear	V72.3	Papanicolaou smear	88150-5	Cytopathology smears, cervical or vaginal
Oral cavity examination	V72.8*	Other specified exam	**	
Palpation for thyroid nodules	V72.8*	Other specified exam	**	
Clinical breast examination	V72.8*	Other specified exam	**	
Nonfasting total cholesterol	V72.6*	Laboratory exam	82465	Cholesterol, serum; total
Fasting plasma glucose	V72.6*	Laboratory exam	82947	Glucose, except urine
			82948	Glucose, blood, stick test

Table 25.5
ICD-9-CM and CPT Codes for Other Preventive Services (*continued*)

Procedure	ICD-9-CM Code	Title	CPT Code[a]	Title
Electrocardiogram	V72.8*	Other specified exam	93000	Routine ECG with at least 12 leads
Mammogram	V72.5*	Radiological exam, NEC	76092	Screening mammography, bilateral
Colonoscopy	V72.8*	Other specified exam	45378	Colonoscopy, fiberoptic
Auscultation-carotid bruits	V72.8*	Other specified exam	**	
Fecal occult blood	V72.6*	Laboratory exam	82270	Blood, occult, feces, screening
Bone mineral content	V72.5*	Radiological exam, NEC	78350	Bone density study
Functional status	V72.8*	Other specified exam	**	
Visual acuity	V72.0	Examination of eyes and vision	**	
Dipstick urinanalysis	V72.6*	Laboratory exam	81002	Urinalysis without microscopy
Sigmoidoscopy	V72.8*	Other specified exam	45330	Sigmoidoscopy, flexible fiberoptic, diagnostic
Glaucoma testing	V72.0*	Examination of eyes and vision	92120	Tonography with medical diagnostic evaluation
ABO typing	V72.6*	Laboratory exam	86900	Blood typing, ABO only
Rh typing	V72.6*	Laboratory exam	86901	Rho (D) only
Other antibody screens	V72.6*	Laboratory exam	86850	Antibody screen, RBC
HBsAg testing	V72.6*	Laboratory exam	86287	HBsAg, RIA or EIA
Counseling:				
Diet	V65.3	Dietary surveillance and counseling	See Table 1	

	Code	Description	
Exercise	V65.41	Exercise counseling	See Table 1
Substance use	V65.42	Counseling on substance use and abuse	See Table 1
Injury prevention	V65.43	Counseling on injury prevention	See Table 1
Dental health	V65.4*	Other specified counseling	See Table 1
Procreation	V26.4	General procreative counseling and advice	See Table 1
Contraception	V25.09	General contraceptive counseling and advice	See Table 1
HIV counseling	V65.44	HIV counseling	See Table 1
Sexually transmitted diseases	V65.45	Counseling on other STDs	See Table 1
Other:			
Passive smoking	V65.4*	Other counseling, NEC	See Table 1
Skin protection from UV light	V65.4*	Other counseling, NEC	See Table 1
Hemoglobin testing	V26.3*	Genetic counseling	See Table 1
Aspirin therapy	V65.4*	Other counseling, NEC	See Table 1
Estrogen replacement therapy	V65.4*	Other counseling, NEC	See Table 1
Genetic counseling	V26.3	Genetic counseling	See Table 1
Amniocentesis counseling	V65.4*	Other counseling, NEC	See Table 1

*Physicians' current procedural terminology, fourth edition. Chicago: American Medical Association, 1994. CPT codes, descriptions, and two digit numeric modifiers only are copyright 1994 American Medical Association. All rights reserved; U.S. Department of Health and Human Services. International classification of diseases, ninth revision, clinical modification, 5th edition, volumes 1 and 2 (CD-ROM format). Washington, DC: Government Printing Office, 1994. Legend: NEC; not elsewhere classified.

*Nonspecific code

**No code available

the World Health Organization's *International Classification of Diseases* (ICD-9). Volumes 1 and 2 of the ICD-9-CM are the Tabular List and Alphabetic Index for the diagnosis codes. The diagnosis codes are used by both physicians and hospitals to report and bill for various diagnostic entities pertaining to both inpatients and outpatients. Volume 3 contains a procedure classification (both a tabular list and alphabetic index) used for hospital reporting and billing of inpatient procedures. HCFA's Diagnosis Related Groups (DRGs), which determine reimbursement rates for hospitalized patients, are based on a combination of ICD-9-CM diagnosis and procedure codes. Because codes from Volume 3 of the ICD-9-CM are used only by hospitals and not by individual practitioners, they will not be discussed further in this chapter.

The ICD-9-CM diagnosis codes may be used to identify patients at higher risk for the development of chronic illnesses, patients in need of specific preventive services, and patients seen for specific procedures. The classification is divided into chapters that are based on organ systems, with separate chapters for infectious diseases, neoplasms, injuries and poisonings, and signs and symptoms. In addition, there are two "supplemental" classifications: external causes of injury ("E-codes") and factors influencing health status ("V-codes").

There are several groups of ICD-9-CM diagnosis codes of special relevance to practitioners of preventive medicine, most of which can be found in the V-code chapter. The V-codes are a supplementary classification of factors influencing health status and contact with health services. This chapter includes codes for contact with or exposure to communicable diseases (V01.0–V01.9), need for prophylactic vaccinations and inoculations (V03–V06—See Table 25.4), personal and family history of diseases and disorders (V10–V19), and "status" codes for postsurgical states (V42–V45). Also included in the chapter are encounters for "persons seeking consultation without complaints or sickness" (V65), "problems related to lifestyle" (V69), "persons without reported diagnosis encountered during examination and investigation of individuals and populations" (V70–V82), encounters for diagnostic testing (V72.0–V72.9), and a series of codes for "special screening" examinations (V73–V82). The use of these screening codes has historically been restricted to screening examinations of defined population groups (such as community testing for glaucoma or tuberculosis) and have not been assigned for screening of individuals. However, there is no prohibition against the use of these codes for screening of individual patients. Table 25.6 lists the screening codes for screening encounters recommended in the 1989 report of the U.S. Preventive Services Task Force. Physicians wishing to use these codes should be aware that they may not be acceptable to all payers. If this is the case, the applicable diagnosis code from Table 25.5 may be used instead.

Table 25.6
Screening Codes Available in ICD-9-CM

Screening Test	ICD-9-CM Code	Code Title (Special screening for . . .)
Hb & Hct	V78.0	iron deficiency anemia
	V78.1	other anemia
Erythro. protoporphyrin	V78.2	sickle-cell
	V78.3	other hemoglobinopathies
Hb electrophoresis	V78.2	sickle-cell
	V78.3	other hemoglobinopathies
T4/TSH	V77.0	thyroid disorders
Phenylalanine	V77.3	PKU
Blood pressure	V81.1	HTN
Eye exam—amblyopia	V80.2*	other eye conditions
Urinalysis—bacteriuria	V74.9	unspecified bacterial disease
PPD	V74.1	pulmonary TB
Testicular exam	V76.49*	malig. neoplasm other site
VDRL/RPR	V74.5*	bact. & spirochete venereal disease
Chlamydia testing	V73.8*	viral & chlamydial dis.
GC culture	V74.5*	bact. & spirochete venereal disease
HIV testing	V73.8*	viral & chlamydial dis.
PAP smear	V76.2	malign. neoplasm cervix
Oral cavity exam	V82.8*	other spec. cond.
Palpation thyroid-nodules	V77.0	thyroid disorders
Clinical breast exam	V76.1	malign. neoplasm breast
Fasting plasma glucose	V77.1	diabetes mellitus
ECG	V81.2*	other cardiovasc. cond.
Mammogram	V76.1	malign. neoplasm breast
Sigmoidoscopy	V76.49*	malign. neoplasm other sites
Colonoscopy	V76.49*	malign. neoplasm other sites
Auscultation-carotid bruits	V81.2*	other cardiovasc. cond.
Fecal occult blood	V82.8*	other spec. cond.
Bone mineral content	V82.8*	other spec. cond.
Dipstick urinalysis	V81.6*	other & unspec. GU cond.
Sigmoidoscopy	V76.49*	malign. neoplasm other sites
Glaucoma testing	V80.1	glaucoma

Adapted from U.S. Department of Health and Human Services. International classification of diseases, ninth revision, clinical modification, 5th edition, volumes 1 and 2 (CD-ROM format). Washington, DC: Government Printing Office, 1994.

*nonspecific code

In addition to the V-codes, there are many conditions coded to the individual organ system chapters of the ICD-9-CM that may identify patients at increased risk of developing chronic illness. For example, substance use and abuse are included in the mental disorders chapter (303–305); hypertension (401–405) is listed in the chapter on diseases of the circulatory system.

Codes in Chapter 16, "Symptoms, Signs, and Ill-Defined Conditions," for abnormal physical and laboratory findings (e.g., elevated blood pressure without diagnosis of hypertension, 796.2) are also useful to practition-

Table 25.7
ICD-9-CM Codes for "High Risk" Individuals

Risk Factor	Code	Title (if different)
Contact with or exposure to infectious and		
parasitic diseases:		
Tuberculosis	V01.1	
Syphilis	V01.6*	venereal diseases
Gonorrhea	V01.6*	venereal diseases
Hepatitis B	V01.7*	other viral diseases
HIV	V01.7*	other viral diseases
Need for isolation and other prophylactic measures:		
Postmenopausal hormone replacement therapy	V07.4	
Asymptomatic infections:		
Asymptomatic HIV infection	V08	
Personal history of:		
Colorectal cancer	V10.05	malignant neoplasm of large intestine
	V10.06	malignant neoplasm of rectum, rectosigmoid junction, & anus
Breast cancer	V10.3	
Endometrial cancer	V10.41	malignant neoplasm of cervix uteri
	V10.42	malignant neoplasm of other parts of uterus
Ovarian cancer	V10.43	
Skin cancer	V10.82	malignant melanoma of skin
	V10.83	other malignant neoplasm of skin
Tuberculosis	V12.01	
Malaria	V12.03	
Cryptoorchidism/Testicular atrophy	V13.2*	other genital system and obstetric disorders
Gestational diabetes	V13.2*	other genital system and obstetric disorders
Perinatal infections	V13.7*	perinatal problems
Congenital malformations	V13.6	
Irradiation	V15.3	
Family history of:		
Familial polyposis	V16.0*	malignant neoplasm of gastrointestinal tract
	V18.5*	other digestive disorders
Breast cancer	V16.3	
Skin cancer	V16.8	other specified malignant neoplasm

Condition	Code	Description
Coronary artery disease	V17.3	ischemic heart disease
	V17.4*	other cardiovascular diseases
Diabetes mellitus	V18.0	
Hearing loss	V19.2	deafness or hearing loss
Social circumstances:		
Homelessness	V60.0	lack of housing
Dilapidated housing	V60.1	inadequate housing
Person living alone	V60.3	
Person living in residential institution	V60.6	
Divorce/Separation	V61.0	family disruption
Unemployment	V62.0	
Imprisonment	V62.5*	legal circumstances
Bereavement	V62.82	
Substance abuse and mental disorders:		
Tobacco use	305.1x	tobacco use disorder
Alcohol use	303.9x	alcohol dependence syndrome
	305.0x	alcohol abuse
Drug use	304.xx	drug dependence
	305.xx	nondependent abuse of drugs
Depression	296.20–296.36	major depressive disorder
	296.50–296.66	bipolar affective disorder
	300.4	neurotic depression
	301.12	chronic depressive personality disorder
	311	depressive disorder, not elsewhere classified
Environmental exposures:		
Blood and blood products	E858.2*	accidental poisoning by agents primarily affecting blood constituents
	E875.0–E875.9*	contaminated or infected blood, other fluid, drug, or biological substance
	E934.7	natural blood and blood products causing adverse effects in therapeutic use
Sunlight	E926.2*	visible and ultraviolet light sources
Noise	E928.1	
Diseases and disorders:		
HIV Disease	042	
Hodgkin's disease	201.0–201.9	

Table 25.7
ICD-9-CM Codes for "High Risk" Individuals (*continued*)

Risk Factor	Code	Title (if different)
Multiple myeloma	203.0	
Inflammatory bowel disease/adenomatous polyps	211.3*	benign neoplasm of colon
Dysplastic nevi/congenital nevi	216.0–216.9*	benign neoplasm of skin
Suspicious oral lesions	210.0–210.9*	benign neoplasm of lip, oral cavity, and pharynx
Diabetes mellitus	250.00–250.91	
Hypercholesterolemia	272.0	
Obesity	278.0	
Hemoglobinopathies	282.0–282.9	hereditary hemolytic anemias
Immunosuppression	279.0–279.3	disorders involving the immune mechanism
Hypertension	401–405	hypertensive diseases
Coronary atherosclerosis	414.0	
Atrial fibrillation	427.31	
Transient ischemic attack	435.0–435.9	transient cerebral ischemia
Chronic obstructive pulmonary diseases	490–496	chronic obstructive pulmonary diseases and allied conditions
Cirrhosis	571.2, 571.5	
Chronic renal disease	581–582, 585–587	
History of fetal death/growth retardation	646.3*	habitual aborter
Drug abuse during pregnancy	648.3	drug dependence
Failure to gain weight during pregnancy	646.8*	other specified complications of pregnancy

From U.S. Department of Health and Human Services. International classification of diseases, ninth revision, clinical modification, 5th edition, volumes 1 and 2 (CD-ROM format). Washington, DC: Government Printing Office, 1994.

*Nonspecific code

ers of preventive medicine. Finally, codes in the supplementary classification of external causes of injury and poisoning (E-code) chapter can be used to identify the external causes of current injuries or poisonings (motor vehicle collisions [E800–E848], accidental lead ingestion [E866.0]), or the late effects of external causes (motor vehicle collisions [E929.0], accidental lead poisoning [E929.2]). The E-codes have not received wide use in the past, but they are now being required for inpatient reporting by several state governments. Use of the E-codes in outpatient settings has been minimal.

Table 25.7 lists a variety of ICD-9-CM diagnosis codes that are available to identify "high risk" individuals as defined by the "HR" groups in the 1989 recommendations of the U.S. Preventive Services Task Force. Table 25.5 contains a list of other ICD-9-CM diagnosis codes for care encounters involving delivery of preventive services. It should be noted that these "encounter for" V-codes should only be used when the patient has no other diagnosis to explain his or her health care encounter.

The ICD-9-CM is updated annually. The Coordination and Maintenance Committee on ICD-9-CM is composed of representatives of HCFA and the National Center for Health Statistics (NCHS). This committee holds public meetings three times a year in which proposed modifications to the classification are discussed. Requests for modifications to Volumes 1 and 2 of the ICD-9-CM should be addressed to the National Center for Health Statistics, which has lead responsibility for the diagnosis classification.

FUTURE DEVELOPMENTS

As the American health care delivery system undergoes change, access to, delivery of, and appropriate reimbursement for effective clinical preventive services should be a fundamental tenet of every "basic benefit package" or reform proposal. The distinction between "preventive," "diagnostic," and "therapeutic" medical services and their differential treatment by payers may become less important as capitated or global health care budget mechanisms replace the traditional fee-for-service model. Improved reimbursement for preventive services should be facilitated by a number of developments set in motion by the important work of such groups as the U.S. Preventive Services Task Force. Innovative strategies to pay for these services should provide the appropriate patient, provider, and payer incentives to promote their use. Increased awareness of their clinical effectiveness should lead to increased demand for their coverage. Continued research on the cost and cost-effectiveness of preventive services relative to other medical services, facilitated by updated diagnostic and procedural codes, should provide a sound data base to design more appropriate reimbursement policies in the future.

SUGGESTED READINGS

Coding clinic for ICD-9-CM. Chicago: American Hospital Association, 1984–1995.

Burchard LL, Jabour M, Michels DE. Tips on getting paid for counseling. Patient Care 1993;27:120–123.

U.S. Department of Health and Human Services. ICD-9-CM official guidelines for coding and reporting. Washington, DC: Government Printing Office, 1991.

REFERENCES

1. U.S. Department of Health and Human Services. Healthy people 2000: National health promotion and disease prevention objectives. (PHS) 91-50212. Washington, DC: Government Printing Office, 1991.
2. Iglehart JK. The American health care system—introduction. N Engl J Med 1992;326:962–967.
3. Davis K, Bialek R, Parkinson M, Smith J, Vellozzi C. Paying for preventive care: moving the debate forward. Am J Prev Med 1990;6(4 suppl.):7–32.
4. Employer-sponsored health insurance in private sector firms in 1992. Washington, DC: Health Insurance Association of America, 1993.
5. GHAA's annual HMO industry survey. Washington, DC: Group Health Association of America, 1992.
6. U.S. Congress, Office of Technology Assessment. Preventive health services for Medicare beneficiaries: policy and research issues (OTA-H-416). Washington, DC: Government Printing Office, 1990.
7. Preventive services in the clinical setting: what works and what it costs. Special report to the National Coordinating Committee on Clinical Preventive Services. Washington, DC: U.S. Public Health Service, Office of Disease Prevention and Health Promotion, 1993.
8. Physicians' current procedural terminology, fourth edition. Chicago: American Medical Association, 1994.
9. U.S. Department of Health and Human Services. International classification of diseases, ninth revision, clinical modification, 5th edition, volumes 1 and 2 (CD-ROM format). Washington, DC: Government Printing Office, 1994.

26. Computer-Assisted Decision Making and Reminder Systems

PAUL S. FRAME

INTRODUCTION

Most health professionals have computer capability in their offices, but the majority use computers only for billing (1). The use of computers for clinical applications, including preventive medicine, is a newly developing field that has seen much research effort but is still evolving into readily available commercial products. Three types of computer applications, health risk appraisal, development of risk-related health maintenance protocols, and health maintenance tracking, are relevant to clinical preventive medicine in the primary care office setting. All of these computer applications have the ability to rapidly sort through large amounts of data and make decisions based on simple or complex algorithms. The weak link in most applications has been the effort, cost, and reliability of data entry (2). A related problem is the need for standard formats and terminology to allow the easy exchange of clinical information between independent computers (3). Significant progress is being made toward overcoming these problems.

HEALTH RISK APPRAISAL

Health risk appraisal tools are the most established preventive computer application. Manual, paper-based health risk appraisal systems have been available since the early 1970s. They are used in many settings, including worksite wellness programs, the assessment of occupational risk, at "health fairs" and other nonmedical settings, as well as by clinicians. See Chapters 1 and 2 for further background on health risk appraisals.

All health risk appraisals involve obtaining a data base of information about a particular patient and using that information to calculate a risk score for the conditions in question. In the example of computerized health risk appraisal, data can be obtained by an interviewer, the patient can fill out a questionnaire, or the patient can enter data directly into the computer.

The health risk appraisal developed by the Carter Center for the U.S. Centers for Disease Control and Prevention (4) is a typical example. The patient completes a four-page, 45-item questionnaire about medical status, including cholesterol level, social status, family history, and lifestyle. This information is then entered into the computer, which applies a multivariate statistical analysis based on a preestablished protocol and determines the patient's relative risk for the 12 leading causes of death. The printout of this information can be used by the clinician or patient to change behaviors, modify risk factors, or initiate treatment.

The computer-generated printout provides specific quantitative information about the patient's risk and is often felt to be more authoritative than a simple verbal statement of risk by the provider. The presentation of risk data may be useful for motivating patients to adopt healthier lifestyles and may alert the provider to risks that were overlooked. Providers should remember, however, that the results generated are valid only if the data entered is complete and accurate and if the algorithms used to calculate risk are valid. As discussed in Chapter 1, questions have been raised about the validity and reliability of health risk appraisal instruments (5). Given these limitations, the relative risks derived from health risk appraisals should be considered estimates rather than precise values.

DEVELOPMENT OF RISK-RELATED HEALTH MAINTENANCE PROTOCOLS

Several computer programs have been created to help clinicians determine which preventive procedures are indicated for a particular patient based on risk status, age, and gender (6, 7). These programs are similar to health risk appraisals in that it is necessary to enter a data base of information about each patient into the computer. The computer then processes that information according to a protocol of risk-related recommendations such as those of the U.S. Preventive Services Task Force (USPSTF) and generates a list of recommended preventive interventions along with a risk profile.

The first edition of the *Guide to Clinical Preventive Services* (8) made approximately 80 health care recommendations for adults that depended on over 100 risk factors or patient conditions. Many of these recommendations apply only to specific high-risk groups. Clearly, it is difficult or impossible for clinicians to remember all the combinations of recommendations and risk factors. The same task is easy for a computer, however, if the appropriate data have been entered. One study (7) found that the average patient had 15.4 risk factors, which generated 24.5 recommendations for preventive services based on the USPSTF guidelines.

Data for health maintenance recommendations can be entered directly by patients or can be obtained by interviews as is done with health risk appraisals. If patients are to answer questions themselves or enter data,

MD Suggestions Report

```
27 year old    Afro-American    Female        ID # 19284    JAN 08, 1993


PATIENT NAME:    _____
```

PART B: SUGGESTIONS

PHYSICAL EXAMINATIONS	Freq	Pri	Note
Cardiac auscultation	once	N	8
Skin examination for early cancer	q1-3y	N	67
Thyroid palpation for masses	q1-3y	N	69

SCREENING TESTS	Freq	Pri	Note
Glucose, random blood	q1-3y	N	29
Mantoux test (PPD) for TB exposure	once	N	75

PROPHYLAXIS/IMMUNIZATIONS	Ready	Pri	Note
Hepatitis B Immunization	L	N	76
Tetanus toxoid booster	L	N	83

COUNSELLING AND REFERRAL	Ready	Pri	Note
Advice about dietary calcium	H	N	18
Advice about dietary fat, fiber, cholesterol, sodium	H	N	19
Exercise counseling for prevention of CAD	L	N	23
Exercise counseling; special considerations	L	N	24
Review of medication use and compliance	N	N	32
Regular tooth brushing, flossing, dental visits	N	N	46
Advise skin protection, teach self-examination	N	N	70
Counsel about dangers of hand weapons\violent behavior	N	H	86

HEALTHQUIZ SUPPORT MODULES			Note
Occupational Health Assessment			31
Dietary Habits Assessment			33

** Please see annotations to Part C

Figure 26.1. Health Quiz II physician suggestion report. Recommendations are based on the patient's risk factors using the U.S. Preventive Services Task Force guidelines from 1989. *Legend: Pri,* priority of the intervention (*H,* high; *N,* routine); *Ready,* patient's willingness to accept an intervention (*H,* interested; *N,* neutral; *L,* possible barrier); *Note,* references for the intervention. (Reproduced with permission of the Anesthesia and Critical Care Research Foundation.)

it is vital that the questions be written so that they are easily understood by the patient and an unambiguous answer can be given. The computer tells the provider what preventive procedures are indicated based on the patient's risk profile. Figure 26.1 shows a sample physician suggestion report from the Health Quiz II system (9), indicating the procedures and interventions that should be considered based on the patient's risk status. The format also includes an indication of the priority of the intervention and the patient's receptiveness to the intervention.

COMPUTERIZED HEALTH MAINTENANCE TRACKING

Health maintenance tracking refers to a system for determining over time what health maintenance interventions a given patient has received and what procedures are currently indicated. Tracking systems can be manual (information is recorded and retrieved from a paper-based system, such as the flow sheets described in Chapter 22) or computerized. Tracking typically includes prompting mechanisms for providers and sometimes for patients. Table 26.1 shows the relative advantages and disadvantages of manual versus computerized systems.

A manual, flow sheet-based health maintenance tracking system has several advantages: It is powerful when used in conjunction with the rest of the patient's chart (e.g., problem list, data base, progress notes). All of these chart contents are readily available, in one place, when the clinician sees the patient. The manual flow sheet is flexible and easy to individualize to a particular patient. The clinician can write notes or comments on the flow sheet and can use extra lines for procedures unique to that patient. Codes for abnormal tests, tests done elsewhere, and tests refused or not in-

Table 26.1
Comparison of Manual and Computerized Health Maintenance Tracking

	Strengths	Weaknesses
Manual Flowsheet	Powerful when used with the problem list data base and progress notes. Flexible, easy to individualize. Inexpensive and technically simple.	Dependent on provider motivation. Recall of patients is difficult. Difficult to change global protocol. Quality assurance requires chart audit.
Computerized Tracking	Less dependent on provider motivation. Easily generates reminders to providers and patients. Global criteria changes are easy. Forces the practice to institutionalize prevention.	Significant cost to operate and maintain. More rigid data-entry requirements. Difficult to individualize for particular clinicians.

dicated can easily be included (see Chapter 22). The manual system is inexpensive and technically simple. Major disadvantages of a manual health maintenance tracking system are that it is dependent on provider motivation and does not easily include a specific recall system for patients who do not have regular office visits.

Computerized health maintenance tracking systems do the same job as manual flow sheet-based tracking systems (10). To be preferred over manual systems, computerized systems must do a better job at an acceptable cost. Several systems have been previously described (11–16). Some are "stand-alone" systems that require separate demographic as well as health maintenance data entry (12, 15), some are part of comprehensive electronic medical record systems (14), and some are designed to be linked to existing billing or demographic data systems (12, 13). In a computerized system, whether freestanding, linked to a billing system, or part of a computerized patient record, data are entered into the computer either directly or by clerical personnel. The computer processes the data according to a predetermined algorithm or protocol and creates a provider and (ideally) a patient reminder of what procedures have already been done and what procedures are indicated. Most systems can also create detailed summary reports for quality assurance and monitoring.

Computerized tracking systems can be powerful, but only if the appropriate data are entered into the system. This data entry can be time-consuming; unless the medical record is totally computerized, it may duplicate information entry into the manual chart. A computerized system is relatively rigid and difficult to individualize to a particular patient or provider. Computerized systems are more expensive and technically more complex than manual systems.

There are major advantages of a computerized tracking system: It is less dependent on provider motivation. Reminders can be generated to recall patients if the provider fails to offer a needed health maintenance intervention or fails to suggest a specific recall date. Initial as well as repeat reminders can be sent to inactive patients, provided their names and demographic data have been entered into the computer system. These reminders can be sent repeatedly regardless of provider or patient compliance.

For a computerized health maintenance tracking system to be an effective, cost-efficient tool for the primary care clinician, it must do more than create a health maintenance status report at the time of acute patient visits. A number of additional features are desirable: (a) Patient demographic data should be obtainable from the same files used for billing and administrative purposes. Duplicate demographic data entry for health maintenance is unacceptably costly. (b) Data entry for all health maintenance procedures done on a given visit should be rapid and, preferably,

HEALTH MAINTENANCE PROCEDURES (N/C)

CODES:

D = DONE	X = ABN.	N = N/I
R = REFUSED	I = INACTIVE	E = DONE ELSEWHERE

REMINDER OVERRIDE (IF OTHER THAN BIRTH MONTH):

CANCEL ☐   START ☐   CHANGE MONTH: _____ *07*

CHG. CODE	SERVICE & FREQUENCY		CODE + DATE DONE MM/YY	ALTERNATE FREQUENCY
1458	HX TOBACCO USE	ONCE	*D 5-88*	
1454	BLOOD PRESSURE	Q2YR	*X*	
1456	WEIGHT	Q4YR	*D*	
1457	SERUM CHOLEST.	Q4YR	*E 6-90*	
1450	GUAIAC	Q2YR 40-50 Q1YR 50+	*R*	
1449	DT (ADULT)	Q10YR	*D 3-82*	
1451	TEACH SELF EXAM	Q4YR	*D*	
1460	PAP SMEAR	Q2YR	*N*	
1461	BREAST EXAM	Q2YR <50 Q1YR >50	*D*	
1462	MAMMOGRAM	Q1YR>50	*D*	*Q2YR*
1463	EVAL OSTEOPOROSIS	45-55	*D*	
1464	REP. POST MENOPAUSAL BLD.	>45y	*N*	
1448	SIGMOIDOSCOPY	0		
1447	FLU VACCINATION	0		
1445	RECTAL EXAM	0		

Figure 26.2. Health maintenance portion of the Tri-County Family Medicine encounter form showing health maintenance data entry. The "alternate frequency" feature allows changing the frequency of a procedure, or cancelling the procedure for a particular patient. Procedures with a "0" frequency (e.g., sigmoidoscopy) are not part of the routine practice protocol, but prompting can be initiated for individual patients by using the alternate frequency feature. The "cancel/start" feature allows cancelling the mailing of direct patient reminders for that patient.

carried out on a single screen. (c) Multiple-entry options for each procedure should be available to encompass the range of provider and patient decision scenarios, including procedure not indicated, patient refused, procedure done elsewhere, procedure done, and procedure not done. (d) The system should be able to generate patient reminders for designated persons, regardless of whether they have been seen recently by the practice. (e) The system should allow providers to specify or cancel the distribution of patient reminders. The provider should be able to specify the month in which reminders should be sent or defer to a default month for sending reminders. A logical default month is the month of the patient's birth. (f) A status report for the chart should be updated periodically and include notations of which procedures are due at that time. (g) The global health maintenance protocol should be modifiable without the assistance of a computer programmer. A detailed list of recommended features that clinicians should consider before purchasing or developing a computerized health maintenance tracking system was developed recently by the American Cancer Society Advisory Group on Preventive Health Care Reminder Systems (17).

The HTRAK system was developed by Tri-County Family Medicine (Cohocton, NY) to include these features and has been shown to achieve superior health maintenance compliance when compared to a flow sheet system (12, 18). Providers enter health maintenance data on the encounter form along with billing and diagnostic data. The health maintenance portion of this form is shown in Figure 26.2. Data entry personnel enter these data into the billing computer at the same time as billing and diagnostic data are entered.

Once a month, demographic and health maintenance data from the practice's billing system are downloaded into a personal computer containing the HTRAK software. A health maintenance status report is created for both the patient and clinician once a year, in the month of the patient's birth (unless an alternate month has been designated), regardless of the patient's appointment status. The provider status report, shown in Figure 26.3, is placed on the front of the patient's chart. It clearly shows the clinician when procedures were done and which procedures are overdue. The patient reminder, Figure 26.4, is designed to be placed in a window envelope for direct mailing to the patient. Patients are encouraged to make an appointment for overdue health maintenance procedures and to show the patient reminder to the clinician at each visit.

A compromise system combining elements of manual and computerized tracking can be created by continuing to use a manual flow sheet tracking system, as described in Chapter 22, but in addition programming the practice billing computer to send a general health maintenance re-

HEALTH MAINTENANCE STATUS PHYSICIAN REMINDER

Office: Dansville   Reminder Status: MB   Geoffrey Wittig, MD

Date of Birth: Guarantor:
December 15, 1992   Sex: F
                                       Age: 64

HM Procedure	Prev Done	Code	Last Done	Code	Over Due	Next Due	Done in Interim
History of Tobacco Use	-		03/91	D			__ __/__
Blood Pressure	08/90	D	03/91	D		03/93	__ __/__
Serum Cholesterol	-		11/90	X		11/94	__ __/__
Fecal Occult Blood Test for Colon C	-		03/91	D	YES	*NOW*	__ __/__
Weight	-		03/91	D		03/95	__ __/__
Tetanus-Diphtheria Immunization	-		-		YES	*NOW*	__ __/__
Teach Self Examination for Lumps	-		01/90			01/94	__ __/__
Pap Smear	-		03/91	N		03/93	__ __/__
Physician Breast Exam	-		01/90	D	YES	*NOW*	__ __/__
Mammogram	-		01/89	D	YES	*NOW*	__ __/__
Reporting Post-Menopausal Bleeding	-		-		YES	*NOW*	__ __/__

Figure 26.3. HTRAK provider health maintenance status report. This report is produced once a year and is placed on the front of the patient's chart. *Legend: D*, done and normal; *X*, done but abnormal; *N*, not indicated for this patient; *R*, offered but the patient refused; *E*, done elsewhere.

minder to all patients who have not had an office visit within a predetermined period of time (probably 1 or 2 years). Use of such a system has not been reported in the literature but, in theory, combines the advantages of computer outreach to inactive patients with the low cost and simple technology of the manual flow sheet.

Clinicians are naturally concerned about the costs of establishing and maintaining a computerized health maintenance tracking system. Computerized systems are more expensive to establish and maintain than manual systems. It may be worth the investment, however, if that cost results in better patient care and reduced malpractice risk. Costs can be divided into start-up costs (hardware, software, training of clinicians and staff, and perhaps programming to link the health maintenance and billing systems) and operating costs (data entry, creation of clinician and patient reminders, system maintenance, and troubleshooting). In general, stand-alone systems will have lower start-up costs but will have higher operating costs, especially for data entry, compared to systems linked to the practice billing system.

The HTRAK system developed at Tri-County Family Medicine uses an IBM-486 computer with a 320-megabyte hard drive linked to the practice billing system. About 100 hours of programming were required to link the two systems. Annual operating costs, including data entry, supplies, creation of clinician and patient reminders, mailing patient reminders, postage, and follow-up clinician and patient reminders, were 78 cents per

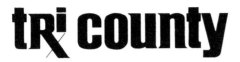

**Tri-County Family
Medicine Program**

Administration/Business/Research Office
P.O. Box 601
Dansville, NY 14437
Administration: (716) 335-3416
Billing: (716) 335-3100
Research: (716) 335-7355

HEALTH MAINTENANCE STATUS REPORT

```
                                        DOB:
                                        Age: 71  Sex: M
                                        Last Visit: 11/18/91


Head of Household:                Phone:
Office: Dansville                 Reminder Status: MB


Dear                              01/93
```

Preventing illness and keeping our patients as healthy as possible is an important part of family medicine.
Our records indicate you had the following health maintenance procedures done on the dates indicated:

```
    History of Tobacco Use                  05/91
    Blood Pressure                          05/91
    Fecal Occult Blood Test for Colon Cancer 05/91
    Weight                                  05/91
    Tetanus-Diphtheria Immunization         05/91
    Teach Self Examination for Lumps        05/91
```

You are overdue for the following health maintenance procedures:

Fecal Occult Blood Test for Colon Cancer

If you do not already have an appointment in the next 2 months, please call the Dansville office at (716) 335-6041 to schedule a health maintenance checkup. Show this letter to your physician at your next appointment.

22 Red Jacket St. Box 339	Park Avenue	61 State Street	North Church Street	East Naples Street
Dansville, NY 14437	Cohocton, NY 14826	Nunda, NY 14517	Canaseraga, NY 14822	Wayland, NY 14572
(716) 335-6041	(716) 384-5310	(716) 468-2528	(607) 545-8333	(716) 728-5131

Figure 26.4. HTRAK patient health maintenance reminder. Reminder fits in a window envelope and is mailed to all patients yearly, regardless of appointment status, unless health maintenance is up-to-date or patient reminders have been canceled. Reminder is sent in the month of the patient's birth unless another month has been specified.

patient in 1992. Two-thirds of this cost related to creating, mailing, and troubleshooting patient reminders (18). Other systems will have widely differing costs depending on the circumstances in which they are used.

In an ideal situation, patients' risk profile data would already be stored in an electronic medical record that could generate health risk appraisals on request, would individualize each patient's health maintenance protocol according to risk profile and concurrent diagnoses, and would track health maintenance, providing prompts for both patients and clinicians on a regular basis. The individual components of such a system are available, as well as the necessary supporting technology; however, the ideal, totally integrated system has yet to be developed.

RESOURCES

Anesthesia and Critical Care Research Foundation
5622 Woodlawn Avenue
Chicago, IL 60637
312-702-2132
    Information about Health Quiz II software.

The Healthier People Network, Inc.
1549 N. Clairmont Road, Suite 205
Decatur, GA 30033
404-636-3127
    Healthier People Network Health Risk Appraisal software.

COSTAR Users Group
348 Rancheros Drive
San Marcos, CA 92069
    Information about COSTAR "Computer Stored Ambulatory Record."

Don Fordham
University of California, San Francisco
Division of General Internal Medicine
400 Parnassus Avenue
San Francisco, CA
415-476-0557
    Information about Check-Up computerized health maintenance tracking system.

Paul S. Frame, MD
Tri-County Family Medicine
Box 112
Cohocton, NY 14826
716-384-5310
    Information about HTRAK health maintenance tracking system.

Jim Medder, MD
Department of Family Practice
University of Nebraska Medical Center
600 South 42nd Street
Omaha, NE 68198
    Information about Health Screen risk-related health maintenance protocols.

Physician Micro Systems, Inc.
2033 Sixth Avenue, Suite 707
Seattle, WA 98121
 Information about Practice Partner.

REFERENCES

 1. Melville SK, Luckman R, Coghlin J, Gann P. Office systems for promoting screening mammography: a survey of primary care practices. J Fam Pract 1993;37:569–574.
 2. Dambro MR, Weiss BD, McClure CL, Vuturo AF. An unsuccessful experience with computerized medical records in an academic medical center. J Med Education 1988;63:617–623.
 3. McDonald CJ, Tierney WM. Computer-stored medical records: their future role in medical practice. JAMA 1988;259:3433–3440.
 4. Health risk appraisal program. Decatur, GA: Carter Center of Emory University, 1987.
 5. Smith KW, McKinlay SM, McKinlay JB. The reliability of health risk appraisals: a field trial of four instruments. Am J Public Health 1989;79:1603–1607.
 6. Hayward RSA, Ford DE, Steinberg EP, Roizen MF. Prevention practice project: information tools for the clinician. Toronto 1991, COACH Conference XVI Proceedings, pp. 79–84.
 7. Medder JD, Kahn NB, Susman JL. Risk factors and recommendations for 230 adult primary care patients, based on U.S. Preventive Services Task Force guidelines. Am J Prev Med 1992;8:150–153.
 8. U.S. Preventive Services Task Force. Guide to clinical preventive services. Baltimore: Williams & Wilkins, 1989.
 9. Health Quiz II Preventive Health Program. Chicago: Anesthesia and Critical Care Research Foundation, 1992.
 10. Frame PS. Health maintenance in clinical practice: strategies and barriers. Am Fam Physician 1991;45:1192–1200.
 11. Frame PS. Can computerized reminder systems have an impact on preventive services in practice? J Gen Intern Med 1990;5(suppl):S112–S115.
 12. Frame PS, Zimmer JG, Werth PL, Martens WB. Description of a computerized health maintenance tracking system for primary care practice. Am J Prev Med 1991;7:311–318.
 13. Harris RP, O'Malley MS, Fletcher SW, Knight BP. Prompting physicians for preventive procedures: a five-year study of manual and computer reminders. Am J Prev Med 1990;6:145–152.
 14. Ornstein SM, Garr DR, Jenkins RG, et al. Computer-generated physician and patient reminders; tools to improve population adherence to selected preventive services. J Fam Pract 1991;32:82–90.
 15. McPhee SJ, Bird JA, Fordham D, Rodnick JE, Osborn EH. Promoting cancer prevention activities by primary care physicians: results of a randomized, controlled trial. JAMA 1991;266:538–544.
 16. Orenstein SM, Garr DR, Jenkins RG. A comprehensive microcomputer-based medical records system with sophisticated preventive services features for the family physician. J Am Board Fam Pract 1993;6:55–60.
 17. American Cancer Society. Advisory Group on Preventive Health Care Reminder Systems. Computerized health maintenance tracking systems: a clinician's guide to necessary and optional features. J Am Board Fam Pract 1995;8:221–229.
 18. Frame PS, Zimmer JG, Werth PL. Controlled trial of a health maintenance tracking system. Arch Fam Med 1994;3:581–588.

27. Ethical Issues in Health Promotion and Disease Prevention

JOHN M. LAST and STEVEN H. WOOLF

INTRODUCTION

Ethics is the philosophical discipline concerned with moral values, with distinctions between what we consider to be right and wrong, with our duties and obligations to others and society at large, and with our fundamental values and beliefs. There is a close relationship between law and ethics, both being founded in moral values; the law tells us what we can (and cannot) do; ethics tells us what we *ought* to do. Concern about ethics has grown in all walks of life in recent decades, perhaps because a combination of declining religious convictions and rising personal expectations in an increasingly complex society have left many people with the need for a stronger moral compass. Moreover, the increasing complexity of society has itself contributed to entirely new ethical and moral problems.

PRINCIPLES OF BIOMEDICAL ETHICS

The branch of ethics that deals with medical problems is called biomedical ethics, and within it, several basic principles are commonly identified. They include respect for persons, beneficence, justice, integrity, loyalty, and truth-telling (Table 27.1). Ideally, we strive to uphold all the principles of biomedical ethics, but sometimes situations arise in which recognition of and response to one ethical principle requires violation of another. We cannot always do good for one person without harming others. We then face the moral and ethical problems that make biomedical ethics so challenging. Ethical issues in health promotion and disease prevention often involve conflicts between the needs of individual patients and those of society. To fully appreciate these conflicts, it is useful to consider the competing agendas of the different interest groups concerned with health promotion and disease prevention.

GROUPS INTERESTED IN HEALTH PROMOTION AND DISEASE PREVENTION

Healthy people often take their own health for granted; or if they care, their concern is confined to circumscribed aspects such as treatment of inciden-

Table 27.1
Basic Principles of Biomedical Ethics

Respect for persons	Embodies two concepts: (a) autonomy, recognition of free will and human rights, dignity, freedom; and (b) special care for persons with diminished autonomy, such as infants and children, the mentally ill, prison inmates, members of armed forces, etc., who are not completely in control of their own lives.
Beneficence	The principle of doing good. Sometimes a separate principle of nonmaleficence, not harming, is identified. This recognizes the ancient medical maxim, *primum non nocere,* first do no harm, which from antiquity to near our own time was often all that physicians could hope to accomplish.
Justice	The principle of equity that regards all persons as equal in rights, dignity, and freedoms, not discriminating in favor of some at the expense or to the detriment of others. This principle becomes particularly important when resources are limited and choices have to be made about allocation: for instance, between using tax dollars to immunize senior citizens against influenza or to provide long-term care facilities for the elderly infirm.
Integrity	Applies to both health workers and their clients or patients. Integrity of health workers can be equated with honesty and is an issue in medical research if allegations of fraud or misrepresentation arise. Integrity has a different meaning when the term is applied to patients and others who use health services. In this context it means recognition that even persons who are not autonomous, such as children and prison inmates, have human rights that must be respected.
Loyalty	Commitment to the needs of those for whom we are caring.
Truth-telling	Honesty; not lying to or deliberately misleading or deceiving people whose health we are endeavoring to protect.

tal symptoms and complaints, and not to measures that might be used to avoid future illness. Healthy people sometimes resent suggestions about ways to promote their good health, regarding these as gratuitous or needlessly intrusive on their autonomy.

Patients, especially if they have long-term disabling disorders, often become concerned about how to promote their return to good health, and about how to prevent their disease or disability from returning. They may also have an interest in how to prevent other people from experiencing the discomfort and distress that they have endured.

Family members and friends of people with distressing diseases (e.g., lung cancer, motor vehicle injuries) sometimes become eloquent advocates for measures that will reduce the risk of others experiencing similar conditions. Many health promotion and disease prevention *advocacy groups* (e.g., non-smokers' rights associations, Mothers Against Drunk Driving) have been born out of this concern. The aims and the political and social agendas of advocacy groups vary greatly. Many are serious participants in the quest for improved health, usually by raising money to support research, sometimes by actively seeking to prevent the disease in question. A few engage in activities that are on the fringes of conventional medical science, and one or two are frankly disreputable.

Physicians and other health professionals care about health promotion and disease prevention. Specialties with a long tradition of assigning a prominent place to health promotion and disease prevention include pediatrics and obstetrics; family medicine joined them at least thirty years ago, and since then an increasing interest in prevention of premature death and disability has penetrated virtually all branches of clinical medical and surgical practice.

Health insurance carriers and managed care plans, concerned about the inexorably rising costs of medical care, have an interest in health promotion and disease prevention. Nevertheless, interventions aimed at promoting health and preventing disease are poorly (or not at all) rewarded with reimbursement under the terms and conditions of many health insurance plans. This is as true in nations that have comprehensive tax-supported health insurance programs as it is in the United States, with its patchwork quilt of private insurance carriers, health maintenance organizations, and other payers. Some of these lapses in coverage relate to payers' concerns about the cost-effectiveness of health promotion and disease prevention programs.

Employers and stockholders in corporations have an interest in health promotion and disease prevention. A healthy work force with low rates of absenteeism due to illness is more productive, and profits are greater, than if large disbursements to cover costs of sick leave have to be deducted before profits and dividends are declared.

Labor unions have a long history of activist interventions aimed at ameliorating unhealthy and dangerous workplace conditions in mines, agriculture, and factories, and some of this has extended to health promotion initiatives such as exercise breaks for sedentary workers and smoking cessation campaigns.

Finally, *governments,* perhaps to a lesser extent in the United States than in most other industrialized nations, have great interest in health promotion and disease prevention. Government interest goes back at least to Bismarck, perhaps as far as the ancient Greeks and Romans, who desired a healthy populace that could defend the homeland and attack its enemies. In many nations, the government is the largest stakeholder in health promotion, which arouses some unease among those who disapprove of governmental social engineering. As a major funding source for health promotion programs, governments often share the same concerns as other payers about the cost-effectiveness of preventive services.

Differing Aims and Agendas

Consider the differing aims and agendas of these interest groups in the dialogue about health promotion and disease prevention. Governments, employers, and stockholders in corporations want workers to be healthy but do not want to spend vast sums of money to achieve this aim. Medical insurance carriers recognize that premiums could be reduced and profits maximized if there were fewer claims for reimbursement of medical and hospital expenses. Insurance carriers therefore might be expected to have greater interest in financially supporting health promotion than appears to be the case. Reimbursement is often inadequate; some health insurance plans barely recognize this activity at all, although this is changing with some managed care programs. Health professionals such as physicians understandably want recognition and adequate financial compensation for the demanding tasks of counseling individuals to achieve better health. Many individuals want good health but are not prepared to make sacrifices, monetary or otherwise (such as giving up pleasurable or profitable habits that are harmful to health). Is it surprising that the dissonance among these interest groups generates some ethical problems?

ETHICAL PROBLEMS IN SOCIAL POLICY

Social policy around health promotion and disease prevention often raises important ethical issues. Because this chapter focuses on issues directly affecting practitioners, social policy problems will be mentioned only briefly, but they have enormous implications for the delivery of preventive medicine. For example, implicit in the concept of health promotion is empowerment, and the notion that people and their medical advisers can form a partnership aimed at promoting better health and preventing illness, disability, and premature death. For this partnership to be successful, financial support is required; the extent to which this actually happens is nowhere adequate. Neither governments nor private insurance carriers have recognized or honored their obligation to provide sufficient financial support to implement the methods and procedures of health promotion and disease prevention in which they claim to believe (1). Some health promotion policies are clearly opposed for financial reasons. For example, certain health protection measures may conflict with the economic interests of business (e.g., the food industry).

In some cases, health promotion policies are opposed because of political or moral concerns. The decision to have or refrain from having a child is private and very personal. However, when a family planning program is paid for by public funds, political leaders of the party in power may seek to impose their ideology on participants in the program, providers and clients alike. Many societies have entrenched or enshrined values and moral standards relating to aspects of human reproduction; the problems that arise were complex and difficult enough already, and they became more troublesome with the advent of new reproductive technologies. The ethical issues are too complex for brief discussion and so are not considered here.

In other instances, social implementation of health promotion programs can have unintended adverse effects. For example, epidemiologists and public health specialists have identified many "unhealthy" industries and communities in which an occupational or environmental health problem is attributable to a dangerous source of pollution in a local industry. In the Eastern Townships of Quebec, where asbestos fibers from local mining and processing were causing both human and animal illness, public health workers and epidemiologists argued that the plants should be closed. The workers and the residents of the townships, however, resisted this, recognizing that it would cause unemployment and economic hardship to the entire community. Similarly, if antismoking campaigns are pursued to their logical conclusion and all Americans refrain from using tobacco, a huge and lucrative industry that is the economic mainstay of several states would be wiped out. What health effects will emerge from the resulting unemployment and lack of access to health care?

ETHICAL PROBLEMS IN CLINICAL PRACTICE

The raison d'être for an ethical approach to medical practice is to avoid doing harm or causing wrong to people. What could be harmful or wrong about such a worthwhile goal as promoting good health and preventing disease, disability, and premature death? Ethical problems can arise because of differences in the aims and agendas of interest groups, because health professionals may fail to take account of the feelings of individuals, and because of dissonance between official policies and the aspirations of individuals and those who are caring for them. The most common ethical problems involve the fulfillment of responsibilities to patients and the conflicting demands of other individuals and society.

Ethical Obligations to Patients

Avoiding Stigmatization

Epidemiological studies have identified categories of persons who are at high risk for certain conditions and who may benefit from health promotion and disease prevention interventions. Sometimes we attach pejorative labels to high-risk individuals. Smokers become tobacco "addicts," fat people are "greedy," people who do not engage in regular daily exercise are "lazy." Our programs "target" these persons. These words and our actions can cause embarrassment or harm by arousing scorn or discriminatory actions. Therefore, a high priority for clinicians engaged in health promotion and disease prevention efforts is to avoid actions and approaches that can stigmatize.

Blaming the victim is a variation on this theme. When people who engage in unhealthful behaviors (e.g., smoking) develop related illnesses (e.g., emphysema), they themselves are often already aware that their unhealthy behavior is a contributing cause. For fear of being blamed, they may be reluctant to seek health care for this and other conditions. Thus, when dealing with patients who engage in unhealthy behaviors, physicians and other health care providers have a special duty to demonstrate that their approach to everyone is nonjudgmental and nondiscriminatory. This can be difficult for those who believe, for instance, that certain diseases result from moral weakness (e.g., alcoholism) or are a punishment for sin. The latter is still a rather common attitude towards sexually transmitted diseases, especially human immunodeficiency virus (HIV) infection, where the negative attitude may be overlaid with homophobia. Such attitudes have no place in modern medical practice.

Having said this, it should be noted that stigmatizing attitudes toward infectious diseases have historical roots. Societies have protected themselves against contagious disease since ancient times by developing methods of identifying and often segregating persons thought to be harboring contagious diseases. The classic example is leprosy: lepers were obliged to carry a bell and wear distinctive clothing so that others would be warned of their passing and could shun them. Thus, the victims of communicable diseases often have been stigmatized by society. The concept of contagion led to the practice of segregating persons with contagious diseases—the use of lazarettos, quarantine (in which healthy contacts, such as family members and passengers on ships, were shut away from the rest of humankind), and sanatorium care for tuberculosis (which had the secondary purpose of providing a setting for focused care but was primarily intended to isolate patients). Thus, persons with contagious or communicable diseases were "punished" by society for the sin of acquiring their disease.

Limiting Inequalities in Health

Whether through community-wide health promotion programs or through personal services obtained from private clinicians, some people are more receptive and responsive to health promotion than others.

Those who are generally the most interested are the well-educated professional and middle class members of society. Those who respond poorly are often the uneducated working class, the unemployed, the working poor and marginally employed, the disenfranchised underclass, homeless persons, and recent immigrants. All of these groups usually have poorer health, even before health promotion is considered. Health promotion tends to aggravate inequalities in health that already exist (2), the opposite of what it is supposed to accomplish. What is required to correct this trend is a greater effort directed toward those social groups that are least receptive to health promotion programs. Clinicians caring for such patients need to use culturally sensitive approaches and speak in the patient's language to explain the importance of healthy behaviors, screening tests, and immunizations (see Chapters 2 and 5). Health professionals who have recognized the difficulty of communicating across a wide social and cultural gulf have attempted to close the gap by recruiting staff from the culture they want to reach.

Screening Tests

Several ethical questions that relate to screening apparently healthy people have long been recognized (3). New ethical questions that arise in relation to prenatal and genetic screening are too complex to discuss here. What is important is for the physician to recognize that it is unethical to order screening tests without considering their potential adverse effects and without sharing this information with the patient.

In a perfect world, screening tests would infallibly sort diseased from nondiseased individuals; in our imperfect world with imperfect screening tests, some diseased individuals are not detected by screening and some healthy individuals are wrongly identified as "diseased" (or at least suspected of being diseased) because the screening test gives a false-positive result. False-negative results of cancer screening can have disastrous consequences if a person with cancer is wrongly reassured that there is no cancer. False-positive tests expose the subject to the expense, anxiety, and potential harm of further investigations made necessary by suspicion of the target condition. See Chapter 4 for further details.

Even accurate screening test results can be harmful. Many patients with hypertension, for example, feel fine until their blood pressure level has been recorded and communicated to them. They are then prescribed antihypertensive drugs that may cause side effects and admonished to change their lifestyle. It has been observed that persons identified as hypertensive, who were never previously absent from work, have increased rates of absenteeism after their condition has been diagnosed, regardless of the clinical status or response to treatment (4). The mere fact of attaching a disease label causes harm.

The treatment that follows screening often brings both benefits and harms. Antihypertensive medication may reduce the risk of cardiovascular disease, but it can also produce side effects that may make the treatment seem worse to patients than the disease. Some drugs can impair sexual potency or affect cognitive function. Persons with hypertension who occupy prominent professional positions where they are responsible for high-level decision making may find that their active leadership role and decision making capability are eroded by the effects of their medication.

Given these complexities, it is unethical for physicians to order screening tests without first advising patients of the consequences, including the potential for inaccurate results, the nature of follow-up tests and their potential complications, the evidence that early detection is beneficial, and the potential harms of treatment (see discussion of "Shared Decision Making" in Chapter 19). Screening should also not be undertaken without considering the cost of confirmatory tests and treatment. Both direct and indirect costs have to be taken into account. Clinicians should be respectful of patients' choices to defer screening based on this information. Women offered breast cancer screening are sometimes reluctant to accept it: they may fear cancer or may harbor guilt that cancer is a punishment for their sins or is preordained by fate. Another powerful reason for reluctance to find out if they have breast cancer is the question of who will care for their family if they have to be hospitalized and then face a long period of convalescence and infirmity due to chemotherapy or radiation.

Another ethical problem can arise in the performance of screening tests in patients with low risk of disease, who are more likely for statistical reasons to receive inaccurate results (see Chapter 4), or when only a small proportion of patients will benefit from early detection. Both problems are illustrated by the debate over breast cancer screening in premenopausal women. No study has demonstrated a statistically significant reduction in breast cancer mortality as a result of screening women under age 50. When such screening is performed, a large proportion of women receive false-positive results and undergo unnecessarily the physical and psychological discomfort of breast biopsy. A small number of women with breast cancer will be detected, however. And although the population of screened women, as a whole, may not benefit from screening, some individual women with breast cancer are likely to benefit greatly from early detection of their disease. This is a variation of what Rose called the "prevention paradox" (5).

Similar issues apply to screening for prostate cancer, a condition for which there is little evidence that early detection improves outcome. Currently available screening tests produce a large proportion of false-positive results, subjecting some men to unnecessary imaging studies and needle-biopsy procedures (see Chapter 21). Ethical arguments against screening emphasize the potential harms of screening and the lack of evidence that treatment is effective. Ethical arguments for screening, on the other hand, note that prostate cancer is the second most common cause of cancer deaths in men and suggest that it is unethical to withhold a potentially life-saving intervention while awaiting the completion of clinical trials.

As discussed in Chapter 17, screening may be unethical if there is no provision for follow-up confirmatory tests or for necessary treatment. Similarly, screening for untreatable conditions or to obtain information that will not influence treatment is often unethical, especially when done to satisfy the physician's curiosity rather than to inform the patient. Testing out of intellectual curiosity is an unfortunately common practice among physicians, who are often unconsciously motivated to order tests to check diagnostic suspicions or to satisfy their curiosity.

A more complex ethical question relates to the appropriateness of such testing when done to satisfy the patient's intellectual curiosity. For example, patients often request screening tests for cancer, even when they are advised beforehand that no effective treatment is available. It was concluded at several consensus conferences, many years ago, that use of such screening tests would be unethical at the population level. On the other hand, ethical decisions to proceed with such screening tests can be made at the individual level. One screening test that falls into this category is to detect Huntington's disease. Studies have suggested that, while a positive test result confers a hopeless prognosis, sufferers generally feel better for knowing rather than not knowing that ultimately they will fall victim to this relentlessly progressive form of dementia and disability (6).

Physicians in the United States order many unnecessary screening tests out of self-interest, to protect themselves legally in the event that they are sued for malpractice. In what has become known as "defensive medicine," the fear of litigation has replaced clinical reasoning as a basis for determining proper indications. There are three obvious problems with this practice. First and foremost, tests ordered to protect the physician may harm the patient, a violation of the ethical principle of nonmaleficence. Second, if the patient experiences complications from the test, the physician can be sued for subjecting the patient to this risk without a legitimate indication. Third, even if there is no direct harm to the patient, the enormous cost of performing millions of "defensive" tests each year, in an era of limited health care dollars, draws resources away from effective and necessary health care services. Finally, if screening for legal reasons is unethical, certainly it is unethical (and often illegal) to order screening tests for financial gain (e.g., self-referral to a physician-owned laboratory).

Health Promotion Counseling

Many behaviors that are harmful to health may also be pleasurable. Examples abound: tobacco smoking, use of alcohol and recreational drugs, eating excessively large and appetizing meals or tasty high-fat foods, extramarital and promiscuous sexual activity, potentially dangerous body-contact sports, and many other socially popular pastimes. Clinicians who seek to dissuade people from taking part in these activities are sometimes perceived as killjoys and interfering busy-bodies. Counseling about dietary fat intake and other lifestyle issues may seem especially misdirected when patients are of advanced age or infirm. When people have few or no other sources of pleasure or solace, clinicians have a responsibility to ensure that patients really will be better off after they have changed their behavior, not merely less prone to a particular risk factor.

Some so-called healthful behaviors are potentially harmful as performed by some persons. For example, although reduction of dietary fat consumption is generally beneficial, low-fat diets in young children may impair growth. In some older adults, reduced intake of fat-containing foods may precipitate nutritional deficiencies (see Chapter 8). Exercise, if improperly performed, can cause musculoskeletal injuries and, in selected patients, myocardial ischemia or infarction. Inaccurate counseling or improper adherence to advice about sexual practices can result in an increased risk of sexually transmitted diseases (e.g., using rubber condoms) or unwanted pregnancy (e.g., switching from oral contraceptives to condoms without spermicide). The clinician has a responsibility to ensure that patients will benefit from the recommended behavior and that accurate instructions about appropriate practices are provided.

Immunizations

No biological preparation used to vaccinate or immunize persons against communicable disease is free of adverse effects. The potential harms that may be caused by adverse effects must be weighed against the benefit of protection against potentially lethal or crippling communicable diseases. Moreover, this benefit has to be seen in the larger social context of herd immunity as well as in the context of personal protection. If a high enough proportion of the population is immunized against a particular communicable disease, the probability of transmission of an infectious agent to a susceptible host falls to a level where the risk of epidemic spread becomes very low, even nonexistent. This introduces an important ethical dilemma when parents object to the immunization of their children.

Faced with an outbreak of smallpox in 1947, the public health authorities in New York City vaccinated about five million people in the space of a few weeks. The harms due to vaccination included 45 known cases of post-

Table 27.2
Estimated Numbers of Adverse Outcomes, Pertussis Immunization Programs

	Number of Cases (per million)	
Effect	With Program	Without Program
Birth–6 mo		
Hospitalization	1,060	11,098
Death	12.5	130.6
Encephalitis	2.4	25.5
Residual defect	0.8	8.5

	Number of Events (per million)	
Event	With Program	Without Program
6 mo–5 yr		
Cases of pertussis	34,048	356,566
Hospitalizations, total	6,529	38,787
Deaths	44	457
Encephalitis	162	87
Residual defect from encephalitis, total	54	29

From Pertussis: CPS, a case study. In: U.S. Department of Health and Human Services, Task Force on Health Risk Assessment. Determining risks to health—federal policy and practice. Dover, MA: Auburn, 1986.

vaccinal encephalitis and four deaths (7). This was an acceptable risk in view of the enormous benefit: the protection of eight million people against a potentially devastating epidemic that would have caused many deaths and much disability and suffering; it was a heavy price, however, for the victims of vaccination and for their next of kin. In more recent years, concerns about the risks of pertussis vaccination have raised similar issues. Table 27.2 shows that the risks of not vaccinating older children (ages 6 months to 5 years) are slightly less than the risk of vaccinating, for one specific adverse effect (encephalitis), but overall the benefits of vaccinating older children are greater than the potential harms. Nonetheless, as discussed in Chapter 18, the potential complications of the vaccine have generated considerable parental anxiety. All clinicians have an obligation, as part of the process of informed consent, to ensure that all persons who are receiving immunizations (and parents or guardians) are made aware of the risk of harm due to the immunizing agent.

Ethical Obligations to the Patient's Family and Friends

Health professionals hold a position of trust. The clinician's confidential relationship with patients or clients is assumed. In some situations, the assumption is made explicit by a statement that information obtained in interviews will be held in confidence. Sometimes these ethical obligations to the patient are challenged by responsibilities to parents or other family members. For example, when the patient is a minor, whether or not there are local laws about informing parents or legal guardians, the clinician must decide whose interests are harmed if the confidentiality of the doctor-patient relationship is violated (e.g., informing parents that a minor is using drugs or is seeking advice about contraception or about a possible termination of pregnancy).

Pediatricians generally agree that children as young as age 10 are mature enough to know that they have a fatal illness. How old must a girl be before she can take responsibility for decisions about her own reproductive life? What is the likely outcome if the clinician violates the confidentiality of a 16 or 17-year-old girl and informs her parents that she has sought advice about contraception? Perhaps the best approach for clinicians in settings where the law requires that they inform parents of minors is to discuss these obligations fully with the patient and to obtain informed consent to discuss the situation with the parents.

As discussed in Chapter 12, the control of sexually transmitted diseases may require the clinician to violate the confidentiality of the doctor-patient relationship to protect the health of spouses or other sexual partners. For patients with gonorrhea, syphilis, and other sexually transmitted diseases, the patient's sexual partner is notified and subject to treatment, often compulsorily. In many public health services, the staff (usually public health nurses) who trace contacts of notified cases of sexually transmitted diseases go about their task with considerable tact and delicacy. Nonetheless, it can be a severe emotional shock if an innocent woman first learns about her husband's marital infidelity from a public health nurse who is tracing the contacts of a man with gonorrhea.

Ethical Obligations to Society and Social Institutions

The legal requirement of physicians to report cases of notifiable communicable diseases to the public health authorities represents an ethical obligation to protect the health interests of society, even if it is against the wishes of the patient. The reasons for notification include the socially imperative function of surveillance, required to protect society as a whole, and application of control measures such as epidemic investigation, provision of vaccines and sera, etc., to control infectious diseases that threaten the community at large. Physicians have an ethical obligation to explain to patients and their families the reasons for reporting infectious diseases and to seek their voluntary consent to disclose necessary information to public health authorities. Reassurance that privacy and confidentiality will be respected is also important.

Another example of the tension between societal and individual needs relates to the refusal of parents to vaccinate their children against dangerous transmissible diseases, such as pertussis, because of religious concerns or the belief that the vaccines are unsafe. Although the clinician has an ethical obligation to respect the parents' wishes, there also exists a responsibility to protect the health of other children who may be exposed to the parents' unimmunized children. Most states have addressed this problem by requiring children to be completely immunized before they can attend school. In these situations, the responsibilities of the clinician, at a minimum, are to educate parents about the true benefits and risks of vaccination and about the impact of their decision on the health risks of other children.

Ethical obligations to the patient are sometimes challenged by the information requirements of other social institutions. For example, what happens when physicians are employed by a government agency or a company that imposes requirements on the physician's behavior? Clinicians in workplace health programs may discover habits or practices that are not in the best interests of the employer, but that are otherwise not harmful, either to the health of the worker concerned, or to others. What should they do? Smoking on the job in areas where smoking is dangerous to the safety and health of others, as well as to the smoker, is commonplace. Workplace health promotion campaigns can make use of this to encourage adherence to a no-smoking policy. Advising the worker concerned to desist is an obvious response, reporting to the employer is not, because even though the clinician may be employed by management, the confidentiality of the clinician's relationship to the worker remains intact.

Legal requirements to report cases to law enforcement agencies can present similar ethical conflicts. If a clinician observes evidence of or suspects child abuse, there is a legal as well as a moral obligation to report this to the appropriate child protective services agency. If the illegal conduct observed were equipment used to forge banknotes, the moral obligation would be less, and perhaps, if the clinician believed it to be more important to preserve the patient's trust, this might not be reported to the police. Similarly, unless the safety of other individuals is in jeopardy, the patient's involvement in other illegal activity (e.g., use of illicit drugs) need not be disclosed to law enforcement officials. See Chapter 13 regarding appropriate counseling and rehabilitation interventions for such patients.

Ethical Problems Associated with HIV Infection

Screening and counseling for HIV infection provide a case study for virtually every ethical issue discussed in this chapter. The emotional impact of coping with infectious diseases is greatest with HIV infection. Not only is the infection lethal, many who are afflicted are already stigmatized. Some, notably members of the gay community and families of hemophiliacs infected with HIV by contaminated blood transfusions, have had powerful support from advocacy groups. Users of illicit intravenous drugs and their children have had less support, often none.

The test for HIV infection is a procedure not to be undertaken lightly: a positive result is not only a virtual death sentence (until effective treatment becomes available) but while still healthy, HIV-positive individuals may encounter discriminatory practices, including restrictions on employment, travel, and eligibility for life and health insurance. Therefore, all persons tested for HIV infection should be counseled before the test and informed about the implications of a positive result (8). See Chapter 12 for a discussion of appropriate pretest and posttest counseling.

Situations have arisen wherein HIV testing is mandatory: many life insurance carriers require a negative HIV test before they will issue policies over a specified amount. In some health care settings, the pressure to perform HIV testing of both patients and providers is growing. In some jurisdictions, anonymous tests give persons who fear that they may have HIV infection the assurance that information will remain confidential, but anonymous testing restricts the scope of counseling and denies public health authorities an opportunity to identify cases and contacts.

For community-wide surveillance, anonymous unlinked HIV testing is practiced. This makes use of aliquots of blood left over from other routine tests, such as screening tests for inborn errors of metabolism in newborn infants. Before the test is done, blood samples are stripped of all personal identifiers. Anonymous unlinked HIV tests are recommended by the expert group of the World Health Organization Global Programme on AIDS (8) and are used in many countries, although in some there were initial ethical objections on the grounds that it would be impossible to identify cases and trace their sexual partners. However, in all nations save the Netherlands, it has now been recognized that the social good of maintaining surveillance outweighs the theoretical harm of unidentified cases at large in the community; the belief is that the positive cases will come to light in other ways.

CONCLUSION

The role of ethics in health promotion and disease prevention, and in medicine generally, can only increase in the future, as society confronts new technologies, moral debates, and health problems. The likely emergence of genetic testing will bring with it complex ethical debates about the appropriateness of using such tests to predict future diseases in adults, children, and, most controversially, the fetus. What benefits, harms, and misinformation will result from such testing? Ethics will also encompass complex social policy issues. In the near future, policy makers engaged in health care reform in the United States must address how to correct inequities in disease risks and health care services while maintaining controls on rising costs.

As an observer of these complex debates, the practicing clinician faces a professional responsibility to set aside personal views and concentrate on what is best for the patient. Inevitably, providing the patient with unbiased information about options, irrespective of the clinician's opinions, and supporting respectfully the patient's choices will, in most cases, satisfy the best principles of biomedical ethics.

REFERENCES

1. Davis K, Bialek R, Parkinson M, Smith J, Vellozzi C. Paying for preventive care; moving the debate forward. Am J Prev Med 1990;6:4 (Suppl).
2. Abelin T. Health promotion. In: Holland WW, Detels R, Knox EG, eds. Oxford textbook of public health, 2nd ed. Oxford and New York: Oxford University Press, 1991.
3. McKeown T, Knox EG. The framework required for validation of prescriptive screening. In: Screening and medical care; a review of the evidence. London: Oxford University Press for the Nuffield Provincial Hospitals Trust, 1968;159–173.
4. Haynes RB, Sackett DL, Taylor DW, et al. Increased absenteeism from work after detection and labeling of hypertensive patients. N Engl J Med 1978;299:741–747.
5. Rose GA. The strategy of preventive medicine. Oxford: Oxford University Press, 1992.
6. Wiggins S, Whyte P, Huggins M, et al. The psychological consequences of predictive testing for Huntington's disease. N Engl J Med 1992;327:1401–1405.
7. Greenberg M. Complications of vaccination against smallpox. Am J Dis Child 1948;76:492–502.
8. WHO Global Programme on AIDS. Guidelines for counseling about HIV infection and disease. Geneva: WHO AIDS Series, No. 8, 1990.

28. Future of Health Promotion and Disease Prevention in Clinical Practice and in the Community

ROBERT S. LAWRENCE

The most reliable guide to predicting future developments in health promotion and disease prevention is a careful examination of current trends in society and progress in research. The information and recommendations presented in this book are based on data acquired over decades. Some of them are now fully assimilated into clinical practice; other elements are still being debated or are diffusing more slowly into practice because of organizational, economic, logistic, or behavioral and attitudinal barriers. To predict what may lie ahead, this concluding chapter will examine current trends in the organization of preventive services and research in fields relevant to health promotion and disease prevention.

It is safe to predict that those clinical preventive interventions and health promotion activities that are currently based on high-quality evidence will eventually be incorporated into practice if the barriers already mentioned can be overcome. It is more difficult to predict the new discoveries in the biologic or behavioral sciences that will influence disease prevention as dramatically as the advances in virus isolation and vaccine development that, many years ago, were made possible by the invention of tissue culture. Similarly, just as the pundits were proven wrong in designating 1994 as the year of health care reform in the United States, many of today's trends influencing health promotion and disease prevention policy are likely to surprise us with new twists and turns. With these caveats, let us first examine current trends in society, then the role of the clinician in the community, and, finally, research possibilities.

CURRENT TRENDS INFLUENCING HEALTH PROMOTION AND DISEASE PREVENTION

Many of today's policy discussions about health promotion were shaped by the 1974 publication of the Lalonde Report, which was commissioned by Health Canada to assess priorities for improving the health status of the

Canadian people (1). The report described the relationships among access to health care services, human biology, environment, and individual behaviors, estimating the relative contribution to outcomes that progress in each of these fields might make. The commission estimated that advances in modifying personal risk, improving the environment, and adding to our knowledge of human biology were more likely to improve health status than further work on the quality and efficiency of the medical care system. The report is now credited with establishing health promotion as a major component of strategies to improve health and for stimulating research on the determinants of health-related behaviors and methods to modify them for risk reduction (2).

Heightened interest in risk reduction paved the way for the creation of the Canadian Task Force on the Periodic Health Examination, whose report in 1979 represented another major contribution to health promotion and disease prevention by introducing a method of applying evidence-based decision rules to setting priorities for clinical preventive services. The task force used data on burden of suffering to determine those conditions or risk factors most needing preventive interventions. Next, the task force conducted a systematic review of the literature and evaluated the quality of evidence regarding the efficacy and effectiveness of preventive maneuvers against each of the priority conditions or risk factors. Finally, the characteristics of the preventive maneuver were assessed in terms of accuracy, reliability, safety, cost, and discomfort to the patient. A recommendation for each intervention was then developed by integrating the quality of evidence with the characteristics of the maneuver. The Canadian approach was adopted by the U.S. Preventive Services Task Force when it began its work in 1984, leading to the publication of the first edition of the *Guide to Clinical Preventive Services* in 1989 (3) and the second edition in 1996 (4) (see the introduction for further details).

Advances in health and the resulting increase in life expectancy in the last 50 years have produced a demographic shift toward an older society, especially in the industrialized countries of North America, Europe, and Japan. An older population has a high burden of suffering caused by chronic conditions, many of them products of multiple risk factors. The magnitude of the shift in the proportion of persons age 65 years and older will change the dependency ratio (the ratio of persons employed to persons not working) from the current 5:1 to a projected 3:1 ratio by 2020. This shift makes it all the more important to promote healthy and successful aging and to reduce the burden of disability in the elderly so that more independent living arrangements can be preserved.

Recent studies have affirmed the value of programs to promote physical activity to increase strength, flexibility, and bone mass; smoking cessation to lower risks of heart disease, emphysema, and cancer; and attention to a balanced diet to avoid malnutrition, overweight, and disorders caused by dietary excesses. The need for health education and other programs to prevent falls, burns, and misuse of prescription drugs will increase. Health professionals committed to preventive care for the elderly will adopt these programs in their own practices and work with community agencies to strengthen regulatory incentives for housing codes that incorporate mandatory temperature controls on hot water systems, safe design of stairways, and adequate lighting.

The relentless increase in the cost of health care has stimulated interest in health sector reform in many parts of the world. Inequities in access to care add to the pressure for reform. Both industrialized countries and developing nations are struggling to achieve the goal of "health for all" by the year 2000, set at the world summit on health in Alma Atta in 1979. In 1993, the World Bank for the first time devoted its annual *World Development Report* (WDR) to health, marking a major shift in thinking about investing in health as an essential component of economic development rather than as a negative input (5). The WDR stressed the need for greater efficiency in the distribution of resources within the health sector, emphasizing the most cost-effective interventions for those conditions responsible for the greatest burden of suffering in each country. Reform was also urged for improving the efficiency of interventions that had passed the test for effectiveness. For the poorest and middle income countries of the developing world, the WDR proposed basic packages of primary and public health services that should be fully implemented before public funds were used for more "discretionary" clinical services or less cost-effective interventions.

While the 1993 WDR is having a profound influence on policy discussions among multinational agencies like the World Bank and the World Health Organization, on ministries of health in the developing world, and on foreign aid programs, it has received little domestic attention in the United States. Only in Oregon, so far, has there been a major effort to set priorities for health expenditures by using the criteria of cost-effectiveness and burden of suffering. We can expect more interest in improving allocative efficiency—whether for clinical preventive services or curative services—as pressures mount to contain costs while increasing access.

The shift away from fee-for-service and toward managed care is another manifestation of efforts to contain costs and improve efficiency in clinical care. An early reluctance by many health maintenance organizations to provide health promotion and disease prevention services has yielded to the growing body of evidence supporting the clinical effectiveness and cost-effectiveness of many clinical preventive interventions as well as to the demands of their members for more health promotion services. The recommendations of the Canadian and U.S. task forces, while not intended to be practice standards, are often interpreted as such.

As managed care spreads to include more of the population, opportunities will increase to combine clinical preventive services with population-based health promotion activities: group smoking cessation programs, health education provided at the worksite or school, and fitness programs. Unfortunately, most geographic sections of the United States have multiple managed care systems competing for patients living in the same area, making true population-based health care difficult if not impossible. A challenge for the health promotion community is to develop new cooperative arrangements among managed care systems, local health departments, and the remnants of the fee-for-service system to provide health promotion services for the entire population at risk. Were universal access to care first achieved at the level of health promotion and disease prevention services, a major gain in equity and allocative efficiency would occur.

Another encouraging trend is the increasing emphasis given to education of new health professionals in health promotion and disease prevention and a growing awareness of the valuable contributions of nonphysician health professionals to health education and the provision of clinical preventive services. The emergence of clinical epidemiology as a respected discipline is helping to reintegrate medical and public health perspectives, to combine the "health of populations" viewpoint of prevention and public health with the "health of the individual" approach of clinical care (6). As we have learned more about the etiology of disease and the multiple contributions to pathogenesis, we have begun to appreciate the importance of interventions that incorporate population-based health education along with individual-based counseling or screening. The Cartesian reductionism of the biomedical model is yielding to a more holistic and integrative notion of human biology and behavior. Advances in social psychology, medical sociology, and anthropology will accelerate this trend; and personality and behavioral profiles will take their place alongside laboratory screening tests as important aids to the practice of clinical preventive medicine.

Recent analyses of the social gradient in health or the correlation of income with health status further demonstrate the importance of taking into account social, economic, and psychologic factors as well as biologic risk in anticipating new opportunities for health promotion and disease prevention. In his studies of British civil servants (Whitehall II), Michael Marmot has demonstrated a social gradient in death rates and sickness absence rates by grades of employment (7). Absence rates due to sickness for both men and women increase markedly from low rates among senior administrators to high rates among office staff in the lower civil service grades.

Similar observations exist for cardiovascular disease rates, even after controlling for differences among civil service grades in such risk factors as smoking, exercise, and blood pressure. Marmot concludes, "Providing more people with fulfilling jobs, adequate compensation, and social environments that foster good relationships may be of crucial importance in reducing inequalities in health." For now the role of the clinician is to inform and counsel patients about the importance of taking stock of job satisfaction and personal relationships and of taking whatever steps are feasible to improve these aspects of daily life to promote better health.

An attractive hypothesis to explain the social gradient is that higher socioeconomic status may provide a greater sense of control over one's fate—a greater sense of self-efficacy—and that self-efficacy may influence the release of neurotransmitters, which in turn may stimulate the production of neurohormones essential to a robust immune system. In the future, as we learn more about the social gradient in health and understand the causal pathways that link higher socioeconomic status to better health status, it may be possible to counsel patients to engage in exercises or other behaviors that will activate the protective biologic pathways, while still striving for greater equity in areas of work, compensation, and control.

Additional insights about the social gradient in health come from Richard Wilkinson's comparisons between countries. These studies have shown a relation between per capita gross national product (GNPpc) and life expectancy for poor countries with GNPpc of less than $5,000 (8). Above $5,000 there is little relation between GNP and life expectancy, but a strong correlation exists between income dispersion and life expectancy. The higher the share of total income going to the bottom 60–70% of the population, the greater the life expectancy for that group. Japan, with the most equitable distribution of income among the wealthy industrialized countries, has the longest life expectancy. The United States and the United Kingdom, with less equitable income distribution, lag behind. In other words, relative deprivation appears to be an important determinant of health inequalities. With our present level of knowledge, however, no interventions appear to be available to the clinician except to act responsibly as an informed member of society. Empirical, and eventually, experimental, data will in the future open new opportunities for health promotion based on the social gradient in health.

The information revolution of the computer age is already having a profound effect on our understanding of human disease and the potential for prevention. Some have argued that the emergence of clinical epidemiology as a discipline was made possible by the developing capacity of the personal computer to analyze large sets of data. The earlier chapter about computer-assisted decision making describes current capabilities. Future systems may offer interactive, multi-media programs for self-assessment of risk factors and guided responses for self-management; educational programs and personal reminder systems for health promotion activities; and on-line communication links between patients and clinicians. Patients will increasingly have access to their medical record or, indeed, be the repository of the medical record via palmtop or smaller computers. Future versions of this book may be distributed on CD-ROM or successors to CD-ROM technology.

ROLE OF THE CLINICIAN IN THE COMMUNITY

Practitioners can play an important role in directing and facilitating many of these encouraging trends. Their primary role, of course, lies in incorporating health promotion and disease prevention into routine patient care, the principal focus of this book. But clinicians who are interested in social change can play a more active role outside the office and clinic by becoming involved in community efforts aimed at health promotion and disease prevention. In many instances, these population-based interventions, on either the local, state, or national level, are more effective and have a broader impact in improving health outcomes than those achieved one patient at a time in the clinical setting. Physicians can play a special role in these community efforts by sharing their medical expertise to improve the quality of programs and by using their credibility to influence policy makers and the public.

Communities deal each day with a broad range of issues of direct relevance to the health promotion and disease prevention topics discussed in this book. The fluoride content of local drinking water, lead levels in aging buildings, and other health risks of concern to the clinician are also the concerns of municipal agencies responsible for ensuring clean and safe air, water, and food supplies. Local school systems struggle with appropriate strategies to educate students about personal health behaviors such as smoking and the importance of exercise; to provide sex education in a manner that is effective and yet acceptable to the community; to ensure adequate nutrition and immunization coverage for the community's children; and to promote injury prevention policies (ranging from sports injury prevention in school athletic activities to the prevention of drinking and driving and the creation of violence prevention programs). Injury prevention is also of direct concern to municipal governments attempting to reduce motor vehicle accidents, promote boating safety, provide bicycle trails to reduce bicycle-related injuries, and control the availability of guns and other weapons. Social service agencies address child abuse and other domestic violence issues. Indeed, most of the preventive interventions discussed in this book depend on an infrastructure of community resources (e.g., public health departments, substance abuse services, mental health agencies, family planning programs, domestic violence crisis shelters) that easily falls victim to financial, administrative, and political threats if active community support is lacking.

Health professionals can intervene when decisions affecting the quality or continued existence of these programs are being made by government agencies, private groups, or the electorate (e.g., ballot issues), or when unrecognized problems need to be brought to public attention. On a limited level, clinicians can play an educational role by simply talking with their patients about these issues. They can act more broadly outside the clinical setting, however, by writing editorials in local newspapers, appearing on local radio or television programs to share their concerns, and participating in other community education efforts. Like other interested citizens, health professionals can join local community action groups or coalitions concerned with correcting the problem. But clinicians are sometimes more effective in influencing public debate when their positions are championed by the local medical society, hospital groups, and local/state chapters of medical specialty societies. Individual clinicians can spearhead these efforts by joining and becoming active in relevant committees in their local medical or specialty society.

Many of the topics addressed in this book fall under the concerns of national health care and public health policy and cannot be adequately addressed on a local level. Most fundamentally, about 40 million Americans without adequate access to health care are unable to benefit fully from most of the clinical interventions discussed in this book. Although efforts to achieve national health care reform in the early 1990s were unsuccessful, many state governments are moving forward with reforms that directly affect the quality of preventive care in their states. National discussions about reducing the size of entitlement programs, such as Medicare and Medicaid, may also influence the delivery of clinical preventive services to a large proportion of patients at risk. Federal and state governments regularly struggle with other programs that affect health promotion and disease prevention, as in debates about what should be taught in public schools, the most effective strategies to control substance abuse, how to prevent the rising death toll from homicide and violence, and funding for continued prevention research.

The action is not limited to the government. Many national trends in health promotion and disease prevention occur in the private sector through changes undertaken by industry. For example, the food industry has both stimulated and responded to the growing public interest in obtaining accurate information about the nutritional quality of food products and in promoting healthier food choices. Through a combination of voluntary and legislated interventions, the automobile industry has introduced new design features and restraint systems to help prevent motor vehicle injuries. Pharmaceutical companies have used child-resistant caps to reduce child poisonings. Alcoholic beverage manufacturers have launched public education campaigns to discourage drinking and driving. The industry with the potential for the greatest impact on the delivery of clinical preventive services, managed care organizations, has assumed a growing role in expanding access to preventive care. These industries, and many others, can go much further in promoting health, but they often require encouragement from health groups and consumers.

Health professionals can help these efforts through the actions of organized medicine and national medical and public health organizations. Clinicians who are interested in becoming more involved with these efforts can join the public health and health promotion committees of state and local medical societies, state chapters and national committees of their medical specialty society, and national organizations such as the American College of Preventive Medicine, American Medical Association, and American Public Health Association.

Public policy regarding health promotion and disease prevention encompasses some of the most controversial issues of our society. Injury prevention and other public health policies often place restraints on the freedom of individuals in order to protect the health of individuals or the health of others. The tension between these social responsibilities is evident in debates about the appropriateness of enforcing tobacco smoke-free areas, requiring motorcyclists to wear helmets, and similar measures. The conflict between individual freedoms and public health is perhaps most strident in the debate over the prevention of firearm injuries through such measures as banning the sale of handguns and assault weapons. Prevention policy often clashes with religious and ethical concerns, as in the debate over the rights of women to have access to a safe, legal abortion if they choose to terminate an unwanted pregnancy.

Health professionals have both an opportunity and a responsibility to participate in these debates. They share the opportunity of all citizens to express their opinions about the appropriateness of different policies. Like other members of society, health professionals are entitled to have different political, religious, and philosophical viewpoints about these contentious topics. Regardless of their personal opinions and beliefs, however, clinicians have a professional responsibility to ensure that such debates are based on accurate information about the public health and clinical implications of different choices. Whether a clinician agrees or disagrees with the appropriateness or effectiveness of handgun legislation, for example, he or she has a professional responsibility to clarify the prominent role of firearms as a leading cause of death and disability in the United States. The medical risks of illegal, "back alley" abortions need to be communicated by health professionals, even if they consider abortion immoral. The public health impact of tobacco use must be emphasized by clinicians, even if they consider the banning of tobacco sales overly restrictive.

RESEARCH OPPORTUNITIES

Despite the great advances in our understanding of the relationship between nutrition and good health, many questions remain unanswered. The role of micronutrients and other dietary supplements such as antioxidants and beta carotene in the prevention of disease is currently being examined. Other investigations to determine the content of a healthy diet should reduce some of the confusion and controversy that still surrounds human nutrition. Further investigation is needed to determine the true causes of weight gain and effective measures for achieving weight loss and healthy weight maintenance.

Vaccine research holds promise for naked DNA vaccines delivered on microspherules into muscle tissue to code for protective antigens, for one-dose nasally or orally delivered vaccines, and for synthetic peptides composed of several different antigens such as that now being tested against malaria. Advances in our understanding of the immune system may permit the development of new approaches to immunization by harnessing lymphokines and cytokines, intercellular messengers, and killer and helper cells to protect against infectious diseases or malignancies.

The mapping of the human genome presents a double-edged sword. On the one hand, risk profiles will be useful to guide patients about special precautions, risk modification, or more intensive screening schedules for genetically linked conditions. On the other hand, as discussed in Chapter 27, great care will be required to avoid stigmatization and other complex ethical ramifications.

Social and behavioral research will expand our knowledge of risk taking and risk-aversive behaviors, prevention of addictive behavior, and motivational factors necessary for adopting health-promoting behaviors. As discussed earlier in the context of the social gradient in health, one of the most important areas for research in the social, behavioral, and biologic domains is the elucidation of the biobehavioral pathway to enhanced self-efficacy. When we understand that central element of our humanity, we will truly enter the golden age of health promotion and disease prevention.

REFERENCES

1. Lalonde M. A new perspective on the health of Canadians. Ottawa: Information Canada, 1974.
2. Pinder L. Medicine in the twenty-first century: challenges in personal and public health promotion. Am J Prev Med 1994; 10(3 Suppl):39–41.
3. U.S. Preventive Services Task Force. Guide to clinical preventive services. Baltimore: Williams & Wilkins, 1989.
4. U.S. Preventive Services Task Force. Guide to clinical preventive services, 2nd ed. Baltimore: Williams & Wilkins, 1996.
5. World development report 1993: investing in health. Washington: World Bank; 1993.
6. White KL. Healing the schism: epidemiology, medicine and the public's health. New York: Springer-Verlag, 1991.
7. Marmot MG. Social differentials in health within and between populations. Dædalus 1994;Fall:197–216.
8. Wilkinson, RG. Income distribution and life expectancy. Brit Med J 1992; 304:165–168.

Appendix

RECOMMENDATIONS OF THE U.S. PREVENTIVE SERVICES TASK FORCE (ABRIDGED)

The following recommendations are excerpted from the *Guide to Clinical Preventive Services*,[a] the report of the U.S. Preventive Services Task Force (1). The excerpted recommendations are drawn from chapters that provide important (and often essential) information to properly interpret the recommendations. Readers are encouraged to refer to relevant chapters in the *Guide* to obtain a better understanding of the task force's scientific rationale and a more detailed explanation of the recommendations. In the interest of completeness, task force recommendations regarding prenatal preventive services are included in this section, although prenatal care is not addressed elsewhere in this book. The following excerpts are provided as a reference and are not necessarily consistent with the recommendations of the editors of this book.

1. *Screening for Asymptomatic Coronary Artery Disease*: There is insufficient evidence to recommend for or against screening middle-aged and older men and women for asymptomatic coronary artery disease, using resting electrocardiography, ambulatory electrocardiography, or exercise electrocardiography. Recommendations against routine screening can be made on other grounds for individuals who are not at high risk of developing clinical heart disease. Routine screening is not recommended as part of the periodic health visit or preparticipation sports examinations for children, adolescents, or young adults. Clinicians should emphasize proven measures for the primary prevention of coronary disease.

2. *Screening for High Blood Cholesterol and Other Lipid Abnormalities*: Periodic screening for high blood cholesterol is recommended for all men ages 35–65 and women ages 45–65. There is insufficient evidence to recommend for or against routine screening of asymptomatic persons over age 65, but recommendations to screen healthy men and women ages 65–75 may be made on other grounds. There is also insufficient evidence to recommend routine

---

[a]The excerpts consist of the "Recommendations" sections at the beginning of each chapter in the *Guide*. This book was published several weeks before the release of the 1996 edition of the *Guide*. The final text of the recommendations was therefore unavailable as this book went to press. The following excerpts are taken from the penultimate draft of the *Guide* and, accordingly, may not reflect late changes in wording. The content of the *Guide* is in the public domain.

screening in children, adolescents, or young adults. Recommendations for screening adolescents and young adults with risk factors for coronary disease, and against routine screening in children, may be made on other grounds. There is insufficient evidence to recommend for or against routine screening for other lipid abnormalities. All patients should receive periodic screening and counseling regarding other measures to reduce their risk of coronary disease.

3. *Screening for Hypertension*: Screening for hypertension is recommended for all children and adults.

4. *Screening for Asymptomatic Carotid Artery Stenosis*: There is insufficient evidence to recommend for or against screening asymptomatic persons for carotid artery stenosis using the physical examination or carotid ultrasound. For selected high-risk patients, recommendation to discuss the potential benefits of screening and carotid endarterectomy may be made on other grounds. All persons should be screened for hypertension, and clinicians should provide counseling about smoking cessation.

5. *Screening for Peripheral Arterial Disease*: Routine screening for peripheral arterial disease in asymptomatic persons is not recommended. Clinicians should be alert to symptoms of peripheral arterial disease in persons at increased risk and should evaluate patients who have clinical evidence of vascular disease.

6. *Screening for Abdominal Aortic Aneurysm*: There is insufficient evidence to recommend for or against routine screening of asymptomatic adults for abdominal aortic aneurysm with abdominal palpation or ultrasound.

7. *Screening for Breast Cancer*: Routine screening for breast cancer every one to two years, with mammography alone or mammography and annual clinical breast examination, is recommended for all women ages 50–69. There is insufficient evidence to recommend for or against routine mammography or clinical breast examination for women ages 40–49 or ages 70 and older, although recommendations to screen high-risk women ages 40–49 and healthy women ages 70 and older may be made on other grounds. There is insufficient evidence to recommend for or against the use of screening clinical breast examination alone or the teaching of breast self-examination.

8. *Screening for Colorectal Cancer*: Screening for colorectal cancer is recommended for all persons ages 50 and older with annual fecal occult blood testing, or sigmoidoscopy (periodicity unspecified), or both. There is insufficient evidence to determine which of these screening methods is preferable or whether the combination of fecal occult blood testing and sigmoidoscopy produces greater benefits than does either test alone. There is also insufficient evidence to recommend for or against routine screening with digital rectal examination, barium enema, or colonoscopy, although recommendations against such screening in average-risk persons may be made on other grounds. Persons with a family history of hereditary syndromes associated with a high risk of colon cancer should be referred to specialists for diagnosis and management.

9. *Screening for Cervical Cancer*: Routine screening for cervical cancer with Papanicolaou testing is recommended for all women who are or have been sexually active and who have a cervix. Papanicolaou smears should begin with the onset of sexual activity and should be repeated at least every three years. There is insufficient evidence to recommend for or against an upper age limit for Papanicolaou testing, but recommendations can be made on other grounds to discontinue regular testing after age 65 in women who have had regular previous screening in which the smears have been consistently normal. There is insufficient evidence to recommend for or against routine screening with cervicography or colposcopy, or for screening for human papilloma virus infection, although recommendations against such screening can be made on other grounds.

10. *Screening for Prostate Cancer*: Routine screening for prostate cancer with digital rectal examinations, serum tumor markers (e.g., prostate-specific antigen), or transrectal ultrasound is not recommended.

11. *Screening for Lung Cancer*: Routine screening of asymptomatic persons for lung cancer with chest radiography or sputum cytology is not recommended. All patients should be counseled against tobacco use.

12. *Screening for Skin Cancer*: There is insufficient evidence to recommend for or against either routine screening for skin cancer by primary care providers or counseling patients to perform periodic skin self-examinations. A recommendation to consider referring patients at substantially increased risk of malignant melanoma to skin cancer specialists for evaluation and surveillance may be made on other grounds. Avoidance of excess sun exposure is recommended for patients at increased risk of skin cancer. Counseling patients at increased risk of skin cancer to avoid excess sun exposure is recommended, based on the proven efficacy of risk reduction, although the effectiveness of counseling has not been well established. There is insufficient evidence to recommend for or against sunscreen use for the primary prevention of skin cancer.

13. *Screening for Testicular Cancer*: There is insufficient evidence to recommend for or against routine screening of asymptomatic men in the general population for testicular cancer by physician examination or patient self-examination. Recommendations to discuss screening options with select high-risk patients may be made on other grounds.

14. *Screening for Ovarian Cancer*: Screening asymptomatic women for ovarian cancer by ultrasound, the measurement of serum tumor markers, or pelvic examination is not recommended. There is insufficient evidence to recommend for or against the screening of asymptomatic women at increased risk of developing ovarian cancer.

15. *Screening for Pancreatic Cancer*: Routine screening for pancreatic cancer in asymptomatic persons, using abdominal palpation, ultrasonography, or serologic markers, is not recommended.

16. *Screening for Oral Cancer*: There is insufficient evidence to recommend for or against routine screening of asymptomatic persons for oral cancer by primary care clinicians. All patients should be counseled to discontinue the use of all forms of tobacco and to limit consumption of alcohol. Clinicians should remain alert to signs and symptoms of oral cancer and premalignancy in persons who use tobacco or alcohol.

17. *Screening for Bladder Cancer*: Screening for bladder cancer with urine dipstick, microscopic urinalysis, or urine cytology is not recommended in asymptomatic persons. All patients who smoke tobacco should be routinely counseled to quit smoking.

18. *Screening for Thyroid Cancer*: Routine screening for thyroid cancer using neck palpation or ultrasonography is not recommended for asymptomatic children or adults. There is insufficient evidence to recommend for or against screening persons with a history of external head and neck irradiation in infancy or childhood, but recommendations for such screening may be made on other grounds.

19. *Screening for Diabetes Mellitus*: There is insufficient evidence to recommend for or against routine screening for diabetes mellitus in asymptomatic adults. There is also insufficient evidence to recommend for or against universal screening for gestational diabetes. Although the benefit of early detection has not been established for any group, clinicians may decide to screen selected persons at high risk of diabetes on other grounds. Screening with immune markers to identify persons at risk for developing insulin-dependent diabetes is not recommended in the general population.

20. *Screening for Thyroid Disease*: Routine screening for thyroid disease with thyroid function tests is not recommended for asymptomatic children or adults. There is insufficient evidence to recommend for or against screening for thyroid disease with thyroid function tests in high-risk patients, but recommendations may be made on other grounds. Clinicians should remain alert to subtle symptoms and signs of thyroid dysfunction when examining such patients. [See Recommendation 45 below.]

21. *Screening for Obesity*: Periodic height and weight measurements are recommended for all patients.

22. *Screening for Iron Deficiency Anemia (Including Iron Prophylaxis)*: Screening for iron deficiency anemia using hemoglobin or hematocrit is recommended for pregnant women and for high-risk infants. There is insufficient evidence to recommend for or against routine screening for iron deficiency anemia in other asymptomatic persons, but recommendations against screening may be made on other grounds. Encouraging parents to breastfeed their infants and to include iron-enriched foods in the diet of infants and young children is recommended. There is currently insufficient evidence to recommend for or against the routine use of iron supplements for healthy infants or pregnant women.

23. *Screening for Elevated Lead Levels in Childhood and Pregnancy:* Screening for elevated lead levels by measuring blood lead at least once at about age 12 months is recommended for all children at increased risk of lead exposure. All children with identifiable risk factors should be screened, as should all children living in communities in which the prevalence of blood lead levels requiring individual intervention, including residential lead hazard control or chelation therapy, is high or is undefined. Evidence is currently insufficient to recommend an exact community prevalence below which targeted screening can be substituted for universal screening. Clinicians can seek guidance from their local or state health department. There is insufficient evidence to recommend for or against routine screening for lead exposure in asymptomatic pregnant women, but recommendations against such screening may be made on other grounds. There is also insufficient evidence to recommend for or against counseling families about the primary prevention of lead exposure, but recommendations may be made on other grounds. Recommendations regarding the primary prevention of lead poisoning by population-wide environmental interventions are beyond the scope of this chapter.

24. *Screening for Hepatitis B Virus Infection:* Screening with hepatitis B surface antigen (HBsAg) to detect active (acute or chronic) hepatitis B virus infection is recommended for all pregnant women at their first prenatal visit. The test may be repeated in the third trimester in women who are initially HBsAg-negative and who are at increased risk of hepatitis B virus infection during pregnancy. Routine screening for hepatitis B virus infection in the general population is not recommended. Certain persons at high risk may be screened to assess eligibility for vaccination.

25. *Screening for Tuberculous Infection (Including Bacillus Calmette-Guerin Immunization):* Screening for tuberculous infection with tuberculin skin testing is recommended for asymptomatic high-risk persons. Bacillus Calmette-Guerin vaccination should be considered only for selected high-risk individuals.

26. *Screening for Syphilis:* Routine serologic screening for syphilis is recommended for all pregnant women and for persons at increased risk of infection.

27. *Screening for Gonorrhea (Including Ocular Prophylaxis in Newborns):* Routine screening for *Neisseria gonorrhoeae* is recommended for asymptomatic women at high risk of infection. All high-risk women should be screened during pregnancy. There is insufficient evidence to recommend for or against screening all pregnant women or screening asymptomatic men. Recommendations to screen selected high-risk young men may be made on other grounds. Routine screening is not recommended for the general adult population. Ocular antibiotic prophylaxis of all newborn infants is recommended to prevent gonococcal ophthalmia neonatorum.

28. *Screening for Infection with Human Immunodeficiency Virus:* Clinicians should assess risk factors for human immunodeficiency virus (HIV) infection by obtaining a careful sexual history and inquiring about injection drug use in all patients. Periodic screening for infection with HIV is recommended for all

persons at increased risk of infection. Screening is recommended for all pregnant women at risk for HIV infection, including all women who live in states,
counties, or cities with an increased prevalence of HIV infection. There is insufficient evidence to recommend for or against universal screening among
low-risk pregnant women in low-prevalence areas, but recommendations to
counsel and offer screening to all pregnant women may be made on other
grounds. Screening infants born to high-risk mothers is recommended if the
mother's antibody status is not known. All patients should be counseled about
effective means to avoid HIV infection.

29. *Screening for Chlamydial Infection (Including Ocular Prophylaxis in Newborns)*: Routine screening for *Chlamydia trachomatis* infection is recommended for all sexually active female adolescents, high-risk pregnant women, and other asymptomatic women at high risk of infection. There is insufficient evidence to
recommend for or against routine screening in asymptomatic men. Recommendations to screen selected high-risk male adolescents may be made on
other grounds. Routine screening is not recommended for the general adult
population.

30. *Screening for Genital Herpes Simplex*: Routine screening for genital herpes simplex virus infection by viral culture or other tests is not recommended for
asymptomatic persons, including asymptomatic pregnant women. There is insufficient evidence to recommend for or against the examination of pregnant
women in labor for signs of active genital herpes simplex virus lesions, although recommendations to do so may be made on other grounds.

31. *Screening for Asymptomatic Bacteriuria*: Screening for asymptomatic bacteriuria
by urine culture is recommended for all pregnant women. There is insufficient evidence to recommend for or against routine screening for asymptomatic bacteriuria in diabetic or ambulatory elderly women, but recommendations against such screening may be made on other grounds. Routine
screening for asymptomatic bacteriuria in other persons is not recommended.

32. *Screening for Rubella (Including Immunization of Adolescents and Adults)*: Routine
screening for rubella susceptibility by history of vaccination or by serology is
recommended for all women of child-bearing age at their first clinical encounter. Susceptible non-pregnant women should be offered rubella vaccination; susceptible pregnant women should be vaccinated immediately after
delivery. An equally acceptable alternative for non-pregnant women of childbearing age is to offer vaccination against rubella without screening. There is
insufficient evidence to recommend for or against screening or routine vaccination of young men in settings where large numbers of susceptible young
adults of both sexes congregate, such as military bases and colleges. Routine
screening or vaccination of other young men, of older men, and of postmenopausal women is not recommended.

33. *Screening for Visual Impairment*: Vision screening to detect amblyopia and strabismus is recommended once for all children prior to entering school, preferably between ages 3 and 4. Clinicians should be alert for signs of ocular mis-

alignment when examining infants and children. Screening for diminished visual acuity in the elderly with Snellen visual acuity chart is recommended. There is insufficient evidence to recommend for or against screening for diminished visual acuity among other asymptomatic persons, but recommendations against routine screening may be made on other grounds.

34. *Screening for Glaucoma*: There is insufficient evidence to recommend for or against routine screening for intraocular hypertension or glaucoma by primary care clinicians. Recommendations to refer high-risk patients for evaluation by an eye specialist may be made on other grounds.

35. *Screening for Hearing Impairment*: Screening older patients for hearing impairment by periodically questioning them about their hearing, counseling them about the availability of hearing aid devices, and making referrals for abnormalities when appropriate, is recommended. There is insufficient evidence to recommend for or against routinely screening older patients for hearing impairment using audiometric testing. There is also insufficient evidence to recommend for or against routinely screening asymptomatic adolescents and working-age adults for hearing impairment. Recommendations against such screening, except for those exposed to excessive occupational noise levels, may be made on other grounds. Routine hearing screening of asymptomatic children beyond age 3 years is not recommended. There is insufficient evidence to recommend for or against routine screening of asymptomatic neonates for congenital hearing loss using evoked otoacoustic emission testing or auditory brainstem response. Recommendations to screen high-risk infants may be made on other grounds. Clinicians examining infants and young children should remain alert for symptoms or signs of hearing impairment.

36. *Screening Ultrasonography in Pregnancy*: Routine third-trimester ultrasound examination of the fetus is not recommended. There is insufficient evidence to recommend for or against a single routine ultrasonographic scan in the second trimester in low-risk pregnant women.

37. *Screening for Preeclampsia*: Screening for preeclampsia with blood pressure measurement is recommended for all pregnant women at the first prenatal visit and periodically throughout the remainder of pregnancy.

38. *Screening for D (Rh) Incompatibility*: D (formerly Rh) blood typing and antibody screening is recommended for all pregnant women at their first prenatal visit. Repeat antibody screening at 24–28 weeks' gestation is recommended for those women found to be negative for D antibodies.

39. *Intrapartum Electronic Fetal Monitoring*: Routine electronic fetal monitoring for low-risk women in labor is not recommended. There is insufficient evidence to recommend for or against intrapartum electronic fetal monitoring for high-risk pregnant women.

40. *Home Uterine Activity Monitoring*: There is insufficient evidence to recommend for or against home uterine activity monitoring in high-risk pregnancies as a screening test for preterm labor, but recommendations against its use may be made on other grounds. Home uterine activity monitoring is not recommended in normal-risk pregnancies.

41. *Screening for Down Syndrome*: The offering of amniocentesis or chorionic villus sampling for chromosome studies is recommended for pregnant women at high risk for Down syndrome. The offering of screening for Down syndrome by serum multiple-marker testing is recommended for all low-risk pregnant women, and as an alternative to amniocentesis and chorionic villus sampling for high-risk women. This testing should be offered only to women who are seen for prenatal care in locations that have adequate counseling and follow-up services. There is currently insufficient evidence to recommend for or against screening for Down syndrome by individual serum marker testing or ultrasound examination, but recommendations against such screening may be made on other grounds.

42. *Screening for Neural Tube Defects (Including Folic Acid/Folate Prophylaxis)*: The offering of screening for neural tube defects by maternal serum alpha-fetoprotein measurement is recommended for all pregnant women who are seen for prenatal care in locations that have adequate counseling and follow-up services available. Screening with maternal serum alpha-fetoprotein may be offered as part of multiple-marker screening. There is insufficient evidence to recommend for or against the offering of screening for neural tube defects by mid-trimester ultrasound examination to all pregnant women, but recommendations against such screening may be made on other grounds. Periconceptional folic acid supplementation to reduce the risk of neural tube defects is recommended for all women who are planning or capable of pregnancy.

43. *Screening for Hemoglobinopathies*: Neonatal screening for sickle hemoglobinopathies is recommended to identify infants who may benefit from antibiotic prophylaxis to prevent sepsis. Whether screening should be universal or targeted to high-risk groups will depend on the proportion of high-risk individuals in the screening area, the accuracy and efficiency with which infants at risk can be identified, and other characteristics of the screening program. All screening efforts must be accompanied by comprehensive counseling and treatment services. Offering screening for hemoglobinopathies to pregnant women at the first prenatal visit is recommended, especially for those at high risk. There is insufficient evidence to recommend for or against routine screening for hemoglobinopathies in high-risk adolescents and young adults, but recommendations to offer such testing may be made on other grounds.

44. *Screening for Phenylketonuria*: Screening for phenylketonuria by measurement of phenylalanine level on a dried-blood spot specimen is recommended for all newborns prior to discharge from the nursery. Infants who are tested before 24 hours of age should receive a repeat screening test by two weeks of age. There is insufficient evidence to recommend for or against routine prenatal screening for maternal phenylketonuria, but recommendations against such screening may be made on other grounds.

45. *Screening for Congenital Hypothyroidism*: Screening for congenital hypothyroidism with thyroid function tests on dried-blood spot specimens is recommended for all newborns in the first week of life.

46. *Screening for Postmenopausal Osteoporosis*: There is insufficient evidence to recommend for or against routine screening for low bone density with bone densitometry in postmenopausal women. Recommendations against routine screening may be made on other grounds. All postmenopausal women should be counseled about hormone prophylaxis and should be advised of the importance of smoking cessation, regular exercise, and adequate calcium intake. For those high-risk women who would consider estrogen only to prevent osteoporosis, screening may be appropriate to assist treatment decisions.

47. *Screening for Adolescent Idiopathic Scoliosis*: There is insufficient evidence to recommend for or against routine screening of asymptomatic adolescents for idiopathic scoliosis.

48. *Screening for Dementia*: There is insufficient evidence to recommend for or against routine screening for dementia in asymptomatic persons. Clinicians should remain alert for possible signs of declining cognitive function in older patients and evaluate mental status in patients who have problems performing daily activities.

49. *Screening for Depression*: There is insufficient evidence to recommend for or against performance of routine screening tests for depression in asymptomatic primary care patients. Clinicians should maintain an especially high index of suspicion for depressive symptoms in those persons at increased risk for depression. Physician education in recognizing and treating affective disorders is recommended.

50. *Screening for Suicide Risk*: There is insufficient evidence to recommend for or against routine screening by primary care clinicians to detect suicide risk in asymptomatic persons. Clinicians should be alert to signs of suicidal ideation in persons with established risk factors. The training of physicians in recognizing and treating affective disorders in order to prevent suicide is recommended. Clinicians should be alert to signs and symptoms of depression and should routinely ask patients about their use of alcohol and other drugs.

51. *Screening for Family Violence*: There is insufficient evidence to recommend for or against the use of specific screening instruments for family violence, but recommendations to routinely ask adults about physical abuse may be made on other grounds. Clinicians should be alert to the various presentations of family violence, including child abuse, spouse and partner abuse, and elder abuse.

52. *Screening for Problem Drinking*: Screening to detect problem drinking is recommended for all adult and adolescent patients. Screening should involve a careful history of alcohol use and/or the use of standardized screening questionnaires. Routine measurement of biochemical markers is not recommended in asymptomatic persons. Pregnant women should be advised to limit or cease drinking during pregnancy. Although there is insufficient evidence to prove or disprove harms from light drinking in pregnancy, recommendations that women abstain from alcohol during pregnancy may be made on other grounds. All persons who use alcohol should be counseled about the

dangers of operating a motor vehicle or performing other potentially dangerous activities after drinking alcohol.

53. *Screening for Drug Abuse*: There is insufficient evidence to recommend for or against routine screening for drug abuse with standardized questionnaires or biologic assays. Including questions about drug use and drug-related problems when taking a history from all adolescents and adult patients may be recommended on other grounds. All pregnant women should be advised of the potential adverse effects of drug use on the development of the fetus. Clinicians should be alert to signs and symptoms of drug abuse in patients, and refer drug-abusing patients to specialized treatment facilities where available.

54. *Counseling to Prevent Tobacco Use*: Tobacco cessation counseling on a regular basis is recommended for all persons who use tobacco products. Pregnant women and parents with children living at home also should be counseled on the potentially harmful effects of smoking on fetal and child health. The prescription of nicotine patches or gum is recommended as an adjunct for selected patients. Anti-tobacco messages are recommended for inclusion in health promotion counseling of children, adolescents, and young adults.

55. *Counseling to Promote Physical Activity*: Counseling patients to incorporate regular physical activity into their daily routines is recommended to prevent coronary heart disease, hypertension, obesity, and diabetes. This recommendation is based on the proven benefits of regular physical activity; the effectiveness of clinician counseling to promote physical activity is not established.

56. *Counseling to Promote a Healthy Diet*: Counseling adults and children over age 2 to limit dietary intake of fat (especially saturated fat) and cholesterol, maintain caloric balance in their diet, and emphasize foods containing fiber (i.e., fruits, vegetables, grain products) is recommended. There is insufficient evidence to recommend for or against counseling the general population to reduce dietary sodium intake or increase dietary intake of iron, beta-carotene, or other antioxidants to improve health outcomes. Women should be encouraged to consume recommended quantities of calcium. Parents should offer breastfeeding to their infants. Providing pregnant women with specific nutritional guidelines to enhance fetal and maternal health is recommended. Although there is insufficient evidence to recommend for or against special assessment of the dietary needs and habits of older adults, recommendations to do so can be made on other grounds, such as the increased prevalence of nutrition-related disorders in this age group. There is insufficient evidence that nutritional counseling by physicians has an advantage over counseling by dietitians or community interventions in changing the dietary habits of patients.

57. *Counseling to Prevent Motor Vehicle Injuries*: Counseling all patients to use occupant restraints (lap/shoulder safety belts and child safety seats) for themselves and others, to wear helmets when riding motorcycles, and to refrain from driving while under the influence of alcohol or other drugs is recommended. There is currently insufficient evidence to recommend for or against counseling patients to prevent pedestrian injuries.

58. *Counseling to Prevent Household and Environmental Injuries*: Periodic counseling of the parents of children on measures to reduce the risk of unintentional household and environmental injuries is recommended. Counseling to prevent household and environmental injuries is also recommended for adolescents and adults based on the proven efficacy of risk reduction, although the effectiveness of counseling these patients to prevent injuries has not been adequately evaluated. Persons with alcohol or drug problems should be identified and counseled, and their progress monitored. Those who use alcohol or illicit drugs should be warned against engaging in potentially dangerous activities while intoxicated. Counseling elderly patients on specific measures to reduce the risk of falling is recommended based on fair evidence that these measures reduce the risk of falls, although the effectiveness of counseling elders to prevent falls has not been adequately evaluated. There is insufficient evidence to recommend for or against the use of external hip protectors to prevent fall injuries, but recommendations for their use in institutionalized elderly may be made on other grounds. More intensive individualized multifactorial intervention is recommended for high-risk elderly patients in settings where adequate resources to deliver such services are available.

59. *Counseling to Prevent Youth Violence*: There is insufficient evidence to recommend for or against clinician counseling of asymptomatic adolescents and adults to prevent morbidity and mortality from youth violence. Adolescent and adult patients should be screened for problem drinking. Clinicians should also be alert for symptoms and signs of drug abuse and dependence, the various presentations of family violence, and suicidal ideation in persons with established risk factors.

60. *Counseling to Prevent Low Back Pain*: There is insufficient evidence to recommend for or against the use of exercise to prevent low back pain, but recommendations for regular physical activity can be made based on other proven benefits. There is also insufficient evidence to recommend for or against the routine use of educational interventions, mechanical supports, or risk factor modification to prevent low back pain.

61. *Counseling to Prevent Dental and Periodontal Disease*: Counseling patients to visit a dental care provider on a regular basis, floss their teeth, brush their teeth daily with a fluoride-containing toothpaste, and appropriately use fluoride for caries prevention and chemotherapeutic mouthrinses for plaque prevention, is recommended based on evidence for risk reduction from these interventions. Educating parents to curb the practice of putting infants and children to bed with a bottle is also recommended based on limited evidence of risk reduction. The effectiveness of clinician counseling to change any of these behaviors has not been adequately evaluated. Appropriate dietary fluoride supplements are recommended for children living in communities with inadequate water fluoridation. While examining the oral cavity, clinicians should be alert for obvious signs of oral disease.

62. *Counseling to Prevent HIV Infection and Other Sexually Transmitted Diseases*: All adolescent and adult patients should be advised about risk factors for HIV

and other sexually transmitted diseases, and counseled appropriately about effective measures to reduce the risk of infection. Counseling should be tailored to the individual risk factors, needs, and abilities of each patient. The recommendation is based on the proven efficacy of risk reduction, although the effectiveness of clinician counseling in the primary care setting is uncertain. Individuals at risk for specific STDs should be offered testing in accordance with recommendations on screening for syphilis, gonorrhea, hepatitis B, HIV, and chlamydial infection. Injection drug users should be referred to appropriate treatment facilities.

63. *Counseling to Prevent Unintended Pregnancy*: All women and men at risk for unintended pregnancy should receive detailed counseling about effective contraceptive methods. Counseling should be based on information from a careful sexual history and should take into account the individual preferences, abilities, and risks of each patient. Sexually active patients should also receive information on measures to prevent sexually transmitted diseases.

64. *Counseling for the Primary Prevention of Gynecologic Cancers*: There is insufficient evidence to recommend for or against routine counseling of women about measures for the primary prevention of gynecologic cancers. Clinicians counseling women about contraceptive practices should include information on the potential benefits of oral contraceptives, barrier contraceptives, and tubal sterilization on risk of certain gynecologic cancers. Clinicians should also promote other practices that may reduce the incidence of certain gynecologic cancers and have other proven health benefits.

65. *Childhood Immunizations*: All children without established contraindications should receive diphtheria-tetanus-pertussis, oral poliovirus, measles-mumps-rubella, conjugate *Haemophilus influenzae* type b, hepatitis B and varicella vaccines, in accordance with recommended schedules. Hepatitis A vaccine is recommended for children and adolescents at high risk for hepatitis A virus infection. Pneumococcal vaccine and annual influenza vaccine are recommended for high-risk children and adolescents.

66. *Adult Immunizations (Including Chemoprophylaxis Against Influenza A)*: Annual influenza vaccine is recommended for all persons age 65 and older and persons in selected high-risk groups. Pneumococcal vaccine is recommended for all immunocompetent individuals who are age 65 and older or otherwise at increased risk for pneumococcal disease. There is insufficient evidence to recommend for or against pneumococcal vaccine for high-risk immunocompromised individuals, but recommendations for vaccinating these persons may be made on other grounds. The series of combined tetanus-diphtheria toxoids should be completed for adults who have not received the primary series, and all adults should receive periodic tetanus-diphtheria boosters. Vaccination against measles and mumps should be provided to all adults born after 1956 who lack evidence of immunity. A second measles vaccine is recommended for adolescents and young adults in settings where such individuals congregate (e.g., high schools and colleges). Hepatitis B vaccine is recommended for all young adults not previously immunized and for all persons at

high risk for infection. Hepatitis A vaccine is recommended for persons at high risk for hepatitis A virus infection.

67. *Postexposure Prophylaxis for Selected Infectious Diseases*: Postexposure prophylaxis should be provided to selected persons with exposure or possible exposure to *Haemophilus influenzae* type b, hepatitis A, hepatitis B, meningococcal, rabies, or tetanus pathogens.

68. *Postmenopausal Hormone Prophylaxis*: Counseling all perimenopausal and post-menopausal women about the potential benefits and risks of hormone prophylaxis is recommended. There is insufficient evidence to recommend for or against hormone therapy in all postmenopausal women. Women should participate fully in the decision-making process, and individual decisions should be based on patient risk factors for disease, clear understanding of the probable benefits and risks of hormone therapy, and personal patient preferences.

69. *Aspirin Prophylaxis for the Primary Prevention of Myocardial Infarction*: There is insufficient evidence to recommend for or against routine aspirin prophylaxis for the primary prevention of myocardial infarction in asymptomatic persons. Although aspirin reduces the risk of myocardial infarctions in men ages 40–84, its use is associated with important adverse effects, and the balance of benefits and harms is uncertain. If aspirin prophylaxis is considered, clinicians and patients should discuss potential benefits and risks for the individual before beginning its use.

70. *Aspirin Prophylaxis in Pregnancy*: There is insufficient evidence to recommend for or against the routine use of aspirin to prevent preeclampsia or intrauterine growth retardation in pregnant women, including those at high risk.

REFERENCE

1. U.S. Preventive Services Task Force. Guide to Clinical Preventive Services. 2nd ed. Baltimore: Williams & Wilkins, 1996.

Index

Page numbers in *italics* denote figures; those followed by "t" denote tables.

childhood schedule for, 391t, 396t,
396–397
contraindications to, 392t
indications for, 395
patient education materials about, 394,
418–419
precautions and contraindications to,
400–401
schedule for children beginning after
age 7, 397t
Divorce, 339
Domestic violence, 34, 243, 245, 501, 587
Down syndrome, 585
Doxepin, 345t
Drinking and driving. See Motor vehicle accidents
Driving habits, xxviii, 32, 237–238, 238t.
See also Motor vehicle injuries
Drowning, 233, 241–242
causes of, 241–242
counseling for prevention of, 242
deaths from, 233, 241
Dry mouth, 330t
Dysthymia, 342

Early and Periodic Screening, Diagnostic,
and Treatment (EPSDT) program,
526
Early detection of disease, 20, 49. See also
Screening tests
Eating. See also Diet; Weight management
approaches to, 226
healthy, 227–230
Ectoparasites, 282t, 285t
Effexor. See Venlafaxine
Elavil. See Amitriptyline
Elderly. See Older adults
Electrocardiography, 85, 90t, 124–126
accuracy and reliability of, 125
counseling about, 125
guidelines for, 124
medical record documentation of, 126
office/clinic organization for routine
screening, 126
patient education materials about, 139
potential adverse effects of, 125
technique for, 124–125
Electroconvulsive therapy, 345
Electronic fetal monitoring, 585
Emergency department prevention programs, 518–522
advantages of, 519–520
basic primary care, 519
counseling, 518–519
disadvantages of, 520–521
role in community-based prevention, 522
screening, 518

Employee fitness programs, 511, 514–516.
See also Worksite health promotion
programs
Employee Retirement Income Security Act
(ERISA) of 1974, 526
Employers' health care costs, 511, 512
Empowerment of patients, xli. See also
Shared decision making
Endep. See Amitriptyline
Endometrial biopsy, 431, 455
Endometrial cancer
estrogen replacement therapy and,
428–429, 455
patient education materials about, 461
Environmental exposures
exploratory questions about, 39–40
primary screening question about, 39
sunlight, 303–314
Enzyme-linked immunoassay (ELISA) test,
for HIV, 101–102
Epididymitis, 112
Ergoloid mesylates, 349
Erythrocyte protoporphyrin, 105–107
Estrogen deficiency, 428
Estrogen replacement therapy, 41,
428–432
benefits of, 428, 430t
compliance with, 429
contraindications to, 431–432
counseling about, 429–431
effect on lipid profile, 428–429
endometrial biopsy for patient on, 431
patient education materials about, 429,
434–435
recommendations for, 429, 590
regimen for, 430–431
risks of, 428–429, 430t
transdermal administration of, 431
vaginal bleeding during, 431
Ethical issues, 449, 554–568
in clinical practice, 558–567
definition of ethics, 554
ethical obligations to patients, 558–564
avoiding stigmatization, 558–559
health promotion counseling, 563
immunizations, 563–564, 564t
limiting inequalities in health, 559–560
screening tests, 560–562
ethical obligations to patient's family and
friends, 564–565
ethical obligations to society and social
institutions, 565–566
groups interested in health promotion
and disease prevention, 554–557
differing aims and agendas of, 557
law and, 554
principles of biomedical ethics, 554, 555t